Informed
D

Other books published by the American Cancer Society

A Breast Cancer Journey: Your Personal Guidebook

American Cancer Society's Guide to Complementary and Alternative Cancer Methods

American Cancer Society's Guide to Pain Control

Cancer in the Family: Helping Children Cope with a Parent's Illness, Heiney et al.

Caregiving: A Step-By-Step Resource for Caring for the Person with Cancer at Home, Houts and Bucher

Colorectal Cancer: A Thorough and Compassionate Resource for Patients and Their Families, Levin

Coming to Terms with Cancer, Laughlin

Consumers Guide to Cancer Drugs, Wilkes et al.

Our Mom Has Cancer, Ackermann and Ackermann

Prostate Cancer: What Every Man—and His Family—Needs to Know, Revised Edition, Bostwick et al.

Women and Cancer: A Thorough and Compassionate Resource for Patients and Their Families, Runowicz et al.

Also by the American Cancer Society

American Cancer Society's Healthy Eating Cookbook: A Celebration of Food, Friends, and Healthy Living, 2nd Edition

Celebrate! Healthy Entertaining for Any Occasion

Kids' First Cookbook: Delicious-Nutritious Treats to Make Yourself!

Informed Decisions

SECOND EDITION

THE COMPLETE BOOK OF
CANCER DIAGNOSIS, TREATMENT, AND RECOVERY

Harmon J. Eyre, M.D., Dianne Partie Lange, and Lois B. Morris

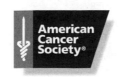

Published by: American Cancer Society–Health Content Products
1599 Clifton Road NE • Atlanta, GA 30329, USA
800-ACS-2345 • www.cancer.org

First published in 1997 by Viking Penguin

ISBN 0-944235-27-1

5 4 3 2 1   01 02 03 04 05

Grateful acknowledgment is made for permission to reprint excerpts or adapt and use selections from the following works:

"How to Perform Skin Self-Examination," information provided by The Skin Cancer Foundation, New York, NY, ©1992.

"My Life as a Runner with Cancer." From *The New York Road Runners Complete Book of Running* by Fred Lebow and Gloria Averbuch, ©1992 by New York Road Runners Club. Used by permission of Random House, Inc.

"Exercises to Do in Bed" by Willibald Nagler, M.D.

"Metamorphosis" from "Beauty Tips for the Dead," 1992 by Judith Hooper.

"The Three-Step Analgesic Ladder," World Health Organization. From Cancer pain relief and palliative care. Report of a WHO Expert Committee. Geneva, Switzerland: World Health Organization; 1990.

"Words for Describing Pain" from "The McGill Questionnaire" by Ronald Melzack, Ph.D., 1970.

"Coping with Disappointment and Frustration" and "Don't Avoid It—Talk About It" from *Cancer and Hope: Charting a Survival Course* by Judith Garrett Garrison, MED, LSW, and Scott Sheperd, Ph.D. (CompCare Publishers, 1989).

"Single with Cancer." Excerpt from *Cancervive: The Challenge of Life After Cancer.* ©1991 by Susan Nessim and Judith Ellis. Reprinted by permission of Houghton Mifflin Company. All rights reserved.

"Becky's Mom Has Cancer," from *An Almanac of Practical Resources for Cancer Survivors: Charting the Journey,* by the National Coalition for Cancer Survivorship, Fitzhugh Mullan, M.D. and Barbara Hoffman, J.D., editors (Consumer Reports Books, 1990) (updated editions published by Chronimed Publishing and John Wiley & Sons).

"To Die in Loving Arms" by Lois B. Morris, originally published in *Sunday Woman*, April 20, 1980.

"Florida Living Will," "Florida Designation of a Health Care Surrogate," and "Artificial Nutrition and Hydration" from "Artificial Nutrition and Hydration and End-of-Life Decision Making" reprinted by permission of Partnership for Caring, Inc., 1620 Eye Street NW, Suite 202, Washington, DC, 20006. 800-989-9455, *www.partnershipforcaring.org.*

Library of Congress Cataloging-in-Publication Data
Informed decisions: the complete book of cancer diagnosis, treatment, and recovery / [edited by] Harmon Eyre, Dianne Partie Lange ; Lois B. Morris, consulting editor.-- 2nd ed.
    p. ; cm.
    Includes index.
    ISBN 0-944235-27-1 (alk. paper)
    1. Cancer--Popular works. [DNLM: 1. Neoplasms--diagnosis--Popular Works. 2. Neoplasms--therapy--Popular Works. QZ 201 I43 2001] I. Eyre, Harmon J. II. Lange, Dianne. III. Morris, Lois B. IV. American Cancer Society.
    RC262 .I4985 2001
    616.99'4--dc21

                                                                                        2001001880

A NOTE TO THE READER

The information contained in this book is not intended as medical advice and should not be relied upon as a substitute for consulting with your physician. This information may not address all possible actions, precautions, side effects, or interactions. All matters regarding your health require the supervision of a physician who is familiar with your medical needs. For more information, contact your American Cancer Society at 800-ACS-2345.

Printed in the United States of America

Line drawings by David Rosenzweig • Design by Mouse Design Studio, Inc. Roswell, GA

This book is dedicated to Gerald P. Murphy, M.D., D.Sc., who was the Director of Cancer Research at the Pacific Northwest Cancer Foundation in Seattle and the former Chief Medical Officer of the American Cancer Society.

Dr. Murphy was a pioneer in developing the PSA test for the early detection of prostate cancer. He was deeply and energetically committed to research and education. His honors are too numerous to mention, but included eight honorary degrees from various colleges and universities, the Papal Medal for distinguished service to humanity, and the Silver Medal from the European Organization for Research and Treatment of Cancer. While Dr. Murphy was serving as the director of Roswell Park Cancer Institute, President Richard M. Nixon appointed him to the National Cancer Advisory Board.

Dr. Murphy conceived of this book, encouraged cancer specialists throughout the country to contribute to it, and ushered the first edition to its completion. He passed away while attending a cancer research meeting in Israel in January 2000.

Managing Editor

Katherine V. Bruss, Psy.D.

Editor

Amy Sproull

Editorial Review

Terri Ades, R.N., M.S., A.O.C.N.
Colleen Doyle, M.S., R.D.
Joy L. Fincannon, R.N., M.S.
Ted Gansler, M.D.
Herman Kattlove, M.D.
Margaret Ney, M.S.N., R.N., A.N.P., O.C.N.

Publishing Director

Emily Pualwan

Production Manager

Candace Magee

CONTENTS

ACKNOWLEDGMENTS

We would like to acknowledge many individuals for their help in preparing the first edition of this book.

Thanks to Terri Ades, R.N., M.S., A.O.C.N.; Robert M. Beazley, M.D.; Don Beerline, M.D.; Foster Boyd, M.D.; Tony W. Cheung, M.D.; Grace H. Christ, D.S.W.; Nessa Coyle, R.N., M.S.; Myles P. Cunningham, M.D.; Jerome J. DeCosse, M.D., Ph.D.; Philip J. DiSaia, M.D.; Robert C. Eyerly, M.D.; Irving D. Fleming, M.D.; Lawrence Garfinkel, M.A.; Gerald Haase, M.D.; George J. Hill, M.D.; Reginald Ho, M.D.; Edward W. Humphrey, M.D.; George W. Jones, M.D.; Rosaline R. Joseph, M.D.; Betsy Jubb, M.L.I.S.; Richard H. Lange, M.D.; John Laszlo, M.D.; Walter Lawrence, Jr., M.D.; Edward R. Laws, Jr., M.D.; Seymour H. Levitt, M.D.; Virgil Loeb, Jr., M.D.; Matthew Loscalzo, A.C.S.W.; LaMar S. McGinnis, M.D.; Robert J. McKenna, Sr.; Willibald Nagler, M.D.; Daniel W. Nixon, M.D.; Darrell S. Rigel, M.D.; Eugene G. Roach, Ph.D., M.D.; Arlene E. Robinovitch, M.S.W.; David S. Rosenthal, M.D.; Richard W. Sayre, M.D.; Wendy S. Schain, Ed.D.; Leslie R. Schover, Ph.D.; Robert J. Schweitzer, M.D.; and Naomi Stearns, M.S.W.

PREFACE

We are making progress in the war against cancer. The cancer incidence and death rates are declining and the quality of life and survival rates of those with cancer are rising.

Estimates indicate that 8.9 million Americans are living with a history of cancer. Yet if more people pursue state-of-the-art screening methods and treatment, this survival rate can be further improved. Studies show that more of us could survive cancer if we took advantage of our increasing knowledge about how to prevent cancer, detect it early, and obtain the highest quality therapy for the disease.

To understand something is to gain knowledge and information, minimizing the mystery and fear that surround it. Educating people about cancer—helping them understand its causes, avoid risk factors, and learn how it can be treated—has been part of the American Cancer Society's mission since the beginning.

Informed Decisions, 2nd Edition marks another milestone in our efforts to provide the public with vital information and emphasize that no one is powerless against this disease.

Informed Decisions, 2nd Edition can enhance your knowledge of the cancer care options to which you're entitled. Here are the facts you need—we hope *Informed Decisions* will also provide you with the peace of mind that comes from having accurate, reliable information at a time when you need it the most.

—**Harmon J. Eyre, M.D.**
Chief Medical Officer
and Executive Vice President for
Research and Cancer Control
AMERICAN CANCER SOCIETY

Introduction

How to Use This Book

Although not so many years ago a diagnosis of cancer resulted in a very different outcome, today more people are living with cancer than ever before. Most men, women, and children who have cancer now also have a future. And they are able to be more in control of their futures than ever before.

No two people or families have the same cancer experience, and there is no master list of "right" choices for someone with cancer. The chapters in this book address the likely day-to-day living concerns faced by people with cancer and their family members. The topics won't affect you in the order you see here, nor will you face only one aspect of cancer at a time—these issues overlap and may affect you for only a short time, repeatedly, or not at all.

Some people are comfortable only when they have a clear understanding of all of their options; others feel safest when following a trusted doctor's treatment recommendation. Even if you choose to leave the decision-making to others, in this book you can find out what is happening and why. You may want to use this book as a starting place for developing questions for your doctor and opening up discussions with your friends and family.

Other ways in which you may want to use this book include:

- to understand the options you have

- to feel secure in your choice of health care professionals and treatment facilities

- to comprehend the recommendations that your health care team provides

- to organize and evaluate the enormous amounts of information and details you will encounter at a time when you are least able to absorb them

- to request additional therapies, services, or programs that may not have been offered to you

- to collaborate with your health care team rather than feel helpless and passive

- to be sure you are receiving the best possible care

- to feel in control of what is happening to you

- to reduce fear and anxiety

- to understand the medical terms and concepts health care professionals use to describe cancer and its treatment

- to appreciate the current state of knowledge about cancer and grasp what is on the horizon

- to be aware of the resources and services available to you and your family, even in this era of managed health care resources

A diagnosis of cancer presents many emotional, physical, and financial challenges. Decisions can be difficult to make, especially if they will influence the course and quality of your life, if they must be made quickly, and if you lack the knowledge to choose wisely. *Informed Decisions* addresses challenges one step at a time and can help you deal with the many complex issues of cancer.

New to This Edition

The new edition of this book has been updated to reflect the most recent developments in cancer diagnosis, care, and treatment. It contains the latest information about every aspect of cancer, from modern methods of detection to the challenges of recovery. It covers a broad range of topics including cancer causes and risk factors, screening and diagnostic tests, treatment strategies, coping tips, and questions to ask your doctor. It also offers tips about how to obtain the most advanced care possible.

In addition, three chapters have been added to this new edition. One new chapter includes information on how to identify symptoms that signal specific cancer emergencies. A separate new chapter has also been included to provide tips on understanding and coping with fatigue. The third new chapter offers information concerning the costs of cancer and includes practical advice about money, insurance, and how to manage the financial burden of cancer.

As always, *Informed Decisions* aims to provide those with cancer and their loved ones with valuable information so they can make decisions that suit their particular needs and desires, feel in control of their situations, and calm their fears and anxieties.

How the Book Is Organized

Early Detection, Diagnosis, and Treatment

You will be better prepared to understand what is happening to you once you're armed with the knowledge about how cancer develops and which tests are used to diagnose the disease. In Part I (*Is It Cancer?*) of this edition, the background about the nature, language, early detection, and diagnosis of cancer is provided. In Part II (*When the Diagnosis Is Cancer*), you'll learn about choosing a doctor and a hospital, talking with your doctor, when and why to consider getting a second opinion, and who you might want to take with you to doctor's appointments.

Cancer is a disease with as many as 100 different forms, so a treatment that is effective in fighting another person's cancer isn't necessarily the best for fighting your cancer. And every person with cancer—even two people with cancer at precisely the same stage—differs from every other. Treatments have different side effects. Choosing and undergoing treatment for cancer is therefore often stressful and even confusing. It's important to learn about options and consult your doctor and health care team about which options may be best suited to your situation.

The latest developments in promising cancer treatments are discussed in Part III (*Treatment Strategies*), whether they are new treatments, new incarnations of existing therapies, or more traditional treatments. Options for the person with cancer may be surgery, radiation, and chemotherapy. They may also include gene therapy, immunotherapy, a clinical trial, or a stem cell transplant. In these chapters you'll find out what the therapies are, how they might help you, and the costs and benefits of each one.

Living with Cancer

Cancer affects your body, but it also affects how you feel emotionally. Part IV (*Living with Cancer*) guides you through the emotional and physical aspects of your cancer. It covers topics including nutrition, body image, sexuality, coping with stress, dealing with coworkers, and challenges in the workplace.

Many people diagnosed with cancer are immediately concerned about the side effects of the disease and its treatment. Part IV offers approaches to controlling side effects such as pain, fatigue, nausea and vomiting, anxiety, fear, depression, and sexual effects.

This section also addresses those issues that affect the family and friends of someone with cancer, outlining what they can expect and how to communicate at this difficult time as well as how to cope with role changes, changes in routine, common stresses, and intimacy issues. It offers information about children with cancer in the family, how to soothe their concerns, and how to keep an eye out for problems as they face this confusing change in their lives and the life of their loved one.

Advanced Illness

Part V (*Advancing Illness*) discusses the important information to know if cancer returns. Included are such topics as hospice and home care at the end of life, advance directives, and living wills.

Overview of Specific Cancers *(formerly called Encyclopedia)*

This section (Part VI) includes informational overviews of some of the most common cancers. It reflects current incidence and survival rates, risk factors, and treatment options. This section of the book is a helpful tool in learning the basics about cancer types.

Resources

The American Cancer Society offers many programs and services that are valuable to the person with cancer. Many other organizations provide medical information and cancer services as well. A list of contact information and overviews of important resources appears in the back of the book.

About the American Cancer Society

Represented in more than 3,400 communities throughout the country and Puerto Rico, the American Cancer Society (ACS) is a nonprofit health organization dedicated to eliminating cancer as a major health problem. This book is just one example of the many ways the American Cancer Society seeks to fulfill its mission: to save lives and diminish suffering from cancer through research, education, advocacy, and service.

The ACS is the largest private source of cancer research dollars in the United States. Founded in 1913 by ten physicians and five concerned members of the community, the organization is now represented by two million Americans. Most offer their time free of charge to the ACS to work to conquer cancer.

PART

Is It Cancer?

Cancer Basics

Each year, over one million Americans are diagnosed with cancer. Their lives are turned upside down in an instant. Their plans and concerns about almost every aspect of life—work, relationships, money, and pleasure—are overshadowed by one question that often goes unspoken, "Am I going to die?"

The answer, statistically speaking, is no. Of all those whose cancers are diagnosed today, more will survive than will die as a result of the disease. Considerable progress has been made in treating many forms of cancer. Most types of cancer are curable if the disease is found at an early stage, and some types are curable even if the cancer has spread. These include Hodgkin's disease, Ewing's sarcoma (a bone cancer), testicular cancer, gestational chorio-carcinoma (cancer that starts in the placenta), rhabdomyosarcoma (muscle cancer), osteogenic sarcoma (a bone cancer), Wilms' tumor (kidney cancer in children), and acute lymphocytic leukemia in children.

We are experiencing the first sustained decline in the population's death rate from cancer since record keeping began in the 1930s. Today, many of those confronting cancer are learning that even when being cured—that is, permanently ridding the body of all cancer cells—is not possible, long-term survival is. In fact, cancer is increasingly being treated as a chronic condition like heart disease or diabetes. With prompt treatment, regular monitoring, and proper psychological and social support, there's a good chance that a person can live a productive life with the disease for many years. Childhood cancers used to almost always be fatal, but 75 percent of children diagnosed with cancer in 2001 will survive five years or more. Childhood cancer mortality rates have declined 50 percent since 1973. The cancer death rate for adults has also begun to decline in recent years.

Changing Views About Cancer

As new discoveries have been made about how the body works, knowledge has evolved regarding the causes of cancer. In ancient Greece, Hippocrates (460–370 B.C.) used words that refer to a crab, "carcinos" and "carcinoma," to describe tumors with their fingerlike projections. At that time, it was believed that an imbalance in body fluids (called the four humors) caused cancer. Some ancient minds thought one of the four humors (an excess of black bile) in a particular body part was the most likely cause of tumor formation.

By 1761 A.D., when Giovanni Morgagni published what he had learned about death by performing autopsies, the humoral theory had given way to the belief that cancer was formed by lymph, a colorless fluid that flows in and out of the blood and circulates around all of the body's cells. In the mid-1800s, the lymph theory was replaced by the blastema theory of German pathologist Johannes Muller. He proposed that cancer did not come from normal cells but from "blastema" between normal tissues.

Later, Muller's student Rudolph Virchow, who has been called the founder of cellular pathology, used the recently invented microscope to determine that all cells, including cancer cells, arise from other cells. He proposed that chronic irritation caused cancer. During the seventeenth and eighteenth centuries, several other theories had their moments in medical history. Some doctors supported the parasite theory that suggested cancer was contagious. Others proposed that cancer was the result of traumatic injury.

Medical historians say that the turning point in understanding cancer was the beginning of the twentieth century, when scientists began to look at life-threatening diseases as solvable problems. Several medical mysteries were unraveled at the time. Mosquitoes were identified as yellow fever carriers, lice were linked to typhus, a treatment for syphilis was found, and the first radical mastectomy was performed. Medical institutions became centers of research, and doctors started to systematically share their knowledge with each other.

Many speculated at this time that cancer was a natural result of aging. As cells degenerated, researchers thought some became malignant. Other scientists believed cancer was hereditary, and investigations into genetics began. Some began to consider chemical links, and still others questioned whether viruses or bacteria were at fault.

But the irritation theory persisted, and researchers began trying to identify irritants such as tobacco and coal tar that caused cancer in laboratory animals. Ultimately, these experts were forced to confront the fact that although these substances might be involved in some cases, none of them invariably caused cancer in humans.

Scientists eventually abandoned the theory that cancer had a single cause, but there was enough truth in the beliefs and speculations of the time to support a range of misconceptions, some of which still persist. For example, despite the fact that scientists have proven that you can't "catch" cancer, many people continue to think of it as contagious. If cancer were infectious, we would have cancer epidemics just as we have flu epidemics, and cancer would spread like measles, polio, or the common cold.

Today's Advances

It has taken approximately 2,000 years for scientists to go from thinking black bile was the cause of cancer to unraveling the mysteries of DNA. Clearly the work is still incomplete. Yet there is excitement in almost every field of biological research because we are on the brink of learning what the many pieces of the puzzle are and how they fit together. Fortunately, each basic discovery also aids scientists who are developing new treatments. Although a cure for all cancers is probably in the distant future, cures for certain types of cancer, ways to slow cancer's progress, and treatments to extend a person's lifespan *with* cancer and improve the quality of his or her life are continually emerging.

Cancer Is a Process

All the diseases we call cancer have one characteristic in common: the out-of-control growth and accumulation of abnormal cells. The development of these abnormal cells is a lengthy, progressive, multistep process called carcinogenesis. It starts with damage to one or more genes that eventually causes a cell to produce more abnormal cells. It ends—sometimes years later—with the formation of a detectable tumor. Carcinogenesis may take ten to twenty years from the time the first abnormal cells begin replicating to the point at which a person notices any sign or symptom of a tumor.

How Healthy Cells Behave

To understand carcinogenesis, it's helpful to know how healthy cells behave. A normal cell divides, matures, dies, and is replaced by another according to a genetic program that is unique to that particular cell type (that is, skin, intestine, blood, etc.). As a cell grows, it takes its proper place among the other cells in its tissue of origin. And when the cell matures, it performs the task it is genetically programmed to do. Eventually it dies and is replaced by a new, younger cell. As the developing cells mature, one cell bumps against a neighboring one and molecular messages are relayed and received, telling the young cell that it's time to stop growing.

All cells are equipped with controls designed to prevent them from making too many copies of themselves or flawed ones. For example, cells are

Age-Adjusted Cancer Death Rates

For Males by Site, US, 1930–1997*

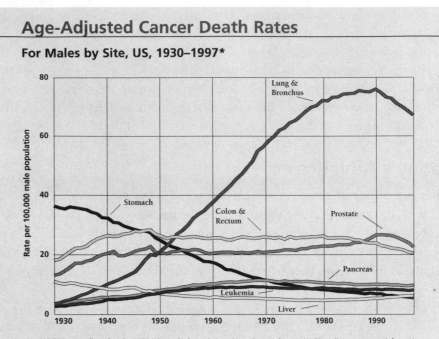

*Per 100,000, age-adjusted to the 1970 US standard population. Note: Due to changes in ICD coding, numerator information has changed over time. Rates for cancers of the liver, lung & bronchus, and colon & rectum are affected by these coding changes.

Source: US Mortality Public Use Data Tapes 1960–1997, US Mortality Volumes 1930–1959, National Center for Health Statistics, Centers for Disease Control and Prevention, 2000. American Cancer Society, Surveillance Research, 2001

For Females by Site, US, 1930–1997*

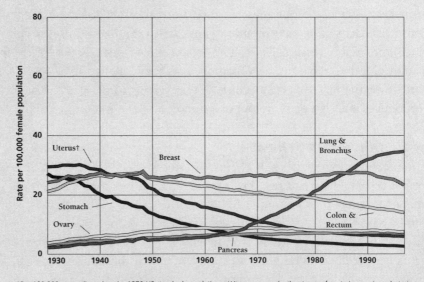

*Per 100,000, age-adjusted to the 1970 US standard population. †Uterus cancer death rates are for uterine cervix and uterine corpus combined. Note: Due to changes in ICD coding, numerator information has changed over time. Rates for cancers of the uterus, ovary, lung & bronchus, and colon & rectum are affected by these coding changes.

Source: US Mortality Public Use Data Tapes 1960–1997, US Mortality Volumes 1930–1959, National Center for Health Statistics, Centers for Disease Control and Prevention, 2000. American Cancer Society, Surveillance Research, 2001

programmed to die after a certain number of replications. This phenomenon is known as apoptosis, and it is an important part of the normal aging process. Certain genes produce substances that are needed for this process to occur. Loss or malfunctions of these genes can cause or contribute to development of some types of cancer.

Recently, it was discovered that every time a cell divides, some DNA, or deoxyribonucleic acid (the body's basic genetic material), is lost from the tips of the cell's chromosomes. Eventually, when these tips (known as telomeres) and their extra DNA are nearly depleted, the chromosomes become unstable. Consequently, the cell cannot duplicate itself, and it ages and dies. Cancer cells, in contrast, produce an enzyme called telomerase that replaces the lost portion of the chromosome tips, which makes the cells immortal.

Cellular Disorder

When a cell has been transformed into a cancer cell, its offspring—the daughter cells—no longer follow the biological rules in an orderly way. They often divide more often than they should. Their growth is disorderly, and they never mature properly. Their offspring, in turn, are similarly abnormal and have a tendency to become even more disorderly. These wayward cells tumble over each other, piling on top of neighboring cells and eventually forming a mass or tumor. Some types of cancer cells don't divide more often than normal, but they do fail to die on schedule.

Cancer cells that don't know when to stop dividing and/or when to die are called immortal. They may destroy normal surrounding tissues and often spread throughout the body, which is a hallmark of malignancy.

Eventually, if the disruptive growth of the cancer cells is not controlled, and the abnormal cells extend to adjacent areas or spread (metastasize) to form tumors elsewhere in the body, the affected organs and systems cannot continue their vital functions (see Chapter 30). Unless the proliferation of cancer cells is arrested, the body cannot survive.

The Cancer Puzzle: What Makes a Cell Go Wrong?

The question that has intrigued minds since Hippocrates is, "How does cancer happen?" In the 1950s, the answer began to surface with the advent of molecular biology. Now researchers could scrutinize cells' DNA and the genes they contain. The period from the late 1970s through the early 1980s was a time of major breakthroughs in understanding the biology of cancer. For example, researchers discovered that as the genetic material in cells is replicated and the information is passed along to subsequent generations of cells, mutations in the genes that can cause cancer are passed along as well.

Over time, as normal cells divide, more and more mutations occur. This discovery was a very important advance in understanding the origin of cancer.

It's expected that the Human Genome Project will continue to provide even greater understanding of how our genes contribute to cancer. This program completed sequencing the DNA of all human genes in 2000. This information will provide an extremely useful reference to all human genetic information, including genes that initiate cancer. However, it will take many years for scientists to learn what all of these genes do and exactly how some play a role in the development of cancer.

Genes are segments of DNA that direct a cell's functions, which are usually aimed at creating a particular protein. Genes contain the cellular blueprint for hereditary characteristics such as hair and eye color, as well as the susceptibility to certain diseases, such as cancer.

The two classes of genes that play a critical role in cancer are oncogenes and tumor suppressor genes. In some cases, tests can detect mutations in oncogenes and tumor suppressor genes. Such tests can help identify a type of cancer, help predict the prognosis of a person with that cancer, or help determine which person is likely to benefit from a certain treatment. Tests can also identify some people who are at high risk for developing cancer because they inherited a mutated oncogene or tumor suppressor gene from one of their parents.

Oncogenes. Genes that normally control how often a cell divides are called proto-oncongenes. When these genes develop mutations they are called oncogenes and are permanently activated, or "turned on." Cells containing oncogenes divide too quickly and eventually accumulate to form a tumor.

Scientists are attempting to learn how to inhibit or turn off oncogenes and thereby stop the cancer process. In 1998, the U.S. Food and Drug Administration approved the monoclonal antibody trastuzumab (Herceptin), a protein that fits like a lock and key with a protein on certain breast cancer cells. (Monoclonal antibodies are antibodies produced in the laboratory. They're designed to react with specific antigens on the surface of certain types of cancer cells.) The protein (antigen) on the breast cancer cells is the *HER2/neu* onco-protein. Having too many copies of the *HER2/neu* oncogene increases the aggressiveness of breast cancers by causing cells to produce too much of the growth-promoting *HER2/neu* oncoprotein. Once trastuzumab attaches to the cells, it prevents the *HER2/neu* oncoprotein from stimulating growth of cancer cells. Trastuzumab may also act as a chemical signal to attract immune cells that help kill the cancer cells. Studies are underway to determine if trastuzumab will be useful in treating people with other cancers.

Ninety percent of people with chronic myelogenous leukemia have experienced a chromosomal translocation, or shifting in chromosomes. This translocation—which is thought to be responsible for the development of this cancer and its malignant behavior—produces an abnormal protein, *bcr-abl*, which causes benign bone marrow cells to become leukemia cells. A drug called STI-571 (Gleevec) inhibits, or represses, the protein created during the shift in chromosomes that results in chronic myelogenous leukemia.

Dozens of other oncogenes have been identified thus far. These include ras, which is mutated in some types of colon and lung cancer and myc, which is activated by chromosomal translocations that lead to some types of lymphomas.

Tumor Suppressor Genes. These genes are involved in slowing cell division; increasing apoptosis, or programmed cell death; and in repairing DNA. When these genes are mutated, they are inactivated or turned off, which causes the cell and its offspring to divide rapidly and grow out of control. Alteration of tumor suppressor genes can occur during the life of the person—a so-called acquired mutation—or the abnormality can be inherited.

Thus far, approximately thirty tumor suppressor genes have been identified, including p53, BRCA 1 & 2 (also known as breast cancer genes), APC, and RB. Mutations in the p53 gene can be acquired or, much less often, inherited and have been linked to over half of the cancers that occur in humans, including brain tumors, breast cancer, and leukemia. Abnormalities in the RB gene can lead to retinoblastoma (a type of eye cancer), osteosarcoma, (a bone cancer), and others. A defective APC gene causes familial polyposis, a condition in which hundreds or thousands of colon polyps develop, and some of them become malignant.

Although there is no treatment currently available to correct mutations in tumor suppressor genes, laboratory experiments and even some clinical trials are being done using gene therapy to replace defective tumor suppressor genes or to destroy cancer cells that have p53 mutations.

Tumor Growth Factors. The chemical messengers that control cell growth are called growth factors. When they attach to receptors on the cell's surface, vital signals are transmitted to the biological machinery within the cell. Some cancer cells produce excessive levels of growth factors. Some have too many growth factor receptors, making them abnormally sensitive to even normal levels of the growth factors. Some cancer cells receive more signals to grow and divide by producing too many receptors and excessive levels of the growth factors.

Drugs that can prevent certain growth factors from promoting cancer cell growth are being tested in laboratory experiments and clinical trials. New drugs that block the extra receptors on cancer cells, causing them to destroy themselves, are also being developed. Another experimental approach is to develop toxins that are carried by naturally occurring growth factors. When the sabotaged growth factors attach to receptors on the cancer cells, the toxin will destroy the cancer cell.

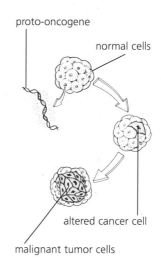

proto-oncogene

normal cells

altered cancer cell

malignant tumor cells

How Cancer Begins

For unexplained reasons, a proto-oncogene in the cell's DNA becomes a cancer gene and causes the cell to behave abnormally and reproduce uncontrollably. The multiplying cancer cells form a tumor.

Carcinogens and Stages of Carcinogenesis

Science has clearly and strongly implicated exposure to certain factors in the development of tumors. For example, a number of agents cause a cell to alter its growth in a cancerous direction: chemicals like benzene; viruses like the human papilloma virus; and radiation from nuclear reactions, x-ray machines, or ultraviolet rays from the sun.

Carcinogenesis is believed to take place in three stages: initiation, promotion, and tumor progression. This view of cancer formation is based on laboratory experiments in which researchers use a series of cancer-causing influences to turn normal cells into cancerous ones. This view is useful in helping scientists understand how cancers form and how they might be prevented. However, for most people with cancer, the exact start and end of each stage can rarely be identified, and the influences responsible for each of these stages are often unknown.

Initiation. During the initiation phase, some critical mutations, usually involving several oncogenes or tumor suppressor genes, alter a cell's genetic programming, transforming it into a cell that will reproduce abnormal versions of itself.

The initial damage done or the cause of the mutations may be inherited or it can be acquired over time by exposure to a class of cancer-causing influences that scientists call initiators. All initiators are capable of causing damage to DNA, although they cause this damage in different ways. The DNA mutations caused by initiators are irreversible. Some of these initiators have been identified; others remain a mystery. Examples of initiators include ultraviolet radiation in sunlight, x-rays, radon gas, vinyl chloride, and many of the substances found in tobacco smoke.

Promotion. The second step, which increases the likelihood of carcinogenesis, is called promotion. Some carcinogens, known as promoters, do not cause DNA damage. But they do increase the likelihood that cells with DNA already damaged by initiators will become cancerous. Promoters are believed to affect how the genes' messages are expressed. Some substances (including many found in tobacco) are both initiators and promoters. Others, especially substances naturally occurring in the body such as bile acids, estrogens, and androgens act only as promoters.

Tumor Progression. When a cancer first forms, its cells may not be able to metastasize, or spread to other tissues and organs. But as cells continue to accumulate new mutations, clones evolve that become progressively more malignant. These new clones develop new features that help them break through the walls of lymph vessels and blood vessels, attach and grow in distant organs, promote angiogenesis (the forming of new blood vessels) more effectively, and better evade recognition by the patient's immune system. Cancer cells can also change to develop resistance to certain chemotherapy drugs or hormonal therapy drugs. All of these changes are examples of tumor progression.

The Body Fights Back

Since genetic alterations or mutations occur throughout life, everyone is at some risk of getting cancer. Whether a malignancy eventually occurs, however, will be influenced by your body's own defenses.

The immune system, for example, is a kind of built-in search-and-destroy system. Cancer cells—like infectious organisms such as viruses and bacteria— contain foreign substances called antigens. Scientists believe that when immune cells circulating in the bloodstream detect these "foreign" antigens, they destroy the invader. Occasionally, though, cancer cells escape detection since their differences from normal cells may be quite subtle. Some researchers think that cancer cells can reduce the number of antigens that alert the immune system or camouflage them. To illustrate just how important healthy immunity is, consider the high cancer risk among people who lack normal immunity because of certain drugs or diseases such as acquired immune deficiency syndrome (AIDS). People with AIDS have almost 200 times more malignancies than the general population. They tend to develop lymphomas, skin cancers, and a few other types of cancers. But the most common cancers (breast, prostate, colon, lung) aren't greatly increased in these individuals, and the role of the immune system in the development of these cancers is not clear.

Learning how the immune system responds and what might stimulate it into action sooner or more forcefully is also an area of intense investigation (see Chapter 13).

The Language of Cancer

The term "cancer" is used to refer to many different diseases. How many types of cancer are there? The answer depends on how you define types and subtypes, and on the purpose of your classification. Let's forget cancer for a moment and think of animals instead. How many kinds of animals can you name? Most of us would probably start with a list that includes insects, amphibians, reptiles, birds, and mammals. We might then list some of the most common members of these categories, like dogs, cats, and cows. But zoologists would point out that there are about 6,000 known species of reptiles and over 800,000 species of insects. They make these subtle distinctions because each animal has a slightly different combination of appearance, behavior, and habitat. These distinctions are of little interest to the average person, but are critically important to zoologists and conservationists. Oncologists and other cancer professionals think of cancers in much the same way. Various types of cancer differ substantially with regard to

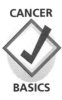

CANCER

BASICS

Cancer Vocabulary

A tumor is any abnormal lump, bump, or mass of tissue. Although calluses, swollen bruises, pimples, and abscesses can all form lumps and bumps, doctors usually use the word tumor to refer to a group of diseases they call neoplasms. A neoplasm is a growth that starts from a single abnormal cell. It may be benign or malignant.

- A benign neoplasm is usually slow growing, doesn't spread or invade surrounding tissue, and can't spread to distant parts of the body, although it may recur if not completely removed. Most benign neoplasms never become malignant, but some kinds may.

- A malignant neoplasm invades surrounding tissue and often spreads to other parts of the body. Even if the original mass is completely removed, a cancer may recur if its cells have already spread to other parts of the body.

  The suffix "-oma" usually refers to benign neoplasms, such as an adenoma (benign tumor of glandular tissue), lipoma (benign tumor of fat tissue), or osteoma (benign tumor of bone tissue). However, there are some confusing exceptions to this rule, such as melanoma (cancer of pigment-producing skin cells). Most cancers have names that include the suffixes "-carcinoma" or "-sarcoma."

their risk factors and causes, how they are diagnosed, their likelihood of spreading, the way they affect the body, the symptoms they produce, and how they are treated. Most of the language that describes cancer relates to these distinctions.

Although medical terminology is used primarily among professionals to communicate details concisely, it is helpful for the layperson to understand the terms in a general way. This helps to comprehend a diagnosis and is invaluable when seeking information about a particular cancer. Although the language medical professionals use often seems unwieldy because the terms include many Greek and Latin words, there is an order and precision to the jargon.

Cancer Classification

Cancer is classified by the part of the body in which it began, and by its appearance under a microscope. Oncologists use terms for different types of cancer, which vary in their rates of growth, patterns of spread, and responses to different types of treatment. Cancer treatment is designed for each cancer's specific combination of tumor type, cancer site, tumor grade, and stage. Here we'll explore the meanings of different terms related to cancer classification.

Types of Tissues. One way in which oncologists refer to cancers is related to the type of tissue where the tumor develops or the type of cell it affects.

- The most common cancers, accounting for 80 to 90 percent of cases, are carcinomas, which originate in epithelial tissue. Epithelial tissue is found throughout the body; it includes the skin as well as the covering and lining of most organs, such as those of the gastrointestinal tract, respiratory tract, and most reproductive organs. Many of these organs, such as the intestines, cervix, and bronchi (breathing tubes), have an obvious lining or covering layer. Other organs that secrete something, such as the breasts, the pancreas, and the thyroid gland, have tiny glands (that can be seen only under a microscope) that are lined by epithelial cells.

- Carcinomas are divided into two main subtypes: adenocarcinoma, which indicates a cancer that develops from the cells of a gland, and squamous cell carcinoma, which refers to a cancer that originates in the flat cells that cover the surface of the skin, mouth, cervix, and several other organs. Some less common types of carcinoma, such as small cell carcinoma and clear cell carcinoma, are named according to the appearance of their cells under a microscope.

- Sarcoma refers to cancer that begins in connective tissue such as bones, tendons, cartilage, muscle, and fat. This category includes osteosarcoma (bone cancer), fibrosarcoma (cancer of tissue that resembles tendons and ligaments), rhabdomyosarcoma (cancer of voluntary muscles), leiomyosarcoma (cancer of involuntary muscles), and liposarcoma (cancer of fatty tissue).

- Leukemias are cancers of the bone marrow, where blood cells are made.

- Myeloma is cancer that originates in the plasma cells, the antibody-producing cells of bone marrow.

- Lymphomas develop in the lymphoid tissue, collections of immune system cells found in lymph nodes (bean-sized immune system organs found in the underarm and groin areas, on the sides of the neck, and inside the chest and abdomen) as well as in other organs (specifically the spleen, tonsils, and thymus). The function of normal lymphoid tissue is to purify body fluids and produce infection-fighting white blood cells, or lymphocytes. One class of lymphoma is known as Hodgkin's disease; all others are called non-Hodgkin's lymphomas.

- Tumors of the nervous system are named after the specific type of cell they affect. For instance, cancer of the glial cells, which surround and nourish nerve cells, is called glioma. A benign tumor on the covering of the brain, the meninges, is labeled a meningioma.

- Tumors of reproductive system cells in the testicles and ovaries that develop into sperm cells and ova (egg cells) are called germ cell tumors.

- Some cancers are named for the person who discovered them or first described them, such as Ewing's tumor or Wilms' tumor.

Cancer Site. The body part in which cancer first develops is known as the primary site. A cancer's primary site may determine how the tumor will behave; whether and where it may spread, or metastasize; and what symptoms it is most likely to cause. The most common primary sites of cancer are the prostate, breast, lung and bronchus, large intestine (colon and rectum), skin, and urinary bladder. A cancer is always described in terms of the primary site, even if it has spread to another part of the body. For instance, advanced breast cancer that has spread to the lymph nodes under the arm and to the bone and lungs is always considered breast cancer. To convey the extent of the cancer, a doctor might say this is "a primary tumor of the breast with regional metastases to the axillary lymph nodes and systemic spread to the bones and lungs."

Tumor Grade. Once a tumor has been detected, some or all of it can be removed for microscopic examination. Once the pathologist determines whether the tumor is benign or malignant and decides what type of normal tissue it most closely resembles (i.e., gives the cancer a specific name), the next step is to determine how closely the cancer cells resemble healthy, mature cells. The tumor grade is a measure of how abnormal the cells appear. If the cells are very similar to normal tissue, the cancer is said to be well differentiated, grade 1, or low grade. Cancer cells that do not look at all like their healthy counterparts are called poorly differentiated, grade 3, or high grade. Cancers with an intermediate appearance are called moderately differentiated, grade 2, or intermediate grade. High-grade cancers tend to grow and spread more rapidly than do low-grade ones. Although most cancers are graded on a scale of one through three, the grading systems for some cancers have one, four, or five categories.

The grade is useful in estimating how successful treatment may be, and sometimes influences how the cancer should be treated. However, in choosing among treatment options, the grade of cancer generally has less impact than its stage (extent of spread).

Tumor Stage. Cancers are further classified according to stage. Staging is the process of finding out how much cancer there is in the body and where it is located. The stage assigned to the cancer as a result of this evaluation is useful to the doctor who is determining the appropriate treatment.

Most types of cancer are classified by five stages, usually labeled 0 to IV. Depending on the type of cancer, stages are sometimes further subdivided, such as IIA and IIB. Simply put, a cancer in its early stage will probably be small and confined to its primary site. In an advanced stage, it will be large and will have spread to lymph nodes or other structures.

Carcinoma in situ refers to cancer that is limited to the layer of cells where it developed. Also known as stage 0, it is the earliest stage of a carcinoma. There is no stage 0 category in classification of sarcomas.

There are different ways to determine the stage of a cancer, depending on its type. Some cancers may be staged with physical examination, x-rays, and laboratory tests; others require surgery to explore the tumor directly and remove tissue from it to examine under the microscope.

The TNM system. Cancers are often classified and staged according to the TNM system of the American Joint Committee on Cancer, which looks at three aspects of a cancer.

From Cell to Tumor

The stages of the TNM system represent a natural progression of cancer. All cancers are thought to develop from a single abnormal cell, which divides into two abnormal cells, which divide into four abnormal cells,

| 1 cell | 2 cells | 4 cells | 8 cells | 16 cells | 1 million cells (20 doublings) undetectable | 1 billion cells (30 doublings) lump appears | 1 trillion cells (40 doublings) 2 pounds |

then eight, then sixteen, then thirty-two, and so on. Some cells divide fairly slowly; others divide rapidly. The rate at which cancer cells grow is called doubling time. It is thought that the doubling process must occur thirty times—which can take months, even years—before a tumor can be detected. At this point it will contain about one billion cells and will be large enough to be felt or seen on an x-ray or with an imaging procedure.

- T indicates features of a primary tumor such as its size and whether it has begun to invade nearby tissues and structures, which may include blood vessels, bones, nerves, and organs.

- N refers to whether the cancer has spread to lymph nodes and, if so, the number of nodes involved and the size of the metastases. The location of the affected nodes may influence the N classification in some cancers.

- M signifies whether a cancer has spread to other organs and the extent to which metastasis has occurred.

Each of these letters is assigned a numerical value, a number that defines the extent to which a primary tumor has grown, invaded lymph nodes, and metastasized. However, TX means the tumor cannot be assessed because information is unavailable, T0 means there is no evidence of a primary tumor, and Tis means carcinoma in situ. NX means the local lymph nodes cannot be evaluated, N0 means cancer hasn't spread to the lymph nodes, and N1 means cancer cells were found in the nodes. N2 and N3 refer to more extensive involvement of lymph nodes. MX means spread to distant sites was not evaluated. M0 refers to cancers that haven't spread to distant parts of the body, and M1 refers to those that have.

Once the T, N, and M categories have been determined, this information is condensed by a process known as stage grouping, and each cancer receives a stage of 0 through IV. The details of stage grouping differ somewhat for each cancer type but in general, T1 or T2, N0, M0 cancers are stage I, and any cancer with distant spread (M1) will be stage IV.

Other staging systems. In addition to the TNM staging systems, several other systems are used for some cancers. Since leukemias usually do not form tumor masses and because their cells freely spread throughout the bloodstream, they are staged by a completely different type of system.

2

Cancer Causes and Risks

Who Gets Cancer?

Today, epidemiologists—scientists who study the frequency and distribution of diseases within populations and the factors that influence those patterns—search for factors that appear statistically linked to a person's risk of becoming ill. Their conclusions provide important clues for other scientists investigating the causes of cancer. The discovery that lung cancer occurs more frequently among smokers, for example, led to research that eventually identified the chemicals in cigarette smoke that damage lung cells. Knowing that a family history of colon cancer increases risk encouraged researchers to seek (and ultimately to find) genes related to certain types of the disease. Epidemiologists have identified factors that strongly influence whether or not a person gets cancer. Risk factors increase a person's chance of getting a disease such as cancer. However, neither a risk factor, nor a combination of risk factors can accurately predict an individual's fate. People may use their awareness of some risk factors to guide their behavior, but it's important to remember that statistical odds say nothing about a specific person or his or her fate.

Age

Age is the single most important risk factor for cancer. Cancer is much more likely to occur as a person's age increases. Therefore, most cases affect adults beginning in middle age. About 85 percent of all cancers are diagnosed at ages 50 and older. Several possible explanations exist as to why older people are more susceptible to cancer. One theory suggests that immune function declines with age, so people may lose some of their ability to fight off malignancies. Another theory proposes that free radicals damage the body's cells a million or more times a day. Though natural bodily defenses repair much of this harm, the ability to repair declines with time, and the damage may accumulate until it leads to cancer. According to another theory, the simple fact that older people have lived longer means they've been exposed to carcinogens longer— long enough for many cancers to develop.

Whatever the reason, most forms of cancer rarely strike before the age of 30. Of course, there are exceptions—such as Wilms' tumor, neuroblastoma, Ewing's tumor, and retinoblastoma—that are virtually always limited to children. In general, the probability of developing cancer rises steadily as a person ages. Among some nonepithelial cancers, such as multiple myeloma and chronic lymphocytic leukemia (CLL), rates increase with age until approximately age 74.

CANCER

BASICS

Cancer Risk and Age

This table lists the percentage of patients by age and type of cancer:

Cancer Type	Age in Years			
	<40	40–49	50–64	>64
Prostate	<1	2	33	65
Breast	5	18	32	45
Lung	1	4	21	74
Colorectal	2	7	20	71
All Combined	5	10	26	59

Gender

Throughout his lifetime, a man has approximately a one in two probability of developing cancer; whereas a woman has approximately a one in three probability of developing cancer. With the exception of skin cancer, the most common malignancies in men and women are prostate and breast cancers. Lung cancer is the most common cause of cancer death among both men and women. Breast and prostate cancers now rank as the second largest cancer killers of their respective sexes, and colorectal cancer is third among both men and women. The good news is that overall, mortality rates from 1990 to 1997 showed a decline for both genders.

Leading Sites of New Cancer Cases* and Deaths—2001 Estimates

Cancer Cases by Site and Sex

Male	Female
Male	**Female**
Prostate 198,100	Breast 192,200
Lung & Bronchus 90,700	Lung & Bronchus 78,800
Colon & Rectum 67,300	Colon & Rectum 68,100
Urinary Bladder 39,200	Uterine Corpus 38,300
Non-Hodgkin's lymphoma 31,100	Non-Hodgkin's lymphoma 25,100
Melanoma of the Skin 29,000	Ovary 23,400
Oral Cavity 20,200	Melanoma of the Skin 22,400
Kidney 18,700	Urinary Bladder 15,100
Leukemia 17,700	Pancreas 15,000
Pancreas 14,200	Thyroid 14,900
All Sites 643,000	All Sites 625,000

Cancer Deaths by Site and Sex

Male	Female
Male	**Female**
Lung & Bronchus 90,100	Lung & Bronchus 67,300
Prostate 31,500	Breast 40,200
Colon & Rectum 27,700	Colon & Rectum 29,000
Pancreas 14,100	Pancreas 14,800
Non-Hodgkin's lymphoma 13,800	Ovary 13,900
Leukemia 12,000	Non-Hodgkin's lymphoma 12,500
Esophagus 9,500	Leukemia 9,500
Liver 8,900	Uterine Corpus 6,600
Urinary Bladder 8,300	Brain 5,900
Kidney 7,500	Stomach 5,400
All Sites 286,100	All Sites 267,300

*Excludes basal and squamous cell skin cancer and in situ carcinomas except urinary bladder.

Economics and Race

Low socioeconomic standing (SES) and race/ethnicity factors are often closely related in the United States to the risk of developing—and especially to dying from—cancer. Variations in genetic susceptibility may account for some of these divergences, but SES differences are clearly important. When African Americans are matched with whites by income and educational level, cancer rates among whites are consistently higher—except for cervical, prostate, and stomach cancers. Furthermore, whites in the lowest socioeconomic group experience 20 percent more cancer than whites in the highest socioeconomic group, with cervical cancer incidence four times more likely to occur among poor women. Incidence of larynx and esophageal cancers (cancers related to tobacco and alcohol use) are twice as likely to occur in low SES white men, compared to white men in the highest SES group of white males.

The influence of education and financial resources on cancer diagnosis and treatment is becoming more obvious. Routine Pap tests and treatment of precancerous lesions have drastically decreased cervical cancer mortality among women receiving adequate medical care. But people who do not have access to health care cannot benefit from early detection. People who are poorly educated about cancer often believe that a cancer diagnosis is always fatal. Thus, they often fail to recognize the potentially life-saving importance of early detection.

Higher-income individuals, though their overall cancer rate is lower, still suffer disproportionately from malignancies of the breast and uterus. This may be due in part to having children at a later stage in life, which in turn increases a woman's exposure to estrogen.

Family History

Some malignancies, such as breast, ovarian, prostate, colon, and some other cancers occur far more often in some families than others. Just as we inherit hair color, eye color, and other attributes in our genes, we may inherit susceptibility to some cancers. A few cancers have been linked to specific genes that can be tracked within a family. For example, approximately 40 percent of children with retinoblastoma (cancer of the eye) have inherited an abnormal Rb tumor suppressor gene from one parent. In some cases, such as the very rare Li-Fraumeni syndrome, particular genes make family members susceptible to a wide variety of malignancies.

A member of a family who knows that a particular cancer has occurred in several generations or who has first-degree relatives with the cancer is said to have a family history of the disease. Family history is such an important clue to one's susceptibility to cancer that a primary health care worker taking a person's health history will spend some time inquiring about the health of other family members. Accurate tests exist that can determine whether or not a gene known to increase the risk of a particular cancer has been inherited (see pages 22–23, *What Is Genetic Testing?*).

Although it is extremely helpful to know your genetic heritage, it's also important to keep in mind that less than 10 percent of all cancers are associated with a family history. Most families, especially large ones, have one or more members who have had a cancer, but relatively few of these families carry inherited cancer predisposition genes.

Shaking the Family Tree

To create a resource that will be useful to you and your relatives, assemble the following facts about your parents, siblings, grandparents, aunts, and uncles. Keep in mind, though, that many factors—environmental as well as inherited—are involved. Being aware of your genetic heritage can help your doctor tailor a cancer prevention and early detection plan for you. Make a chart that indicates the following information about your relatives: cause of death—that is, the cause given on the death certificate; serious illnesses, including age of onset; and behavioral risk factors, such as smoking and drinking.

If elderly relatives are reticent about discussing cancer, a taboo subject a generation or two ago, explain how the information will help you. Next, make sure to let your doctor know your findings and share them with those relatives who may also be affected.

INFORM

YOURSELF

Heredity and Cancer. Between 10 and 15 percent of all cancers are thought to have a familial basis. That means that the cancer tends to occur among members of a family. Much of the time, different types of cancer occur apparently by chance, or in association with common family habits such as cigarette smoking. However, studies have suggested that certain cancers can occur to excess in some families. For example, a woman whose mother and/or sisters (first-degree relatives) had breast cancer is two to three times more likely to develop breast cancer than a woman whose close female relatives have not had breast cancer.

In some families, cancers of one or more types develop in several family members significantly more often than the average cancer occurrence. Families with above average occurrence of breast cancer, for example, have been observed to have more cancers of the ovary, prostate, and pancreas than expected. Scientists are studying members of some of those families, seeking genetic changes that might explain why the cancers develop. (For more information about genes and cancer, or for information about the Human Genome Project, see Chapter 1.)

Genetic Counseling. A gene is a segment of DNA that contains information on hereditary characteristics such as hair color, eye color, and height, as well as susceptibility (likelihood of being affected) to certain diseases. Some genes, called oncogenes, contribute to the development of cancer. Other genes may protect individuals from cancer. Genes that suppress or stop cancer growth are called tumor suppressor genes (see Chapter 1).

If an inherited cancer gene is suspected, a genetic counselor is immediately consulted. Genetic counselors often have specialized training or master's degrees in their field. Advanced practice oncology nurses may also provide genetic counseling with specialized training. The philosophy of genetic counseling has typically been to present information in an unbiased or neutral fashion to allow the patients to make their own decisions about genetic testing. Sometimes, however, the indications are clear-cut enough that the doctor will make a recommendation about the testing and follow up care.

Issues you may want to discuss with a genetic counselor include:

- the way in which families inherit cancers and how genes are transmitted

- the types of cancer seen in your family

- which family members should be tested

- individuals' estimated risk

- the benefits, risks, costs, and limitations of testing

- effective ways to manage the risk, such as lifestyle changes, early detection practices, watching for signs and symptoms of cancer, chemo-prevention, and preventive surgery

Many issues require a counselor's expertise. The risk of disease for children and the potential for discrimination can be frightening. A genetic counselor can help you explore fears and concerns as well as coping strategies. He or she can also explore with you how to discuss the test results and what they mean with other family members. A positive result on a genetic test does not mean that you will inevitably develop the cancer for which you are at increased risk. Meeting with a genetic counselor at this time will help you understand exactly what your cancer risk is and what you need to do to reduce the risk as well as detect cancer early, should it occur.

What Is Genetic Testing? Some gene mutations can be inherited from parents and cause a person to have a greater risk of developing certain cancers. Inherited mutations affect all cells of a person's body. These inherited mutations can often be identified by genetically testing blood samples. Genetic counseling and testing may be recommended for some people with a strong family history of cancer.

Genetic testing may be conducted to see if a person has a certain gene change (mutation) known to increase the risk for a specific condition or disease (such as cancer), or to confirm a suspected mutation in an individual or family. Such testing is not recommended for everyone, but doctors will sometimes recommend patients undergo genetic testing if there is a strong family history of a disease. If you have more than two first-degree relatives (mother, father, sister, brother) with cancer, family members who developed cancer at a young age, relatives with rare cancers, or a known genetic mutation in the family, you might consider genetic testing.

The Risks and Benefits of Genetic Testing. Genetic analysis is an area of intense research interest. For example, researchers have isolated gene mutations associated with familial adenomatous polyposis, a familial form of colorectal cancer. They believe that if preventive measures are not taken, up to 95 percent of people with these gene mutations will eventually develop cancer of the colon.

Similarly, certain mutations of the BRCA1 and BRCA2 genes indicate that a woman has a 50 to 85 percent chance of developing breast cancer.

Despite the seemingly beneficial potential of identifying genes associated with increased cancer risk, genetic testing is controversial because:

- Genetic tests provide limited answers. These tests do not provide perfect answers for those concerned about inherited diseases. A positive test result does not necessarily mean that a disease will occur. On the other hand, a negative result does not mean that you have no risk.

- Genetic testing can have immense and complex psychological impact. Learning that you have or might develop a serious disease is frightening and can affect entire families. Positive results may be upsetting, and the implications of these results are not precise, which may cause confusion. Many results may require additional testing and create significant anxiety for a family.

- Genetic testing involves privacy issues. Most people who are concerned about privacy issues and genetic information are concerned about how the information may harm them.

Furthermore, there is a concern about who beyond the individual is entitled to genetic information and who has access to it. Many fear that health and life insurers might use such data to deny coverage to those at higher than normal risk or that potential employers would avoid hiring anyone who might one day face a devastating illness. There are serious concerns about the medical, scientific, ethical, legal, and social issues raised by the development of and use of genetic tests.

The American Cancer Society supports the National Institutes of Health–Department of Energy Working Group on Ethical, Legal and Social Implications of Human Genome Research and the National Action Plan on Breast Cancer (NAPBC) recommendations on genetic information and health insurance and employment. Among the various recommendations are that insurance providers and employers should be prohibited from using genetic information to deny or limit coverage or increase the cost for it, employers cannot request this information or use it to affect the hiring of a person, and holders of genetic information (apart from research settings governed by the Federal Policy for the Protection of Human Research Subjects) should be prohibited from releasing genetic information without prior written authorization of the individual.

QUESTIONS

TO ASK

Before You Have That Test

If you suspect that you are at increased risk of a particular cancer, it's helpful to discuss your concerns with a genetic counselor before you have the test. Talking over answers to the following questions will help you make an informed decision.

- What are the benefits of this test for me and my family?

- What are the drawbacks?

- Will a positive result affect my ability to keep and get life, disability, and health insurance?

- Will the test results influence my job or my future prospects?

- Is it possible to keep the results of the test confidential?

- If the test result is positive, is there anything that can be done to lower my risk? To improve the possibility of early detection?

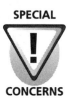

SPECIAL

CONCERNS

Do You Need Extra Tests?

If you have a family history of a particular cancer or if your lifestyle, environment, or occupation has exposed you significantly to a carcinogen, you may be at high risk for a type of cancer for which routine screening is not recommended.

If you want a test that is not routinely recommended, your doctor should explain the costs, risks, and benefits of the procedure under the principle of informed consent.

If you want such a test but your doctor disagrees with your choice, you have two options: (1) the doctor may proceed with the test after explaining his or her misgivings, or (2) the doctor may refuse to perform the test and you can seek a second opinion (see Chapter 7).

Environment

The term environment refers not only to the natural world, but to every outside influence on the body. Thus, to say that environmental factors account for cancers doesn't mean that epidemiologists exclusively blame industrial chemicals seeping into drinking water or wastes contaminating the air. Rather, it means that cancers may arise from countless outside forces, including viruses and other infectious agents; x-rays, sunlight, and other sources of radiation; and substances encountered in the home or workplace. It is estimated that three-fourths of all cancers in the United States arise from tobacco and alcohol use, diet, and reproductive and sexual behavior. Contrary to most people's perceptions, exposure to occupational and industrial hazards and pollution probably accounts for fewer than 10 percent of all cancer cases.

Tobacco. Tobacco is an environmental factor that accounts for at least 30 percent of all cancer deaths affecting users—smokers—as well as nonsmokers who breathe in second-hand smoke.

Lung cancer, which strikes smokers nearly twenty times more often as nonsmokers, overwhelmingly results from cigarette smoking. Cancers of the mouth, throat, larynx, esophagus, bladder, kidney, colon, pancreas, cervix, and other organs are also related to use of tobacco products. Smoking also triples the risk of squamous cell skin cancer. In the case of cancer in organs along the airway—including the mouth, throat, and lungs—direct exposure to smoke is to blame. But the carcinogens in cigarette smoke can be swallowed, contributing to esophageal and colon cancers. The carcinogens also enter the bloodstream from the lungs and circulate to distant organs. For instance, carcinogens from tobacco smoke are filtered by the kidneys and concentrated in the urine, which damages the cells that line the bladder. In fact, the greatest risk factor for bladder cancer is smoking.

Pipes and cigars, though less likely to cause lung cancer than cigarettes, are implicated in tumors of the mouth, throat, and lip. More than 200 years ago, smokeless tobacco (snuff and chewing tobacco) was tied to mouth cancer. More recently, scientists have established that passive smoking—inhaling others' cigarette smoke without smoking oneself (second-hand or environmental tobacco smoke)—also increases the risk of developing lung cancer. A nonsmoker married to a smoker has a 30 percent greater risk of developing lung cancer than if he or she were married to a nonsmoker.

Alcohol. Alcohol works in partnership with tobacco, increasing the chances that smokers who also drink will develop mouth, throat, larynx, stomach, liver, and esophageal cancer. Heavy drinking will lead to liver cirrhosis, causing scarring that obstructs blood flow in the liver and increases the risk of cancer.

Use of alcohol is clearly linked to increased risk of developing breast cancer. Compared with nondrinkers, women who consume one alcoholic drink a day have a very small increase in risk, and those who have two to five drinks daily have about 1.5 times the risk of women who drink no alcohol.

Diet and Physical Activity. A diet high in animal fat and low in vegetables and fruits and a sedentary lifestyle may account for approximately one-third of the 500,000 cancer deaths that occur in the United States each year. These include types of food, food preparation methods, portion sizes, and food variety. Obesity, which can result from a sedentary lifestyle as well as consuming too many calories, is a lifestyle factor that is linked to cancer of the endometrium, cervix, uterus, ovary, and gallbladder among women; cancer of the breast in postmenopausal women; and colon and prostate cancer in men.

Fat and cancer. Limiting high-fat foods, particularly from animal sources, may lower your risk of developing cancer. A high-fat diet is believed to be a cancer promoter. Whether risk is influenced by the total amount of fat, the particular type of fat (saturated, monounsaturated, or polysaturated), the calories contributed by fat, or some other factor in food fats has not yet been determined. Consumption of meat, especially red meat, has been associated with increased cancer risk at several sites, most notably colon and prostate. Dietary fat also seems to be involved in the production of free radicals, which play a role in many types of cancer.

Additives and preparation methods. An estimated 2,300 "flavoring agents" are added to foods to preserve them and to enhance color, flavor, and texture. Additives are usually present in very small quantities in food, and no convincing evidence exists that any additive at these levels causes human cancers.

Pesticides and herbicides. The term pesticide covers a wide range of biologically active chemical compounds intended to kill pests: insects (insecticides), fungi (fungicides), rodents (rodenticides), and plants or weeds (herbicides). The health hazards of pesticides are primarily connected to direct contact with the chemicals at potentially high doses, for example, farm workers who apply the chemicals and work in the fields after the pesticides have been applied, and people living near aerially sprayed fields. In contrast to occupational and environmental health hazards, pesticide residues in marketed foods pose negligible risks to human health. Government regulations establish safety standards and provide inspection procedures to guard against violation of those standards. Tolerance levels for pesticide residues in food are set far below levels at which toxicity occurs in experimental animals and far below levels at which many natural carcinogens already exist in food. The benefits of a balanced diet rich in fruits and vegetables far outweigh the largely theoretical risks posed by occasional, very low pesticide residue levels in foods.

Natural carcinogens. Although naturally occurring carcinogens do not present much of a problem in the United States, they do exist. One of the most notable is aflatoxin, one of the most potent liver carcinogens known. Aflatoxins are chemicals produced by fungi that grow on moldy grains, corn, peanuts, cottonseed, or other crops. Long-term exposure to it contributes to the high rates of liver cancer in Africa.

Although much attention has been paid to food additives and preservatives, many epidemiologists now believe that perhaps more attention should be focused on dietary habits than on particular chemical carcinogens.

INFORM

YOURSELF

American Cancer Society Nutrition Guidelines*

1. Choose most of the foods you eat from plant sources.
   - Eat five or more servings of fruits and vegetables each day
   - Eat other foods from plant sources, such as breads, cereals, grain products, rice, pasta, or beans several times each day

2. Limit your intake of high-fat foods, particularly from animal sources.
   - Choose foods low in fat
   - Limit consumption of meats, especially high-fat meats

3. Be physically active: achieve and maintain a healthy weight.
   - Be at least moderately active for thirty minutes or more on most days of the week
   - Stay within your healthy weight range

4. Limit consumption of alcoholic beverages, if you drink at all.

For persons who are two years old and older

Sexual and Reproductive Behavior. Reproductive and sexual behavior—including number of sexual partners, exposure to sexually transmitted viral infections, and age at which a woman first gives birth—also influences cancer risk. People's choices regarding sexuality and reproduction affect their cancer risk in a variety of ways.

Sexually transmitted infections. Because exposure to the sexually transmitted human papilloma viruses has been strongly associated with cervical cancer, women's risk of contracting the disease rises when they have many sex partners, when they have sex with men who have had many sex partners, or when they become sexually active early in life (see *Infectious Agents,* page 28).

Delaying or avoiding childbearing. Women who don't have children or who have them later in life are at increased risk for both breast and ovarian cancer. This is because a high cumulative exposure to estrogen is a major risk factor for these cancers. When a woman has a child at a later stage of life, her exposure is greater than that of women who have children when they're younger. When a woman has no children, her exposure to estrogen continues until menopause.

Infectious Agents. Because viruses can invade and alter cells' genetic material, viral infections are implicated in some cancers. The Epstein-Barr virus, for example, is associated with Burkitt's lymphoma, a tumor found mainly among children in Africa. Epstein-Barr has also been linked to nasopharyngeal cancer. Hepatitis B and C viruses are responsible for much of the world's liver cancer that often results in death. The human papilloma viruses that cause genital warts also play important roles in cervical cancer and to a lesser extent contribute to vaginal, vulvar, and penile cancers. The human T-cell leukemia/lymphoma virus—a close relative of the human immunodeficiency virus or HIV that causes acquired immune deficiency syndrome (AIDS)—is associated with a type of leukemia found most often in the Caribbean and Japan. Scientists have found that most tumors in people with Kaposi's sarcoma contain a virus they have named Kaposi's sarcoma-associated herpes virus, or human herpesvirus-8 (HHV-8). Since the virus has also been found in people who do not have Kaposi's sarcoma, researchers think it leads to the development of the cancer in people who have other conditions such as HIV infection, AIDS, or whose immunity has been suppressed by drugs taken to facilitate organ transplantation.

Recently bacteria, one-cell organisms that are larger than viruses, have also been implicated in cancer risk. For example, a long-standing stomach infection with *Helicobacter pylori* damages the inner lining of the stomach and seems to create a precancerous condition. Animal studies have shown that these bacteria convert nitrates and nitrites into compounds that cause stomach cancer. It's believed that dietary factors—such as eating a lot of smoked and salted foods and starches and few fruits and vegetables—also influence stomach cancer risk.

People with cancer of the stomach have a higher rate of *Helicobacter pylori* infection. The infection is also linked to some types of lymphoma of the stomach. However, having the infection does not mean one will develop cancer. In fact, most people who carry the bacteria in their stomachs never develop cancer.

Parasites, organisms that live in or on other organisms, are associated with an increased risk of certain cancers. *Opisthorchis viverrini*, a liver fluke in East Asia, causes an infection that is associated with increased risk of cancer of the bile ducts. Chronic infection with another parasitic worm found in Asia, called

Clonorchis sinensis, increases the risk of liver cancer. *Schistosoma haematobium*, which is found in Africa and Asia, is linked to bladder cancer.

Other Carcinogens in the Environment. Environmental factors include smoking, diet, and infectious diseases as well as chemicals and radiation in our homes and workplaces. We've discussed the first few factors in earlier sections; here we'll address the trace levels of pollutants that may sometimes be present in food, drinking water, and in the air. Keep in mind that the degree of risk from pollutants depends on their concentration and intensity, as well as people's exposure to the pollutants. Strong regulatory control and attention to safe occupational practices, drug testing, and consumer product safety play an important role in reducing risk of cancer from environmental exposures. The U.S. Food and Drug Administration (FDA), the Environmental Protection Agency (EPA), and the Occupational Safety and Health Administration (OSHA) develop safety standards and apply laws and procedures aimed at controlling risk for Americans.

Radon. This radioactive gas is produced by the natural breakdown of uranium, and it cannot be seen, tasted, or smelled. Outdoors, there is so little radon that it is not a danger. But indoors, radon can be more concentrated and can become a possible risk for cancer. In recent years, concerns have been raised about houses in some parts of the United States built over soil with natural uranium deposits, which can create high indoor radon levels. High radon levels in some mines can increase the lung cancer risk for miners. An unknown but substantial number of homes and office buildings contain radon.

Ultraviolet (UV) light. The main source of UV radiation is sunlight. Tanning lamps and booths are another source. UV radiation poses a definite danger, especially to light-skinned people, and this hazard increases as one approaches the equator.

People who are often exposed to strong sunlight without protection have a greater risk of skin cancer, including melanoma and nonmelanoma skin cancer. The amount of UV exposure depends on the strength of the light, the length of exposure, and whether the skin is protected.

People who live in areas with year-round, bright sunlight have a higher risk. For example, the risk of nonmelanoma skin cancer is twice as high in Arizona as compared to Minnesota. Spending a lot of time outdoors for work or recreation without protection with clothing and sunscreen increases your risk. Tanning lamps and tanning booths are other sources of UV radiation that may produce a greater risk of nonmelanoma skin cancer.

People who suffer severe, blistering sunburns, particularly in their childhood or teenage years, are also at increased risk of developing melanoma. Intermittent, intense exposures are associated with melanoma risk more than lower level, chronic exposures, even if the total dose of UV is the same.

CANCER

BASICS

Evaluating Carcinogenic Substances and Cancer Risk

Risks are assessed to protect people against unsafe exposures and to set appropriate environmental standards. The first step in risk assessment is identifying the chemical or physical nature of a hazard and its cancer-producing potential through research. Special attention is given to any evidence suggesting that cancer risk increases with increase in exposure. The second step is measuring levels of hazard in the environment (air, water, or food) and the extent to which people are actually exposed (how much they eat of a particular food, use a particular water source, and so on). Knowledge of how the body absorbs chemicals or is exposed to radiation is essential for such dose measurements.

Unfortunately, evidence of risk for most potential carcinogens is usually the result of high-dose experiments on animals or observations where high-dose exposures have occurred in humans. To use such information to set human safety standards, scientists must extrapolate from animals to humans and from high-dose to low-dose conditions. Because both extrapolations involve much uncertainty, conservative assumptions are used so that risk assessment will err on the side of safety. For cancer safety standards, only increased risks of one case or less per million persons over a lifetime are usually acceptable.

Safety standards developed in this way for chemical or radiation exposures are the basis for federal regulatory activities. The organizations on page 31 provide information about potentially carcinogenic substances to regulatory and research agencies and the public. These groups often identify *potential cancer hazards*, or substances that are *reasonably thought to be carcinogens*, as well as *known carcinogens*. It is important to understand that a substance's appearance in one of the organizations' reports on carcinogens does not necessarily mean that the substance presents a cancer risk to an individual in daily life.

It is also important to note that listings of carcinogenic substances do not always address or attempt to balance potential benefits of exposures to certain carcinogenic substances in special situations. For example, numerous drugs used to treat cancer have been shown to increase the occurrence of secondary cancers. In these instances, the benefits of exposure to the drugs for treatment or prevention of a specific disease have been determined by the FDA to outweigh the additional cancer risks associated with their use.

Decisions about the use of a given drug or any other agent should be made only after consulting with a doctor or other appropriate specialist about both risks and benefits.

Contact the organizations on the next page for a current list of carcinogenic substances (see *Resources* for contact information).

The U.S. Department of Health and Human Services' **National Toxicology Program (NTP)** consists of work by the National Institutes of Health's National Institute of Environmental Health Sciences (NIH/NIEHS), the Centers for Disease Control and Prevention's National Institute for Occupational Safety and Health (CDC/NIOSH), and the FDA's National Center for Toxicological Research (FDA/NCTR).

The NTP's *Report on Carcinogens (RoC)* identifies substances—such as metals, pesticides, drugs, and natural and synthetic chemicals—and mixtures or exposure circumstances that are *"known"* or are *"reasonably anticipated"* to cause cancer, and to which a significant number of Americans are exposed.

The *RoC* is published every two years. The 9th edition of the *RoC*, published in 2001, contains 218 entries. The new listings in the 9th edition include some agents and substances to which large numbers of people are exposed including tobacco, alcohol, diesel exhaust, UV solar radiation, and use of sun lamps and sun beds.

The listing of a substance in the *RoC* is not a regulatory action, but listing may prompt regulatory agencies to consider limiting exposures or uses of a substance. In addition, the U.S. Congress, Federal and State Agencies, businesses, unions, and the general public all use the *RoC* to ensure that reasonable precautions or regulations are in place.

The International Agency for Research on Cancer (IARC) is part of the World Health Organization, which is involved in cancer research. The IARC coordinates and conducts research on the causes of human cancer and the mechanisms of carcinogenesis.

The *IARC Monographs* are critical reviews and evaluations of scientific evidence on the cancer-causing effects of a wide range of human exposures. These evaluations represent only one source of information on which regulatory measures may be based. Because priorities and socioeconomic factors vary from country to country, no recommendations for regulations are given. Legislation is the responsibility of individual governments and/or other international organizations.

The **U.S. Environmental Protection Agency (EPA)** implements the federal laws designed to promote public health by protecting U.S. air, water, and soil from harmful pollution. The EPA conducts research, monitors and enforces activities, and sets standards. The EPA also coordinates and supports research and anti-pollution activities of state and local governments, private and public groups, individuals, and educational institutions. The EPA also monitors the operations of other federal agencies with respect to their impact on the environment.

Occupation. Occupational exposures to chemical carcinogens contribute to approximately 4 percent of cancers, and scientists have identified a number of occupations that increase risk.

Industries whose workers may face increased cancer risks include transportation, chemicals, rubber, shipbuilding, hairdressing and cosmetology, agriculture, electric equipment manufacture, health care, and farming. Such materials as asbestos, petroleum, benzene, styrene, formaldehyde, solvents, dyes, cadmium, lead, cotton and wool dust, the disinfectant ethylene oxide, diesel exhaust, radioisotopes, flame retardants, fertilizers, and pesticides may all contribute to cancers. But keep in mind that although cancer risk may increase when these substances are encountered frequently and at high levels, when the general public encounters low-level exposures in the environment there is often little impact on cancer risk.

Medical Treatments. Ironically, some of the treatments that doctors use to restore health can increase the risk of cancer. For example, some cancer chemotherapy drugs are carcinogenic. Immunosuppressive drugs used in conjunction with organ transplants reduce the body's ability to fight off malignancies. Estrogen may be prescribed following the removal of the ovaries and to replace the estrogen no longer produced by a woman's body after menopause. It may also increase a woman's risk of endometrial cancer. The radiation from radiation therapy can damage cells, and when that damage is extensive, it may cause cancer. Several types of cancer chemotherapy drugs also increase the risk of developing a second cancer, especially in patients who also receive radiation therapy.

However, the benefits of these treatments far outweigh the slightly increased risk of cancer they may cause. The low risk of developing cancer as a result of undergoing treatment pales in comparison to the danger involved with not treating existing cancer at all. Although doctors are careful to avoid prescribing any more radiation or chemotherapy than is absolutely necessary, patients concerned about second cancers should not hesitate to ask their oncologists about this issue.

Fear of Cancer

People's perceptions of cancer risk do not always match the true level of danger. Although approximately half of all smokers die from diseases caused by smoking, millions of people continue to puff away, either undeterred by the fact that stopping would lower their risk of developing cancer or not caring. On the other hand, a great deal of media attention has been paid to the potential cancer risk of living near high-tension electrical power lines or utility substations. Yet after years of deliberation, the American Physical Society, representing the

Can Emotions Make You Sick?

For some years now, the suspicion has been growing that the mind may play a role in influencing who gets cancer. One popular theory suggests that emotional states like depression can encourage the growth of a malignancy. Another holds that stress and negative feelings suppress the immune function, which is believed to be crucial to preventing the disease.

A veritable industry now churns out books, articles, tapes, lectures, and workshops dedicated to the proposition that positive emotions, thoughts, and attitudes can keep cancer at bay and even defeat it should it strike.

Some psychological researchers seek the traits that add up to a "cancer-prone" personality. Others map mental strategies to defeat malignancies. In fact, some of the more extreme mind-body approaches come perilously close to "blaming the victim" for either becoming sick or failing to conquer an aggressive, potentially fatal disease. Others more circumspectly observe that social support seems to help many people cope with the severe stress of having cancer and undergoing its treatment.

The scientific verdict on this work is mixed. Although some studies support a relationship between mental factors and either the onset or course of cancer, others do not. Critics, furthermore, discount as poorly designed some of those studies claiming a connection. Recent large, well-designed studies have found no relationship between emotions and cancer onset. But there is one way that emotions can affect cancer risk more directly: smoking, drinking, and other behaviors known to be linked to cancer often represent an attempt to cope with stress or depression.

world's largest group of physicists, has found no scientific evidence that the electromagnetic fields radiating from the power lines cause cancer.

Behavior Impacts Risk

Although many Americans fear cancer more than any other disease, some studies suggest that people more readily accept risks that they choose voluntarily, like smoking, than they do risks imposed on them without their consent, like air pollution. This may explain why people greatly overestimate the proportion of the nation's cancers that arise from involuntary exposure to industrial chemicals and pollution. Although some environmental factors do pose serious hazards to people working in particular industries or living in certain areas, these represent only a small portion of Americans' total cancer risk. Rather, those elements of lifestyle like smoking, diet, and reproductive practices that are theoretically changeable but deeply embedded in people's habits account for the great majority of cancers. A rational view of risk must be at the heart of any sensible prevention program. Indeed, research shows that the less people know about cancer, the more they fear it. Fearful people are less likely to take effective action to protect their health and to follow guidelines for early detection of cancers that are most easily treated before they produce noticeable symptoms (see Chapter 4). A practical approach to cancer prevention thus demands an understanding of what does and does not cause the disease and awareness that there remain many unknown factors.

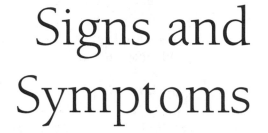

CHAPTER

3

Signs and Symptoms

A symptom is an indication of disease, illness, or injury, or simply that something is not right in the body. Symptoms can be felt or noticed by a patient. For example, symptoms that might indicate pneumonia are chills, weakness, achiness, shortness of breath, and coughing.

A sign is also an indication of illness, injury, or that something is not right in the body. But, signs are defined as observations made by a doctor, nurse, or other health care professional. Signs that may indicate pneumonia are fever, rapid breathing rate, and abnormal breathing sounds heard through a stethoscope.

The presence of one symptom or sign may not provide enough information to suggest its cause. For example, a rash in a child could be a symptom of a number of things, including poison ivy, a generalized infection like rubella, an infection limited to the skin, or a food allergy. If the rash is associated with a high fever, chills, achiness, and a sore throat, the combination of symptoms provides a better picture of the illness. But in many cases, a patient's signs and symptoms do not provide enough clues to determine the cause of an illness, and medical tests such as x-rays, blood tests, or a biopsy may be needed.

As untreated cancer progresses, it goes through many stages, producing an array of symptoms and signs along the way. Some occur early and are caused by a tumor growing within a single organ or structure. If a cancer spreads, it may produce entirely new symptoms and signs as other organs, structures, and systems become involved. As the immune system fights to rid the body of malignant cells, still other symptoms and signs arise.

Effects of Primary Tumor Growth

The signs and symptoms caused by a primary tumor vary greatly, depending mostly on the tumor's location. If a tumor arises near the surface of the body, the patient or a health care professional may notice a lump, thickening, or swelling. Many skin, thyroid, salivary gland, breast, and testicular cancers are found this way. But the situation is different for tumors that develop deep inside the body. These tumors generally cannot be felt until they are very large, and they are often found because their growth affects the functioning of the organ they develop within or that of nearby organs, nerves, and blood vessels. This pressure creates some of the earliest warning signs of cancer, especially when a tumor is in an area of the body with little room for expansion. For instance, even a small tumor in the brain can cause headaches by pressing on blood vessels and nerves or blocking the flow of spinal fluid. A growth inside the esophagus, the passageway between the throat and stomach, may cause dysphagia, or difficulty swallowing.

Cancers of the head of the pancreas next to the bile duct may block the flow of bile while they are still quite small. This blockage causes bile to accumulate in the blood and tissues, resulting in jaundice, a yellowing of the skin and eyes. However, if the tumor is in the tail of the pancreas there is no blockage, and jaundice is unlikely. In this case, the tumor will usually grow quite large before causing any symptoms. Pain or backache, which occur if the tumor grows around nearby nerves, may be one of the first symptoms of this tumor. For this reason, tumors in the tail of the pancreas are usually found later than those of the head, and tend to have a worse prognosis.

Growing tumors can also erode blood vessels. This usually results in bleeding from an orifice near the tumor. Common examples are blood in the stool caused by a tumor rupturing blood vessels in the colon, blood in sputum caused by ruptured vessels of a lung cancer, and a blood-tinged vaginal discharge in women with cervical or endometrial cancer.

Effects of Metastatic Tumors

As a cancer spreads to distant organs and tissues, additional signs and symptoms often develop. For example, the spread of cancer to bones may cause pain over the affected bone. Brain metastases may cause neurological symptoms such as weakness or paralysis, or problems with speech or thinking. In most metastatic cancer cases, the patient's diagnosis is already known. Sometimes, however, the primary cancer may be very small. In these cases, the symptoms resulting from metastatic tumors are the first indication of a cancer.

Paraneoplastic Syndromes

Cancers occasionally cause symptoms by interfering with the functioning of organs far from the primary or metastatic tumors. These remote effects are called paraneoplastic syndromes, and are due to biologically active substances produced by the cancer cells and released into the bloodstream.

Many of these syndromes are caused when cancer cells release hormone-like substances. For example, some small cell lung cancers produce high levels of antiduretic hormone (ADH), a substance normally produced by the pituitary gland to help regulate water balance in the body. The high levels of this hormone released by these cancers may cause serious water retention and dilution of the blood, leading to weakness and even coma. Squamous cell lung cancer and, less often, cancers of the kidneys, ovaries, pancreas, or other organs can release hormone-like substances that interfere with normal calcium balance in the body. These substances cause excessively high calcium levels in the blood, leading to such symptoms as weakness, dizziness, confusion, and other nervous system problems, as well as constipation and frequent urination.

Other cancers, especially those of the pancreas and stomach, may release substances that cause blood clots in veins or arteries of the arms, legs, or lungs.

The body's immune system often recognizes cancer cells as abnormal but, unfortunately, is usually unable to effectively destroy the malignant cells (see Chapter 1). Sometimes an immune response against the cancer cells runs awry and the immune system starts to attack normal cells. The immune systems of patients with lung, breast, and ovarian cancers sometimes produce antibodies which, although ineffective against the cancer cells, can damage cells of the cerebellum, the part of the brain responsible for balance and coordination.

Although paraneoplastic syndromes are relatively uncommon, they are important for two reasons. The first is that their symptoms can have a significant and adverse impact of the patient's quality of life. The second is that they may initially suggest that the patient has a condition other than cancer, causing a delay in accurate diagnosis and effective treatment.

The Body Goes to War

The immune system is like an elaborate military force. Each of its several components has a different and highly specialized function. As the immune system battles cancer cells, the consequences of this internal war may become obvious. For example, immune system cells release cytokines, hormone-like substances that cause a variety of symptoms, such as chills and fever, loss of appetite, fatigue, and other problems similar to the flu. People with cancer also may find they are more susceptible to infectious diseases as the immune system directs much of its energy to killing the cancer.

General Signs and Symptoms of Cancer

It is important to be aware of some of the general (nonspecific) signs and symptoms of cancer. They include unexplained weight loss, fever, fatigue, pain, and changes in the skin.

Weight Loss

Most people with advanced cancer will lose weight and may develop a related condition called cachexia, which refers not only to the loss of fat and muscle, but also to the wasting away of organs. The heart, liver, and brain are usually spared the effects of cachexia (see Chapter 18). But unexplained weight loss can also be an early sign of cancer. Unexplained weight loss means the scale may register a five-pound loss within two weeks or a ten-pound loss within a month or so, even though the person has not dieted or increased the amount of his or her exercise.

Fever

About 30 percent of people with cancer experience fever at some point in the course of their disease. There are many causes of fever in people with cancer, such as infections, reactions to medications or blood transfusions, and production of fever-causing substances by the cancer cells themselves. A cancer patient's white blood cell count is the best predictor of how likely he or she is to develop a serious infection. Among patients with low white blood cell counts, two-thirds of fevers are due to infections. When the patient's white blood cell count is not low, about one-fifth of fevers are due to an infection. Kidney cancer, liver cancer, Hodgkin's disease, and non-Hodgkin's lymphoma are the cancers most likely to cause fever by releasing fever-causing substances.

Fatigue

Fatigue—having less energy to do the things you normally do or want to do— is the most common side effect of cancer treatment, but it can also occur before treatment is ever started. Usually fatigue is not a significant symptom until a cancer is fairly advanced, unless the person is experiencing chronic blood loss. (Often stomach or colon cancer causes blood loss.) Cancers that replace normal blood-forming cells of the bone marrow may lead to a shortage of red blood cells. This, in turn, may cause weakness and low energy levels. For reasons that are still not understood, some cancer patients have severe fatigue even when they have no shortage of red blood cells.

Pain

Pain is a symptomatic wild card. It may result from many aspects of the disease. Most often, discomfort suggests advanced disease. Usually it's the result of the destruction of healthy tissue by a tumor or infection, pressure on nerves, stretching of internal organs and other structures, or the obstruction of an organ.

Most early cancers cause masses that are painless, but pain is occasionally among the first signs of cancer. For instance, sarcomas are often painful early

SPECIAL

CONCERNS

Can Your Mood Be a Cancer Symptom?

By influencing hormones and brain chemicals, physical illnesses such as cancer can produce anxiety and depression. In other cases, cancers can cause physical symptoms such as fatigue and loss of appetite that are interpreted by patients and doctors as being caused by a mood problem. Of the cancers that can produce such symptoms, pancreatic cancer seems to be the most common. In many cases, symptoms of depression, anxiety, insomnia, and feelings of impending doom appear before any physical symptoms of cancer. Since cancer of the pancreas often produces no specific bodily signs and symptoms until the illness is quite advanced, symptoms of mood changes could be an important early warning sign in some cases.

Pay attention to depression, anxiety, or other emotional symptoms that seem to appear from nowhere. Like most of the other early warning signs of cancer, the mood symptoms could also indicate a number of other problems, or nothing at all. If your feelings of depression or anxiety don't go away within a few weeks, see your doctor. Regardless of whether your emotional symptoms occur before or after a diagnosis of cancer, or whether they result from hormonal, nervous system, or other causes, it is important to remember that talking to your doctor is the first step toward finding treatments that can help you feel better.

on; testicular cancer can cause pain in the scrotum; bladder cancer can make urination uncomfortable; and certain lung tumors can cause discomfort in the arm, shoulder, and upper back and chest on the side where the growth is located. Growths that are confined to small spaces—such as the brain, eye, or sinuses—may cause pain by pressing on nearby blood vessels or nerves.

Cancer pain does not always occur at the site of the tumor. Because the body is linked by a network of nerves that feed into the same system for interpretation by the brain, pain in one part of the body may be perceived as originating in another. This phenomenon is known as referred pain. For example, pain produced by a tumor of the esophagus is often felt in or near the shoulder, and stomach cancers often cause pain in the chest.

Although the pain of advanced cancer can be intense and persistent, progress in pain management now means that unremitting suffering can be avoided (see Chapter 23).

Skin Clues

Cancer can cause dozens of visible signs of its presence. Some of the most obvious are cancers of the skin. A skin tumor often starts as a small growth that eventually ulcerates, bleeds, and doesn't scab over and heal. A mole that becomes malignant (that is, a melanoma), initially exhibits subtle but significant changes. It may change from having a definite border to looking as if it is spreading in all directions. It may change in color or size.

Although rare, a metastatic growth on the skin can result from a primary tumor of the lung, breast, colon, ovary, stomach, or kidney. Such a growth on the skin is usually a firm flesh-colored, reddish, or bluish nodule. Sometimes these tumors arise on the scalp and cause patchy hair loss.

Among the other signs of cancer that appear on the skin are:

- darkening of the skin, or hyperpigmentation
- reddening of skin, or erythema
- itching, or pruritus
- excessive hair growth, or hirsutism

INFORM YOURSELF

When to See a Doctor

A good rule of thumb when trying to decide whether to make an appointment with your doctor is to ask yourself if the symptom has been bothering you for a while. Symptoms that linger—even those that are only a mild annoyance—are especially important cancer warnings. Although they may turn out to be false alarms, it is best to have these symptoms checked.

Since it is impossible for you to remember all the symptoms of the more than one hundred different cancers, the American Cancer Society (ACS) established the following seven symptoms that are common cancer clues.

1. A change in bowel habits or bladder function. Chances are you are at least vaguely aware of when and how often you move your bowels and how often during a normal day you need to urinate. A change in either routine might be a sign of cancer. Chronic constipation or, conversely, long-lasting diarrhea may indicate cancer of the colon or rectum.

See a doctor about these symptoms immediately, because waiting until the constipation becomes so severe that even laxatives don't help or stools become pencil thin often means allowing the cancer to become dangerously advanced.

You should also see a doctor immediately if you notice blood in your stool.

See your doctor if passing urine is painful or difficult, if blood appears in your urine, or there is a change in bladder function. These are potential signs of prostate or bladder cancer.

2. Sores that do not heal. Cancers of the skin may bleed and resemble sores that never heal. They can crop up anywhere on the body, including the genitals. Such sores may also form in the mouth and should be evaluated as soon as they are noticed; this is particularly true of people who smoke, chew tobacco, or frequently drink alcohol because their use of these substances increases the chance that the lesions in their mouths may be malignant.

3. Unusual bleeding or discharge. Unusual bleeding can occur in early or advanced cancer. Coughing up blood is a sign of lung cancer. A woman who has vaginal bleeding between periods or anytime after menopause should see a doctor immediately. Cancer of the lining of the uterus (the endometrium) or of the cervix can cause vaginal bleeding. Blood in the stool may indicate cancer of the colon or rectum. Blood in the urine can mean cancer of the bladder, kidneys, or prostate. A bloody discharge from the nipple may be a sign of breast cancer.

4. Thickening or lump in the breast or elsewhere. Many tumors can be felt through the skin, particularly in the breast, testicles, or soft tissues of the body. You can also sometimes feel lumps in certain lymph nodes, such as the axillary nodes under the arm. The best ways to catch these palpable cancers are by having the checkups and exams and performing self-exams recommended by the ACS (see Chapter 4). In general, any thickening or a lump should be reported to your doctor promptly. You may detect a primary tumor in an early, operable stage, before it has metastasized.

5. Indigestion or difficulty in swallowing. These two symptoms are also known as dyspepsia and dysphagia, and they may indicate cancer of the esophagus, stomach, or pharynx (the tube connecting the mouth with the esophagus). Usually by the time these symptoms occur, the cancer is fairly advanced.

6. Recent change in a wart or mole. A doctor should immediately examine warts or moles that change color, lose their definite borders, or grow. The skin lesion may be melanoma or other types of skin cancer, which are often curable if attended to early.

7. A nagging cough or hoarseness. If you develop a cough that lingers for two weeks or more, see a doctor. Along with persistent hoarseness, this may be an indication of a malignancy of the lung, larynx (voice box), or thyroid. It often suggests an advanced stage of cancer.

The best way to find cancer early is to have regular checkups and tests before any symptoms occur. Even though these tests greatly improve your chances of finding a cancer before it has spread, they cannot find early cancers of certain organs. For this reason, it is still important to be aware of these symptoms and seek medical attention without delay.

Tumor Sizes

Tumors are typically measured in centimeters, sizes that are sometimes hard to visualize. The size of a quarter is a helpful comparison. These circles will give you a rough idea of how large some tumors are relative to a quarter.

Quarter

0.3 cm or 1/8 inch

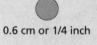

0.6 cm or 1/4 inch

1.2 cm or 1/2 inch

2.4 cm or 1 inch

4.8 cm or 2 inches

The Power of Denial

Denial is a very common response to the suggestion of cancer. Many people who notice something amiss in their bodies often attempt to make sense of the symptoms or find some less serious cause. "That nagging cough is just part of a bad cold," they might say. Or, "I'm constipated because I haven't had time to eat properly." Or, "That headache won't go away because my workload is so intense right now." People may deny that something serious might be wrong, and because many of the warning signs of cancer mimic symptoms of less serious illnesses, or even of stress, it is easy to postpone a checkup.

Some people are as frightened of the loss of independence that goes with serious illness as they are of the sickness itself. They hate the thought of being dependent on family, friends, and doctors. They may also be afraid of what their disease will mean to others. A woman may fear that losing a breast to cancer will affect her husband's feelings for her. A young parent may worry about how his or her children will deal with the realities of the disease. Rather than denial, some people respond with guilt, anger, depression, or panic. Most of the time, these reactions serve as delay tactics. It isn't until a symptom arises that seriously interferes with day-to-day life that some people are spurred into action. Pain is a major motivator for seeking medical help, for instance.

The problem with putting off medical care, of course, is that time is of the essence when it comes to fighting cancer. Cancer waits for no one. With the passage of time, a tumor grows and the cancer can spread. On the other hand, it is quite possible to stop many tumors before they have time to do lasting damage. Knowing the signs and symptoms can help even the most fearful person act and get help.

4

Detecting Cancer Early

For most of human history, people have gone to healers and doctors when they felt sick. But as the practice of medicine has become more sophisticated, we have learned how to detect many serious illnesses even before symptoms occur. Early detection and intervention is one of our most effective tools in saving lives and containing health care costs.

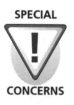

SPECIAL

CONCERNS

Too Scared or Embarrassed to Get Tested?

Detecting life-threatening illness as early as possible offers the greatest opportunity for survival with the best quality of life. Cancer doesn't stop developing just because you aren't ready to deal with it, and what you don't know *can* hurt you.

If you are embarrassed about having any of the early detection examinations recommended by the American Cancer Society (ACS), keep in mind that the only people who will be present during the examination are you and your doctor and/or nurse. The goal of these health care professionals is to keep you as healthy as possible. Checking your mouth, ears, or heart is no different to a health care professional than doing a pelvic, rectal, or skin examination—in each case, they are examining parts of your body in order to make sure you are healthy.

The vast majority of people screened are free of illness, and normal test results are an enormous relief. Indeed, for those at normal or increased risk of various cancers, the best way to escape worry and concern is to regularly undergo screening tests.

If you think that psychological barriers such as fear of cancer or embarrassment are preventing you from having a recommended test, talk to your friends, family, and certainly your doctor. The support and encouragement of others can help you begin to take loving care of yourself.

The first and oldest early detection method, the cancer-related checkup, consists of discussing your health history and undergoing a physical examination in a medical setting. Supplementing the checkup are numerous early detection tests used to find abnormalities in people who have no symptoms or who don't recognize a symptom as being associated with cancer.

If Your Doctor Doesn't Follow the American Cancer Society Guidelines

INFORM

YOURSELF

Guidelines are recommendations, not rules. Some doctors believe that some tests should be done more or less often than the ACS suggests, and the interval with which they are done may vary depending on your health and family history.

You may never have had a "cancer-related checkup" because your doctor calls this examination by another name. Or your doctor may give you different parts of the checkup when you come in for health problems rather than scheduling a visit specifically to conduct screening tests and examinations.

But doctors can overlook some tests or wrongly assume that another doctor is doing them. For instance, your primary care doctor may assume that your dentist examines your mouth, tongue, and throat as part of your annual dental checkup. If you are a woman, your internist or family doctor may assume that you see a gynecologist regularly for a Pap smear and pelvic examination.

Take responsibility for your health. Ask your doctor whether you should have the cancer-related checkup and other tests and examinations at the intervals suggested by the ACS. If your doctor believes that other intervals are appropriate, find out what he or she suggests and why. If you are unsatisfied with the explanation, get a second opinion (see Chapter 7).

The Cancer-Related Checkup

The ACS recommends a cancer-related checkup every three years for asymptomatic men and women who are 20 to 39 years of age and an annual exam for those 40 and older. Since the risk of cancer increases with age, the frequency of checkups also increases at age 40. If you are at high risk for certain cancers, your doctor may suggest a more frequent checkup schedule.

The checkup may be performed by your primary healthcare provider—usually a family doctor, an internist, a gynecologist, or a nurse practitioner. Some women may visit their family doctor for all aspects of the checkup except the breast and pelvic exams, which may be done by their gynecologist or nurse practitioner.

Health History and Counseling

The checkup begins with a review of family and personal health histories. The doctor or nurse practitioner asks about your prior illnesses and those of close family members. A history of cancer in any first-degree relative (parent, sibling, or children) is especially important. Next comes a review of your lifestyle, focusing on any factors that may increase the risk of cancer (see Chapter 2). Based on this review of your lifestyle-related risk factors, your doctor or nurse practitioner will discuss topics such as nutrition, physical activity, and how to quit smoking. The ACS recommends beginning testing earlier and having tests more often if you have a strong family history of certain cancers or some other cancer risk factors. The checkup also offers the health care provider an opportunity to teach self-examinations of the breasts and skin (see *Guidelines for the Early Detection of Breast Cancer* and *ACS Guidelines for the Early Detection of Other Cancers: Skin Cancer* later in this chapter).

The Physical Examination

The physical examination relies on the doctor's ability to both see and feel different body parts and organs and thereby identify variations from normal size, surface texture, and sensitivity.

The Oral Cavity. Focusing a light into your mouth, the doctor or dentist inspects and feels the lips, gums, tissues lining the mouth, the hard palate on the roof of the mouth, the tongue, and the throat. (Dentures are removed before the examination.) He or she looks for abnormalities in color, moisture, surface texture, and symmetry, and for areas of thickening, sores, or discharge. After observing tongue movement, the doctor or dentist depresses the tongue with a flat instrument to see the back of the mouth and throat. The doctor or dentist will also check the salivary glands next to the ears, under the jawbone, and under the tongue for enlargement or nodules.

The Thyroid Gland. The thyroid is a butterfly-shaped gland located at the base of the neck, in front of the larynx or voice box. It secretes a hormone that controls many aspects of metabolism.

The doctor observes the front of the neck for any swelling. The doctor asks you to swallow a sip of water, and he or she watches for any abnormal movement in the neck. Then the doctor gently manipulates the structures in your neck and palpates the front and side surfaces of the thyroid gland, noting any tenderness, discomfort, or nodules.

The Lymph Nodes. The lymphatic system is a network of tissues and organs that produce infection-fighting cells called lymphocytes and channels that carry lymph fluid throughout the body. Round or bean-shaped lymph nodes or glands are located along the lymph channels. Waste products, bacteria, and other microorganisms are filtered by these nodes, as well as cancer cells that have spread into the tissue surrounding a tumor.

Many illnesses, particularly infections, can lead to temporarily swollen lymph nodes. Cancer spread may be suspected when nodes remain enlarged yet the body shows no sign of an infection. Lymph nodes are located throughout the body, including behind the knees, around the elbows, around the lungs and aorta, and in the gastrointestinal system. However, nodes of normal size can be effectively palpated only in three areas where sufficiently large masses of them occur: in the neck, under the arms (axilla), and in the groin. The neck nodes are palpated at the same time as the thyroid examination, the nodes in the armpit are checked as part of the breast examination in women, and the groin nodes are checked at the same time as the pelvic examination in women. The doctor feels the nodes with the fingertips, using a circular motion. Normal nodes are movable and soft.

The Skin. A thorough skin examination requires the removal of clothing so that every inch of the body can be examined. Some doctors will ask you to stand and turn slowly for the examination; others perform the examination while you recline and ask you to turn as needed. Photographs may be taken for comparison in following years if someone is at high risk for skin cancer, particularly if he or she has many moles. In addition to simple observation, the doctor usually spreads the buttocks to view inner skin and raises a man's testicles or spreads a woman's legs to examine the genital area.

Many doctors use an ABCD mnemonic (memory aid) as a guide for spotting malignant melanoma, the most severe type of skin cancer. These lesions tend to

(A) be **A**symmetrical.

(B) have irregular **B**orders.

(C) vary in **C**olor from one area to another.

(D) have a **D**iameter greater than 6 millimeters (that is, larger than about one-quarter of an inch, or the size of a pencil eraser).

The doctor also looks for signs of nonmelanoma skin cancer: a sore that has been present for more than three weeks that bleeds, oozes, or crusts; any irritated red patches that may or may not itch or hurt; and any change in long-standing skin markings, such as elevation, change of color, growth, tenderness, or pain.

The Female Pelvis. The pelvic examination is used to detect cancers of the female reproductive system, specifically the ovaries, endometrial lining of the uterus, cervix, vagina, and vulva. Unfortunately, a pelvic examination is not highly effective in detecting these cancers in their early stages. (The exception is cancer of the cervix, which can be detected by a Pap test.) Despite the limitations of this examination, it is recommended because it poses no risks and is one of the few methods available for cancer detection of a woman's reproductive organs.

A woman should avoid sexual intercourse for twenty-four hours before a pelvic examination, and should avoid douching and taking any medication, including vaginal contraceptives, for three days before the test. She should urinate immediately before the procedure, and if necessary, move her bowels. After removing her clothing from the waist down, the woman reclines on a special examining table that has stirrup supports to keep her legs raised and spread.

First, the doctor visually inspects the external genitalia: the vulva, labia majora and minora, clitoris, and anal region, looking for any sores, swellings, or other abnormalities. Then he or she palpates the lymph nodes in the groin (inguinal lymph nodes).

Next, the vagina and cervix are inspected using a speculum—a metal or plastic instrument with two paddle-like extensions. The speculum is inserted into the vagina, and the paddles are opened to expose the inside walls of the vagina and the cervix. After a visual inspection in which the doctor looks for abnormal discharge, sores, erosion, or growths, a Pap test (see page 64 for *Guidelines for the Early Detection of Cervical Cancer*) may be performed.

The third part of the pelvic exam is the bimanual examination. The doctor uses gloved hands to palpate the internal pelvic organs in the following manner: the lubricated index and middle finger of one hand are inserted into the vagina while the other hand is placed on the abdomen. By pressing the fingers and hand together, the doctor can palpate the size, shape, and position of the uterus and ovaries and may be able to detect abnormal masses.

The final segment of the pelvic exam is the recto-vaginal exam. One gloved finger is inserted in the vagina and another is inserted into the rectum. Again, as the fingers press together over the back wall of the vagina and the front wall of the rectum, the doctor can feel local structures and abnormalities.

Physical Examination: Does It Hurt?

None of the physical examinations recommended in the cancer-related checkup should cause pain or serious discomfort. Although the doctor often applies a very firm hand when palpating an organ or area, this pressure should not cause pain. If you experience unusual discomfort or tenderness, speak up. It could be an important warning sign.

Your own level of tension or a doctor's lack of dexterity may contribute to discomfort during a pelvic examination. If you can relax your vaginal and rectal muscles by breathing deeply and slowly, and the doctor works quickly but gently, the only sensation should be moderate pressure. Many people feel squeamish about the digital rectal examination. The examination should not be painful, because the doctor's entering finger is far smaller than the size of typical exiting bowel movements. Entry may be easier if you bear down, as if moving your bowels, but then try to relax for the few seconds it takes for the examination.

The Testicles. The egg-shaped testicles are the male reproductive glands that produce sperm and male sex hormones, such as testosterone. The two testicles hang outside the body in a small pouch called the scrotum, located below and behind the penis.

The testicular exam is relatively brief. With the man standing, the doctor observes the genital area, looking for any signs of swelling or other abnormalities. Then the doctor raises the scrotum, observes the underlying skin, and palpates lymph nodes in the groin and along the upper inner thigh. Using both hands, all surfaces of each testicle are palpated for any lump, thickening, or other abnormality. The doctor also notes any significant differences in the size, weight, and firmness of the testicles.

American Cancer Society Guidelines for Testing for Early Cancer Detection

The cancer-related checkup is a general screening examination. But early detection (sometimes called secondary prevention or screening) also involves other examinations and tests intended to find specific cancers as early as possible—ideally, before symptoms develop—when it can be treated most effectively and with the fewest possible side effects. These tests include self-examinations as well as clinical examinations.

Many screening tests are performed in conjunction with the cancer-related checkup, but they may be done at any time. All adults, regardless of whether they are at risk, should be tested periodically for early cancer detection, and some tests are particularly important for people at high risk for certain cancers. These include men and women who:

- have a strong family history of certain cancer types.

- have had disorders that predispose them to certain cancers, such as chronic inflammatory bowel disease (colitis), which increases their risk of colorectal cancer.

- have been exposed to carcinogens, such as those whose occupations put them in contact with known cancer-causing chemicals.

- have already had one cancer, in which case screening tests can help detect another cancer of the same type and check for other cancers for which the person may be at higher risk. For example, women who have had breast cancer are at increased risk of cancer in the other breast as well as cancer of the ovaries.

Based on scientific research and expert opinion, the ACS has established recommendations to detect cancer early in asymptomatic people (people without symptoms of cancer). The ACS suggests more frequent and extensive screening tests for people with risk factors for certain cancers. Those at higher risk for any reason should discuss with their doctor whether more frequent physical examinations and/or screening tests are needed and which other tests not routinely recommended might be added to their cancer checkup.

INFORM

YOURSELF

Can a Screening Test Tell If You Have Cancer?

Most screening tests cannot tell for certain whether you have cancer. Rather, they indicate an abnormal result that may be caused by cancer, may be a precursor to cancer, or may be due to some benign condition.

A positive screening test requires a more complete diagnostic evaluation. Further tests are performed to find the cause of the positive result and determine whether cancer is present (see Chapter 5). A diagnostic test confirms the presence and location of a specific type of cancer. For example, a breast lump found by your doctor or an abnormal area on your mammogram may be a cancer or a benign lump. In some cases, a biopsy will be needed to be certain. Likewise, a high blood prostate-specific antigen (PSA) level may be due to prostate cancer or to benign enlargement of the prostate gland, and a biopsy may be necessary to decide which is present.

ACS Recommendations for the Early Detection of Cancer

INFORM YOURSELF

For Average Risk, Asymptomatic People

Cancer Site	Population	Test or Procedure	Frequency
Breast	Women, age 20+	Breast self-examination	Monthly, starting at age 20
		Clinical breast examination	Every 3 years, ages 20–39
			Annual, starting at age 40*
		Mammography	Annual, starting at age 40
Colorectal	Men & women, age 50+	Fecal occult blood test (FOBT) & flexible sigmoidoscopy† -or-	Annual FOBT and flexible sigmoidoscopy every 5 years, starting at age 50
		Flexible sigmoidoscopy -or-	Every 5 years, starting at age 50
		FOBT -or-	Annual, starting at age 50
		Colonoscopy -or-	Colonoscopy every 10 years, starting at age 50
		Double contrast barium enema (DCBE)†	DCBE every 5 years, starting at age 50
Prostate	Men, age 50+	Digital rectal examination (DRE) & prostate-specific antigen test (PSA)	The PSA test and DRE should be offered annually, starting at age 50, for men who have a life expectancy of at least 10 years.‡
Cervix	Women, age 18+	Pap test and pelvic examination	All women who are, or have been, sexually active, or have reached age 18 should have an annual Pap test and pelvic examination. After a woman has had 3 or more consecutive satisfactory normal annual examinations, the Pap test may be performed less frequently at the discretion of the physician.
Cancer-related checkup	Men & women, age 20+	Examinations every 3 years from ages 20 to 39 years and annually after age 40. The cancer-related checkup should include examination for cancers of the thyroid, testicles, ovaries, lymph nodes, oral cavity, and skin, as well as health counseling about tobacco, sun exposure, diet and nutrition, risk factors, sexual practices, and environmental and occupational exposures.	

* Beginning at age 40, annual clinical breast examination should be performed prior to mammography.

† Flexible sigmoidoscopy together with FOBT is preferred compared with FOBT or flexible sigmoidoscopy alone.

‡ Information should be provided to men about the benefits and limitations of testing.

Guidelines for the Early Detection of Breast Cancer

The ACS recommends the following examinations for women at average risk for breast cancer:

- Women aged 40 and older should have a screening mammogram every year.

- Between the ages of 20 and 39, women should have a clinical breast examination by a health professional every three years. Starting at age 40, women should have a breast exam by a health professional every year.

- Women aged 20 or older should perform breast self-examination (BSE) every month.

The ACS believes the use of mammography, clinical breast examination, and breast self-examination, according to the recommendations outlined above, offers women the best opportunity for reducing the breast cancer death rate through early detection. This combined approach is clearly better than any one examination. Without question, breast physical examination without mammography would miss the opportunity to detect many breast cancers that are too small for a woman or her doctor to feel but can be seen on mammograms. Although mammography is the most sensitive screening method, a small percentage of breast cancers do not show up on mammograms but can be felt by a woman or her doctor.

Mammography. A mammogram is an x-ray of the breast. Diagnostic mammography is an x-ray examination of the breast in a woman who either has a breast complaint (for example, a breast mass or nipple discharge) or has had an abnormality found during screening mammography. But screening mammography is also used to look for breast disease in asymptomatic women.

Many people are concerned about exposure to x-rays, and rightly so, but the very low levels of radiation in up-to-date mammograms do not significantly increase the risk for breast cancer. Strict guidelines are in place to assure that mammography equipment is safe and uses the lowest dose of radiation possible. To put dose into perspective, consider the fact that a woman who receives radiation as a treatment for breast cancer will receive several thousand rads. If a woman had yearly mammograms beginning at age 40 and continuing until 90, she will have received about 20 rads. One mammogram exposes a woman to roughly the same amount of radiation as flying from New York to California on a commercial jet (the earth's atmosphere filters out some of the cosmic radiation from outer space, so radiation levels are greater at very high altitudes).

A woman can shower or bathe the night before or on the morning of the test, but she should avoid using deodorant, powder, cream, or other substances on the breasts or underarm areas. These products may interfere with the quality of the mammogram and obscure the image.

Clothing is removed from the waist up. One breast is placed on a flat plastic plate while another plate presses against it, flattening the tissue so it is of uniform thickness.

During a mammogram, the breast is compressed to flatten and spread the tissue. Although this may be temporarily uncomfortable, it is necessary in order to produce a good image. The compression only lasts a few seconds. Two different views of each breast are taken, then the procedure is repeated on the opposite breast. The entire procedure for screening mammography takes approximately twenty minutes. This procedure produces a black and white image of the breast tissue on a large sheet of film that is "read," or interpreted, by a radiologist.

Only accredited facilities are allowed to perform the test. To be accredited, a breast center, radiologist's office, or clinic must have dedicated mammography equipment, the personnel performing the x-ray must be licensed or certified, the doctors interpreting the mammograms must be certified, and the x-ray and film-processing equipment must be inspected annually. Furthermore, clinics must mail women an easy-to-understand report of their mammogram results within thirty days—sooner if the results suggest cancer is present. In the past, results were sent only to the woman's doctor.

In 2000, the U.S. Food and Drug Administration (FDA) approved digital mammography for routine breast cancer screening. This is similar to standard mammography, but the image is recorded electronically and viewed on a computer monitor instead of being viewed on a sheet of x-ray film. Consequently, the image can be magnified, made brighter, and the contrast can be changed to allow greater accuracy. The digital images can also be transferred to x-ray film. They can also be transmitted by computer so that experts in distant centers can be consulted. Although digital mammography is not widely available yet, it's expected to become more popular over time.

Radiologists look for masses and calcifications on the film. Calcifications, tiny mineral deposits within the breast tissue, appear on the film as small single white spots or clusters of white. They are a sign of changes within the breast that can either be monitored by additional, periodic mammograms, or can be examined by biopsy. They may be caused by benign breast conditions, or less often, by breast cancer. Another important change that can be seen on a mammogram is a mass, which may occur with or without calcifications. Masses can be due to many things, including cysts and benign tumors such as fibroadenomas, but may be cancer and usually should be biopsied if they are not fluid-filled cysts.

Keep in mind that a mammogram, while suggestive, cannot prove that an abnormal area is cancer. To confirm whether cancer is present, a small amount of tissue must be removed and examined under a microscope. Women at high risk for breast cancer and women who have undergone breast conserving treatment or lumpectomy should discuss appropriate screening intervals with their doctors.

Mammography: Does It Hurt?

If mammography is done properly and at the appropriate time in the menstrual cycle, most women will feel only minimal discomfort when their breast is pressed onto the x-ray plate. Of course, individuals may vary in their perception of the discomfort involved. A small percentage of women who have especially dense breasts do find that mammography can be painful.

Because your breasts are likely to be most tender just before or during your menstrual flow, try to schedule your appointment for two weeks after menstruation. If your cycle suddenly changes, don't hesitate to reschedule the appointment.

Clinical Breast Examination. A clinical breast examination (CBE) is an examination of your breasts by a health professional, such as a doctor, nurse practitioner, or doctor's assistant. For this examination, you undress from the waist up and sit or stand with your hands on your hips. The health professional will first look at your breast for changes in size or shape. He or she will look for any marked unevenness, imbalance, or abnormal breast contour and for unusual nipple position, discharge, retraction (or turning inward), and skin changes such as puckering, dimpling, discoloration, or scaling. Then, using the pads of the fingers, the examiner will gently palpate (feel) your breasts. He or she will pay special attention to the shape and texture of the breasts, location of any lumps, and whether such lumps are attached to the skin or to deeper tissues. The lymph nodes in the armpits are also palpated. Some doctors may gently squeeze each areola (the pigmented area around the nipple) to check for nipple discharge. The CBE is a good opportunity for you to ask your doctor or nurse to teach you breast self-examination.

Breast Self-Examination. The ACS recommends that all women aged 20 and older should examine their breasts monthly. Monthly examination increases the likelihood that a small abnormality, which might appear between professional examinations, will be noticed. Cancers found by breast self-examination (BSE) tend to be less advanced than symptom-causing cancers found by women who do not do BSE. The major risk of BSE is that a woman may believe that self-examination can replace a clinical breast examination or mammogram.

A woman may miss a tumor that a doctor or nurse can feel or that will appear on an x-ray. Some women experience considerable anxiety when they examine their breasts for cancer. If this anxiety keeps you from doing monthly self-examinations or prevents you from doing them thoroughly, more frequent clinical breast examinations may be necessary.

By regularly examining your own breasts, you are likely to notice any changes that occur. The best time for breast self examination is about a week after your period ends, when your breasts are not tender or swollen. Performing BSE monthly will allow you to become familiar with the appearance and feel of your breasts and enable you to detect any changes. Postmenopausal women may find it easier to remember to do BSE if they examine their breasts at the same time each month. Women who are pregnant or breast-feeding need to regularly examine their breasts, too.

- Lie down with a pillow under your right shoulder and place your right arm behind your head.

- Use the finger pads of the three middle fingers on your left hand to feel for lumps in the right breast.

- Press firmly enough to know how your breast feels. A firm ridge in the lower curve of each breast is normal. If you're not sure how hard to press, talk with your doctor or nurse.

- Move around the breast in a circular, up and down line, or wedge pattern. Be sure to do it the same way each month, check the entire breast area, and remember how your breast feels from month to month.

- Repeat the exam on your left breast, using the finger pads of the right hand. (Move the pillow to under your left shoulder.)

- Repeat the examination of both breasts while standing, with your one arm behind your head. The upright position makes it easier to check the upper and outer part of the breasts (toward your armpit). This is where about half of breast cancers are found. You may want to do the standing part of the BSE while you are in the shower. Some breast changes can be felt more easily when your skin is wet and soapy.

For added safety, you can check your breasts for any dimpling of the skin, changes in the nipple, redness, or swelling while standing in front of a mirror right after your BSE each month.

If you develop a lump or swelling in the breast or underarm area, skin irritation or dimpling, nipple pain or retraction (turning inward), redness or scaliness of the nipple or breast skin, or a discharge other than breast milk, see your health care provider as soon as possible for evaluation. However, remember that most of the time, these breast changes are not cancer.

INFORM

YOURSELF

How to Perform Breast Self-Examination

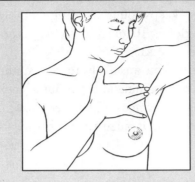

By making small circular motions or following another pattern along a particular grid, you can examine the entire area from collarbone to below the breast and from the breastbone to the armpit.

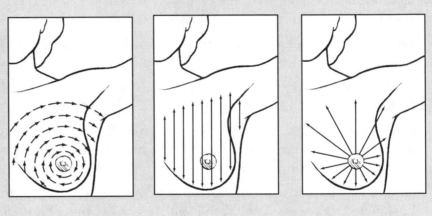

Guidelines for the Early Detection of Colorectal Cancer

Adenomatous polyps, also known as colorectal adenomas, are benign growths of glandular cells that are the precursor lesions (abnormal tissue areas) for almost all colorectal cancers. Colorectal cancer screening saves lives in two ways. First, the tests find early cancers that are often curable. Second, the tests can find adenomatous polyps. Removal of these polyps can prevent them from changing into a cancer. It usually takes several years for adenomas to change into cancers, and most adenomas never become malignant. But there is no way to determine which will progress and which will not, so the best strategy is to remove them.

The ACS guidelines offer a set of screening recommendations for different levels of colorectal cancer risk. When determining which of these screening methods to pursue, discuss with your doctor accuracy, prevention potential, costs, and risks.

Approximately 70 to 80 percent of all colorectal cancers occur among people at "average risk." Although the incidence of colorectal cancer is low in people at age 50, about 25 percent of adults at age 50 will have adenomatous polyps. Beginning screening at age 50 raises the potential to detect and remove precancerous lesions. Therefore, the ACS recommends that by age 50, both men and women at average risk should follow one of the five screening options below:

- Yearly fecal occult blood test (FOBT)*

- Flexible sigmoidoscopy every five years

- Yearly fecal occult blood test plus flexible sigmoidoscopy every five years**

- Double contrast barium enema every five years

- Colonoscopy every ten years

A colonoscopy should be done on any person with a positive FOBT, flexible sigmoidoscopy, or double contrast barium enema result.

People should begin colorectal cancer screening earlier and/or undergo screening more often if they have any of the following colorectal cancer risk factors:

- A strong family history of colorectal cancer or polyps (cancer or polyps in a first-degree relative younger than age 60 or in two or more first-degree relatives of any age). Note: a first-degree relative is defined as a parent, sibling, or child.

- Families with hereditary colorectal cancer syndromes (familial adenomatous polyposis and hereditary non-polyposis colon cancer).

- A personal history of colorectal cancer or adenomatous polyps (adenomas).

- A personal history of chronic inflammatory bowel disease.

Based on your individual situation and preferences, you and your doctor can decide which of the screening options above is best for you.

Approximately 15 to 20 percent of colorectal cancers occur among people at "increased risk" (approximately twice average risk), and approximately 5 to 10 percent of all colorectal cancers occur among people at "high risk," defined as much greater than twice the average risk. For screening guidelines for women and men at increased risk or high risk, refer to pages 58–59, *ACS Guidelines on Screening and Surveillance for the Early Detection of Colorectal Adenomas and Cancer.*

---

*For FOBT, the take-home multiple sample method should be used.
**Of the first three options above, the American Cancer Society prefers yearly FOBT and flexible sigmoidoscopy every five years, rather than either test alone.

INFORM

YOURSELF

ACS Guidelines on Screening and Surveillance for the Early Detection of Colorectal Adenomas and Cancer

For Women and Men at Increased Risk or at High Risk

Risk Category	Age to Begin	Recommendation	Comment
INCREASED RISK			
People with a single, small (< 1 cm) adenoma	3–6 years after the initial polypectomy	Colonoscopy*	If the exam is normal, the patient can thereafter be screened as per average risk guidelines.
People with a large (1 cm +) adenoma, multiple adenomas, or adenomas with high-grade dysplasia or villous change.	Within 3 years after the initial polypectomy	Colonoscopy*	If normal, repeat examination in 3 years; If normal the patient can thereafter be screened as per average risk guidelines.
Personal history of curative-intent resection of colorectal cancer	Within 1 year after cancer resection	Colonoscopy*	If normal, repeat examination in 3 years; If normal, repeat examination every 5 years.
Either colorectal cancer or adenomatous polyps, in any first-degree relative before age 60, or in two or more first-degree relatives at any age (if not a hereditary syndrome).	Age 40, or 10 years before the youngest case in the immediate family	Colonoscopy*	Every 5–10 years. Colorectal cancer in relatives more distant than first-degree does not increase risk substantially above the average risk group.
HIGH RISK			
Family history of familial adenomatous polyposis (FAP)	Puberty	Early surveillance with endoscopy, and counseling to consider genetic testing	If the genetic test is positive, colectomy is indicated. These patients are best referred to a center with experience in the management of FAP.
Family history of hereditary non-polyposis colon cancer (HNPCC)	Age 21	Colonoscopy and counseling to consider genetic testing	If the genetic test is positive or if the patient has not had genetic testing, every 1–2 years until age 40, then annually. These patients are best referred to a center with experience in the management of HNPCC.

Risk Category	Age to Begin	Recommendation	Comment
HIGH RISK (cont'd)			
Inflammatory bowel disease, Chronic ulcerative colitis, Crohn's disease	Cancer risk begins to be significant 8 years after the onset of pancolitis, or 12–15 years after the onset of left-sided colitis	Colonoscopy with biopsies for dysplasia	Every 1–2 years. These patients are best referred to a center with experience in the surveillance and management of inflammatory bowel disease.

* If colonoscopy is unavailable, not feasible, or not desired by the patient, double contrast barium enema (DCBE) alone, or the combination of flexible sigmoidoscopy and double contrast barium enema are acceptable alternatives. Adding flexible sigmoidoscopy to DCBE may provide a more comprehensive diagnostic evaluation than DCBE alone in finding significant lesions. A supplementary DCBE may be needed if a colonoscopic exam fails to reach the cecum, and a supplementary colonoscopy may be needed if a DCBE identifies a possible lesion, or does not adequately visualize the entire colorectum.

Fecal Occult Blood Test. The fecal occult blood test (FOBT) is used to find occult (hidden) blood in feces. Blood vessels at the surface of colorectal adenomas or cancers are often fragile and easily damaged by the passage of feces. The damaged vessels may release enough blood to change the color of the stool. More often, the damaged blood vessels release only a small amount of blood into the feces. This small amount of blood does not change the appearance of the stool, but can be detected by tests for fecal occult blood. The FOBT alone has been shown to reduce risk of death from colorectal cancer by about one-third when repeated annually.

People having this test will receive a test kit with instructions that explain how to take a stool or feces sample at home. The kit is then returned to the doctor's office or a medical laboratory for testing. Fecal occult blood tests are also being sold in drugstores and on the Internet. Before purchasing a home test, discuss your screening options with your doctor. If you decide to buy a test rather than getting a test kit from your doctor, be sure the test is approved by the FDA and follow the instructions carefully. Report your test results to your doctor and schedule additional screening tests based on the ACS guidelines. If you are having symptoms of colorectal cancer, you should notify your doctor instead of relying on a home test because false negative results may occur (some people with colorectal cancer have a negative result).

Ask your doctor if there are foods or medications that you should avoid that may interfere with test results. You may be asked to avoid:

- nonsteroidal anti-inflammatory drugs such as ibuprofen, naproxen, or aspirin (more than one adult aspirin per day) for seven days prior to testing.

- vitamin C in excess of 250 mg from either supplements or citrus fruits and juices for three days before testing.

- red meats for three days before testing.

Sometimes people are not able to stop taking medications even for a short time, so be sure that you understand which medications you need to continue taking before and during the test.

If this test result is positive, additional testing is needed to find the source of the bleeding and its cause. Colorectal cancer is not the only condition that can cause blood in the stool, so a positive test result does not necessarily indicate that a polyp or cancer is present. Other causes of bleeding include hemorrhoids and diverticulosis.

Digital Rectal Examination. A digital rectal examination (DRE) refers to the palpation of the anus and lower rectum by a health practitioner using a gloved finger. Although DRE is useful in identifying tumors in the anal canal or lower rectum, the area examined is quite limited. Therefore, while DRE is often included as part of a routine physical examination, it is not recommended as a stand-alone screening test for colorectal cancer. However, DRE should be performed prior to insertion of a sigmoidoscope or colonoscope.

Sigmoidoscopy. Evidence from case control studies has shown notable drops in the death rate from cancers within reach of the sigmoidoscope, as well as a lower incidence of colorectal cancer associated with a history of screening with sigmoidoscopy.

A sigmoidoscopy allows a doctor to look at the inside of the sigmoid colon (the lower part of the large intestine or colon) and the rectum. The doctor will use a sigmoidoscope (a slender, flexible, hollow, lighted tube) to do the test. A sigmoidoscope is about the thickness of a finger and is inserted through the rectum up into the colon. The sigmoidoscope is connected to a video camera and a video display monitor. This allows the doctor to look for bleeding, cancer, and polyps (small growths that can become cancerous). The length of a sigmoidoscope is about 60 centimeters (about 2 feet), allowing the doctor to see one-third to half of the colon. A sigmoidoscope is shorter in length than a colonoscope. A sigmoidoscopy may be somewhat uncomfortable, but it should not be painful.

You may be asked to use two enemas prior to the exam or to drink only clear liquids (water; any Jello except red; and grape, apple, or cranberry juice) for a day or two before the exam in addition to an enema prior to the exam. Your doctor will give you specific instructions for cleansing the bowel.

A sigmoidoscopy takes ten to twenty minutes. Bleeding and puncture of the colon are possible complications of sigmoidoscopy. However, such complications are uncommon. You may receive medicine before the test to help you relax, but you will be awake for the test. You may be placed on your side or on your back with your knees positioned near your chest. Your doctor may also have a special table that rotates to ease positioning.

To ease discomfort and the urge to have a bowel movement, it is helpful to breathe deeply but slowly through your mouth. The sigmoidoscope may stretch the wall of the colon so you may feel muscle spasms or lower abdominal pain. Air will be placed into the sigmoid colon through the sigmoidoscope so the doctor can see the colon better. During the procedure, you might feel pressure and slight cramping in your lower abdomen. You will feel better afterward, when the air leaves your colon.

Barium Enema with Air Contrast. A barium enema with air contrast, also called a double contrast barium enema or lower GI series, uses x-rays to view the large intestine. The procedure takes about thirty to forty-five minutes to perform. The process of cleansing the bowel usually includes a liquid diet for two days before the procedure and clear liquids the day before the procedure. Avoid eating or drinking dairy products the day before the test, and don't eat or drink anything after midnight the night before the procedure. A laxative or enema may be given before the procedure to make sure your colon is empty. Check with your doctor for specific instructions.

Barium sulfate, a chalky substance, is used to partially fill and open up the colon. The barium sulfate is given in the anus. When the colon is about half full of barium, the patient is turned on the x-ray table so the barium spreads throughout the colon. Then air is inserted to cause the colon to expand. This allows good x-ray films to be taken. You may be asked to change positions so that different views of the colon and rectum can be seen on the x-rays. The doctor can then see the size and shape of the colon and rectum. The barium can cause constipation and your stool may appear gray or white for a few days after the procedure.

Colonoscopy. A colonoscope is a slender, flexible, hollow lighted tube about the thickness of a finger. It is inserted through the rectum up into the colon. A colonoscope is much longer than a sigmoidoscope (about four feet long), and in most cases allows the doctor to see the lining of the entire colon. The colonoscope is connected to a video camera and video display monitor so the doctor can closely examine the inside of the colon.

Preparation for the test usually includes the following:

- You will need to drink only clear liquids. Do not eat or drink anything after midnight the night before your test. Check with your doctor for specific instructions.

- The large intestine must be cleaned out so that it is visible during the test. Your doctor will prescribe a laxative to do this.

Colonoscopy may be done in a hospital outpatient department, in a clinic, or in a doctor's office, and usually takes fifteen to thirty minutes, although it may take longer if polyp removal is involved. You will get an intravenous (IV) line so that medicine can be given through a vein. The medicine will relax you and make you feel sleepy, but you will be awake. You should arrange for someone to drive you home from the test because the sedative can affect your ability to drive.

INFORM

YOURSELF

Advantages and Disadvantages of Early Detection Tests for Colorectal Cancer

Tests	Advantages	Disadvantages
Fecal Occult Blood Test	No direct risk to the colon. No bowel preparation. May do sampling at home. Inexpensive. Proven effective in clinical trials.	May miss many polyps and some cancers. May produce false-positive test results. Pre-test dietary limitations needed. Should be done annually or in addition to a flexible sigmoidoscopy every 5 years.
Flexible Sigmoidoscopy	Fairly quick and safe. Minimal bowel preparation. Only done every 5 years. Not that uncomfortable. Doesn't require a specialist.	Views only about a third of the colon. Can't remove all polyps. Very small risk of infection or bowel tear. Should be done every 5 years, alone or in addition to an annual fecal occult blood test.
Barium Enema	Can usually view entire colon. Relatively safe. Only done every 5 years. No sedation needed.	Can miss small polyps. Full bowel preparation needed. Some false positive test results. Cannot remove polyps during testing.
Colonoscopy	Can usually view entire colon. Can biopsy and remove polyps. Only done every 10 years. Can diagnose other diseases.	Can miss small polyps. Full bowel preparation needed. Can be expensive. Sedation of some kind is needed. You miss a day of work. Small risk of bowel tears or infection.

During the procedure, you will be placed on your side with your knees flexed and a drape will cover you. Your blood pressure, heart rate, and breathing rate will be monitored during and after the test. Although uncommon, bleeding and puncture of the colon are possible complications of a colonoscopy.

The colonoscope is lubricated so it can be easily inserted into the rectum. Once inserted into the rectum, the colonoscope is passed through the transverse colon and into the ascending colon and rectum. You may feel an urge to have a bowel movement when the colonoscope is inserted or pushed further up the colon. To ease any discomfort, it is helpful to breathe deeply but slowly through your mouth. The colonoscope will deliver air into the colon so that it is easier to see the lining of the colon and use the instruments to perform the test. Suction will be used to remove any blood or liquid stools.

If a polyp is found, the doctor may remove it. Polyps, even those that are not cancerous, can cause bleeding and may become cancerous. For this reason, they are usually removed. This is done by passing a wire loop through the colonoscope to sever the polyp from the wall of the colon using an electrical current. The polyp can then be sent to a lab to be checked under a microscope to see if it has any areas that have changed into cancer.

If the doctor sees anything else abnormal, a biopsy may be done. Colonoscopy usually does not cause pain, although it may be uncomfortable. If a polyp is removed or a biopsy is done during the colonoscopy, you may notice some blood in your stool after the test.

New Colorectal Cancer Screening Methods. Several new methods are being developed and tested that may be useful for future colorectal screening.

Computed tomography colonography (virtual colonoscopy). This promising imaging technology for colorectal cancer screening creates detailed x-ray images of the colon and rectum. After a bowel cleansing similar to that used before a barium enema or colonoscopy, the patient is given an especially thorough and detailed computed tomography (CT) scan of the pelvis and abdomen. Special computer software transforms the CT scan image into a three-dimensional view of the inside of the colon and rectum. This view resembles what a doctor would see looking through an actual colonoscope. But with virtual colonoscopy, no tubes are placed into the colon, making this test quicker and less uncomfortable. So far, it is still less accurate than real colonoscopy and is not recommended for routine use. But, as CT scanning and computer technologies continue to improve, the accuracy of virtual colonoscopy may eventually be enough to justify routine use.

Molecular genetic screening. Researchers have recently found DNA mutations that often affect certain genes (such as the K-ras oncogene and p53 tumor suppressor gene) of colorectal cancer cells. Studies are testing new diagnostic ways to recognize these DNA mutations in cells found in stool samples to see if this approach is useful in finding colorectal cancers at an earlier stage. Cells from the lining layer of the colon and rectum are constantly shed into the stool and replaced by new cells. The cells that slough off of the lining typically undergo apoptosis, a specific type of cell death that causes recognizable changes in the cells' DNA. Cells that slough off from the surface of colon cancers do not usually undergo these changes. Finding DNA that appears intact (DNA that lacks the changes of apoptosis) in stool samples appears to be useful in finding colorectal cancers. Recent studies that have combined DNA tests to look for gene mutations and for intact-appearing DNA have shown promising results. Nonetheless, more research is needed to confirm the accuracy of these tests before widespread use can be recommended.

Guidelines for the Early Detection of Cervical Cancer

Cervical cancer was once one of the most common causes of cancer death for American women, but it much less common today. Between 1955 and 1992, the number of cervical cancer deaths in the United States declined by 74 percent. The main reason for this change is the increased use of the Pap test, a screening procedure that permits diagnosis of pre-invasive and early invasive cancer.

Cervical cancer can usually be found early by having regular Pap tests (see page 65) and pelvic examinations (see page 48 of *The Physical Examination* section). Early detection greatly improves the chances of successful treatment.

Despite the recognized benefits of Pap test screening, not all American women take advantage of it. Between 60 and 80 percent of American women with newly diagnosed invasive cervical cancer have not had a Pap smear in the past five years, and many of these women have never had a Pap test.

The ACS recommends that all women begin yearly Pap tests and pelvic examinations at age 18 or when they become sexually active, whichever occurs earlier. If a woman has had three satisfactory negative annual Pap tests in a row, this test may be done less often at the judgment of a woman's health care provider. But the annual pelvic exam should be continued, regardless of how often the Pap test is done.

This recommendation also applies to women who are past menopause (no longer having periods) and past childbearing. If a hysterectomy was done for cancer, more frequent Pap tests may be recommended.

Women who have had a hysterectomy (surgery to remove the uterus, including the cervix) should talk with their doctor about whether to continue to have regular Pap tests. If the hysterectomy was performed for treatment of a precancerous or cancerous condition, the end of the vaginal canal still needs to be sampled for abnormal changes. Some doctors recommend that if the uterus (including the cervix) was removed because of a noncancerous condition such as fibroids, routine Pap tests may not be necessary. However, it is still important for a woman to have regular gynecologic examinations as part of her health care.

It is important to remember that while the Pap test has been more successful than any other screening test in preventing a cancer, it is not perfect. Because some abnormalities may be missed (even when samples are examined in the best laboratories), it is not a good idea to have this test less often than the ACS guidelines recommend.

Pap Test (Papanicolaou Smear). A Pap test or Pap smear involves removing cells from a woman's cervix and examining them under the microscope to detect abnormal cells. While the Pap test is done primarily to detect cervical cancer, it can find some endometrial cancers and advanced ovarian cancer. It is named after Dr. George N. Papanicolaou, the researcher who developed the technique more than sixty years ago. The test is usually performed during a complete pelvic examination (see page 48 of *The Physical Examination* section).

The vagina is held open by the paddles of a speculum and a sample of cells and mucus is lightly scraped from the ectocervix (outer area of the cervix) using a small spatula. A small brush or a cotton-tipped swab is used to take a sample from the endocervix (inner part of the cervix). The specimen is then smeared on a glass slide, which is sprayed with or dipped in a preservative and sent to a laboratory. The cells are usually screened for abnormalities by a cytotechnologist.

To help ensure the test's accuracy, intercourse should be avoided for twenty-four hours before the exam and douching and any medications, including vaginal contraceptives, should be avoided for three days before the test. Since menstruation interferes with recognition of abnormal cells, it's best to schedule during the middle two weeks of the menstrual cycle.

False-negative Pap test results are not rare. A woman can improve her chances of obtaining an accurate result by following the preceding directions. It is helpful to inquire about the laboratory to which specimens are sent. It should be certified by the College of American Pathologists, the American Society of Cytolopathology, or both.

Because of the estimated eight to nine year lead time before precancerous changes evolve into invasive carcinoma, almost all false-negative results can be caught at an early stage by repeat testing within one to three years.

New Cervical Cancer Screening Methods. The following methods are being developed in the hope of improving the accuracy of cervical cancer screening.

Computerized screening and rescreening. One approach to Pap test improvement is the use of computerized instruments that can recognize abnormal cells in Pap tests. Two instruments, the PAPNET and the AutoPap, are currently approved by the FDA for use in addition to examination by technologists and doctors. The instruments can be used for retesting Pap smear samples that were interpreted as normal by technologists. (AutoPap is also approved by the FDA for initial screening of Pap smears, but a technologist would still examine all smears identified as abnormal by the AutoPap.) The current instruments sometimes identify samples as abnormal when the woman has a normal cervix, and they increase the cost of the Pap test. Use of computerized instruments has been increasing during the past few years. Although there is some debate among doctors as to whether current instruments should be used for Pap testing, many agree that technical improvements in the near future will improve their accuracy and lower the cost of testing.

ThinPrep. Another new approach to improving Pap test accuracy, called the ThinPrep, changes how cells are placed on the microscope slide and spreads them more evenly on the slide. Recent studies indicate that it can slightly improve detection of cancers, significantly improve detection of early precancers, and reduce the number of tests that need to be repeated. Whether or not this method has a significant impact on preventing cancer and whether it is the best approach to improving the Pap test needs to be studied further. This method is not used by most laboratories and is more expensive than a usual Pap test.

HPV testing. Infection with some human papillomavirus (HPV) types can greatly increase a woman's risk of developing cervical cancer. Tests are now available that can identify DNA from these HPV types. Some doctors recommend using this test for women whose Pap test results are uncertain. If the HPV test result is positive, they recommend colposcopy (viewing the cervix through binocular magnifying lenses), but if it is negative, the woman may be able to continue routine annual Pap tests without undergoing colposcopy.

Guidelines for the Early Detection of Endometrial Cancer

At this time, no early detection tests or examinations are recommended for women without symptoms who are at average endometrial cancer risk. Although endometrial cancer is now the most common female genital cancer, no screening test or examination currently exists that can reliably detect endometrial cancer in women who have no symptoms.

The ACS recommends that women at increased risk for endometrial cancer due to increasing age, history of unopposed estrogen therapy (estrogen without progestin), late menopause, tamoxifen (a drug used in treating breast cancer and for risk reduction in women at increased breast cancer risk) therapy, nulliparity (never giving birth), infertility or failure to ovulate, obesity, diabetes, or high blood pressure should be informed about endometrial cancer early detection testing. However, there is no indication that screening for endometrial cancer should be recommended for women at increased risk for endometrial cancer because of a history of these conditions. These women should be informed about the risks and symptoms of endometrial cancer, and should be informed about potential benefits, risks, and limitations of testing for early endometrial cancer detection.

Hereditary nonpolyposis colon cancer (HNPCC) is an inherited condition that greatly increases a man or woman's risk of developing colon cancer. It also increases a woman risk for developing endometrial cancer. Women with a family history that suggests they might have this condition and women with positive genetic tests for HNPCC should be offered annual testing for endometrial cancer with endometrial biopsy beginning at age 35. Because of the high risk of endometrial cancer in this group and because of the potentially life-threatening nature of endometrial cancer, screening is recommended.

Endometrial Biopsy. An endometrial biopsy is an office procedure in which a sample of endometrial tissue—the lining of the uterus—is obtained through a very thin flexible tube inserted into the uterus through the cervix. The tube removes a small amount of endometrium using suction. The suctioning takes about a minute or less. The discomfort is similar to severe menstrual cramps and can be helped by taking a nonsteroidal anti-inflammatory drug such as ibuprofen an hour before the procedure.

Guidelines for the Early Detection of Prostate Cancer

The ACS recommends that health care providers should offer the prostate-specific antigen (PSA) blood test and DRE yearly, beginning at age 50 years, to men who have at least a ten-year life expectancy.

Men at high risk, such as African Americans and men who have a first-degree relative (a father, brother, or son) diagnosed with prostate cancer at an early age, should begin testing at age 45.

Prostate-Specific Antigen (PSA) Test. Until the 1980s, the digital rectal examination was the only technique available to screen men for prostate cancer. Now the PSA blood test has proven to be helpful in estimating how likely a man is to have prostate cancer. It has been in increasingly widespread use since 1985.

Measurement of serum PSA level (a protein which is made by prostate cells) is the most accurate method for the detection of prostate cancer. Nevertheless, DRE should also be included in testing.

It is important to understand how the PSA blood test is used in early detection of prostate cancer. PSA levels estimate how likely a man is to have prostate cancer but the test does not provide a definite answer. Conditions such as benign prostatic hyperplasia (noncancerous prostate enlargement) and prostatitis (inflammation of the prostate) can cause a borderline or high PSA result.

On the other hand, some men with prostate cancer have negative or borderline PSA results. Certain measures are recommended by many doctors to make PSA testing as accurate as possible. Because ejaculation can cause a temporary increase in blood PSA levels, some doctors suggest that men abstain from sexual activity for two days before testing. Several medications and herbal preparations can lower blood PSA levels. Men having the PSA blood test should tell their doctors if they are taking finasteride (Proscar or Propecia) or PC-SPES (an herbal mixture). It is not known if saw palmetto (an herb used by some men to treat benign prostate enlargement) interferes with the measurement of PSA.

Since doctors started using the PSA blood test, the percentage of prostate cancers found at an early, curable stage has increased. And since most men have normal test results, they can be reassured that they are unlikely to have prostate cancer, especially if their DRE result is also negative.

The PSA test involves drawing a blood sample from a vein in the arm. The blood is analyzed in a laboratory to determine the level of PSA, a protein made by prostate cells. The higher the PSA level, the more likely a man is to have prostate cancer. Still, 40 percent of those with cancer do not have an elevated PSA.

A result over 10 ng/ml is definitely considered abnormal, and should be evaluated by a biopsy. Values between 4 and 10 are often evaluated by a percent free-PSA test, although some doctors routinely biopsy men with results in this range. The patient's risk factors (family history and race) may be considered in this decision. Results under 4 ng/ml are usually considered normal, unless the patient's PSA velocity is high. If the DRE result is abnormal, a biopsy is recommended regardless of the PSA levels.

The percent free-PSA test. This test indicates how much PSA circulates alone in the blood and how much is bound together with other blood proteins. For PSA results in the borderline range, a low percent free-PSA means that a prostate cancer is more likely to be present and suggests the need for a biopsy. A recent study found that if men with borderline PSA results had prostate biopsies only when their percent free PSA was 25 percent or less, about 20 percent of unnec-essary prostate biopsies could be avoided. Although this test is widely used, not all doctors agree whether 25 percent is the best value to use.

The PSA velocity. This measure of how quickly the PSA level rises over a period of time is another way to evaluate a man with borderline PSA values.

Since the PSA blood test will need to be repeated the next year to determine PSA velocity, this approach does not provide an immediate answer. A PSA velocity of 0.75 ng per ml per year is usually considered high. Even when the total PSA value is normal, a high PSA velocity suggests that a cancer may be present and a biopsy should be considered.

The PSA density (PSAD). The PSAD is determined by dividing the PSA number by the prostate volume (its size as measured by transrectal ultrasound). A higher PSAD indicates greater likelihood of cancer.

Age-specific PSA reference ranges. This is another way to interpret PSA results. It is known that PSA levels are normally higher in older men than in younger men, even in the absence of cancer. For this reason, some doctors have suggested comparing PSA results for individual patients with results from other men the same age. In practice, a PSA result within the borderline range might be very worrisome in a 50-year-old man but causes less concern in an 80-year-old man. This is because 80-year-old men without cancer are often found to have borderline PSA test results. Because cancers missed in older men (when using age-specific PSA reference ranges) may be lethal, this practice has not gained widespread acceptance.

Not all doctors agree on how to use these additional PSA tests. If your PSA test result is not normal, ask your doctor to discuss your cancer risk and need for further tests.

SPECIAL

CONCERNS

If Your Doctor Does the Exam Differently

The instructions your doctor gives you on how to prepare for a test and the way he or she performs a particular examination may differ slightly from what you read here and elsewhere.

To reassure yourself, discuss the screening examination with your doctor. You might bring a copy of the information you have read when you have your checkup and share it with him or her. Don't be hesitant to ask questions about how to prepare for a test. If you are not satisfied with the instructions you get or have questions that are not answered by the office or clinic staff, ask to speak to the doctor.

If you think that an aspect of the examination has not been done or has been performed differently from what you expected, ask why. Usually there is a logical explanation that will set your mind at ease. If you are still not satisfied, consider having the test or examination repeated elsewhere.

Early Detection of Other Cancers

In addition to screening tests recommended in the ACS guidelines, other tests are available to screen for different types of cancer. Some are controversial, and some are appropriate only for those at high risk for certain cancers.

Oral Cancer. An examination of the oral cavity should be part of the cancer-related checkup (see page 46).

Some doctors and dentists recommend oral self-examination (OSE) to people at high risk of oral cancers because of a history of smoking, using smokeless tobacco products, or prior tissue abnormalities in the mouth.

No research is available to document the potential benefits or risks of the procedure, but the American Dental Association encourages self-examination.

Oral self-examination. Using a mirror, check the lips, gums, cheek lining, and tongue, as well as the throat and floor and roof of the mouth. Look as best you can for any of the following signs and symptoms:

- color change of the oral tissue

- a lump, thickening, rough spot, crust, or small eroded area

- pain, tenderness, or numbness anywhere in the mouth or on the lips

- difficulty chewing, swallowing, speaking, or moving the jaw or tongue

- a change in the way the teeth fit together

- a lump or thickening in the cheek

- a white or red patch in the gums, tongue, tonsil, or lining of the mouth

- loosening of the teeth or pain around the teeth or jaw

- swelling of the jaw

If you notice any of these signs or symptoms, contact your dentist or doctor immediately for an examination.

Skin Cancer. Examining the skin for abnormalities should be part of the cancer-related checkup (see pages 47–48).

Although the ACS has made no formal recommendations about skin self-examination (SSE), the Skin Cancer Foundation suggests that parents begin examining their children when they're young so that by their teens, people can perform SSE. The Foundation currently advises self-examination every three months, which should supplement an annual skin examination by a doctor, though the frequency of this recommendation may change in the near future.

Skin self-examination. Your SSE should take place with all of your clothes removed, in a well-lighted room, and in front of a full-length mirror. You should have a hand mirror so that you can see the back of your body.

You will slowly examine every visible area of your skin, including body crevices, between your legs, under your arms, and under the hair on the back of your neck.

The first time you do SSE, it may be useful to draw a rough sketch of your body, front and back, and to note the locations of any moles or skin lesions

How to Perform Skin Self-Examination

INFORM

YOURSELF

The illustrations below will help you notice a suspicious lesion that may be skin cancer.

Examine your face, especially the nose, lips, and mouth, and the front and back of the ears. Use a hand mirror or floor-length mirror or both to get a clear view.

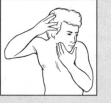

Thoroughly inspect your scalp, using a blow dryer and mirror to expose each section to view. Get a friend or family member to help, if you can.

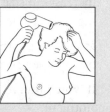

Check your hands carefully: palms and backs, between the fingers, and under the fingernails. Continue up the wrists to examine both the front and back of your forearms.

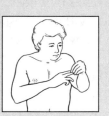

Standing in front of a full-length mirror, begin at the elbows and scan all sides of your upper arms. Don't forget the underarms.

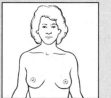

Next focus on the neck, chest, and torso. Women should lift breasts to view the underside.

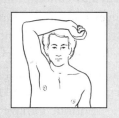

With your back to a full-length mirror, use a hand mirror to inspect the back of your neck, shoulders, upper back, and any part of the back of your upper arms you could not view earlier.

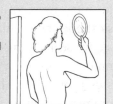

Still using both a hand mirror and a full-length mirror, scan your lower back, buttocks, and backs of both legs.

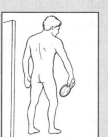

Sit down; prop each leg in turn on a stool or chair. Use a hand mirror to examine the genitals. Check the front and sides of both legs, thigh to shin, ankles, tops of feet, between toes, and under toenails. Examine the soles of feet and heels.

you have, as well as their size and color. Then refer to your sketches to check for changes.

You can use the ABCD method described on page 47, though this technique applies mainly to screening for malignant melanoma. The following guidelines recommended by the Skin Cancer Foundation will help you scrutinize your body for all types of skin malignancies. Look for:

• any skin growth that increases in size or becomes pearly, translucent, tan, brown, black, or multicolored.

• any mole, birthmark, beauty mark, or brown spot that changes color, increases in size or thickness, changes texture, has irregular borders, or is bigger than the size of a pencil eraser and appears after age 21.

• any spot or sore that continues to hurt, itch, crust, scab, erode, or bleed, or any open sore that does not heal within three weeks.

If you observe any of these changes, call your doctor for a prompt appointment.

Testicular Cancer. An examination of the testes by a doctor as part of a routine cancer-related checkup is recommended by the ACS, since many men with testicular cancer do not have any of the known risk factors.

Young men at high risk for testicular cancer are sometimes encouraged to practice testicular self-examination (TSE) regularly. Those at high risk include men whose testes did not descend into the scrotum until after the age of 6 or who continue to have one or both testes undescended.

The issue of regular testicular self-examination for men who are not at increased risk is more controversial. The ACS believes it is very important to make men aware of testicular cancer and remind them that any testicular mass should be evaluated by a doctor without delay. Some doctors feel that delay in seeking medical attention after discovering a mass is the most common reason for a delay in treatment. Other doctors feel that not noticing masses promptly is also an important factor in delaying treatment and they recommend monthly testicular self-examination by all men after puberty. The ACS does not feel that for men with average testicular cancer risk, there is any medical evidence to suggest that monthly examination is any more effective than simple awareness and prompt medical evaluation. However, the choice of whether or not to perform this examination should be made by each man, so instructions for testicular examination are included on page 73.

Lung Cancer. Because lung cancer usually spreads beyond the lungs before causing noticeable symptoms, an effective program for early detection of lung cancer could save many lives. Three tests have been put forward as potential screening procedures. They are the chest x-ray, sputum analysis, and spiral or

How to Perform TSE

The best time to perform a self-exam is during or after a warm bath or shower, when the scrotal skin is most relaxed. Although the two testicles are encased in a single scrotal sac, each should be examined separately. Hold the testicle between your thumbs and fingers with both hands and roll it gently between your fingers. Then stand in front of a mirror, holding your penis out of the way, and observe the testicles.

You are looking for any hard lumps or smooth round masses or any change in the size, shape, or consistency of your testes. If you notice any abnormalities, see your doctor promptly. Also call your doctor if you experience any other signs of testicular cancer, such as a dull ache or a sensation of dragging and heaviness in the lower abdomen, groin, or both.

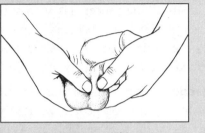

helical low dose CT scanning. The screening tests below have been evaluated for their ability to help save lives of people with lung cancer, and the findings have not resulted in the tests' inclusion in the ACS recommendations for cancer screening. New tests continue to be evaluated in the hopes that they may one day save lives, such as tests designed to detect early lung cancers by recognizing changes in the DNA of bronchial cells. However, these tests are still not routinely used.

Chest x-ray. The use of chest x-rays for early lung cancer detection was tested several years ago. Most studies concluded that these tests could not find many lung cancers early enough to improve a patient's chance for a cure. X-ray diagnosis in people without symptoms only seemed to generate a lead-time bias—that is, although the time from detection to death was lengthened, the outcome remained the same. In other words, people learned they had lung cancer sooner, but they didn't live any longer. For this reason, lung cancer screening is not a routine practice for the general public or even for people at increased risk, such as smokers.

Sputum cytology. The use of sputum cytology—in which sputum is analyzed for abnormal cells in a manner similar to analyzing Pap smears of the cervix—presents different problems. A coughed-up sputum sample provides a collection of cells that can come from anywhere in the lung. Although dysplasia (abnormal cells) and lung cancer may be detected in this way, subsequent attempts to find exactly where the cancer cells came from can be very tedious and costly. Sputum testing of large numbers of asymptomatic people was not found to reduce the mortality rate from lung cancer either. This test is not recommended for lung cancer screening by the ACS.

Spiral or helical low dose computed tomography. Recently, a new x-ray technique called spiral or helical low dose CT scanning has been successful in detecting early lung cancers in smokers and former smokers. Whether this new kind of x-ray will actually save lives has not been proven and studies to answer this important question are in progress. The ACS recommends that people at increased lung cancer risk who seek screening should be informed by their doctors about the benefits, limitations, and risks of testing. People who choose to undergo testing should be encouraged to do so in a setting that is linked to a multispecialty group for diagnosis and follow-up.

Bladder Cancer. Tests intended specifically for bladder cancer detection are not recommended for people without symptoms who do not have strong risk factors for this disease. Risk factors that would justify screening include proven exposure to cancer-causing chemicals, earlier bladder cancers, or certain birth defects of the bladder.

Urinalysis. Many people are screened for bladder cancer when they have a routine urinalysis (laboratory test of urine). Although urinalysis is usually done to check for other conditions, such as diabetes and noncancerous kidney diseases, the test can uncover small amounts of blood in the urine. Such small amounts do not change the color of urine, but can be detected by chemical tests by viewing the urine under a microscope, and are often the first sign of bladder cancer. However, urinalysis is not recommended as a screening test for bladder cancer because of its high false negative and false positive rates.

Cytology and cytoscopy. People who have a high risk of developing bladder cancer may be advised to have certain tests. These could include periodic urine cytology and cystoscopy (see Chapter 5). In urine cytology, the urine is examined under a microscope to find any cancerous cells. In cystoscopy, a slender tube with a lens and a light is placed into the bladder through the urethra. This allows the doctor to check the bladder and urethra for possible cancers. Small tissue samples can also be removed during cystoscopy so they can be checked under a microscope for signs of cancer. This procedure is usually done using a local anesthetic but some patients may require general anesthesia. Your doctor will let you know what to expect before and after the procedure.

Ovarian Cancer. Currently there are no recommended screening tests for ovarian cancer in women who are not at high risk for the disease. In preliminary studies of women at average risk of ovarian cancer, transvaginal sonography and the CA 125 blood test did not make any difference in the number of deaths caused by ovarian cancer. For this reason, these tests are not recommended for ovarian cancer screening of women without known strong risk factors. However, some recent studies found that cancers detected by these tests tend to be somewhat less advanced than cancers of women who did not have any screening tests. Additional research is in progress to improve ovarian cancer screening tests. It is hoped that further improvements will make these tests effective enough to lower the ovarian cancer death rate.

Women with a family history of ovarian cancer or who are at high risk for other reasons—for example, if they have breast, endometrial, or colon cancers or know they carry the breast cancer susceptibility gene (BRCAl)—might want to discuss periodic CA 125 screening and periodic transvaginal sonography evaluations with their doctors.

Transvaginal sonography. Women with a high risk of developing epithelial ovarian cancer, such as those with a very strong family history of this disease, may be screened with transvaginal sonography (an ultrasound test performed with a small instrument placed in the vagina). Transvaginal sonography is helpful in finding a mass in the ovary, but it does not accurately predict which masses are cancers and which are due to benign diseases of the ovary.

CA 125 test. Blood tests for ovarian cancer may include measuring the amount of CA 125. The amount of this protein is increased in the blood of many women with ovarian cancer. However, some noncancerous diseases of the ovaries can also increase the blood levels of CA 125 and some ovarian cancers may not produce enough CA 125 to cause a positive test result. Thus, the test is not recommended for routine screening of women at average risk of developing ovarian cancer. Some doctors recommend this test for women at increased ovarian cancer risk. And, the test is often used to detect recurrence after ovarian cancer treatment.

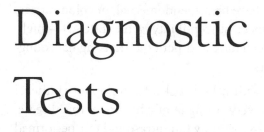

5

Diagnostic Tests

Many signs and symptoms of cancer resemble those of other conditions. Weight loss and abdominal pain may be caused by an ulcer or by stomach cancer. Pink or reddish urine may be caused by a bladder infection, certain noncancerous kidney diseases, or bladder cancer.

Screening test results may raise the possibility of a cancer being present, but doctors can't always be sure that the cause of a positive result is cancer. For example, a positive fecal occult blood test can indicate a variety of intestinal problems and an elevated blood PSA level may be due to prostate cancer or to benign enlargement of the gland. The only way to confirm—or rule out—cancer as the cause of a suspicious symptom or screening test result is to undergo diagnostic testing.

The specific tests that are ordered depend on a number of factors, including the symptoms, location of the abnormality, type of suspected tumor, and preferences of the doctor and person being tested.

Many times the doctor will order more than one test because no single one—except a biopsy—supplies all the information required both to confirm a cancer diagnosis. The least costly and/or least uncomfortable or invasive tests are done first. For example, to detect a mass that cannot be felt, the doctor may order an ultrasound exam to find out if it is solid or filled with fluid. This test is relatively inexpensive, safe, painless, and noninvasive. Then, if the situation warrants it, the doctor may order more costly imaging procedures, such as computed tomography or magnetic resonance imaging exams. Finally, if a mass is found, the most definitive test, a biopsy of the mass, is done.

Is This Test Necessary?

When diagnostic tests are ordered, ask your doctor these questions:

- Why are you recommending this test? What will you learn from it?

- What are the alternatives to the test? Do any less invasive or less costly procedures provide the same information?

- What are the possible side effects, complications, or risks of the test?

- What are the risks of not having the test?

- Will I be hospitalized? For how long? Can the test be done on an outpatient basis?

- How much will the test cost? Is it covered by my health insurance or health care plan?

- Does a certified technician or a board-certified doctor perform the test? Does a board-certified doctor interpret and evaluate the test results?

- Where will the specimen be tested? Will it be done at a hospital with a certified laboratory, accredited by the College of American Pathologists?

- When will I get the results? How accurate will they be? Who will explain the results to me?

- What further tests will be necessary if the results are positive? What if they are negative?

Diagnostic tests attempt to locate an abnormality and then determine whether it is a malignancy or not. The following are the tests most commonly used to provide a complete inner picture of the body. However, at times, nothing short of surgery will enable a doctor to make an accurate diagnosis.

Imaging Examinations

Conventional x-rays have been available for almost a century. They are the most familiar, inexpensive, and accessible imaging exams. Newer imaging exams, such as computed tomography (CT scan), magnetic resonance imaging (MRI), and ultrasound are based on computers. In most body regions, these techniques provide more information than standard x-rays and may detect tumors not seen on an x-ray.

Using imaging techniques, a doctor can sometimes pinpoint the location of a suspicious mass, even if it is deep within the body. Often these techniques allow the doctor to precisely place a biopsy needle in a mass or suspicious lesion, thus avoiding exploratory surgery. However, even the most sophisticated imaging exams cannot always distinguish between benign and malignant tumors with certainty, so further diagnostic tests may be required.

After a diagnosis is made, imaging exams may be used to stage the disease. Following treatment, they may help determine whether therapy has been successful.

A certified technician, radiologist, or other doctor performs imaging exams in a doctor's office, outpatient facility, or hospital. A radiologist (a doctor who specializes in imaging techniques) interprets the exams.

QUESTIONS

?

TO ASK

What Is This Test Like?

Studies show that diagnostic tests may be less stressful if you know exactly what to expect. Here are some questions to ask so that you'll be prepared:

- What happens during the test? What will I feel, see, smell, and hear during the procedure?

- Is the test invasive? That is, will anything be inserted or injected into my body?

- Is any part of the test painful or uncomfortable?

- Can anything be done to prevent or lessen the discomfort? Will I be given a sedative or local or general anesthesia?

- How long does the test take?

- Does this test have any side effects or complications?

Conventional Radiography

Because x-rays are painless, quick, easily accessible, and relatively inexpensive, and because they require little, if any, preparation, they are often used for the initial evaluation.

X-rays are high-energy beams of radiation. When they pass through the body, they create shadows on a sheet of film, called a radiograph. A radiograph is commonly referred to as an x-ray or film. The x-rays pass through soft tissue more readily than through dense tissue, such as bone. Since the soft tissue absorbs fewer x-rays than dense tissue, it appears darker on the film, whereas bones are white.

Tumors are usually denser than the tissue that surrounds them, which can make them noticeable on the radiograph or x-ray. Other tumors are less dense than the surrounding tissue, so they appear as very dark areas on the film.

Contrast Studies. To improve and increase the information obtained from conventional x-ray techniques, air or an iodine-based dye or barium sulfate may be used as a contrast medium to outline, highlight, or fill in parts of the body. X-rays with a contrast medium can be used to detect tumors in organs deep within the body, such as in the kidneys, stomach, and colon. Depending on the dye and the part of the body examined, the contrast medium may be introduced in the following ways:

- By enema, as in a barium enema, which is used to study the large intestine and rectum.

- Swallowed, as in an upper GI (gastrointestinal) series, used to study the upper digestive tract, including the esophagus, stomach, and upper small intestine.

- Injected into an artery, as in an arteriogram, or into a vein for an intra-venous pyelogram (IVP), also known as an intravenous urogram (IVU). Since the kidneys remove and concentrate the dye and then excrete it so that the dye is carried away in the urine, an IVP is used to study the kidneys and urinary tract.

- Inserted through a catheter into a natural opening, as in a hysterosalpin-gogram, in which dye is injected into the uterus through a slender tube that has been passed through the vagina and cervix into the uterus to study that organ and fallopian tubes.

A special diet, enema, or other preparation measures may be required when a contrast medium is used. Eventually, the material will be eliminated by the body.

These tests may be uncomfortable. Dye may cause a warm or burning sensation as it enters the tissue. It may also cause nausea and vomiting, flushing, itching, or a bitter or salty taste in your mouth. However, the discomfort is usually brief and sedatives may be administered before certain tests.

Most contrast studies involve little risk, including risk of allergic reaction, but complications can occur when a dye is used. If you have a history of allergies or sensitivity to iodine or seafood (which is high in iodine) or any medication, tell the radiologist. The test may still be done with a different dye and medication that reduces the chance of an allergic reaction.

A few contrast studies are considered high-risk procedures, but for most people the risk of a serious complication is less than 2 in 100 procedures.

It is important that procedures such as a cerebral angiogram, also called arteriogram (an x-ray of the blood vessels in the neck and brain that requires injecting dye into neck arteries), be performed by skilled and experienced technicians and doctors. Safer, less invasive tests—such as CT scans, ultrasounds, or nuclear scans—may substitute for some contrast studies.

QUESTIONS

TO ASK

Getting a Safe, Accurate Test

Ask your doctor the following questions to prepare for a diagnostic imaging test:

- Should I curtail my activity, restrict my diet, or refrain from smoking or ingesting alcohol or caffeine before the test or immediately afterward?

- Should I decrease the dose of or stop taking over-the-counter or prescribed medications, such as aspirin, vitamins, painkillers, or oral contraceptives?

- Will I be able to drive myself home after the test?

- When will I be able to resume my usual activities?

Tell your doctor if you:

- are pregnant or think you may be.

- currently have any illness.

- have had a serious illness in the past.

- have taken any prescription or over-the-counter medications, including contraceptives, hormones, vitamins, aspirin, laxatives, or cough medicine within the past few days, weeks, or months.

- have any allergies, especially to x-ray dye or shellfish.

- have a pacemaker.

- had surgery to repair an aneurysm.

- have any metal clips, pins, or implants in your body from surgery or any metal fragments in your eyes from accidents.

- smoke.

- have not had adequate rest lately.

- feel nervous, anxious, or upset.

- are claustrophobic.

Digital Radiography

Instead of using film, digital radiography records x-ray images as electronic data that can be viewed on a monitor and stored on computer disks. The technique allows specific areas of the image to be enlarged, and the contrast of the image can be adjusted to allow greater visibility, thus reducing the amount of radiation required for a clear image. Most large hospitals have digital radiography equipment.

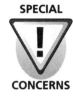

SPECIAL

CONCERNS

Is Radiation Risky?

Radiation can damage cells, causing them to reproduce abnormally. Usually the damaged cells simply die or the body's immune system destroys them with no ill effects. In most cases, the risk that diagnostic x-rays will cause enough damage to induce cancer is far outweighed by the diagnostic benefits, especially when the x-ray is taken with modern equipment that emits low doses of radiation.

But since the effects of even low-level radiation are cumulative and the risk of cancer grows with the amount of radiation a person is exposed to over a lifetime, x-rays should not be done indiscriminately.

If your doctor recommends that you have an x-ray, you can minimize the amount of radiation exposure by taking the following steps:

- Have your x-rays done in a medical center, hospital, or office of a board-certified radiologist, where x-ray machines are more likely to be regularly calibrated and inspected and where skilled, accredited personnel perform the exams.

- Ask for your x-ray report and keep track of x-rays you have had to avoid needlessly repeating the same exam. Many doctors accept x-rays taken by others. Repeat exams are sometimes needed, however, to assess the effectiveness of treatment or evaluate new symptoms.

- Stay still when the x-ray is being taken to avoid a blurred image, which will require a repeat exam.

- Before having an x-ray, be sure to tell the doctor if you are pregnant or think you may be.

Computed Tomography (CT Scan)

The CT scan, also known as computed axial tomography or CAT scan, is a sophisticated x-ray procedure that relies on a computer to create clear slices or cross-sectional images of internal structures. It offers much more information than conventional x-rays. Unlike a conventional x-ray exam, which directs one broad x-ray beam over an area, a CT scan is produced by numerous pencil-thin rays passing through the body from various angles and levels.

While you lie on a table, a scanner rotates around you and directs thousands of x-ray beams at a particular region of your body. A computer generates a two-dimensional picture or slice from these images. Individual slices are displayed on a computer screen.

A technician usually performs a CT scan and a radiologist evaluates the results. No hospitalization is required. The image may clearly show a tumor's size, shape, volume, and location.

The test usually takes about fifteen to thirty minutes, but it's even faster when the latest equipment is used. It is painless, although there may be some discomfort when holding still in certain positions for a long time. An intravenous dye may be used to provide contrast. Fasting or an enema may be necessary before the test.

The technique has some limitations. Very small tumors may not be visible, and the scan may not show how far a cancer has spread. Also, the radiation exposure is higher than that of a conventional x-ray. Another disadvantage of the test is its cost, which may run six to ten times that of a conventional x-ray.

Magnetic Resonance Imaging

Magnetic resonance imaging (MRI) uses radio waves and a strong magnetic field to penetrate the body and generate high-quality, two-dimensional images of almost every organ in the body. MRI can provide views from all directions. The procedure is especially useful for areas that are difficult to visualize with standard x-rays, such as the brain, spinal cord, pelvis, and musculoskeletal system. Indeed, almost all body parts can be visualized, and new applications are being developed every day.

An MRI image can display images more easily in three dimensions than a CT scan, and is better at recognizing and characterizing some kinds of tumors. An MRI also distinguishes between tumors and cysts.

There are limitations to MRI. It doesn't detect calcifications (tiny calcium deposits that can signal cancer in the breast tissue) as clearly as a CT scan or conventional x-ray. MRI is also more expensive than CT, and may not be covered by your insurance or health plan.

An MRI takes about an hour. It is painless, but because the test requires complete enclosure in a narrow, tubular machine, it can be uncomfortable and even frightening for some people. Children and those who are very large or claustrophobic may have difficulty lying still for the time required. It is important to remain as still as possible, because movement during the test will make the images less sharp. Some people complain of the continual loud thumping and pounding of the machinery.

Some facilities offer "open" MRI, which reduces the feeling of claustrophobia. This design has open sides, no pounding noise, and can accommodate very large people. However, open MRIs are not widely available, and because they are less powerful, they do not produce the clearest image.

MRI is usually not recommended for pregnant women. Anyone wearing a pacemaker or who has internal clips, metal implants, joint replacements, and other medical devices or who has metal fragments in the eye may be unable to have an MRI because the strong magnetic field can disrupt or dislodge the devices or fragments.

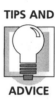

TIPS AND

ADVICE

Having an MRI?

Before having an MRI tell your doctor if you:

- cannot comfortably lie flat.

- are severely claustrophobic.

- are pregnant or think you may be.

- have any medical devices, such as a cardiac pacemaker, aneurysm clip, implants, or hearing aid.

- have any metal shrapnel in your body from an old war wound or an auto accident or any metal fragments in the eye.

- have any tattoos (some tattoos contain metallic particles).

Nuclear Medicine

Nuclear medicine involves the use of radioactive substances, called radionuclides or tracers, to create images of organs and detect masses in areas that are not visualized by standard x-rays.

The radionuclides are administered orally or intravenously. A machine (called a rectilinear scanner, gamma ray camera, or scintiscope) produces a two-dimensional image (except for SPECT, which is three-dimensional), or scan, showing how and where the radioactive compound travels in the body and where it accumulates.

Radionuclides appear on the scan as spots of light. Depending on the organ being scanned and type of radionuclide used, a tumor may be detected as an area of either increased radioactivity (a "hot spot") or decreased radioactivity.

One disadvantage is that a very small tumor cannot be detected through a nuclear scan, nor can the scan distinguish between tumors and cysts.

Although nuclear medicine procedures do not provide as much detail as CT or MRI scans, they can provide information not available from other scans.

They provide information about how an organ is functioning, while most other imaging tests only display its shape and size.

The procedure causes little discomfort. The radioactive substance used is weak, so the risks are not greater than those of a conventional x-ray. Also, the scanning machine emits no radiation, and most of the radioactive substance introduced into the body is eliminated within a day or so.

Positron Emission Tomography (PET Scan). The PET scan conveys the metabolic activity of organs as well as a slice or cross-sectional image of internal structures. A radioactive form of sugar is injected into a vein and absorbed by the body's cells in varying amounts, depending on their rate of metabolism. Cancer cells tend to have more active metabolism than benign cells and absorb more of the radioactive sugar. A special camera records the location of radioactivity leaving the body and a computer uses the information to produce an image. PET scans are especially useful for images of brain tumors. The technique is still relatively new, and is becoming more widely used to assess the spread of lymphomas and cancers of the breast, colon, rectum, ovary, and lung. Before the test, you should not eat anything for at least four hours and you may be asked to fast overnight. Let your doctor know if you are diabetic or have some other condition that would make fasting unsafe. The doctors can then make other arrangements.

The test takes about an hour, plus the waiting time after the radioactive material is given. After the injection, you rest quietly for thirty to sixty minutes, while the sugar circulated throughout your body and is absorbed by your cells. You will then lie down on the scanner table and will be positioned inside a large donut-shaped camera. You will need to remain still while you are inside the camera, usually about thirty to sixty minutes.

Single Photon Emission Computed Tomography (SPECT). SPECT is similar to other nuclear medicine procedures in that a radioactive substance is injected into the body and becomes more concentrated in tumors than in normal tissues. Several different radioactive substances can be used, depending on what type of cancer is suspected.

Unlike usual nuclear medicine images, which are two-dimensional, SPECT produces images that resemble the body slices of a CT scan. This is done by using a scanner that rotates around the body and by analyzing the data with computer software similar to that used in CT imaging. Although this test is relatively new, its use is increasing in oncology, especially in imaging lymphomas inside the abdomen and looking at bone metastases. The scanning may be repeated several times over a period of a few days.

Ultrasonography

Ultrasonography, or diagnostic ultrasound, is effective, painless, noninvasive, readily available, and relatively inexpensive. The procedure involves no radiation and is considered safe enough to examine fetuses during pregnancy. Consequently, it is sometimes recommended as the initial diagnostic method, particularly when a positive screening test raises a suspicion of cancer. And in some people at high risk of certain cancers—such as ovarian cancer—doctors use it as a screening test.

Ultrasound uses sound waves and their echoes to create a picture of the interior of the body. A microphone-like instrument, called a transducer, emits and receives sound waves as it is passed over the part of the body being examined. The echo patterns are converted to a detailed computer image that is viewed on a monitor.

In most cases, little preparation is required for an ultrasound. Depending on the organ being examined, it may be necessary to fast overnight, take a laxative, have an enema, or consume large quantities of water before the test. It is usually performed on an outpatient basis in a hospital, but some specialists do have ultrasound equipment in their offices.

Ultrasonography, which can differentiate cysts from solid masses, can visualize soft tissues that don't show up well on x-rays, so it is often used to detect tumors in the liver, pelvis, and abdominal area. The procedure has also been used to detect prostate cancer, ovarian tumors and, along with mammography, to determine if a breast lump is a fluid-filled cyst or a solid mass. It may also be helpful in guiding needle aspirations or needle biopsies.

Ultrasound cannot penetrate bone or gas-filled spaces, so it is ineffective for detecting tumors in the brain, lungs, or intestines. It may be inaccurate when used in obese people, because fat cells interfere with the sound waves.

The long-term effects of ultrasound are unknown, but no harmful effects have been detected.

Blood Tests

While there is no single "blood test for cancer" yet, there are tests for specific substances produced by cancer cells and sometimes by normal cells that may be detected in the blood or urine. These substances are called tumor markers. For example, a substance called carcinoembryonic antigen (CEA) is usually found in the blood of those with colon cancer. Determining the CEA level was the first blood test for a common cancer. But thus far, the only marker that has been found useful for widespread cancer screening is prostate-specific antigen (PSA).

Blood tests can also reveal how well various organs are functioning by measuring the levels of normal chemicals in the body. For example, the levels of particular enzymes may reveal a liver abnormality and indicate that further diagnostic tests to evaluate the organ are needed.

Most blood tests are easy to perform, usually inexpensive, and virtually risk-free. The blood sample is obtained by a lab technician, nurse, or doctor inserting a needle into a vein and is relatively painless. The only preparation may be the need to fast for several hours.

INFORM

YOURSELF

Blood Tests for Cancer

Everyone hopes that someday a simple, inexpensive blood test will reveal whether a person has cancer. Since cancer is actually a group of more than a hundred different diseases, it is unlikely that one test will screen all types of malignancies. However, tests can now detect certain molecules—often a type of protein—produced by specific types of cancer. These molecules are called tumor markers.

Tumor markers are most useful to monitor the effectiveness of treatment, to follow the course of a disease, and to detect recurrent disease after treatment. Some tumor markers can also help predict the stage of the disease, since the higher the tumor marker level, the greater the likelihood that the disease has metastasized. With a few exceptions, tumor markers are not widely used to screen or diagnose disease because noncancerous conditions can sometimes produce a positive result.

Some of the most common tumor markers are the following:

- Carcinoembryonic Antigen (CEA). This substance is elevated in the blood of people with colorectal and, less often, some types of thyroid, breast, pancreatic, and lung cancers. Cigarette smoking and several benign disorders also cause elevated CEA levels. The test is not specific enough for diagnosis, but it is used to detect tumor recurrence or to monitor treatment of colorectal cancer.

- Carbohydrate Antigen 125 (CA 125). Over 90 percent of women with advanced ovarian cancer have elevated levels of this antigen in their blood, but it may also be elevated when the cancer is contained within the ovary. Therefore, it is sometimes used as a screening test in women at high risk for this cancer. CA 125 is also sometimes elevated in endometrial, pancreatic, stomach, and colorectal cancers, especially when they are widespread. But a high level is not proof of cancer, because CA 125 is elevated in women with endometriosis and other benign conditions. A low CA 125 level does not exclude malignancy, and about half of women with stage I ovarian tumors do not have an elevated CA 125 level. Therefore, the test is not reliable for detecting early-stage ovarian cancer. It is most valuable when combined with a careful pelvic exam and ultrasonography or when used to detect recurrent disease in women who have been treated for ovarian cancer (see the *Ovarian Cancer* section of Chapter 4).

- Carbohydrate Antigen 19-9 (CA 19-9). Originally used to detect colorectal cancer, CA 19-9 is useful in diagnosing pancreatic cancer and detecting its recurrence after treatment. The marker is also elevated in some other forms of digestive system cancer, especially cancer of the bile ducts.

- Carbohydrate Antigen 15-3 (CA 15-3). This antigen is elevated in 75 percent of women with widespread breast cancer. However, it is often elevated in healthy women as well. The test is sometimes used to detect recurrence, but its routine use is not recommended by the American Society of Clinical Oncologists or by the National Comprehensive Cancer Network.

- Prostate-Specific Antigen (PSA). This antigen, produced by the prostate gland, is elevated in many men with prostate cancer. However, prostatitis (an inflamed prostate), benign prostatic hyperplasia (an enlarged prostate), and recent ejaculation also cause elevated PSA levels. In addition, the PSA test is not sensitive enough to detect all prostate cancers and may miss about a third of them. Nevertheless, PSA is currently the most accurate method available for early detection of prostate cancer the only tumor marker currently recommended for early detection of cancer by the American Cancer Society (see the *Guidelines for the Early Detection of Prostate Cancer* section of Chapter 4).

   The PSA test is most valuable when combined with a digital rectal exam. Together, the two tests find more cases of prostate cancer than either test alone. The PSA test is also used to monitor men who are being treated for prostate cancer and to check for recurrent cancer following treatment.

- Human Chorionic Gonadotropin (HCG). Pregnant women normally have high levels of this hormone, but when it remains high in the months after delivery, it is a strong indication of a rare condition called gestational trophoblastic neoplasia. Cancers of the testicles and ovaries and some lung tumors can also cause elevated HCG levels. HCG can be used to monitor success of treatment and detect recurrence of cancers that produce this substance.

- Alpha-Fetoprotein (AFP). Elevated levels of this substance can indicate acute and chronic hepatitis and also occurs in many people with liver cancer. The higher the AFP level, the greater the likelihood of cancer, so an abnormal AFP level should be followed with ultrasonography. AFP is also produced by a rare type of testicular and ovarian cancer called yolk sac tumor or endodermal sinus tumor. This test can be used to detect recurrence of these liver, testicular, and ovarian tumors after treatment.

Endoscopy

If the tumor is in an internal internal organ, an endoscopy may be recommended. This allows the outside or inside surfaces of the organs to be viewed directly. Tissue from organs can also be removed through the endoscope for biopsy.

An endoscope is a lighted, hollow magnifying instrument narrow enough to pass through one of the body's natural openings, such as the nose, mouth, anus, urethra, or vagina. Some endoscopes are made of flexible materials and use fiberoptic technology to see around turns and bends in the intestines, lungs, and other organs.

An endoscope may also be inserted through a small incision into the abdomen (laparoscopy) or chest (thoracoscopy). These procedures are sometimes called "Band-Aid" surgery because the incision is small enough to be covered by a small bandage.

The examining doctor can see deep inside the body and, with the aid of an attached brush or cutting instrument, remove tissue samples for biopsy. Some endoscopes have a tiny camera built onto the tip that transmits images to a television monitor.

Endoscopy is often recommended to evaluate an abnormality detected on an x-ray or other exam. It may also be used before surgery to pinpoint the exact site of a tumor.

There are many different types of endoscopes, all of which can be identified by how they are used. For example, a cystoscope is used to inspect the urinary tract, a colonoscope is used to examine the colon, and a bronchoscope is used to look inside the lungs.

Depending on the type of endoscope and the part of the body being examined, a special diet or enema may be required. The procedure may be performed on an outpatient basis in a doctor's office, or it may require an overnight stay in the hospital. Recuperating time varies according to the procedure.

Some endoscopies are uncomfortable, but they are usually not painful, especially with anesthesia or a sedative. Many people are exhausted after an endoscopic procedure and might want to curtail some activities for a while, depending on the body part examined.

Complications of endoscopy include the rare risk of perforation of the area being examined, infection, and excessive bleeding.

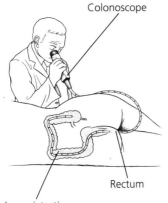

A colonoscope allows the doctor to examine the rectum and colon.

Colonoscope

Rectum

Large intestine (colon)

Cytology

The examination of cells under the microscope is called cytology or cytopathology. Cytologic tests may be used in two ways—for diagnosis or for screening. For example, the Pap test is used as a screening test for cervical cancer and a biopsy is used to confirm the presence of cancer before treatment is started. On the other hand, cytologic testing of bronchial brush samples is considered a diagnostic test for lung cancer and, in the context of a malignant-appearing mass on a chest x-ray, a cytology positive result justifies starting chemotherapy or removing all or part of a lung.

Cell samples can be obtained in several ways—some are simple and painless, and others require more complex equipment and procedures. The best known technique for cytological sampling is to gently scrape or brush some cells from the organ or tissue being tested. For example, Pap test samples are taken by using a small spatula and/or brush to remove cells from the cervix (the lower part of the uterus, or womb). By using an endoscope, cell samples can be taken by brushing the lining of the esophagus, stomach, bronchi (breathing tubes that lead to the lungs), bile ducts, and other areas deep inside the body.

Cancer can also be diagnosed by examining cells found in body fluids such as sputum, urine, and spinal fluid. The fluid that surrounds the lungs, heart, or abdominal organs can be withdrawn through a needle to check for cancer cells.

Fine needle aspiration biopsy (FNA) is usually considered a cytology test even though its name includes the word "biopsy." FNA uses a very thin needle and a syringe to withdraw a small amount of fluid and small tissue fragments from a tumor mass. The doctor can aim the needle while feeling a suspicious tumor or area near the surface of the body. If the tumor is deep inside the body and cannot be felt, the needle can be guided while it is viewed by imaging procedures such as an ultrasound or a CT scan. The main advantage of FNA is that it does not require an incision (cutting through the skin). The disadvantage is that in some cases this thin needle cannot remove enough tissue for a definite diagnosis.

The accuracy of a cytologic diagnosis depends on the skill and experience of both the person obtaining the sample of cells and the technologist or pathologist examining them.

Biopsy

A biopsy is the removal of tissue from a suspicious mass or lesion for microscopic examination. Since it provides the most accurate analysis of tissue, it is considered the gold standard of cancer diagnostic tests.

The tissue may be obtained by a core needle biopsy, through an endoscope, or by surgical removal. Depending on how the tissue is removed, the location and size of the tumor, and the amount of tissue taken, the biopsy may be done in a doctor's office, an outpatient surgical facility with local anesthesia, or a hospital under general anesthesia.

Needle Biopsy

There are two main types of needle biopsies, a fine needle aspiration biopsy (FNA) and a core needle biopsy. The former is generally considered a cytology

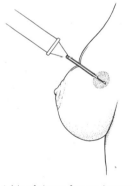

A bit of tissue from a breast lump can be obtained by using a special needle. This needle biopsy can be done in a doctor's office under local anesthesia.

procedure because it removes individual cells and very small groups of cells. The core biopsy removes a cylinder of tissue, usually about an inch long. The core is usually $\frac{1}{16}$ to $\frac{1}{8}$ inch in diameter. Although the core biopsy is a little more uncomfortable than the fine needle biopsy and takes longer to process, the larger amount of tissue makes interpretation by the pathologist easier. For some types of tumors, the accuracy rates are similar; for others the core biopsy is much more effective. Needle biopsies are more easily performed for tumors close to the skin surface, but they can also be used on tumors of internal organs such as the prostate, pancreas, or lung, thus dramatically reducing the need for exploratory surgery. A simultaneous imaging test may help visualize the needle placement, ensuring that it reaches the precise location of the tumor. There is always a risk, however, that the needle will miss a very small tumor or indistinct lesion. Even placing a needle in a large mass can be difficult.

The discomfort and the type of anesthesia needed depend on how close to the surface the suspected tumor is. Local anesthesia may be sufficient when the area from which a biopsy is needed is near the body's surface. Sedation is often needed when the needle must penetrate an organ to reach a deeper tumor. A biopsy gun is used for needle biopsies of the prostate and some other organs. This device inserts and removes the needle in a fraction of a second, making the procedure much more bearable.

It may take only fifteen minutes to obtain a tissue sample of a superficial, easily felt tumor, such as one in the breast. On the other hand, if the tumor is located deep within the body, it may be more difficult to place the needle precisely, and the procedure may take an hour or more.

Endoscopic Biopsy

Small biopsy samples can be taken by using instruments operated through an endoscope. Doctors often use small biopsy forceps with tiny "jaws" that take a $\frac{1}{8}$-inch bite from the tumor. These procedures are often used for lung biopsies and for biopsies of the digestive and urinary tracts.

Surgical Biopsy

A surgical biopsy is more invasive and expensive than a needle or endoscopic biopsy, but it allows more tissue to be removed more precisely. And with more tissue to analyze, the pathologist can make the most accurate diagnosis possible.

Surgical biopsies fall into two broad categories: incisional and excisional. Incisional biopsy is the removal of a piece of the suspicious mass. If a malignancy is confirmed, the entire tumor can be removed later in another operation. Incisional biopsies involve the remote risk that cancer cells, if present, may scatter into normal tissue and cause cancer to spread. This is

Before Having a Biopsy

Always clarify the reasons for a biopsy. Ask any questions about the technique and how the sample will be handled well before the actual procedure begins. You might ask your doctor:

- Are you going to biopsy a portion of the tumor or remove it completely? Why?

- If you biopsy just a portion of the mass, will I need another operation to remove the entire tumor?

- Will the biopsy be examined as a frozen section or fixed-tissue specimen? Why?

- Can the mass be sampled by fine needle or core needle biopsy? If not, why not?

- Will the biopsy be examined by a board-certified pathologist?

- Will the report be confirmed by a second pathologist? (Some cancer centers recommend a second opinion before patients are treated. See Chapter 7.)

- Will you consult personally with the pathologist(s)?

- Will the biopsy leave a scar? Where will it be?

called cancer seeding. It is extremely rare for most types of cancer, but it can happen in both incisional and needle biopsies of some cancers, such as testicular cancer.

Excisional biopsy is removal of the entire tumor, preferably along with a margin of surrounding normal tissue. The goal is to simultaneously establish a diagnosis and treat the primary tumor. Excisional biopsies are usually performed on small, easily accessible tumors that have not begun to spread and do not include vital tissue. For example, an entire suspicious skin lesion or lump in the breast may be removed at once.

Tissue may be prepared for examination by frozen or permanent sections. A frozen section is obtained during surgery and prepared within minutes while the patient is on the operating table. The surgeon removes tissue from the tumor and immediately sends the sample to a pathologist. The pathologist quickly freezes the tissue in a special machine, slices it into very thin sections, places it on slides, stains it by dipping the slide into a series of dyes so that the cells can be clearly seen, and examines it under a microscope. The pathologist then makes a diagnosis and reports it to the surgical team.

If cancer is confirmed and the tumor can be removed, it is excised immediately. Because the biopsy, diagnosis, and surgery all take place at one time (called a one-step procedure), frozen sections most often eliminate the need for a second operation (called a two-step procedure). A disadvantage of the one-step procedure is that freezing distorts the cells, making analysis difficult and resulting in a small risk of error. However, a skilled, experienced pathologist can diagnose a frozen section of most cancers with more than 98 percent accuracy. (To verify the accuracy of the frozen-section diagnosis, tissue is also examined as a fixed-tissue specimen the following day.)

A two-step procedure means that the biopsy and tumor removal take place at different times. A permanent, fixed-tissue section is prepared for the biopsy. Tissue processed this way is placed in a special preserving solution, embedded in paraffin, sliced, placed on a slide, and stained in a more time-consuming procedure that yields a higher-quality slide and a diagnosis with 99 percent accuracy. However, the process takes one or more days. This means if cancer is confirmed and is operable, a second operation is necessary.

A two-step procedure allows time for further testing and second opinions, though. Moreover, you can participate in decisions about immediate treatment. However, if the tumor is deep inside the body, a second major operation may be too risky, and a one-step procedure may be preferable.

If a one-step procedure is preferred or is only a possibility, the surgeon should explain all the options in advance and obtain appropriate patient consent (see Chapter 10).

Sometimes it is known that the tumor is malignant and a biopsy is done to check whether cancer is present in the tissue adjacent to where the tumor is. This area is called the surgical margin. Frozen sections of the surgical margins help the surgeon decide how much tissue must be removed to completely excise a cancer.

Exploratory Surgery

Exploratory surgery allows a doctor to inspect internal organs directly to evaluate a mass and, if necessary, obtain tissue for further study. Depending on what is found, the surgeon may estimate how far the disease has spread, remove lymph nodes that may be affected, and obtain fluid and tissue samples.

The operation, which usually follows imaging exams and other diagnostic tests, is performed in a hospital by a surgeon.

Surgery always involves some risk and chance of complications, such as excessive bleeding and infection. Hospitalization for several days may be necessary, and recovery may require weeks. Postoperative pain and discomfort are common.

Diagnosis by Surgery

Before undergoing surgery, ask your doctor these questions:

- Describe the procedure you are recommending. What will be done and why?

- Why is this surgery necessary?

- What are the risks of this procedure, and how likely are they?

- What are the possible side effects and complications?

- Can I arrange to have my own blood drawn and stored in advance in case I need it?

- Is the procedure covered by my insurance or health care plan? How will I be billed? Will I receive separate bills from the hospital, surgeon, anesthesiologist, pathologist, and radiologist?

- Are there any other diagnostic tests that can be performed instead of surgery?

- Will a board-certified surgeon who specializes in oncology perform the procedure?

- How experienced is the surgeon in performing this type of operation?

- How long will I be hospitalized? How long will the recovery period be?

- When can I return to my daily routine?

Bone Marrow Analysis

Bone marrow aspiration is the removal of a sample of bone marrow for laboratory analysis. It is done to diagnose leukemia, a cancer that begins in the marrow, and to detect the spread of other cancers to the bone marrow.

After the skin and tissue surrounding the area to be penetrated are anesthetized, a long needle is inserted into the hipbone, pelvis, or breastbone. Fluid from the bone marrow (a soft substance at the center of the bone that produces blood cells) is withdrawn and examined microscopically.

A bone marrow biopsy is usually performed in conjunction with a bone marrow aspiration. With the needle still in place, the doctor removes a cylinder-shaped core of bone and its marrow.

Bone marrow aspiration and biopsy are virtually risk-free and take less than an hour to perform in a doctor's office or hospital. However, even though sedatives and local anesthetics are given, the procedure is painful. A sharp jolt and a sensation of intense pressure can be felt when marrow is withdrawn. The puncture site may be bruised and tender for a few days.

The tests are performed by a doctor, and the tissue is examined microscopically by a pathologist or hematologist (a doctor who specializes in blood disorders).

When the Diagnosis Is Cancer

6

Cancer Care:
A Team Approach

From diagnosis to treatment to recovery, cancer care can involve a legion of health care professionals who provide a range of specific skills. The places where care is offered can also vary widely, from the doctor's office to a hospital, from a specialized cancer care center to your own home.

Among all these people and places is an extraordinary breadth of expertise and technology to meet your medical, emotional, and practical needs as well as those of your family. Finding out the available options and orchestrating all of these resources into a functioning system can be a challenge. As more care providers become involved, the need to communicate effectively with them grows even more important.

The Team Concept

Until the last few decades, cancer care was a relatively straightforward process. Perhaps during a routine visit to the family doctor, someone might report a disturbing symptom or the doctor might detect a troubling sign of disease. The person was then referred to a specialist. If cancer was detected, the only treatment available was surgery (and, later, radiation or chemotherapy). After the procedure, the person usually would be sent home—with fingers crossed.

Patient advocacy has changed with advances in treatment, with the development of the medical specialty of oncology (cancer care), and with a vastly greater appreciation of the daily needs of the person with cancer and his or her family. Health concerns are only part of the picture, however. People with cancer need help for psychological, social, financial, and occupational concerns as well. From diagnosis through recovery, the best cancer care today requires far more expertise

INFORM

YOURSELF

Getting the Best Cancer Care from Managed Care

Increasing numbers of people receive medical care through health maintenance organizations (HMOs) and similar managed care plans designed to control health care costs. Typically these plans require that each person be cared for by a primary doctor, the "gatekeeper," through whom all referrals to specialists are made. The specialists usually must also be members of the plan.

The push to control costs has also led to guidelines for the treatment of illnesses and referral to specialist care that in some cases severely restrict the consumer's choices. The doctors in the managed care plan may be limited in what they can do or recommend on their patient's behalf, and a case manager's approval of any recommendations is often required. Some plans offer financial incentives to their doctors to keep costs down, a controversial policy that may be at odds with the best quality of care.

Although not-for-profit HMOs have existed for years, no system is yet in place to assure that this rapid shift to for-profit managed care delivers the diagnostic, treatment, supportive care, and follow-up care opportunities to everyone with cancer. Many state governments are beginning to regulate some HMO practices.

The American Cancer Society (ACS) feels an obligation to assist the managed care industry in understanding the requirements for appropriate care. The ACS is collaborating with numerous medical specialty organizations related to cancer care, patient advocacy groups, and insurance organizations, among others, to develop cancer treatment and care guidelines and accountability practices.

Here's what you can do now to get the most out of your managed care plan:

- Insist on knowing how cancer is managed in your plan. What are the plan's restrictions on your choices of doctors, including specialists? Will you have prompt access to a team of cancer providers in many disciplines—for example, medical, surgical, and radiation oncology; oncology nursing; social work—to help plan your treatment?

- Ask about limitations to screening, diagnostic tests, and treatments.

- Does the plan offer access to clinical trials and investigational treatments?

- Are your doctor or others in the plan experienced in detecting and treating cancer generally or your type of cancer particularly? Ask whether the primary care doctors have specific training in cancer diagnosis and are required by the plan to stay abreast of new developments.

- Does the plan allow its primary care doctors to refer you to doctors outside the network or to specialized facilities if necessary? For example, if your child has cancer, does the health plan permit referral to a specialized pediatric cancer center?

- Will you have final say in all decisions? Will all options be presented to you?

- During the course of your illness, does your primary doctor have to approve treatments, procedures, or tests, or can a specialist assume the role of principal caregiver?

- Can you get rehabilitation, counseling, supportive services, and adequate pain relief as needed?

The more you know about the current standard of care for your particular cancer, the better you will be able to understand your needs and insist on state-of-the-art treatment. Although not all the answers to all your questions may be to your liking—for example, the HMO may delay referrals to necessary specialists—you will have information you need in order, perhaps, to change plans. Certainly you will have grounds for informed complaint, to the primary care doctor, to the managers through the plan's grievance procedures, to the benefits manager at work, or to your state insurance regulatory board, if need be. And by all means, seek the help of your local ACS chapter (see *Resources*). Patient advocacy is one of our most important missions.

than any single caregiver can provide. Thus, many medical professionals and support people are involved in coordinating and providing your care.

Increasingly, experts in cancer care recognize that the person with cancer is best served when all these many helpers function as a unified team, managed by one professional team leader. The reasoning is that by working together, people with cancer, their loved ones, and their caregivers can pool all their strengths and resources to achieve a common goal: survival that offers the highest quality of life for the longest amount of time.

This unity of care and caregivers—in which someone is always available to assess everyone's individual needs and see that they are met—is the ideal scenario. Some hospitals and cancer centers do have formal teams to coordinate and provide care, and many oncologists have at least some of the necessary caregivers on their staffs. Most common, however, is the informal network of care providers and resources to whom your doctor refers you or that you discover through other sources, such as cancer survivors, the American Cancer Society (ACS), other organizations, and books such as this one.

You should be aware, however, that some insurance companies and prepaid or managed health plans discourage the input of more professionals than *they* deem essential to cancer care.

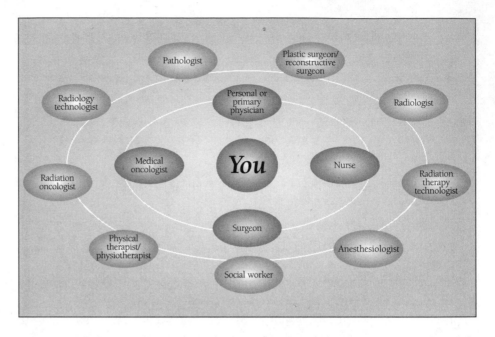

Selecting a Care Coordinator

Most people are best served by a doctor whom they trust who coordinates their care or at least advises on the process and helps evaluate the results. Otherwise, patient and family members will likely be overwhelmed by the numbers of professionals with whom they become involved over the course of the illness. Identifying who will serve this role of care coordinator may be the most important decision in managing your illness.

Some people prefer to work with their primary doctor: the general practitioner, family practitioner, internist, gynecologist, pediatrician, geriatrician, or primary care provider in a health maintenance organization (HMO) whom you consult when earliest symptoms arise or who discovered signs of cancer in a checkup. Primary doctors can help choose an oncologist to manage the cancer treatment, who will keep them informed throughout the treatment. This doctor is often in the best position to provide continuing care, as he or she is likely to have known you before the symptoms emerged and will be involved in your health care after the active cancer treatment ends. This long-term perspective can be extremely valuable in making the most appropriate choices during treatment and recovery.

Your primary doctor may offer to assume this adviser role or agree to provide such a service when asked. But not everyone has a regular doctor, and indeed, that doctor may not be comfortable serving in that capacity.

For many people, oncologists assume the doctor-coordinator role, and their practices are set up to provide many types of services. Of course, they won't necessarily have the detachment from their role of providing your cancer care directly. Still, oncologists are informed about the latest treatments, are aware of the multifaceted needs of people who have cancer, and are familiar with the resources available for follow-up care. Some people prefer to have their surgeon assume the doctor-coordinator role.

Regardless of who assumes the role of professional adviser or coordinator, it is essential that you, the patient, feel comfortable with the choice. If your team leader seems cold and uninvolved or if you are made to feel less like a human being and more like a collection of symptoms, you may need to find someone else to take charge.

When making a decision, it is important to consider your coordinator's qualifications, indeed those of all your caregivers. Suggestions for evaluating doctors' qualifications and behavior, and other factors to consider before committing your care to a person or facility are provided later in this chapter.

Who's on the Team

If you have a doctor adviser or team leader, that person will remain constant throughout your illness and recovery. Other cancer care professionals and support personnel come and go as your needs change throughout your illness and recovery. Often, most of the team is replaced as the process moves from diagnosis to different treatments or to different care settings.

TIPS AND

ADVICE

What's *Your* Role on the Cancer Team?

For the team to provide the best care for you throughout your illness and recovery, you should view yourself as the team's star player—but not necessarily its coordinator or manager. That role you should consider delegating to your chosen doctor adviser.

As the key team member, you will decide which procedures or treatments offer you the best chance for recovery and the highest quality of life. Others will provide information, describe alternatives, and make recommendations. Your authority is to say yes or no or to grant another member of the team (possibly a family member or close friend) the authority to make such decisions for you.

Do not think that to be a "good" team player you must either be exceedingly active in your care, participating in even the most minor decisions, or remain passive and let those in authority have their way. Everyone has his or her own way of coping with the crisis of illness (see Chapters 26 and 27). As long as your style does not prevent you from proceeding with treatment—by denying that you are really sick, for example, by insisting on collecting opinions long after all options have been determined, or by accepting only those caregivers who tell you what you want to hear—you should function in the way that works best for you.

Some people cope by taking control of all their care and learning about every detail. As soon as they hear the diagnosis, they do as much research as time allows into the types of care and doctors and facilities available to provide it. They seek multiple opinions from different specialists until they find one whose philosophy fits their own. Other people, however, feel better relying on the advice of the expert or experts to whom they have entrusted their care. They may feel ill equipped to absorb all the details needed to make major decisions and are satisfied to let others evaluate the technicalities and present them with recommendations from which to choose. It is usually to your advantage to take your time in making a decision about your treatment. Rather than making a quick choice and later wishing you had chosen differently, get as much clear information as you need and make a decision based on an understanding of the risks and benefits.

No matter what role feels right for you, you *always* have the right to state your needs, express your preferences, and obtain the information you require for making informed decisions—indeed, that is your responsibility. A diagnosis of cancer often makes people feel that their bodies —even their entire worlds—are out of control. Recognizing that it is appropriate for you to take an active part in medical decisions may help restore a sense of power over the situation, which can be therapeutic in its own right.

Diagnosis

Cancer may be detected by a primary care doctor, by a specialist, or perhaps by a doctor in a hospital in which you are being treated for a medical emergency. This "first-line" doctor will either order diagnostic tests or make a referral to one or more specialists who can provide these tests. When the test results are available, the doctors involved will confer and, if necessary, consult with other experts.

Unless a care coordinator is already in place, the primary care doctor— the person you tend to think of as "my doctor"—is generally the appropriate person to discuss the diagnosis with you. For example, a man suspected of having prostate cancer may be referred to a urologist, who specializes in the urinary and male reproductive systems, for a prostate biopsy. If the diagnosis is cancer, the urologist may accept responsibility from then on, may collaborate with the primary doctor, or may refer the man to yet another specialist, such as a radiation oncologist.

In any event, no matter who is "in charge" of the case, it is reasonable to expect all doctors who have participated to be available to answer questions.

Treatment

Once the diagnosis is confirmed, the focus will shift to designing the treatment plan. If you are going to work with a doctor who will coordinate your care, now is the time to select him or her.

Most commonly, some combination of surgery, radiation, and chemotherapy is recommended, and the choices you make will determine which doctors will become involved next. In many cases, the treatment begins in a hospital or clinic. Depending on how the hospital or clinic is organized, your inpatient or outpatient care will be coordinated by an attending doctor, resident doctors (doctors who are completing advanced training), and other members of the medical staff.

Depending on your needs during treatment, other professionals may be brought in at the request of the attending doctor. For example, a nutritionist may be consulted about your diet while undergoing chemotherapy, or a mental health professional may be called in to help evaluate and treat depression.

Hospitals also offer the services of a nurse or social worker who direct cancer patients and their families to appropriate sources of help in dealing with insurance companies, financial problems, personal issues, and other practical tasks. Nurses or social workers may also serve as leaders of discussion or support groups and provide education on coping strategies for living with a cancer diagnosis. Another important person is the case manager or discharge planner, again a nurse or a social worker, who coordinates plans for your return home to make sure needed services or equipment will be available.

Depending on the type of cancer involved, the treatment may continue for an extended time following your discharge from the hospital. Nurses working in clinics or doctors' offices frequently administer chemotherapy. Home care nurses, respiratory or other therapists, social workers, or other providers may provide help in the home or in a private or clinic office.

Rehabilitation and Recovery

Recovery from the illness and any side effects of the treatment requires a new or expanded team of cancer care professionals. These may include physical therapists who are specialists in regaining the use of muscles that have been weakened, adjusting to the loss of body parts, and coping with the tasks of life and the practical and emotional consequences of illness. Care is often given in the home or coordinated through available resources in the community.

For those who wish it, social workers, psychologists, psychiatrists, and psychosocial or psychiatric nurses provide counseling and supportive care for individuals or groups. Organizations of people who have had cancer—cancer survivors—provide useful information, practical and emotional support, and sometimes, political activism. Social workers affiliated with hospitals or voluntary organizations offer needed assistance in locating community health and social service organizations and in gaining placement in a rehabilitation center, among many other services.

Advanced Illness

Recurrent or advancing illness calls forth many of the professionals who took part in the earlier diagnosis and treatment. Sometimes the goal of treatment is to control the disease. When this is not possible, the primary goal of treatment may focus on providing the highest quality of life through supportive care. Research centers can provide experimental treatments to aid in patient comfort and to maintain or improve quality of life. Experts in pain management (including pain specialists, physiatrists, anesthesiologists, psychiatrists, psychologists, behavioral medicine specialists, social workers, and nurses) may be called in for consultation. Hospice care professionals offer practical help, comfort, and care for those who are approaching death. Patients and families often wait until death is imminent (less than two weeks), but hospice care can be very beneficial to patients and families for many months before death and can provide bereavement care for their families afterward.

Types of Medical Doctors

People being treated for cancer encounter numerous types of doctors throughout all phases of their cancer care. The following is a guide to medical doctors and their specialties:

- To earn a medical degree and a license to practice, doctors complete four years of college plus four years of medical school and, in most states, an additional year of internship. Doctors with this basic level of training are often referred to as generalists or general practitioners (GPs).

- Many doctors undergo two to five years of additional training to become specialists in one of about two dozen specialties recognized by the American Board of Medical Specialties. A doctor who is board certified has passed certification exams in a specialty. Some qualified and experienced specialists, however, do not elect to apply for board certification. To maintain their certification, doctors must undergo continuing education after passing the exam. To find out whether a doctor is board certified, call the American Board of Medical Specialties at 866-ASK-ABMS (866-275-2267) or visit their web site at www.abms.org.

- In recent years, family medicine has developed into a specialty of its own; those who complete the additional training are usually called family practitioners.

- Collectively, GPs, family practitioners, and doctors who specialize in pediatrics, obstetrics/gynecology, geriatrics, and internal medicine (known as internists) are considered to be primary care doctors. The term primary care reflects the fact that these doctors are usually consulted first when a medical need arises. Some primary care providers are advanced practice nurses who work collaboratively with a doctor. Subscribers to HMOs and other pre-paid health plans are usually required to visit a primary care provider doctor before receiving a referral to a specialist.

- An oncologist specializes in cancer care. A medical oncologist provides chemotherapy, hormone therapy, and other nonsurgical, nonradiation treatments. Medical oncologists often serve as the primary or coordinating doctor for people with cancer. A radiation oncologist specializes in using radiation to treat cancer, and a surgical oncologist performs operations to diagnose and remove cancer. As their titles indicate, gynecologic oncologists and pediatric oncologists subspecialize in treating women's and children's cancers, respectively. Specialists in other areas also provide many of an oncologist's functions.

Other Doctor Specialists

Virtually any type of medical or surgical specialist may be directly involved with cancer care or indirectly if you have additional health problems. Some of these specialists include the following:

- Radiologists specialize in the use of x-rays, ultrasound, computed tomography (CT scans), magnetic resonance imaging (MRI), and other diagnostic imaging techniques. Radiation oncologists are medical doctors specializing in treating cancer with radiation.

- Hematologists specialize in blood disorders and are consulted in cases of cancer of the blood, bone marrow, and lymph system.

- Medical oncologists are medical doctors who prescribe chemotherapy, hormone therapy, and other anticancer drugs.

- Neurologists specialize in disorders of the brain and central nervous system.

- Pathologists study tissue samples to determine the type and extent of disease.

- Gastroenterologists specialize in disorders of the digestive system.

- Endocrinologists specialize in disorders of the glands (thyroid, adrenal, and so on) of the endocrine system.

- Dermatologists specialize in diseases of the skin.

- Nephrologists specialize in kidney disorders.

- Anesthesiologists specialize in administering anesthesia during surgical procedures; they may also be consulted for pain relief.

- Physiatrists specialize in physical medicine or rehabilitation medicine, which in cancer care generally means the diagnosis and treatment of a physical disability.

- Psychiatrists specialize in mental health and mental disorders. In cancer care, psychiatrists are consulted in regard to symptoms—including depression, anxiety, confusion, and dementia—that sometimes occur in people with cancer, occasionally as a direct physical result of the disease.

- Urologists specialize in disorders of the urinary system and the male genitourinary system.

- Obstetricians/gynecologists specialize in diseases of the female reproductive system. Obstetricians deliver babies.

About Surgeons and Their Specialties

Surgeons are doctors who receive additional training in operating on the body for diagnostic and treatment purposes.

- General surgeons or surgical oncologists perform surgical diagnostic procedures to determine the location and extent of disease. They also remove tumors and, if necessary, the surrounding tissue. Some of the specialists listed earlier, such as obstetricians/gynecologists and urologists, also are trained in surgical techniques.

- Some other surgical specialties encountered in cancer care are thoracic surgery (chest), reconstructive/plastic surgery (reconstruction of removed or injured body parts and correction of appearance), neurosurgery (brain and nervous system), and orthopedic surgery (bone and connective tissue).

Types of Nurses

Nurses are vital members of the cancer team and are crucial to the planning and delivery of daily care. They educate patients about their illness, administer medications, monitor responses to treatment, manage side effects, run support groups, and generally administer the treatment plan. Often the most accessible caregivers on the team, nurses are the people patients frequently turn to first to identify problems and find solutions to a range of medical, emotional, and social problems.

Nurses are found in all cancer care settings. Ambulatory care nurses, who work in outpatient clinics or offices, often prepare and administer chemotherapy.

In the hospital, nurses tend to immediate needs in addition to administering many treatments. Nurses also care for patients in their homes or in hospices. Nurses have different degrees of training and experience:

- To earn a nursing degree and a license to practice nursing, registered nurses (RNs) earn an associate degree (two years) or a bachelor's degree (four years) in nursing from a school accredited by the National League for Nursing and pass a state licensing exam. Nursing focuses on the human experience of illness and health. Nurses use the scientific knowledge of diagnosis and treatment and provide a caring relationship that promotes healing. They monitor patients' conditions, provide treatment, and help people with cancer and their families adjust physically and emotionally to illness.

- Advanced practice nurses (APNs) are registered professional nurses with a master's or doctoral degree and are recognized as such by their State Board of Nursing. APNs exercise specialized judgment and skill to work independently and collaboratively with doctors and other health care professionals. Their scope of practice is to provide expert, quality, and comprehensive nursing care to patients. The APNs that can help take care of you if you have cancer are nurse practitioners and clinical nurse specialists.

- Nurse practitioners have additional training in primary care and other specialties, like oncology (cancer care) and acute care, and share many tasks with doctors, such as taking patient histories, conducting physical exams, coordinating the care of and teaching the patient with cancer, and prescribing medications within their scope of practice.

- Clinical nurse specialists are registered nurses with a master's or other advanced degree who specialize in the direct care of patients in specific areas, such as oncology or mental health nursing (Psych CNS). They can also be excellent cancer care resources for patients and families. They usually work in institutions such as hospitals or long-term care facilities.

- Oncology-certified nurses (OCNs) are registered nurses who are clinical specialists in cancer care. They have passed certification and licensing exams qualifying them to administer chemotherapy, manage side effects, administer pain control medications, handle emergencies, and provide long-term care and support. In large facilities, some oncology-certified nurses, like some doctors, subspecialize in such areas as breast cancer or radiation oncology. Advanced practice nurses can become advance oncology certified nurses (AOCNs).

- Licensed practical nurses (LPNs) assist RNs in their duties. LPNs have had one year of nursing education and provide limited routine care.

- Nurses' aides train for a few months to meet patients' needs, such as changing linen and giving baths.

Other Members of the Cancer Care Team

In addition to doctors and nurses, numerous other health care professionals provide help during illness and recovery.

The Medical Support Team

All the following people must be specially trained and often licensed, depending on a state's requirements. Anyone with doubts about a provider's qualifications should ask for proof.

- Radiation technologists assist radiologists with diagnostic and therapeutic services.

- Dietitians/nutritionists design optimal nutrition to improve recovery. Because cancer can affect appetite and changes in weight and treatment can trigger nausea and vomiting, nutritional counseling is often essential. Dietitians and nutritionists also manage tube feedings or IV nutrition for both inpatient care and in the home.

- Physical therapists (sometimes called physiotherapists) work with the body to restore strength, function, flexibility, and muscle tone.

- Speech therapists and speech pathologists work with people who have lost the ability to speak or to speak clearly. They also help with diagnosing and treating functional problems, like swallowing.

- Occupational therapists work with people who have become disabled to help them relearn how to perform daily activities at home and at work.

- Respiratory therapists provide inhalation treatments, deep suctioning, oxygen, and other techniques to aid or strengthen breathing.

- Enterostomal therapists teach people how to care for an ostomy (a surgically created opening into the urinary or gastrointestinal canal).

The Psychosocial Support Team

Although they are not licensed to prescribe medication, the following professionals may offer counseling services:

- Psychologists, who hold a Ph.D., Psy.D., or Ed.D. degree (those with a master's degree also may provide some services), address personality issues, relationship problems, emotional issues, and other psychological concerns. They often suggest behavioral or cognitive approaches to dealing with pain and the side effects of cancer treatment.

- Social workers have a degree in social work (B.S.W, M.S.W, or D.S.W) and in most cases must be licensed or certified by the state in which they work. They are trained to help people with cancer and their families deal with a range of emotional and practical problems related to the illness and its treatment, such as child care, finances, emotional issues, family concerns and relationships, transportation, and problems with the health care system.

- Some social workers (oncology social workers) specialize in cancer-related problems. They counsel people concerning fears, answer questions about diagnosis and treatment, locate care facilities and community service programs, lead support groups, and help people and families overcome communication problems and other relationship issues. Social workers may be involved in care during the hospital stay, but they also may see clients on an outpatient basis in hospitals and clinics, through social service agencies, and in private practice settings.

Choosing and Evaluating a Doctor

Informed consent is critical to today's health care system. The term usually refers to the permission you give to a doctor or hospital to administer medications or to carry out procedures after you receive information about their risks and benefits. Informed consent also relates to your selection of the caregivers themselves. You and your family have the right to know about the training, expertise, and philosophy of treatment of those responsible for delivering care. If you do not feel comfortable with the answers, you have the right to look elsewhere.

Often, however, people are intimidated by the health care system, regarding doctors as all-knowing, all-powerful beings whose word is law. You may hesitate to ask "dumb" questions for fear of taking up the doctor's valuable time, or you may fear you may not understand or remember the doctor's answer. Furthermore, if the doctor has an unpleasant manner or prescribes a course of treatment you find objectionable, you may feel you have no right to protest or to request another approach.

To get the best out of the health care system, you often need to act like a consumer, asking questions until you understand, exploring alternatives, and demanding quality.

Finding a Doctor

Many people already have a relationship with at least one primary care doctor, often the doctor who first discovers evidence of cancer. To find a specialist in cancer diagnosis and treatment, that doctor will supply the names of colleagues in the area. Members of HMOs or similar health plans may be assigned to a primary care doctor or may be asked to select one from a list.

Usually, the members of these plans need written referrals from their primary caregiver before they can see a specialist.

To conduct your own search, two important resources are the toll-free telephone information numbers of the ACS (800-ACS-2345) and the National Cancer Institute (NCI) Cancer Information Service (800-4-CANCER). The NCI is the federal government's principal agency for research on cancer prevention, diagnosis, treatment, and rehabilitation and for dissemination of cancer information. A call to the ACS will yield helpful information as well (see *Resources*). Some hospitals advertise numbers to call for referrals, although such services include only those doctors who have admitting privileges at that facility.

Many libraries carry the *Directory of Medical Specialists*, which lists those doctors who have had additional training and who have passed special qualifying tests. Anyone who has the time or expertise to research specialized on-line consumer databases such as Medline (available through some computer networks and at larger libraries) might look for those doctors who have published journal articles on specific types of cancer or whose work is most often cited. To simplify this process, a trip to a medical library can be helpful. The NCI also maintains an on-line computer database called PDQ, or Physician Data Query (http://cancernet.nci.nih.gov/pdqfull.html), and can provide information from it for callers to the Cancer Information Service toll-free line (see *Resources* for more specific information). Among other things, the database contains a directory of doctors whose practices center on cancer treatment.

State, county, and local health departments or medical societies maintain lists of doctors. A call to the department of oncology or internal medicine at a major medical school or teaching hospital in your area is another option.

Asking friends or family members who have had experience with cancer for names of doctors who have been helpful to them is yet another approach.

Assessing Your Doctor's Qualifications

You should never commit yourself to a doctor's care before determining that he or she is qualified and able to deliver the type of care you require. A simple but effective strategy is just to ask your doctors about their qualifications.

- *Experience* is an essential clue. Years in practice are one measure, but the number of procedures performed or people treated for cancer also is significant. You should ask about the doctor's patient load, percentage of cancer patients, and the types of cancer he or she is experienced in treating. Because doctors doing research usually have published their findings in medical journals, you might ask for copies of articles in order to learn about their philosophy and approach.

Qualifying Questions

- Are you board certified?

- What is your specialty? Do you have a subspecialty?

- What training have you had in treating my type of cancer?

- How long have you been in practice?

- How many patients with my illness have you treated in the past year?

- Are you or others in your practice involved in clinical trials of new treatments?

- What are your office hours?

- How can you be contacted outside those hours?

- Who supervises your patients when you are on vacation?

- What hospitals are you affiliated with?

- Which hospital do you prefer to admit your cancer patients to? Why?

- May I tape-record our conversations so that I can review the details later?

- May I bring someone with me to appointments?

- Who besides you will be on my care team?

- Consider *the nature of the doctor's practice.* A solo practice means that patients see the same doctor on each visit, which provides continuity. A group practice, on the other hand, may offer more resources, expertise, and availability of care. A multispecialty group includes doctors with different areas of knowledge, whereas a single-specialty group may have more experience in a particular field.

- *Hospital affiliations* are important. Because doctors can send patients only to those facilities where they have admitting privileges, people seeking treatment should know where they will go for surgery or other care.

- A *teaching affiliation,* especially with a prestigious medical school, may indicate that the doctor is a respected leader in the field. Academic doctors who maintain practices are often in close touch with experts around the country and may be well versed in the latest therapies.

- A *doctor's reputation* is less easily evaluated. Sometimes asking others in the community can reveal a doctor's standing.

QUESTIONS

TO ASK

Evaluating Practice Style

- Are appointments easy to make? Is your doctor readily available if he or she is needed before the next appointment?

- Is the office environment clean and comfortable, conveying a sense of both efficiency and concern?

- Does the doctor's staff treat you courteously and respectfully?

- Is the doctor reasonably punctual? Does he or she apologize for any long waits?

- Do examinations and conversations take place in private? Do they seem rushed?

- Does your doctor appear open to the contributions of other health professionals, such as social workers, nurses, home care providers, or physical therapists? Will he or she make referrals?

- Do nurses and other assistants seem well trained? Are they willing to take time to answer your questions and to provide instruction and education as needed?

- Does the office staff help with insurance documents? Are they willing to negotiate terms of payment?

- Are phone calls returned quickly? By whom?

- Are the results of lab tests reported promptly?

Other Factors Related to Choosing a Doctor

Assuming that your doctor's qualifications are adequate, you now will want to consider other factors in your choice of caregiver.

- *Location* is important, especially when dealing with a long-term illness like cancer. Doctors whose offices are hard to get to, or hospitals that are inconvenient, may add an unnecessary complication.

- *Length of time in practice* can be relevant. Newly trained doctors may have little hands-on experience treating a particular type of cancer, although they may be more aware of modern techniques of cancer diagnosis and treatment than are some doctors who trained years ago.

- *Style of practice* can be difficult to assess unless you already have been under that doctor's care. Nonetheless, certain elements quickly convey a sense of the doctor's style, as noted in the box at the top of this page.

- A *doctor's personal manner* is perhaps harder to quantify than his or her practice style, although it may be even more relevant—especially if the doctor is serving as your care coordinator. A good communication style is critical. Empathy may not always be obvious, but concern, understanding, and support should be readily evident. For the doctor-patient relationship to succeed, most people need a doctor who will take time to answer questions and to recognize that for anyone with cancer, learning about the disease is an essential part of making informed treatment decisions.

How you weigh each of these various factors is an individual matter, but remember that doctors are human and that few can live up to the ideal image some people have of them.

Do You Have to Like Your Doctor?

TIPS AND

ADVICE

It helps to like your doctor, but it's trust that is essential. A lovable person can be a poor caregiver, and a seemingly uninterested doctor can be quite able. Your focus needs to be on getting well, so if you believe that your doctor's skills will serve that purpose, that's good. If you also like the doctor, that's a bonus.

An exception, perhaps, is the doctor who serves as your care coordinator. A strong bond between you and the person guiding your recovery can be potent medicine. Empathy can also be transformed into advocacy. The doctor who cares about you as a person will make sure that everything possible is being done on your behalf.

Because several doctors may be involved at various stages of your illness, the odds are slim that all of them will meet all of your needs. When dealing with doctors on the team other than the doctor adviser, confidence in their ability is probably more important than rapport. Evaluating doctors ahead of time to the extent possible should help weed out those you simply cannot work with.

If you find that an uncomfortable relationship with a certain provider is interfering with your care, speak up. Talk to the doctor, head nurse, social worker, or other team member you trust and express your concern. Sometimes the problem is merely one of communication.

Sometimes the difficulty results from expecting too much from one person. It is not uncommon to pin all hopes for cure, information, professional support, and 24-hour-a-day concern on the doctor and then to feel disappointed when he or she does not come through in some way. When evaluating a problem with any doctor, always consider whether there is someone else on your care team, or in your doctor's office, who can come through for you in ways that your doctor necessarily cannot.

If the issues between you and your doctor run deeper, however, switching caregivers, though sometimes difficult, is always an option.

In sum, you don't have to like all your doctors, but you do have to trust their strategy for your recovery.

Care Settings

Depending on the specifics of your situation, cancer diagnosis and treatment take place in a variety of settings and facilities. Threading your way through this maze can sometimes be bewildering and discouraging. Knowing what to expect—and where to expect it—can help reduce your anxiety and enable you to take full advantage of the services offered.

During the diagnostic phase, the process usually begins in a primary care doctor's office. Pap smears, biopsies, and certain other procedures and lab tests may be done here. If more tests are needed, you may be referred to a specialist's office, a diagnostic facility (such as a radiology office), or, in some cases, a hospital.

Once the diagnosis is confirmed, the care team or the doctor in charge develops the treatment plan, which may begin with a stay in the hospital. Fortunately, today many people with cancer spend comparatively little time there. Advances in medicine and technology mean that more types of surgery and other procedures can be delivered on an outpatient basis. For example, many chemotherapy regimens are now administered and monitored in doctors' offices or clinics. Also, the advent of managed care has meant tighter controls on hospital admissions and lengths of stay.

Which facility is used depends on a number of factors. As mentioned, the doctor must have admitting privileges at a hospital before he or she can send patients there. Also, people who subscribe to certain HMO or managed care plans may use only those hospitals and other facilities authorized by the insurer.

National Cancer Institute–Designated Centers

The NCI supports academic and research institutions across the country. These institutions are part of the NCI Cancer Centers Program, which is dedicated to cancer research. In order to be eligible for the program, a center must submit to a peer review process that evaluates and ranks the center according to its scientific merit.

An NCI center is appropriate for second opinions, consultation on difficult cases, or for experimental treatments that may not be available elsewhere. The actual physical location of the center may be an entire hospital or a unit within a community or teaching hospital.

There are three types of NCI-designated cancer centers that receive grants based on the degree of specialization of their research: generic, clinical, and comprehensive cancer centers.

Generic cancer centers focus on a narrow area of research. There are ten of these centers across the country.

Clinical cancer centers usually integrate basic science research with patient care. Although they offer fewer services than comprehensive centers (see below), they do investigate new forms of treatment, participate in clinical trials, and some have limited public outreach and education programs. Currently, twelve institutions have this designation.

Comprehensive cancer centers combine several areas of research—basic sciences, clinical research, cancer prevention and control, and epidemiology—with patient care. They have a broader mandate than clinical cancer centers and do more community outreach and public education. In addition to the peer review process, an institution must go through an extra extensive evaluation. Thirty-eight institutions have achieved this designation. Not all facilities that call themselves cancer centers or clinical cancer centers have NCI designation. It does not mean that they provide inadequate care; it does mean that such a hospital or cancer center (which may advertise itself in the popular media) should be evaluated on its own merits. Since the list changes every three to four months, you can confirm that a center has NCI designation by calling the National Cancer Institute at 800-4-CANCER or looking at their web site (www.nci.nih.gov/cancercenters/centerslist.html).

Types of Hospitals

There are many different types of cancer care settings, and where you go will depend largely on where your doctor is affiliated and what your health care plan covers. The following is a list of the major types of hospitals available to most people.

Community Hospitals. Community hospitals with a clinical oncology program or cancer unit often provide highly competent care, even though they may not offer treatment involving high-tech devices or high-risk procedures. Some community hospitals offer investigational therapies. In fact, many national studies are run in part through local oncologists who may work out of community hospitals. Examples include the National Surgical Adjuvant Breast and Bowel Project (NSABP), the Southwest Oncology Group (SWOG), and the Eastern Cooperative Oncology Group (ECOG). In recent years, community hospitals have become increasingly important care sites, owing to the rising numbers of cancer specialists, easier access to up-to-the-minute cancer research databases, and other developments.

Teaching Hospitals. Teaching hospitals have residency and fellowship programs for training new doctors. The best are teaching hospitals directly attached to medical schools. Others may be affiliated with (but not controlled by) medical schools and may have less extensive facilities than an academic institution. Still others have residency programs but no connection with a medical school.

As a rule, teaching hospitals provide a wide range of quality care, in part owing to the leading clinicians, researchers, and educators on their staffs. Because of the hospitals' teaching role, patients are seen by many doctors (and sometimes by medical students). Patients generally receive a lot of attention.

Government-Supported Hospitals. Public hospitals, such as Veterans' Administration (VA), city, county, or state hospitals, chronically suffer from limited funding. Although some may not offer state-of-the-art cancer treatment, others do have excellent cancer programs. These hospitals and programs must be evaluated individually.

Proprietary Hospitals. For-profit hospitals, which are generally owned by large corporations, vary widely in their services. Some prefer to treat patients with less serious, shorter-term, more profitable conditions. Others have excellent cancer programs, and some are NCI-designated cancer centers. Each hospital and program must be evaluated individually.

Some HMOs own their own hospitals, most of which are run similarly to community hospitals. Some HMO-owned hospitals act as cancer centers and conduct clinical research in preventing and curing cancer.

Nonhospital Treatment Settings

In many areas, diagnostic and treatment services are offered in so-called free-standing outpatient centers, meaning that they are not housed in hospitals. These may be privately run, for-profit centers or affiliated with nonprofit institutions. The facilities and care vary, so each must be evaluated on its own merits.

Home Care. Following discharge from a hospital or conclusion of treatment in a freestanding center, some types of care, such as intravenous infusions or feeding via a tube, may be administered by nurses or therapists who come to your home. Home care is becoming a more popular alternative, since it allows people with cancer to be treated in comfortable, convenient, and familiar surroundings. Furthermore, in many cases, home care costs far less than treatment delivered elsewhere (see also Chapter 31).

Hospice Care. Sometimes cancer advances to such an extent that treatment is concentrated primarily on maintaining comfort and quality of life. In such cases, the inpatient hospice may become the care setting, or more likely, hospice care may be provided at home. This type of care is designed to help people with cancer, as well as their families, during the final stages of the illness (see Chapter 31). The few freestanding hospice facilities are usually connected with a hospital.

Getting Quality Cancer Care

There are several ways to confirm the quality of care at a health care facility. Much of the information is online and/or available from the ACS and other organizations.

Evaluating Hospitals

The easiest way to assess a quality hospital informally is by determining which well-respected doctors work there. Good doctors are seldom affiliated with substandard hospitals. After you have selected skilled doctors whom you trust and respect, the choice of a hospital usually follows automatically. Probably the simplest way to evaluate a hospital is to ask doctors in the community what they think of it.

The extent and variety of services available in a facility is a key criterion. The best hospitals offer:

- a postoperative recovery room
- an intensive care unit
- anesthesiologists
- a pathology lab, diagnostic lab, and blood bank
- 24-hour doctor staffing
- a tumor board
- social work services
- respiratory therapists, physical therapists, and other professional support personnel
- advanced diagnostic and therapeutic equipment (CT scans, MRI, interventional radiology, radiation therapy, etc.)

When you are offered a choice of hospitals where your doctor treats patients or when you are deciding among doctors, you should consider other factors. For example, hospitals with more than 500 beds often provide more services and have more experience dealing with cancer of various types. As a rule, hospitals with fewer than 100 beds lack the facilities for complete and adequate cancer care.

Assuming they offer equivalent levels of care, a hospital close to home is usually preferable to one far away. Sometimes the best treatment strategy is to arrange a consultation at a distant comprehensive cancer center, followed by the delivery of care in a local facility.

You might want to choose a hospital because of a certain policy, such as whether or not children are allowed to visit. Such seemingly minor details can take on enormous importance to the person with cancer and the family.

INFORM

YOURSELF

Resources

There are two major organizations that monitor the quality of cancer care provided by their membership. At the very least, a quality hospital is accredited by the Joint Commission on Accreditation of Healthcare Organizations (JCAHO, 630-792-5000 or www.jcaho.org). Accredited hospitals are listed in the *American Hospital Association Guide to the Health Care Field*, found in many public libraries. Surprisingly, about one hospital in four fails to earn accreditation. However, accreditation does not necessarily indicate expertise in cancer care.

Commission on Cancer of the American College of Surgeons
A cancer diagnosis and treatment program that has been approved by the Commission on Cancer of the American College of Surgeons (COC) has met stringent standards and offers total, quality cancer care, including lifetime follow-up. More than 1,450 hospitals and treatment facilities nationwide, ranging from NCI-designated facilities to community hospitals to freestanding diagnostic and treatment centers, meet these standards.

The COC includes members from about thirty-seven professional organizations who set guidelines for cancer diagnosis and care. An approved cancer program must provide specific state-of-the-art diagnostic and treatment services in all medical disciplines—not just surgery—that a person with cancer may require. Each facility must also try to follow up with every patient treated there, to ensure that each receives continuing care and, of course, to detect recurrences or new cancers as early as possible. These are only the minimum requirements. The commission also encourages approved programs—which it regularly reviews and recertifies—to offer prevention, screening, nutritional counseling, community out-reach, and support services. Each facility must have a tumor board, consisting of representatives from a range of cancer care disciplines that meets regularly to confer on individual cases and, if possible, improve care. There is never a charge to patients for this multidisciplinary consultation process (see the *In the Hospital* section of Chapter 7 for more information about tumor boards).

For a list of all Commission on Cancer–approved programs, write the American College of Surgeons at 633 N. Saint Clair Street, Chicago, IL 60611-3211 or visit their web site at www.facs.org.

The program's leadership consists of representatives from all health care disciplines involved directly or indirectly with cancer patients at that location. Among their responsibilities are monitoring and evaluating patient care, which includes maintaining a database on care and outcomes.

Many of the programs share these data with the National Cancer Data Base, which monitors treatment and outcome patterns regionally and nationally for over 1,500 hospitals and about 60 percent of all cancer cases the United States. The National Cancer Data Base's Patient Care Evaluation Studies, which report on varying types of cancer, are available on the Internet (http://www.facs.org/dept/cancer/ncdb/index.html). A list can also be obtained by writing the American College of Surgeons at 633 N. Saint Clair Street, Chicago, IL 60611-3211.

Association of Community Cancer Centers

This membership organization serves U.S. doctors, cancer centers, and hospitals. The Association of Community Cancer Centers' (ACCC) web site (www.accc-cancer.org/main2001.shtml) offers a state-by-state guide that profiles cancer programs for over 500 member institutions.

Communicating with Caregivers

Good communication is crucial to good care. People with cancer need to feel they can speak openly and honestly with their doctors and other providers. Caregivers must also be able to talk to patients clearly and directly.

Talking, though, is only one part of effective communication. The other part is listening. The best doctors are those who: 1) give their full attention to what's being said, 2) ask questions to fill in blanks, 3) don't interrupt, and 4) resist making judgments before the whole story has been told. By the same token, people undergoing care need to listen carefully so they can understand the nature of their disease and treatment and make informed decisions each step of the way.

Even in ideal circumstances, good communication can be hard to achieve, and in a medical crisis, the obstacles to communication multiply. Some of the difficulties in communication are listed below.

- Fear—of disease, of treatment, of outcome—can interfere with your ability to think clearly or hear what is being said. Fear of what the answer might be can also prevent you from asking or even remembering important questions.

- The amount of detailed medical information can be too much to absorb and remember.

- Many people stand in awe of their doctors, resisting the urge to question what they're told.

- Some people remain silent because they lack self-confidence, believing that their questions are stupid or that they will be unable to understand the answers.

- Many doctors contribute to the problem by using technical terms.

- The need for many players on the health care team, located at different sites and possessing varying levels of expertise, increases the risk of mis-communication.

TIPS AND

ADVICE

Overcoming Obstacles to Communication

There are many techniques for overcoming—or, better yet, preventing—barriers to communication. Rather than waiting for providers to sharpen their skills in this area, if you want the best care, consider how you can improve the lines of communication.

Decide how much information you want to be told directly and at what level of detail. Let members of your care team know. If you don't tell them, they are apt to take their cue from how you seem to be communicating with them. For example, if you ask, "I don't have cancer, do I?" your doctor may conclude that you are not ready to hear the truth.

Establish who else should be told what information about your illness and treatment and at what level of detail: a family member, friend, or whomever.

Take notes and/or bring another person along with you. It may be helpful to tape-record your appointments with your doctor, as well as consultations and second opinion sessions. Tape-recorded sessions allow loved ones to hear accurate details after the fact. Taped sessions also prevent calls to the office to have information repeated or reworded, as much of your confusion can likely be cleared up if you review the taped material again. Ask to tape important sessions for later review. You may want to ask to record phone conversations as well. Tape-recording medical conversations can improve a person's ability to understand treatment, especially concerning tests and their results. Inform all parties that you will be recording the conversation. If your caregivers are uncom-fortable allowing you to tape-record your meetings, explain your reasons. You may need to explore other options instead, such as having someone accompany you and take detailed notes.

If you don't understand something, ask that it be repeated, rephrased, or explained. You might say, "I'm having trouble grasping what you said—would you mind telling me again, and could you put it another way?" Another tactic is to repeat what was said and ask for confirmation "Let me see if I have it right. You're saying that..."

Ask questions—lots of them.

Prepare questions ahead of time, asking the most important ones first.

Arrange for office visits or phone calls that allow adequate time for discussions. Tell your doctor at the beginning of the visit that you have questions. If you still have questions at the end of the visit, say so and schedule another appointment or phone call to address them.

Assess your attitudes to see whether they are interfering with your treatment: are you angry, hostile, or afraid? If so, express your emotions directly, "I'm afraid of what might happen," or "I'm angry at being kept waiting so long." Doing so will help clear the air and keep your treatment from getting sidetracked.

Be aware that your doctor isn't the only source of information. Ask questions of office staff, nurses, or other specialists caring for you. Emotional and practical issues may be best addressed by social workers or psychologists. Identifying which members of the team can answer which questions, and how they can be reached, is a vital part of the treatment plan.

7

Getting a Second Opinion

I t can be much simpler to take the advice of the doctor diagnosing your cancer and start the recommended treatment than to seek a second opinion. But it may not always be the best choice. People often seek second opinions, and they do so for many reasons.

If you feel your doctor is not taking your condition seriously or is unable to find the cause of your symptoms, it's helpful to consult another doctor. There are many medical and psychological reasons for seeking consultations before, during, or even after treatment. There also may be financial reasons to consult another doctor, since some health care plans require a second opinion. Here we review some of the reasons people explore second opinions and discuss the issues involved in the process.

Why Get a Second Opinion?

It is a good idea to get additional opinions whenever you feel uncertain about the advice you have been given. Doctors agree on well-established and proven treatments for some cancers, but expert opinions about the treatment of choice differ for other cancers. Even when everyone acknowledges that a particular approach is likely to arrest the cancer, questions may arise about your ability to tolerate the treatment's immediate and long-term side effects or how it will affect your quality of life in the long run. For these reasons, cancer specialists suggest second opinions. You may even need three or four consultations before you're assured that the treatment option selected is the right one for you and your cancer.

Is the Diagnosis Correct?

Confirmation of the diagnosis itself occasionally requires a second opinion. This may mean having a second pathologist review slides or having another radiologist look at x-rays or other images to be certain that the diagnosis is accurate.

What Treatment Is Best?

Many people seek another opinion to help them choose among their doctor's suggested options or to learn about other possibilities. Because therapies that are successful in treating cancer can cause long-lasting consequences, such as changes in appearance, infertility, or the need to wear an ostomy bag, the benefits of a particular treatment must always be balanced against its drawbacks. Different therapies present various advantages and disadvantages that you must weigh against your life stage, career needs, family demands, hopes, and dreams. Even though two therapies may present equal opportunities for getting rid of the cancer, they may have very different effects on your life. Consequently, you need to gather as much information as possible before making any decisions.

Second Opinions During Treatment

The decision to seek additional opinions is not only made before treatment. You may want another opinion in the midst of treatment if, for example, the tumor is not responding as expected. Or you may want a consultation at the end of a particular course of treatment to assess the need for further therapy.

In the Hospital

Getting other opinions while you're staying in the hospital may be difficult because you are physically confined and are usually limited to doctors associated with that hospital. Also, the admitting doctor usually must order a consultation if it is to be done in the hospital.

However, most hospitals—even smaller community hospitals with an organized cancer program—have a tumor board, a team of experts representing several medical disciplines. The doctor presents the patient's case to this group of specialists and the board uses its collective expertise in designing a treatment plan.

For example, a radiologist on the tumor board may review a patient's x-rays and scans. A pathologist may review the pathology slides and use a projection microscope to discuss his or her findings with the other doctors. A surgeon, an oncologist, and other specialists also participate in the discussion. And, depending on the hospital, a psychologist or social worker may be part of the group. In large teaching hospitals, medical students and junior staff members attend as well, since the tumor board meetings serve an educational purpose.

In nonacademic settings such as a small community hospital, the doctor presenting a case—particularly if he or she is a general practitioner or family practitioner—usually delegates the management of the cancer patient's care to the appropriate specialist. Sometimes, the primary care doctor oversees the treatment prescribed by an oncologist.

According to the American College of Surgeons, tumor board conferences should focus on problem cases as well as on pretreatment evaluation, staging, treatment strategy, and rehabilitation. Although the conference is usually confidential, the doctor presenting a case may be willing to share with you the important points of the discussion and the rationale for the treatment recommendations.

TIPS AND

ADVICE

Second Opinion Checklist

A second opinion is important if:

✓ your doctor cannot determine the cause of your symptoms.

✓ your health care plan requires it.

✓ you want to confirm the first treatment recommendation offered to you.

✓ your doctor is not an oncologist.

✓ your doctor is not experienced in treating your type of cancer.

✓ you want reassurance that you are getting the most current treatment.

✓ you are concerned about the side effects and/or long-term effects of the recommended treatment.

✓ you are interested in experimental therapies.

✓ you have trouble communicating with your doctor.

✓ you have read about treatments with which your doctor is not familiar.

✓ your doctor has not asked about your lifestyle, family demands, and/or professional commitments and desires.

✓ the recommended treatment interferes with the way you lead your life and you want to know if there are other options.

✓ you are not confident in your doctor's knowledge, experience, or judgment.

✓ you feel uncomfortable with your doctor's recommendation.

✓ your doctor is underestimating the seriousness of your condition or concerns.

Is There Time?

Arranging appointments, consulting with other doctors, and perhaps having additional tests takes time. Some people fear that if they delay the beginning of treatment, their condition may get worse. In the past, many doctors and patients believed that time was of the essence, but as more has been learned about how cancer develops, most experts agree that in most cases, getting more opinions does not create dangerous delays.

As one oncology nurse puts it, "The first thing I tell a patient is to do nothing." What she means is that people need time to adjust to the shock of being told that they have cancer. Then, as soon as they can think clearly, they can take necessary action. Cancer is a serious illness with far-reaching effects on your life. You and your family need to feel confident that you have made the right decisions about your treatment.

Seeking endless consultations, postponing treatment indefinitely, or refusing to make any decisions at all does waste time, however. Indeed, seeking more and more opinions and thereby postponing the beginning of treatment may mask an underlying fear of making the wrong choice. Continuing to seek opinions can also be a way of "wishing" that you will find a doctor who will say only what you want to hear.

Setting a date to talk over your options with your primary care doctor or another doctor is one way to make sure that the opinion- and information-gathering process will be efficient and productive.

Cost

At one time, health insurance companies required second opinions in an attempt to curtail costs, and they paid for the additional consultation. The companies reasoned that they could avoid unnecessary tests and surgery by having doctors serve as a check on one another. But second opinions did not lower costs, so many insurers stopped requiring them. Since health care insurers and organizations vary in their requirements for and coverage of second opinions, it's important to ask your insurance company exactly what, if any, consultation costs are covered.

When you make an appointment for a consultation, ask about the cost. Some doctors do not charge as much for a consultation as for a first visit, since much of the initial work-up, including laboratory and imaging tests, has been done.

Finding the Right Consultant

Your primary doctor or oncologist is the best person to begin with when requesting other specialists in your community. Most doctors are accustomed to furnishing names of potential consultants and are not defensive or insulted when asked for recommendations. In fact, your primary doctor will have to provide the consulting doctor with your medical history and diagnostic test results.

You may also conduct an independent search for a specialist. You may have a friend or family member who has been treated for a similar type of cancer and can suggest a doctor. The American Medical Association (AMA) has a locator service on its web site that (www.ama-assn.org) that provides background information about doctors, including confirmation on board certification (see Chapter 6 for more information on board certification and specialists). The American Society of Clinical Oncology (ASCO), an international medical society representing cancer specialists who do research as well as care for patients, has a web site (www.asco.org) that provides a directory of their members. Most hospitals provide a referral service. So do local medical societies and health departments. You can also contact the nearest cancer center for a recommendation to a specialist in your type of cancer.

Although some doctors will provide a second opinion only if you have been referred by another doctor, most will, regardless of the referral source. If your insurer or health plan covers consultations only with specialists enrolled in their plan, ask for a list of those doctors.

CASE HISTORIES

TRUE STORIES

How Far To Go

Conflicting and highly technical data about cancer and your particular diagnosis can be overwhelming. In the first few weeks after his diagnosis, Isaac, then 38, who had a rare form of leukemia, was eager to learn everything he could about his illness. On the recommendation of his primary care doctor, he consulted two major research centers about bone marrow transplantation. After he had found a marrow donor and chosen a center for the transplant, however, he found that all the statistics relating to his prognosis and chances for long-term survival only made him more anxious. Since transplant was his best chance for cure, once the treatment began, Isaac chose not to investigate every conceivable side effect or long-term consequence. He had learned enough to give his consent for the procedure; he felt confident that he had made the right decision and asked that his family not continue to explore every possible scenario or complication.

The Process of Getting a Second Opinion

The more you know about your cancer and the issues that are important to you and your family, the more you will learn from the consultation. Being prepared also enables you to efficiently use the limited amount of time you have with the consulting doctor and ensures that you ask the necessary questions. Therefore, when seeking a second opinion, prepare for the visit by completing and reviewing your research. You could ask a friend or family member to do the background research if you are unable to do it.

Who Knows Best?

The most important question to ask when making an appointment with a consulting doctor is, "Do you have experience treating my type of cancer?"

Keep in mind that oncologists can have subspecialties. They may also be, for example, surgeons, gynecologists, urologists, or radiation therapists. Even if you don't choose to be treated by a subspecialist, it's wise to consult one for a second opinion. This subspecialist may work with your referring doctor to design a treatment plan.

When Opinions Conflict

One doctor may advocate treating your cancer with a combination of radical surgery or radiation and/or aggressive chemotherapy. Another may prefer a more conservative approach, such as limited surgery with or without radiation afterward. Based on current studies and their own experience, both specialists' opinions may be equally valid, but their disagreement puts you in a quandary. How can you decide which is best?

At this point, an oncologist should be able to explain to you the pros and cons of each approach. Your referring doctor can help you weigh the advantages and disadvantages of the conflicting recommendations. Don't feel forced to make a decision until you're satisfied that you have adequate information.

Along with gathering brochures, books, and information from credible web sites (see *Resources*), it can be helpful to talk with other health care professionals like nurses and social workers. Some people also seek out others with cancer to ask about their treatment experience.

If all of your pertinent records are in your referring doctor's office, copies can be sent to the consulting doctor. It may also be helpful to obtain your own copies of all medical records, as some cancer advocacy groups recommend. Copies of x-rays and laboratory results may be expensive, but complete, up-to-date reports facilitate the consultation process.

During the visit, the consulting doctor reviews your history, laboratory tests, and imaging examinations. Additional tests may be ordered if needed. Finally, the doctor offers his or her recommendations. The same advice given when discussing the diagnosis with the original doctor applies here: take notes or use a tape recorder and bring a friend or family member (see Chapter 6).

After the consultation, the consulting doctor sends a written report to the referring doctor and/or directly to you.

Comfort and Confidence

Trust is an intangible component of the relationship between you and your doctor, and it must be factored into the final decision-making process. You must feel confident that what your doctor advises is truly the best option.

People with cancer can expect to have a range of emotional responses to treatment recommendations, but it's essential that you feel reasonably comfortable with the treatment decision. Some people feel more at ease with a treatment that has somewhat high risks but offers an opportunity to pursue life goals, such as having a family. Others prefer the choice that offers the best chance of survival, even though the side effects could affect their quality of life more severely. Rarely are there "perfect" solutions, and the ultimate decision must always be a personal one.

By seeking second opinions, you and your family can ensure you've done all you can to participate in the information-gathering and decision-making process. On the other hand, if trusting the first opinion makes you most comfortable, you may not need to consult with another doctor.

CASE HISTORIES

TRUE STORIES

Going with the First Opinion

Mike, aged 50, was diagnosed with Hodgkin's disease in the early 1990s. He did not seek a second opinion regarding treatment for his cancer because he said he felt "fairly comfortable" with the treatment recommended by his doctor. "The cancer specialist came highly recommended," Mike recalls, "and I liked his whole demeanor and the way he explained things clearly to me. I more or less just put myself in his hands. He had given me the prognosis, which I was really pleased with, and I was ready to get involved in the treatment and get on with getting well."

Now, healthy and almost five years in remission, Mike is satisfied with the choice he made. "The doctor told me he had never given anyone such a large dose of chemotherapy, but I tolerated it well. My constitution was pretty strong. That and the fact that I got so much chemo make me pretty relaxed in terms of making it to the sixty-month mark. I was lucky to have found the right professional, and I just went with that gut feeling."

8

Your Support Network

N o one is born knowing how to deal with a serious illness or how to solve the emotional and practical problems it creates. Nor are most people equipped to cope with these matters on their own. Beginning at the time of diagnosis, the support of other people—family, friends, colleagues, religious groups, those who have or have had cancer, and/or helping professionals, and advocacy organizations—is paramount. Together, medical and social support systems address not just the disease but also the needs of the whole person.

Studies have long shown that men and women who have strong bonds with others endure crisis best. Support takes many forms, depending on the people or group involved. It can be as basic as someone offering a ride to the doctor's office or help with the shopping. Or it may mean talking about treatment and recovery with someone with the same illness. Often support means venting deep feelings among a group of people in similar circumstances. It can mean having a place to turn for advice and information. Support of any kind fulfills the basic need to remain connected to human society—a connection that may in itself promote healing.

Those who benefit from others' assistance discover ways in which they can in turn help others. Such reaching out restores a sense of self-worth and self-esteem. Cancer is a life crisis and one that no one would willingly seek out. Still, many people discover that the experience presents an opportunity to rediscover the importance of connections to other people and even to society as a whole.

This chapter describes the support network and ways of using it to achieve the highest quality of life during treatment and recovery. It also offers advice to those who want to help people with cancer. The *Resources* at the end of this book provide more information about particular organizations and services and how to get in touch with them.

Why Is Social Support Important?

Dealing with cancer produces enormous stress, not only for those with the disease, but for everyone who cares about them. Roles and relationships—indeed, your whole outlook on life—change suddenly and dramatically. You and your family must wrestle with social, physical, and financial upheaval and may experience fear, anger, guilt, and hopelessness, among other powerful feelings (see Chapters 26 and 28).

When you first learn of your diagnosis, you and your loved ones may feel as if your lives are collapsing and you have lost all control over your future. During your treatment, you may continue to feel frightened and exhausted as you struggle to cope with the changes in your body, the side effects of the treatment, the complexities of the health care system, the financial impact of the disease, and the challenge of maintaining healthy relationships with your family and friends. After the treatment ends, you may still be grappling with the long-term consequences of a devastating disease, but you will no longer have the daily hands-on care of doctors and nurses. You may feel as if you have been set adrift, even abandoned.

Taking an active step such as creating or tapping into a support network helps you recognize and conquer these and other challenges. This can provide a sense of empowerment.

Making use of the people in your own life as well as the support and self-help groups, advocacy organizations, and helping professionals described in this chapter can lead to additional positive results:

- *Counteracting fear.* Being diagnosed with cancer and treated for it can be extremely frightening. It may be difficult for you to share your feelings about cancer with family, friends, and even caregivers. Finding support by participating in a support group of people in similar circumstances, for example, can help you realize that your emotions are natural and that it's safe to express them. In turn, feeling that you are not alone in your reactions can allow you to focus on other important issues. Fear can make pain and discomfort worse, so relieving your fear may also lessen your physical discomfort.

- *Reducing isolation.* Having a serious illness can be very lonely, even for those with many people in their lives. You may find that some people may not know how to be helpful or may even withdraw from you out of fear or ignorance. Or you may find that despite being surrounded by family, friends, and colleagues, you feel profoundly alone in your experience and reluctant to share what you're really going through. Helping professionals and/or a group of others who understand the experience can lessen this sense of ostracism and isolation. Group experiences can also lead to new friendships built on mutual concern and caring.

- Outside support can also *counteract the isolation* that occurs even in well-meaning families, who may attempt to "protect" you by not talking about your illness. As Chapter 28 explains, family members may try to insulate themselves from their own overwhelming feelings and reactions to having to deal with a crisis by remaining silent about it. Over time, family members may stop communicating and may become cut off just when they need one another most. A group support or counseling program may offer problem-solving strategies for such situations.

- *Keeping your spirits up.* People in your extended support network can help you recognize the signs of depression and get appropriate help (see Chapter 27).

- *Encouraging you to take good care of yourself.* Someone who feels that people understand and care is more likely to try to stay healthy by eating well, getting enough sleep, and exercising. The influence of others also helps discourage destructive habits such as smoking or drinking alcohol that can damage the body and slow the recovery process.

- *Helping the whole family.* So much attention may be focused on the per-son with cancer that the well members of the family, especially children, may feel neglected. Recruiting extended family members or close friends to take over some responsibilities can provide great relief. In addition, support groups and counseling for families, including children, address their own special concerns, fears, worries, and practical problems.

- *Providing practical information.* Support and self-help groups are forums in which to share knowledge and strategies that can help you cope. This information can include advice on dealing with health care professionals and questions to ask; managing pain and side effects; and even where to go to get hats, hairpieces, and prostheses at the best price.

- *Finding out about treatment sources and services and protecting your rights.* Helping organizations often can connect people to relevant clinical trials, sources of funding, and information about how to preserve insurance coverage, deal with managed care, and prevent illegal discrimination at work.

Making the Most of Your Support Network

Informal support comes from family, friends, neighbors, social acquaintances, colleagues, and coworkers—the people you probably turn to first in times of trouble or in whose presence you ordinarily feel comfortable or safe. Given the immense disruptions that cancer can cause in your life, tapping into this network can help you maintain some of your normal life. For example, a cancer survivor who belongs to a square dance club might get tremendous support simply from attending the club's weekly gatherings even if he or she can't participate fully in the activity.

Family and friends can help in any number of ways, depending on their abilities and interests. In practical terms, they can provide child care, act as a "call broker" to handle phone calls from concerned people, arrange transportation, or assist with cooking, housecleaning, shopping, or other errands. You could ask others to look up books or articles in the library or to walk your dog. Ask for what you need. Many people are happy to find out that there's something they can do for you.

Informal support has some limitations. Loved ones may become overwhelmed by the changes in family life and by their concerns about you. Also, if you typically conceal your needs because you don't want to be a "burden" to others, you may push away the support you really want.

Spouses or partners are usually the most important part of the informal support network, but a diagnosis of cancer can present a challenge to the stability of a couple's relationship. Some couples experience increased conflict and struggle with communication problems.

Another reason not to seek all your support from an informal network is that during a crisis not everyone can come through in ways that you would like. Although you might appreciate their efforts, members of the square dance club, for example, may not feel comfortable visiting a casual acquaintance in the hospital. Similarly, squeamish friends may not be the ones to ask to do library research about your disease.

Getting the Support You Need

Formal support, which is provided or overseen by people trained in providing support, is not a replacement for informal support. Instead, it complements the informal support network in a number of ways. Types of formal support include support and self-help groups; psychotherapy or counseling; professional help from religious institutions; political and advocacy organizations; and coordinated volunteer efforts.

Even the most thoughtful and loving friends and relatives cannot offer the same type of empathy and help as can people who, like you, have cancer or are recovering from cancer. For this reason, participation in groups of people with the same illness has been an increasingly recognized element of the recovery process since the mid-1970s.

Support and self-help groups enable the exchange of information, which increases participants' knowledge, dispels myths, and helps people cope with the intricacies of the health care system. Some groups also serve as advocacy organizations for people with cancer by raising public awareness of the disease and the rights and needs of people who have it, campaigning for funding in support of research, and lobbying for changes in the health care system.

Perhaps most important, groups offer their members an opportunity to voice concerns openly and honestly and, in doing so, to come to terms with their illness. People with cancer often dread a recurrence of the disease and must come to grips with their mortality. They fear the changes their bodies are undergoing, including disfiguring surgery or unseen internal damage. They worry that they will be abandoned by their caregivers, by society, and even by their loved ones. The stories of struggle and survival exchanged in a group help the participants recognize the reality—and the validity—of their own deepest feelings.

In 1989, psychiatrist David Spiegel conducted an influential study of support groups for women with metastatic breast cancer. After eighteen months of following these women, Dr. Spiegel found that women who participated in the support group lived longer than those who did not participate in the support group. Since Spiegel's work, several studies exploring this question have reported conflicting results.

Many believe that support groups can improve a person's quality of life. Research has shown that people with cancer are better able to deal with their disease when supported by others in similar situations. Although more research is needed to determine what types of groups are most effective with what type of people, support groups may be useful for some people with cancer. It must be stressed that groups are not a substitute for medical treatment. Any group that contradicts or otherwise interferes with ongoing treatment in any way should be avoided.

Not everyone feels comfortable in a support group, and some people find it especially difficult to reveal aspects of their illness to others. There are also times when a support group is not helpful. You may be so upset that the thought of discussing your illness feels overwhelming. Don't force yourself to take part in a group. It may be better to participate in a group later, when you feel less anxious. Some problems, such as marital difficulties, require professional one-on-one counseling.

People who are uncertain or uneasy about support groups may find it useful to try two or three different types of groups before rejecting the idea entirely. In most areas, a variety of groups are available so you are likely to find one in which you feel comfortable. For instance, a person who is concerned about privacy may desire a group that focuses on education rather than one in which emotional issues are addressed. Professionals such as oncology social workers or nurses, psychologists, psychiatrists, or members of the clergy lead some groups. A person who wants the reassurance of knowing a professional is in charge may find these groups more appealing. Cancer survivors run other groups. Many people prefer cancer survivor–run groups because they know the group leader has personal experience with the disease. Your personal comfort level is your best gauge of whether or not a support group will be truly supportive. If none of the groups sampled feel right to you, another type of support may be helpful.

Educational Workshops or Groups

Educational groups inform their participants about various aspects of cancer. They are often sponsored by hospitals or cancer treatment centers and are usually led by a professional and possibly a layperson. They offer lectures or other types of presentations followed by question-and-answer sessions. The goal of an educational group is to discuss the facts of the disease and its treatment. This type of group is not typically a forum for emotional sharing. People with cancer are encouraged to attend along with concerned family members or friends. Compared with the face-to-face encounters of support groups, educational workshops offer relative anonymity.

Research published in a cancer journal in the early 1990s underscores the importance of such mutual participation. People with cancer and their significant others were invited to watch an educational program together. The program conveyed the message that coping with chemotherapy can be difficult and emphasized that everyone with cancer needs support in finding ways to manage any side effects. The researchers found that watching the program together enhances the ability of couples who participated in the study to talk about the disease and its treatment and that effective communication raises the self-esteem of the person with cancer.

Support Groups

Support groups may be open-ended or closed. Open-ended groups allow people with cancer or their family members to attend when they need to, dropping in and out as they want. An open-ended group can be helpful when there is a decision about a new treatment. A closed group runs for a prescribed period of time with the same group members. Some closed groups are organized for people with the same diagnoses or by the kind of treatment they are receiving. There are women's groups and men's groups. Some people join both types of groups since they satisfy different needs. Support groups fall into two categories: those that are organized and run by one or more professional facilitators and those that are organized and run by the members themselves, usually referred to as self-help groups. In both cases, the focus is on the day-by-day adjustment to living with a serious illness.

Professionally Led Support Groups. Professionally led support groups serve people with certain types of cancer or with other specific needs. For example, there are groups for parents of children with cancer, for women with breast cancer, for people in advanced stages of the disease, or for bereaved family members. Other groups might be tailored to adolescent survivors, outpatient chemotherapy recipients, people undergoing long-term hospitalization, or at-risk populations (such as daughters of women with breast cancer).

In large metropolitan areas you can usually find a group whose participants' situation closely resembles your own.

Some groups charge fees to cover costs of the meeting room and to reimburse professional leaders, but many groups are subsidized by health care facilities or national organizations and do not charge participants.

Self-Help Groups. Also referred to as peer-support networks, self-help groups differ from support groups principally in that they do not involve professional leaders and may concentrate more on practical, how-to issues. They also are operated and are often founded by the members themselves. Sometimes advisers such as oncology social workers are consulted on strategies for group leadership and development, but for the most part the agenda is set and carried out by the members.

Self-help groups may welcome people with any kind of cancer, with specific cancers, or with particular rehabilitative needs. For example, ostomy groups include people with intestinal disease, such as colon cancer, who have had surgery that requires them to wear special bags to collect body wastes. Laryngectomy groups are available for those whose voice boxes have been surgically removed. Groups might address practical problems (managing the ostomy bag, for example, or relearning ways of speaking), or they might deal with the emotional aspects of recovery, depending on their members' needs.

Some self-help groups are local units of national organizations and are affiliated with medical institutions, and others are grassroots groups meeting in homes, churches, or community centers. Self-help groups are usually free, although they may collect voluntary contributions to defray costs.

Group Factors to Consider

The group you end up choosing depends on your own needs and interests, as well as on what is available in your community. The more alike the people in the group are, the more quickly its members will find cohesion and supply mutual aid.

Many people feel more comfortable addressing private issues if the groups are limited to their own sex and to similar diagnoses. For example, women recovering from breast surgery commonly have concerns about their body changes, their feelings of femininity, and the impact of the disease on their sexuality. Similarly, men recovering from prostate cancer may feel more comfortable in groups limited to men, where they can discuss more freely their concerns about impotence or incontinence.

Groups offer a variety of structures. Some meet weekly, twice a month, or monthly for sessions lasting one to two hours. Many groups work best with perhaps six to eight members, although group sizes range from a handful of people to nearly forty; the larger groups tend to be more structured.

Groups for Family Members

Although many groups are open only to people with the illness, others invite family members or close friends to take part either with the person who is ill or on their own. In support or self-help groups organized around the issues and challenges facing the loved ones of people with cancer, participants have an opportunity to share their concerns about diagnosis and treatment, vent their own feelings, share their experiences caring for and communicating with someone with cancer, and discover strategies for meeting the needs of the entire family.

Groups for young children of people with cancer can teach them about cancer and allow them to ask questions and express their feelings in a safe place. It's important that an experienced professional facilitate a children's group. Many groups also offer a corresponding group for parents.

INFORM

YOURSELF

Is Group Support Right for You?

Whether you are alone and need a sense of community or are surrounded by others, as long as you are curious about your illness and are eager to learn ways of managing it, group support may be ideal for you.

Although some people may be reluctant to share their intimate thoughts and feelings with people whom they do not know well, participation does not mean you must talk. Indeed, a well-facilitated group puts no pressure on its members to open up. Even if you are shy in groups, you can gain much from just listening.

When deciding whether to take part in a group, consider the following:

- Attend one or two group meetings on a trial basis. If you don't find it useful, don't go back.

- You may prefer the focus and direction offered in support groups led by professionals. Or you may enjoy the camaraderie and peer support available in a self-help group. If you find both approaches valuable, consider joining one of each. Tell the facilitator of the professionally led group if you also are participating in a self-help group.

- Groups that have an open structure generally allow participants to choose whether or not to attend a particular session.

- Groups don't always focus on feelings. Often a lot of solid information, including survival strategies, is exchanged.

- You have the "right to remain silent." Remember, though, that others may benefit from what you have to say.

- If you have specific needs you want addressed, you should bring them up. You might want to share your concerns with the group's leaders or organizers and tell them what you hope to get from the group.

- Consider taking part in educational workshops, where you can listen but won't be called on to speak or discuss your emotions. Keep in mind that such workshops are primarily for learning, not sharing.

- If you decide not to join a group just now, you can always change your mind. Keep any information you have gathered about group support. At a later stage of recovery, you may decide to give groups another look.

Organized Volunteer Visitation

One kind of formal support is volunteer visitation such as the American Cancer Society's *Reach to Recovery* and *Man to Man* programs (see *Resources*). In such programs, people who have had breast or prostate cancer are trained to interact on a one-to-one basis with other people who have the disease. Volunteers may visit people in their homes or in hospitals to provide understanding, encouragement, educational materials, and rehabilitation counseling. Such direct contact with caring, sympathetic people who know what you are going through and who have been trained to address your needs can make a world of difference in the quality and course of your recovery.

Religious/Spiritual Support

Seeking the formal or informal support of your faith or religious community can provide solace and strength and help you adjust to your illness and changed circumstances.

Most religious institutions provide pastoral counselors for people in need. Besides offering spiritual guidance, such counselors are often in close touch with community and volunteer organizations offering services such as transportation or *Meals on Wheels*. Some religious communities may even help raise funds on your behalf.

Psychotherapy and Counseling

People with cancer and their families who are struggling with emotions like fear and depression (especially over a period of weeks) may benefit from sessions with a mental health professional. The counselor may be a social worker, psychologist, psychiatrist, psychiatric nurse, or member of the clergy. It's important that he or she have at least a master's degree in counseling and experience working with people with cancer. The type of care provided in such cases is generally called supportive psychotherapy, in which the therapist or counselor helps facilitate coping rather than personality change. Psychotherapy can be delivered in a group or individually, or with one or more family members taking part. Therapists are skilled in recognizing the fundamental issues in a problem and exploring approaches to resolving them. The cost of psychotherapy may not be covered by insurance or other health plans.

Private sessions offer the chance to express feelings and thoughts that may not emerge in other settings. Those in individual therapy also have the full attention of the professional for the length of the session. The confidentiality and objectivity available in therapy call be valuable, and a skilled therapist can offer feedback and suggest coping strategies.

Joint therapy sessions, in which couples or other family members participate, provide an opportunity for airing concerns in a focused way. For example, marital conflicts often are put on hold while the couple deals with the needs of treatment and recovery. In time, however, those conflicts may reemerge and require the attention of a therapist. Similarly, families organized to "protect" themselves against the reality of cancer (through silence, avoidance, or denial) may need guidance in ending the secrecy and reopening the lines of communication. Children may benefit from therapy to help them deal with the changes in the family structure caused by a serious illness. In joint sessions, the therapist serves as a moderator who can keep the discussion on track and help resolve emotions that get in the way of effective dialogue.

Mental health professionals also evaluate and treat severe distress (such as anxiety and depression) and help teach specific techniques that will help you better tolerate the symptoms, side effects, and long-term consequences of treatment (see Chapter 27).

The social work department at your hospital can provide counseling, therapy, and/or referrals to trained, licensed psychotherapists who are experts in treating people with cancer.

What Should You Look for in a Cancer Counselor?

QUESTIONS

TO ASK

An experienced cancer counselor will know to anticipate certain emotional reactions from patients. For example, cancer patients often feel more distressed when treatment is over. This is because the person sees the medical treatment team and the facility as a safe place where treatment is fighting the cancer. When that stops, people with cancer have a period of adjustment as they figure out how to live without the safety net of constant clinic visits and medical care.

Counselors can come from the fields of social work, psychology, psychiatry, psychiatric nursing, and pastoral counseling. They should have a minimum of a master's degree in one of the counseling fields. Often they will have a doctoral degree. While credentials will demonstrate a person's formal education in their chosen field, they ideally should be combined with their experience. Professionals who are secure in their abilities know that people need this information and will gladly provide it.

Sometimes people feel that unless a counselor has had cancer or actually "been there" they will not be helpful. While a personal experience can add to a counselor's perspective, it is not essential. If a counselor is skilled in working with crisis and loss, he or she should be able to help you.

Finding a counselor that meets your needs may take more than one try. Trust your instincts. You'll know when you've made the right match. You should feel safe in sharing your concerns with your counselor and feel that he or she will be able to help you. You should also feel that your personality "fits" well with the counselor. After meeting once or twice with a counselor, ask yourself the following questions:

- What are the counselor's credentials?

- Has the counselor ever worked with cancer patients?

- Does the counselor work in a cancer center?

- Do I feel safe sharing my concerns with this counselor?

- Do I trust that this counselor can help me?

- Is the counselor able to listen to me and understand me as an individual?

- Does the counselor seem active, interested, and involved with me and my concerns?

- Is the counselor nonjudgmental?

- Does the counselor seem supportive?

- Does the counselor seem to respect me?

- Could my family relate well to this person?

Finding Sources of Support

The *Resources* at the end of this book list numerous organizations you may consult. In addition, the following people and organizations should be able to tell you what support is available in your area:

- Local chapter of the American Cancer Society.

- Oncologists or oncology nurses on your team.

- Social workers in the hospital's social work or social service department.

- Hospital chaplain.

- Local YMCA, YWCA, or YMHA.

- Local United Way information and referral services.

- Church or synagogue.

- Community centers and senior centers.

- Clinic or hospital nurses.

- State, county, or United Way family agencies and community mental health centers.

- National Self-Help Clearinghouse. This organization provides a listing of self-help groups. Call 212-817-1822 or visit their web site for more information (www.selfhelpweb.org).

- The Internet. Modern computer technology has provided a new source of support for people with cancer. Not only can you get information via the Internet, but you can also tap into a community of others who are ready and willing to talk with you about the disease. You may want to explore the *Resources* listed at the end of this book, including the American Cancer Society's web site (www.cancer.org).

TIPS AND ADVICE

Some Support Dos and Don'ts for People Who Want to Help

- Suggest specific ways of helping. Instead of saying, "Is there anything I can do?" say, for example, "I'm going to the supermarket this morning. If you'd like to give me your list, I can pick up some things for you." Or even, "I'm roasting a chicken and I'll bring it over." You might say, "I have to drop some things off at the library. Would you like me to see if they have any new mysteries?"

- One of the best things you can do is simply to be there. This may mean visiting someone in the hospital or at home, but even more important, it means being there emotionally: listening, avoiding judgments, responding to the person's needs at that moment. Even if you are a casual acquaintance, knowing that you care is extremely important to the person with cancer. Sometimes a quick call or note is enough to show your support. If you are unsure whether a hospital visit would be welcome, call first.

- The support you offer should be based on your relationship. For example, if you have never spent time with the person's children, your offer to "keep the kids for a few hours" may not be appropriate. If you hate driving, offering transportation may make both of you uncomfortable. If you haven't seen the person for a long time, don't expect deep emotions to be revealed in your conversation.

- Remember the others in the family. Sometimes the best thing you can do is to help the spouse or the children.

- Be sensitive to the person's situation. Don't bring a huge houseplant to someone living in a tiny apartment; don't bring food without first knowing tastes or dietary preferences.

- Give the person an out by suggesting alternatives, "I'd like to drop by for a few minutes. Is this afternoon okay, or would tomorrow be better?"

- Don't be offended if your offer of help is rejected. The person may have someone else to handle that need or may get genuine benefit out of doing a certain task himself or herself.

- Resist the temptation to tell the person you are helping about other people you know who have had serious illnesses or to question his or her medical treatment.

- Don't be afraid to discuss cancer directly, but follow the person's lead. If he or she changes the subject, respect that.

- Be aware of your own needs. Are you offering to visit because you want to make the person with cancer feel better, or because you want to make yourself feel better?

- Don't overdo it. Calling every day may be a burden to the person in recovery.

- Read Chapter 28, *Issues for Families and Friends*.

PART III

Treatment Strategies

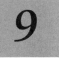

9

Principles of Treatment

Treatment Evolution

Excising (removing) a malignancy had been done since ancient times, but it wasn't until the development of anesthesia in 1846 that surgery became an important treatment for cancer. Today, surgical excision is still the most effective curative cancer therapy for most cancers. However, the possibility of cure is also enhanced by other, additional approaches.

During the early years of organized cancer research, doctors began investigating nonsurgical therapies. Scientists had explored the ability of chemicals to treat infections. "Magic bullet" drugs such as those made of organic mercury were used to treat syphilis. But the foundation for today's anticancer drugs was developed during World War II when it was discovered that the chemical in mustard gas could shrink cancers. When x-rays and radium were discovered at the end of the nineteenth century, the value of radiation therapy in treating cancer soon became clear. Although there were start-up problems in learning how to use this new treatment, by the 1920s it had come into general use for treating some cancers.

After World War II, research efforts to find effective treatments for cancer escalated dramatically. Radiation therapy and chemotherapy were refined (see Chapters 11 and 12), and surgery became safer (see Chapter 10). Today each of these therapies continues to be fine-tuned, leading to more successful results and fewer complications.

The Aims of Treatment

Decisions concerning how best to treat a cancer are based on many aspects of a person's life, but the main concern and primary goal is choosing what will work. What will obliterate the tumor? What will rid the body of any wandering cancer cells? What will prevent the cancer from returning? And what will accomplish these goals with minimal side effects?

In some cases the treatment choice is clear. For example, in the case of a small, localized melanoma skin cancer, surgical removal is effective. The best treatment of some other cancers, however, is still being evaluated. For example, doctors may recommend that a small malignancy in the prostate of an elderly man be treated by radiation alone. Another doctor might argue that removing the prostate is the best approach. Still others might suggest more radical surgery, regardless of the man's age. And, if the cancer is small and contained within one area of the prostate, some may recommend regular observation and monitoring rather than immediate treatment.

You alone must decide how far you want to go in understanding your treatment options and how involved you want to be in treatment. But keep in mind that the more you learn about your condition and the treatments for it, the easier it may be to cope with the challenges of the disease. Experience has shown that knowledge helps reduce fear in people with cancer.

It's also important that you understand your rights as a patient. The American Hospital Association adopted *A Patient's Bill of Rights* in 1973 and revised it in 1992 in hopes that hospitals and health care institutions would support the rights in the delivery of patient care. Several of those rights deal specifically with treatment issues. For example, according to the *Bill of Rights,* a patient has the right to make decisions about the plan of care prior to and during the course of treatment, to refuse a recommended treatment or plan of care (to the extent permitted by law and hospital policy), and to be informed of the medical consequences of this action.

The goal of cancer treatments is to improve survival and quality of life and is based on the following principles:

* to remove or destroy all known tumor

* to prevent the recurrence of the primary cancer

* to balance the likelihood of a cure of the cancer against the side effects of the treatment

The principles for treatment shift slightly if the cancer has recurred after one or more curative therapies, the person is in poor health and cannot tolerate anticancer therapy, or the cancer has spread widely at the time of diagnosis. In such cases the objectives include:

- a direct, antitumor approach to controlling the cancer as long as possible

- the treatment and relief of symptoms if all reasonable curative approaches have been exhausted

Assessment of the Cancer

Although you will have already undergone many tests for purposes of diagnosis, new or repeated tests may be needed to determine the tumor's characteristics and the extent of disease (see Chapter 5). This additional testing phase may take one or two weeks and can include blood tests, x-rays, a CT scan, and even surgery to obtain additional tissue samples.

Critical questions your doctor is attempting to answer in order to plan treatment are: How aggressive is the cancer? (In other words, how likely is it to grow and spread rapidly?) What is the extent of the cancer at the present time?

Cancer specialists evaluate aggressiveness using the following indicators:

- the size of the tumor

- how long it seemed to take to grow to that size

- how far it has spread

- how quickly it recurs (if it does recur) after treatment

How Treatment Is Planned

When weighing the options, your doctor considers the following factors. He or she will address such factors when discussing treatment with you.

Cancer Type

All cancers—even cancers that affect the same organ or system—are not alike. Because of this people with cancers arising in the same organ may treated very differently.

Cancer Stage

The method of treatment your doctor recommends depends on the size of the tumor, whether or not it has spread, and how aggressive it is.

Overall Health

Your health status is a determining factor in how aggressively the cancer will be treated. Among the many factors that the doctor evaluates are:

- *Age.* The general rule has been that children and young adults tend to handle the stress of aggressive treatments better than older people do, but recent studies suggest that many elderly people can tolerate such treatments.

- *General activity level.* People who are able to be active are better able to cope with various therapies than can those whose activity is limited. One system for assessing activity is called performance status (PS), which rates activity on a scale from 0 (normal) to 4 (bedridden). People who are 3 or 4 usually cannot tolerate much treatment.

- *Condition of specific organs and systems.* Kidney, heart, and lung function must be assessed before the treatment begins. Certain chemotherapeutic agents and radiation therapy can damage these organs. Also, older people may have other serious illnesses that may affect their ability to tolerate certain treatments.

Quality-of-Life Issues

In order to tailor the treatment to your individual needs and help you make the right choice in light of all the circumstances of your life, doctors must ask many personal questions. Both you and your family need to consider the answers to these questions and talk about your hopes and concerns. Don't be surprised if your doctor wants to know:

- What are your hopes and dreams at the time the illness is diagnosed?

- What are your plans for marriage or hopes for bearing children?

- How will you take care of young children or other family members?

- Is extending your life worth the side effects of treatment to you?

- Are you frightened of cancer treatments and apt to reject suggestions that might be most likely to help?

- Do you have a strong support system?

Financial Status

In a perfect world, the issue of finances would not be such a crucial part of health care. However, in these times of shrinking insurance coverage, larger copayments for third-party reimbursements, restrictive health plans, and life circumstances that sometimes catch people without adequate health insurance, expense is a factor. For many people, whether they have coverage for a given treatment will be a deciding factor. Cancer treatment can be financially devastating to a family, so information about treatment costs, insurance coverage, and health plan particulars must be obtained, and the way in which the family plans to meet the uncovered costs needs to be discussed. Many states will pay for cancer treatment for people with no insurance and limited financial resources through the Medicaid program (see Chapter 29).

Talk About It!

The period between diagnosis and the beginning of the treatment is one of uncertainty and ambiguity. Feelings of isolation, vulnerability, helplessness, and fear are common. The most valuable coping skill at this time is communication: talk to your family, your doctor, and your close friends. No concern is too insignificant for discussion.

The reason for airing your feelings is not just to "get them off your chest." Many important decisions must be made right now, and emotions can distort your ability to determine what is best for you. For example, like many people, you may fear that the treatment of cancer is worse than the disease. Indeed, you may become so frightened that you decide you would rather let the cancer take its course than try to combat it. Sharing these fears can allow your doctors to give you up-to-date information, help you separate the actual from the imagined risks and benefits, and make your family members feel better prepared. Most important, you will be able to choose a course of action that you will not regret later.

You are less likely to have second thoughts about such important decisions if you make clear all your priorities—to yourself, your family, and your doctors—before embarking on a particular course of treatment. Likewise, informing your doctors and significant others about what you want from life now and in the future will let everyone know exactly where you stand. Your doctor will be able to determine a treatment plan that you will find acceptable, and the other people in your life will be in a better position to support you (see Chapter 26).

Treatment Logistics

Sometimes the type of therapy recommended is appropriate for all reasons except one: you cannot get to the hospital or clinic. This is a common problem for elderly people who live alone or for people who must travel long distances to treatment centers that offer newer options or to research institutions for experimental therapies. For instance, if you live in a rural area far from a radiation therapy facility, traveling there on a daily basis for treatment may be difficult.

Will the Treatment Work?

Your doctor may offer you one or more treatment choices based on the therapies' track records in large clinical trials, current reports in the scientific literature, the most up-to-date standard of care, and his or her own training and experience. In some cases, the likelihood of a treatment's curing your particular kind of cancer is well established. In others, the odds of cure are still under study. Along with knowledge of the healing potential of the various options, your doctor also weighs specific information about your particular type and stage of cancer and your physical condition. For example, you may not be able to tolerate the most effective therapy for your condition because you are in a poor physical state.

Because every person's cancer is unique, exactly how your tumor will respond to any therapy is not entirely predictable. Doctors balance the pros and cons of many treatment possibilities, narrowing the possibilities down to those they believe offer the best chance of extending your life and improving its quality.

QUESTIONS

TO ASK

Treatment Away from Home

If you are considering a treatment that requires traveling a significant distance, you may want to discuss the following questions with your doctor or the hospital or clinic social worker:

- How frequent are the treatments, and how much time does each one take?

- Will I be able to return home immediately after receiving treatment?

- Is any transportation, such as a shuttle bus, provided by the clinic or hospital?

- Is any financial aid available for me or my family when long-term hospitalization is necessary? (For instance, some treatment centers offer low-cost housing adjacent to the hospital to spouses and relatives so they can be nearby.)

Side Effects

Some cancer treatments have uncomfortable, sometimes toxic, side effects. The more common ones, such as hair loss and nausea following chemotherapy, are temporary; and new antinausea drugs have made chemotherapy treatment much more comfortable. However, occasionally some side effects last longer and may be permanent. The possible loss of lung function after radiation doses for a person preparing for a bone marrow transplant, for instance, must be weighed against the consequences of less intensive therapy.

Conventional Approaches to Treatment

When considering different treatment approaches, it is helpful to keep in mind the general principles discussed at the beginning of this chapter: to remove the entire primary tumor, if possible; to prevent its recurrence; and to preserve as much integrity of your organs, physical functions, and immune system as possible.

Most cancer treatments include surgery to remove a tumor and often radiation or chemotherapy as well. Many people with cancer receive some combination of treatments, as either the primary therapy or the therapy for a recurrent tumor. For example, 15 percent of people with breast cancer have surgery, chemotherapy, and radiation therapy as a first course of treatment. Doctors have found that a combined approach best prevents the recurrence of certain cancers (see Chapter 15).

Surgery

The era of the surgeon was launched with the development of anesthesia in 1846. During the last decade of the nineteenth century, William Stewart Halsted developed the radical mastectomy while he was professor of surgery at Johns Hopkins University. Halsted shared with London surgeon W. Sampson Handley the belief that cancer extended outward from the original growth and was not usually spread through the bloodstream. Therefore radical surgery such as removal of the breast and skin, the underlying muscle of the chest, and lymph nodes under the arm became the treatment of choice for breast cancer. From the late 1800s until 1970 surgery was quite radical, typically removing the tumor and many of the surrounding tissues. In fact, until the mid-1970s, approximately 90 percent of women with breast cancer had the Halsted or radical mastectomy.

Because we have learned that bigger operations don't necessarily prevent the cancer from coming back, the radical approach to removing cancer has been replaced in recent years by operations that aim to spare organs and limit the impact on body functions and appearance. At one time, there were no effective treatment options besides radical surgery. But because of years of testing new treatments in clinical trials, we can now use chemotherapy and/or radiation therapy (to shrink tumors before the operation or destroy stray cells left after less radical operations) combined with surgery. Dogmatic assumptions about how to choose treatment have been replaced by knowledge based on the results of clinical trials.

Exploratory surgery (operating in order to look for a growth) also happens far less often than fifteen years ago (see Chapter 5). Improved biopsy techniques and ways to see inside the body, such as computed tomography (CT scan), magnetic resonance imaging (MRI), and ultrasound, have improved the accuracy and ease of diagnosis.

Most people with cancer have surgery, either to obtain a biopsy, or to determine the stage of a particular cancer, or sometimes simply to remove a tumor and some surrounding tissue. Many times, surgery for an early tumor is curative—the procedure both determines the stage of the cancer and removes the tumor.

The recovery and adjustment period after surgery depends on how large the tumor is, where it is located, and how much normal tissue must be removed along with the malignancy. Occasionally the surgery is so extensive that it affects the function of certain organs and interferes with normal life. Rehabilitation and some adjustments in your daily life may be necessary. Sometimes, the surgery is disfiguring, and psychological support may help acceptance of the change.

Because most serious and/or long-term or permanent effects can be predicted, considering these factors is part of the decision to have surgery or not. In the event that the extent of the surgery is unknown beforehand, talking about all possible outcomes is part of the informed consent process.

Chemotherapy

During World War II, U.S. Army researchers were looking for a more effective chemical weapon than the widely used mustard gas. They knew from studies of soldiers gassed in World War I that the agent called nitrogen mustard lowered white blood counts by killing bone marrow cells. They then reasoned that it might be useful against cancers of the white blood cells—leukemias and lymphomas. So-called "alkylating" agents evolved from this first anti-cancer chemical. These drugs kill rapidly growing cells by damaging their genetic material, DNA.

Two years later, researchers found that cancer cells could be destroyed by blocking cellular functions involved in replicating the genetic material of the cell. The drug that resulted—Aminopterin—was a predecessor of methotrexate, which continues to be widely used.

These advances initiated the third most commonly used cancer therapy: chemotherapy, treatment with anticancer drugs that are injected into the bloodstream or taken by mouth and circulate throughout the body. The drugs target critical metabolic processes within cancer cells and cause the cells to stop growing and eventually to die (see Chapter 12). This systemic approach has led to the cure of several types of childhood cancer, Hodgkin's disease, and others. Malignant cells divide more rapidly than do most normal cells, and chemotherapy works by destroying cancer cells during their dividing phase when they are more vulnerable. Unfortunately, however, the cells of some organs (such as hair follicles; the lining of the mouth, stomach, and intestines; and the bone marrow that produces blood cells) also divide rapidly, so these organs are susceptible to side effects of the anticancer drugs.

Today, there are new ways of countering some of the problems associated with chemotherapy. For example, sometimes chemotherapy initially causes the tumor to shrink but then the cells resist the drug(s) and cancer recurs. New drugs, specifically designed to prevent adaptive metabolic pathways from developing, have been partly successful. They prevent cancer cells from escaping the lethal effects of chemotherapy.

A major discovery was the use of more than one anticancer drug at a time or in sequence. Because some cancer cells are vulnerable only at certain points in their metabolic pathway, using different drugs with different actions increases the chance that the cells will be killed. Some very fast-growing types of cancer, particularly those that involve the bone marrow and lymph nodes, respond particularly well to multiple drugs or combination chemotherapy.

An exciting new approach to chemotherapy, called antiangiogenesis therapy, is using drugs that disrupt blood vessel growth in tumors. Another promising approach is selectively blocking a certain enzyme that makes cancer cells immortal. Using chemotherapy in these innovative ways should have little or no harmful effect on normal cells, at least in adults, and so minimize side effects (see Chapter 12).

More than 100 anticancer drugs are now in use. They are given by mouth or injected into muscle or directly into the bloodstream. Chemotherapy is used alone as a definitive treatment for cancers such as lymphomas, in combination with another approach such as radiation, or as an adjuvant therapy (meaning that it is "added" before or after surgery or radiation therapy) to deal with any known or suspected spread of the primary tumor.

One of the advantages of treating people with a combination of drugs, designed to target the malignant cells at specific points in their division cycles, is that in addition to increasing the effectiveness of the chemotherapy, it minimizes the toxic side effects of each particular drug.

The maximum chemotherapy dosage is based on the amount needed to destroy cancer cells versus the amount of damage that the rapidly dividing healthy tissues in the body can sustain.

Informed Consent

Discussing the risks and benefits with the surgeon is part of a process called informed consent, which is a legal standard that means a person has been told enough about the risks and benefits of a treatment or procedure to decide whether he or she wants to proceed. If the person cannot sign a written consent form, permission can be granted by the court or by someone that person has designated. This is called durable power of attorney for health care. (Informed consent is required before you undergo any cancer treatment, as discussed in each of the following chapters in this section.)

INFORM

YOURSELF

Radiation Therapy

At the close of the nineteenth century, Wilhelm Conrad Roentgen announced his discovery of the x-ray, so named because "X" is the algebraic symbol for an unknown quantity. Within months, systems were devised to use x-rays for diagnosis, and three years later radiation was used to treat cancer. It would soon be discovered that, unfortunately, radiation could also cause cancer. In subsequent years, devices and new sources of radiation, such as radium, were developed that delivered safer doses. Now radiation is delivered with great precision to destroy malignant tumors while minimizing damage to adjacent normal tissue.

One in three people newly diagnosed with cancer receive radiation therapy during their treatment. Like surgery, radiation therapy is considered a local treatment. A precise dose of radiation is targeted to a specific tumor to destroy the cancer cells while sparing the surrounding healthy tissue. Radiation damages the diseased cells' DNA, making them less able to reproduce. Because cancer cells divide more quickly than do those of healthy tissue, they are more vulnerable to radiation, just as they are to anticancer drugs.

Radiation may be used alone, as the primary therapy, or following surgery, as a way of eliminating any stray cancer cells in the area and preventing the local recurrence of a tumor.

The equipment used to deliver radiation therapy has become quite sophisticated in recent years, allowing tumors deep within the body to be targeted without damaging the surrounding tissues. Dosages are calculated according to the tumor's sensitivity to radiation and the normal, adjacent tissue's ability to tolerate exposure to radiation.

Investigational Therapies

Some people initially choose to try an investigational treatment, especially when they have a type of cancer that has not responded well to conventional therapies. Doctors often recommend this option for treating recurrent cancer or advanced disease, especially when standard treatments have failed.

New therapies, including new drugs or combinations, and other agents, are studied in clinical trials, which are studies carried out at medical schools, community cancer centers, treatment facilities, or in one of the NCI's comprehensive cancer centers. Clinical trials are designed to incorporate the best available care with new approaches in cancer treatment (see Chapter 16).

Some of the following therapies are better established than others. Some appear to be so promising for certain cancers that they may already be considered "conventional" treatment for them, but are still under study for other types of cancer.

Immunotherapy
The objective of immunotherapy is to use the immune system to kill cancer cells. Sometimes the treatment consists of giving the patient preformed antibodies (called monoclonal antibodies) that attack the cancer. Disease-fighting

monoclonal antibodies—antibodies that seek out cancer cells—are being studied as both diagnostic tools and delivery systems that can carry anticancer drugs directly to the target.

Other times, treatment is directed towards "turning on" the patient's own immune system. This is now a frequently used treatment for melanoma and renal cell cancer.

Other agents now being used for other cancers are biological response modifiers (BRMs), which include interferons and interleukin-2. These agents are not without temporary side effects, however, and can cause severe fatigue, fever, rashes, and diarrhea (see Chapter 13).

Stem Cell Transplant

Stem cells are immature blood cells that will eventually become fully functioning red and white blood cells and platelets. Transplanting stem cells from one person to another was first done to treat people with leukemia (which directly affects the bone marrow) after they first received radiation and high doses of chemotherapy. Now, it's also done to treat cancer that doesn't affect the bone marrow directly, such as lymphoma, and to replace stem cells that cancer therapies such as chemotherapy and radiation therapy have destroyed. Sometimes, for example, in lymphomas, a person's own stem cells can be used. They are removed, stored, and returned after a course of high-dose chemotherapy.

The original method for transplanting stem cells—immature blood cells that will develop red and white blood cells and platelets—was to transplant the spongy tissue from within bones where blood cells are made (bone marrow). Today, another method known as peripheral blood stem cell transplant (PBSCT) is possible. In this procedure, which is typical of a blood transfusion, the stem cells that enter and circulate in the blood are removed and stored until they are needed. For instance, they may be removed before high-dose chemotherapy and given back after the treatment is complete (see Chapter 14).

Manipulating Hormones

In 1896, University of Edinburgh researcher Thomas Beatson reported that removing the ovaries (oophorectomy) in women with advanced breast cancer often improved their condition. Eventually he discovered the stimulating effect of the female ovarian hormone (estrogen) on breast cancer. We know that women who have their ovaries removed while they are young have a lower risk of ever developing breast cancer. Treating women with an estrogen-blocking drug (tamoxifen; Nolvadex) also reduces incidence of the disease in women over 50 at high risk for the disease and can prevent it from coming back after surgery. Some people think it is the single most important anticancer drug ever developed. However, tamoxifen does have some serious side effects. Scientists are currently studying the ability of another estrogen-blocking drug, Raloxifene, to reduce breast cancer incidence. See the *Breast* entry in the *Overview of Specific Cancers* section (pages 569–575) for more information.

A half-century later, University of Chicago urologist Charles Huggins noted that prostate cancer regressed when the testes, which produce the male hormone testosterone, are removed. Later it was found that testosterone-blocking drugs could accomplish the same effect.

In men with prostate cancer, synthetic hormone-blocking drugs can accomplish the same effects as surgical removal of the testes, or orchiectomy. See the *Prostate* entry in the *Overview of Specific Cancers* section (pages 689–692) for more information.

Chemoprevention

One active area of research in which some clinical trials are underway is the prevention of cancer with surgery, chemicals, and supplements of vitamins or minerals. An example of preventive surgery is the removal of an accumulation of abnormal (though not malignant) cells called a precursor lesion.

In 1998, the U.S. Food and Drug Administration (FDA) approved a drug—tamoxifen citrate (Nolvadex)—for the first time for the prevention of cancer in those at high risk for the disease (see the *Manipulating Hormones* section on page 155).

Recently, celecoxib (Celebrex), a nonsteroidal anti-inflammatory drug (NSAID), was approved by the FDA for reducing polyp formation in people with a condition that runs in families known as familial adenomatous polyposis (FAP). It is believed that benign polyps in the large intestine may lead to cancer. Researchers are trying to determine whether certain antioxidants, such as retinoids, vitamin E, and beta carotene, may prevent some cancers. Today, some of the genetic mutations that set the stage for cancer are rapidly being identified, such as for the hereditary forms of breast and colon cancer. Scientists expect to build on that knowledge and devise treatments for reversing the mutation and/or halting carcinogenesis well before cancer cells proliferate and invade healthy tissue.

Looking into the Future

Today's new research frontier is biological therapy: the use of natural, biological materials to stimulate the body's own cancer-fighting mechanisms. Some of these agents also alter cancer cell growth. Looming on the horizon are some exciting possibilities of genetic engineering, such as developing a means to selectively destroy cancer cells regardless of where they are in the body.

Some of the advances mentioned on the following page are still in the early, basic science stage and are not likely to be practiced soon, but they are signs of progress and hope.

Cancer vaccines, which contain cancer cells, parts of cells, or chemically pure antigens (substances foreign to the body), cause the body's immune system to attack cancer cells present in the patient's body.

Antiangiogenesis therapy is the use of drugs or other compounds that interfere with the development of new blood vessels that feed a tumor. This therapy can "starve" tumors by cutting off their blood supply (see Chapter 12).

STI-571 (Gleevec) is the beginning of a new approach to killing cancer cells. The drug interferes with the action of the abnormal enzyme produced by the genetic abnormality in a kind of leukemia, which eventually leads to the death of these cells and disappearance of the leukemia. Because it only targets the leukemia cell, it has no side effects. Researchers are looking at other cancers caused by defects in genes to develop drugs to block their actions.

Non-myeloablative transplants are a new approach to donor stem cell transplants. These procedures use much lower doses of chemotherapy or radiation therapy than standard transplants. Patients are given drugs that suppress their immune reaction, which allows the donor cells to grow and partly take over the patient's immune system. The donor cells then begin reacting against the cancer cells and killing them.

Immunotoxins are made by attaching toxins (poisonous substances from plants or bacteria) to monoclonal antibodies. Immunotoxins studied in clinical trials have shown some early promise in shrinking some cancers, particularly lymphomas.

Psychoneuroimmunology is the intricate link between the mind and immunity. The clinical aspect of mind-body interactions, called mind-body medicine, has produced dramatic results in specific arenas. It is forming the basis for a new perspective on medicine and healing—that every interaction between doctors and patients may affect the mind and in turn the body of the patient.

Living Well with Cancer

The importance of not only living longer but living well has become a top priority among both caregivers and scientists, as it always has been for people with cancer. Drugs and psychological techniques that make the side effects of chemotherapy more tolerable are now available (see Chapters 12 and 27).

Pain is now managed both with medication and mind/body therapies, making this greatly feared aspect of cancer tolerable for most people (see Chapters 23 and 27). The importance of support groups and better coping strategies is being recognized, and ways to measure their impact scientifically are being evaluated (see Chapters 8 and 26). Physical symptoms due to the cancer and to stress, anxiety, and depression can be managed. When they are controlled, the lives of people with cancer are immeasurably improved.

Information about new treatments and how to participate in clinical trials is accessible to everyone and is widely available (see Chapter 16). Regardless of how aggressive you choose to be in seeking treatment, today you have more options than ever before. Now you can make choices suited to your individual physical condition, your emotional needs and comfort level, and the feelings and concerns of those close to you. Living with cancer is a serious, demanding challenge, but the resources for coping well and maintaining an acceptable quality of life exist.

CASE HISTORIES

TRUE STORIES

The Right to Choose

Peter, 63, had been relatively healthy throughout his life. But during his yearly physical exam, his doctor felt a suspicious lump on his prostate, which turned out to be cancerous. Fortunately, further tests showed that the cancer was still small and had not spread outside of the prostate gland. Peter was surprised to learn that he had several treatment options to choose from and that they all gave him about the same chance for long-term survival. He first spoke with a urologist, who recommended surgery to remove the cancer, but a radiation oncologist suggested he consider brachytherapy (radioactive seed implants), which might cause him fewer side effects. After reading up as much as he could on his situation and talking with men who had faced similar choices, he decided on surgery. In the end he felt it was more important to "have it out of there as quickly as possible" and deal with some of the side effects, rather than facing a recurrence years later and realizing that he could have been more aggressive at the start. And, he made the right decision—*for him.* His choice wasn't "right" or "wrong," but it was an informed one.

10

Surgery

S urgery is not only the oldest form of cancer treatment in use today, it's also often the most successful way of achieving a cure for most types of cancer. However, surgery is done for a variety of other reasons as well. It's estimated that about 60 percent of people with cancer will have some type of operation.

Surgery to treat cancer has evolved into a subspecialty called surgical oncology. Modern surgery still uses scalpels, but there have been many advances such as lasers, electrocautery devices (instruments heated with electrical current), and special viewing instruments called endoscopes, laparoscopes, and thorascopes, through which some procedures are done. These slim tubes can be inserted through tiny incisions, and specially designed instruments and even a tiny video camera are inserted through them. Now automatic stapling devices sometimes replace handstitching with suture material to close a skin incision and, especially, for operations to remove tumors of the lungs or digestive system.

Significant improvements have been made in postoperative care in the past few decades, including pain management, infection prevention, and the replacement of lost fluids and nutrients.

Preventive Surgery

One of the most common examples of preventive or prophylactic surgery is the removal of a precancerous lesion, a suspicious area with cells that are likely to become malignant over time. For example, certain abnormalities in the cells of the cervix are detectable on a Pap test and can be removed under local anesthesia with a scalpel (conization), vaporized with a laser, coagulated with an electric current (electrocauterization), or frozen with liquid nitrogen (cryosurgery). Precancerous colon polyps and atypical or suspicious moles on the skin can also be removed to prevent cancer from developing.

In addition, certain benign diseases that are risk factors for cancer can be treated surgically. For example, ulcerative colitis, an inflammatory condition of the large intestine, may warrant removal of the colon. Since people with diffuse colon involvement due to ulcerative colitis have a greatly increased risk of developing colon cancer, doctors often take colon biopsies at regular intervals to check for precancerous areas. If changes likely to progress to cancer are found, removal of the colon is usually recommended, and the small intestine will be connected to the rectum or to a colostomy, a surgically created opening through which intestinal waste exits the body. Likewise, some women with the cancer susceptibility genes BRCA1 or BRCA2 may benefit from a prophylactic mastectomy, removal of the breast.

Diagnostic and Staging Surgery

The most definitive way to diagnose cancer is to remove a sample of tissue and examine it under a microscope. This procedure is called a biopsy (see Chapter 5). Sometimes this can be done by inserting a needle into the suspicious area, but other times the only way to gain access to an area is through an operation that allows the surgeon to directly inspect the internal organs and obtain a tissue sample for biopsy at the same time.

Surgery also is often the best way to determine how advanced a cancer is and whether it has spread from the primary site to other parts of the body. Surgical staging involves examining the internal organs. An example is the laparotomy, which involves opening the abdomen and looking at the liver, spleen, and other organs. Some diagnostic tests, such as ultrasound, may be done with the organs thus exposed.

A less invasive procedure is a laparoscopy. An endoscope inserted through a small incision in the abdomen transmits images of the organs onto a video monitor. When done to look inside the chest, the procedure is called a thoracoscopy. In both laparoscopy and thoracoscopy, tissue may be removed through the endoscope for testing.

After a cancer has been treated, retreatment staging, also known as second-look surgery, allows doctors to determine how successful the therapy has been. This is not done routinely, but in some situations the surgeon may need to re-examine the affected organs to make sure there is no more tumor in the primary site or in nearby areas.

Curative Surgery

The surgical treatment of cancer involves removing, or resecting, the tumor to cure the disease. Typically, an area of normal-looking tissue surrounding the tumor called a margin is removed also to ensure that no cancer cells remain in the immediate vicinity. Because tumor cells commonly spread via the lymphatic system, nearby lymph nodes may be examined and/or excised as well. When cancers of most organs are small and have not spread to other parts of the body, surgical removal is usually curative. Even after spread has occurred, some patients are cured by the combination of surgery together with chemotherapy and/or radiation therapy.

The trend in recent years has been to remove as little tissue as possible in order to spare body parts. For instance, a surgeon treating breast cancer may excise only the tumor with clear margins rather than perform a mastectomy. Radiation therapy often follows to destroy any malignant cells that remain in the breast. Along with these local treatments, chemotherapy is an option (see Chapter 15) to destroy cancer cells anywhere in the body. Use of chemotherapy and/or radiation therapy to shrink a cancer before surgery often permits surgeons to completely remove it without taking out the whole organ. This approach is especially useful for some cancers of the rectum, breast, and bones.

Cytoreductive Surgery

Sometimes a tumor is so advanced that it cannot be removed entirely. For example, malignant cells can invade the area around the primary tumor so extensively that too much tissue would have to be removed for the organ to function properly. In this case, a doctor may consider cytoreductive or debulking surgery, removing as much of the cancer as possible and then treating the remaining cells with radiation therapy, chemotherapy, or both.

Most experts feel that cytoreductive surgery should be undertaken only if there is a good chance that some other form of treatment will be able to destroy the residual cancer cells or at least destroy enough of the remaining cancer to significantly influence the patient's lifespan or quality of life.

Removing Metastases

Removing cancer cells that have migrated from the primary tumor can be a step toward cure for some patients. This is particularly true if the primary tumor has been completely removed and the metastatic cells have settled in only one spot. For instance, colon cancer often spreads to the liver, and removing some metastasis from this organ, followed by chemotherapy to remove any remaining deposits of cancer cells too small to see, may sometimes lead to a cure.

Metastatic cells in the bone, liver, lungs, and brain from other primary sites may occasionally be removed successfully, helping the patient live longer with fewer symptoms, and occasionally increasing the odds of a cure.

Palliation

Palliative surgery attempts to correct a problem that is causing discomfort. It is not intended to cure the cancer. For instance, a tumor in the abdominal area may grow so large that it presses on and blocks a portion of the intestine, interfering with digestion and causing pain and/or vomiting. Debulking surgery, which removes a large portion of the tumor, may relieve the blockage. Or an operation that allows an obstruction to be bypassed may relieve symptoms and allow vital life processes to continue. All or a portion of a tumor that presses painfully on a nerve may be removed.

Supportive Surgery

Surgery to implant devices that aid other therapies is considered supportive. For instance, malnutrition, weight loss, and weakness that sometimes accompany cancers of the throat and esophagus may be improved by inserting a temporary or permanent feeding tube directly into the stomach.

Surgery also is used to implant a device, called a vascular access device, for chemotherapy injections to avoid multiple needle sticks (see Chapter 12).

Restorative Surgery

Sometimes a treatment that cures the cancer causes other problems that make additional surgery necessary or desirable. Merely removing a tumor is not enough. Many experts consider a treatment to be truly successful only if it also restores bodily function and/or appearance. For example, skin, muscle, and bone grafts, dental implants, and surgery to implant a valve between the esophagus and trachea (windpipe) can help head and neck cancer survivors eat and speak more easily.

Breast reconstruction has become increasingly sophisticated as well. Breasts can be rebuilt with implants or with tissue taken from the woman's abdomen, buttock, or back. New types of continent ostomies allow greater control and freedom for survivors of rectal and bladder cancer (see Chapter 22).

The Operation: Before, During, and After

Most operations include preoperative testing and preparation; the actual surgery, which requires some type of anesthesia; and a recovery period. In addition to these physical phases, there also are emotional issues to consider, such as anxiety about the surgery and its aftermath. Knowing what to expect can help relieve some of your fear and nervousness. An "Informed Consent" form must also be signed, which gives the surgeon permission to perform the operation.

QUESTIONS

TO ASK

Questions to Ask Your Doctor About Surgery

Before undergoing surgery, you will want to find out all you can about the benefits, risks, and side effects of the operation. You should understand the goals of the treatment and what your doctor predicts the benefits will be. Answers to the following questions will help you feel comfortable about your decision:

- Why will I have this operation? What are the chances of its success? Is there any other way to treat this cancer?

- Are you certified by the American Board of Surgery and/or other appropriate specialty or subspecialty boards?

- Is the hospital where the operation will be performed accredited by the Joint Commission on Accreditation of Healthcare Organizations and by the Commission on Cancer of the American College of Surgeons?

- How many operations like the one you are suggesting have you done? Are you experienced in operating on my kind of cancer?

- Exactly what will you be doing—and removing—in this operation? Why?

- How long will the surgery take?

- What can I expect after the operation? Will I be in a great deal of pain? Will I have drains or catheters?

- Will I need a blood transfusion?

- How will my body be affected by the surgery? Will the operation affect my mobility, bowel or bladder control, speech, or sexuality?

- How long will it take for me to recover? Will any of the effects be permanent?

- Other than my cancer, am I healthy enough to tolerate the stress of the surgery and the anesthesia?

- How long will I be in the hospital after the surgery?

- What are the potential risks and side effects of this operation? What is the risk of death or disability as a result of this surgery?

- What will happen if I choose not to have the operation?

- What are the chances that the surgery will cure my cancer?

- Do I need to decide about treatment right away? Do I have time to think about options or get a second opinion?

Informed Consent

Even though surgery can accomplish so much, opening the body to the outside environment and inserting instruments into it is a serious invasion. Therefore, surgery is not a step to be undertaken without careful deliberation and discussion of its advantages and disadvantages. Anesthesia also involves some risks, and postoperative discomfort is inevitable.

The physical inactivity that follows surgery can create problems as well. Thus, anyone deciding to have an operation should be fully aware of all the risks of the procedure and why, despite the hazards, surgery is recommended.

In some states, doctors of breast cancer patients are required by law to inform women of all their treatment options, in addition to surgery, and provide them with a written summary on medically acceptable treatment alternatives. State legislatures are considering similar disclosure laws with regard to prostate cancer.

INFORM

YOURSELF

Informed Consent for Surgery

A written consent form must be signed before surgery is performed. It contains a statement about what the operation is and its risks and benefits, such as the reason you are having the surgery (is it to cure you, to relieve symptoms, and/or as part of another type of treatment?); the chances that the operation will achieve this goal; the risk of disfigurement, disability, or death; the benefits and risks of not having the surgery; and any available alternative treatments.

It is important that you read and understand each of these issues, not just sign on the dotted line. If you are feeling too nervous before the surgery to concentrate fully on the form, have a family member or close friend go over it carefully with you.

Planning the Surgery

The surgical team must make many decisions before operating, such as what type of anesthesia to use; the size, location, and extent of the incision; whether it will be possible to remove all of the tumor or only a part of it; whether to use stitches or staples to close the incision; and whether or not to perform an ostomy, breast reconstruction, or other restorative procedures. Each consideration is a potential topic for discussion, depending on how involved you want to be in the planning.

Several tests are necessary to determine your general health and ability to withstand the rigors of surgery and recovery, and some tests are needed to assess the cancer.

In preparation for a major operation, the surgeon must determine whether you have any medical conditions such as diabetes, hypertension (high blood pressure), heart or lung disease, or an infection. Urine analyses, blood tests, chest x-rays, and electrocardiograms to evaluate heart function usually reveal any serious ailments.

The older a person is, the more comprehensive the preoperative testing will be, since the conditions that can interfere with recovery are more common later in life. If possible, certain medical problems are treated before surgery. For example, antibiotics can combat an active infection; hypertension may respond to medication. Chronic illness such as heart disease or diabetes can affect the anesthesia used. Often a specialist in that particular condition consults with the treatment team and is available during the surgery and immediately afterward in case of an emergency.

There are some things you should do before surgery to help it go smoothly. If you smoke, stop—at least for the time being. By clearing your lungs of smoke before your surgery, you diminish the chances of developing lung and breathing problems afterward. Smoking can also affect blood vessels and reduce supplies of oxygen and nutrition to healing tissues. Likewise, avoid junk food and eat a well-balanced diet, because good nutritional status helps recovery.

Preparing for Surgery

Depending on the type of operation you are going to have, your body will be prepared (or prepped) inside and out to ensure that the surgery and recovery from anesthesia go smoothly.

Cleaning the Skin. To cut down on the risk of infection, the hair must be removed from the area surrounding the incision site. In the case of abdominal surgery, the entire abdomen, genital area, and upper legs may be shaved; for a brain operation, the head is shaved. You will shower or bathe the night before surgery. A technician or nurse will clean your skin with antiseptics the day before surgery, and the surgeon will repeat the procedure in the operating room.

Emptying the Digestive Tract. Vomiting during anesthesia is especially dangerous because the material may enter the lungs and lead to pneumonia. If you will be asleep during surgery or there is any possibility that unexpected events during surgery might require a change in anesthetic plans, your upper digestive tract must be empty before the operation; therefore, you cannot eat or drink anything for about twelve hours beforehand. You may be advised to have a light dinner the night before your operation and then to eat nothing else. When surgery involves the colon, the bowels cannot handle the movement of waste material for several days after surgery. Therefore, you will be given a laxative, and your colon will be cleaned out with enemas and/or laxatives and a liquid diet the day or night before surgery.

Rest. It helps to have a good night's sleep before an operation. But since you may be nervous, your doctor may prescribe a sleeping pill.

Special Preparations. For surgery on the digestive tract, a tube may be inserted through your nose into your stomach to keep it and your bowels empty and free of gas. Although stomach tubes do not hurt when inserted, this is usually done after you have been anesthetized.

A catheter (a thin, flexible tube) is often placed into the bladder to keep it empty during surgery. A doctor or nurse may insert the catheter before or during surgery.

Blood Transfusions and Fluid Balance. You may receive a blood transfusion before, during, and/or after surgery, depending on the type of operation and your condition. The blood you receive may come from a donor, in which case it is thoroughly tested for viruses and bacteria, such as those that cause AIDS, hepatitis, and syphilis. You may also store your own blood before surgery. This is called predeposit autologous donation and may be permitted as long as you do not have a serious heart condition or are anemic (have an insufficient number of red blood cells). Up to four units of blood may be collected five or six weeks before surgery and transfused during or after the operation.

The body can recover from the trauma of surgery when the blood contains healthy amounts of its various components, such as water, salt, sugar, protein, potassium, calcium, and vitamins. To keep these substances in balance, you may receive some or all of them intravenously before and/or after surgery.

Anesthesia

Anesthesia temporarily makes the body unable to feel pain. Typically, an anesthesiologist (a doctor who specializes in anesthesia) administers the drugs and monitors your vital signs—pulse, heart rhythm, and breathing rate—during the surgery and observes you after the operation while you regain consciousness. Anesthesia may also be administered by a nurse anesthetist, who has received special training and works under the direction of a doctor.

Local Anesthesia. Minor surgery, such as the retrieval of cells near the skin's surface for biopsy, requires numbing only the area involved, or local anesthesia. A drug to temporarily deaden the nerves supplying the area is injected near the site. You remain awake and usually feel little more than some minor pressure.

Another type of local anesthesia is called topical, in which a numbing agent is sprayed or painted onto the skin's surface or a mucous membrane such as the throat.

Regional Anesthesia. When it is necessary to interfere with sensation in a larger part of the body without affecting consciousness, a regional anesthetic or nerve block is used. For example, an anesthetic agent injected into the fluid surrounding the spinal cord can numb the pelvic region and legs for surgery on the lower body. The drug may be given in a single injection or continuously through a small catheter placed under local anesthesia directly into or near the spinal canal. Although you remain awake, usually you will receive medication to help you relax.

There are several types of regional anesthesia. High spinal anesthesia is used when organs in the middle or upper stomach are being treated. A low spinal, or a saddle block, is used when the surgical site is the rectum or genitals. An epidural, or caudal anesthesia, is injected into the area outside the spinal cord. Anesthetic drugs may also be injected around nerves in the limbs.

General Anesthesia. The purpose of general anesthesia is to put you to sleep so that surgery can be performed. It may be administered via a facemask through which an anesthetic gas flows. As you inhale the gas, it gradually enters the bloodstream, where it is carried to the brain. Or the anesthetic is injected directly into the bloodstream, bringing on almost immediate deep sleep.

Recovery

The recovery room is for people regaining feeling from regional anesthesia or waking up from general anesthesia following surgery in the postoperative (postop) phase. Recovery rooms are outfitted with equipment for monitoring the heart, assisting breathing, and intravenously administering fluids, such as blood and painkillers.

It typically takes one to three hours for regional anesthesia to wear off. The time it takes to regain consciousness after general anesthesia varies according to how deep a sleep was induced. Because vision, hearing, and balance may be affected, things often seem hazy; voices appear to be coming from far away; and people may seem to move strangely.

Whether you've had a regional or a general anesthesia, you'll probably receive medication to ease pain once you're out of the recovery room and in your regular hospital bed. Pain medication ranges from analgesics like aspirin (and other nonsteroidal anti-inflammatory drugs, or NSAIDs) and acetaminophen to opioids (narcotics) such as codeine in pill form, or morphine, which is injected or given orally. A nurse may administer these drugs at set intervals, or you may be outfitted with a patient-controlled analgesia (PCA) pump device, which allows you to self-administer the drug by pressing a button (see Chapter 23). Medication may also be given by means of an epidural, just like that used for anesthesia. The drug you're given will depend on the type of operation you had and how uncomfortable you are.

Getting Back to Normal

In the hours and days following surgery, pain relief is only one concern. Another is regaining the full function of other body organs such as those of the gastrointestinal and urinary tract and the return of muscular activity and strength. There are ways to cope with the common aftereffects of surgery so that your body recovers as quickly and completely as possible.

Mobility. Discomfort in the area of the incision can make walking difficult, but it's important to get moving as soon as is safely possible, because movement stimulates circulation and prevents blood clots. Turning from side to side, getting out of bed into a chair, and walking also encourage deep breathing, which helps restore the lungs to full capacity and prevents pneumonia (see Chapter 19). You may be given a special device to blow into to encourage deep breathing.

Intestinal Function. Walking is also an antidote to stomach and intestinal gas, a frequent side effect of surgery to the abdominal region. Gas pains may persist for up to three days. If they don't subside naturally, a tube can be inserted through the nose and the esophagus into the stomach or into the lower intestine through the rectum to help expel the gas.

Similarly, nausea and vomiting are common after surgery but can usually be relieved with medication given by injection or in a suppository. Frequently, eating and drinking are prohibited for twenty-four hours to allow the digestive tract to regain its ability to digest food.

Urination. Some people find it difficult to empty their bladder after an operation if a catheter is not in place. In that case, medication to stimulate urination may be prescribed, or a catheter may be inserted into the bladder to empty it.

Caring for the Wound

A dressing usually covers the actual wound or incision. Drains—very thin, soft, rubbery tubes, which may or may not be attached to a collecting device—may be placed into the wound to allow fluid to drain. Hospital personnel trained in sterile technique will care for the wound until healing is ensured. This may mean simply changing the bandage periodically. Some stitches gradually dissolve as the wound heals; other types of stitches and staples are taken out by a doctor. As long as the wound heals normally and is not complicated by infection, little specialized care is needed after you leave the hospital.

In some cases, wound care is not so simple, and healing is not uneventful. When specialized care is needed after you return home, nurses provide instruction before you leave the hospital, and visiting nurse appointments may be arranged to monitor your, or your family's, ability to care for the incision site and to avoid complications such as infection.

Permanent Changes

Sometimes the surgery to treat cancer makes it necessary to change how the body works. For instance, after radical surgery for bladder or bowel cancer, it may be necessary to redirect urine or solid wastes. Typically, an opening, or stoma, is created on the surface of the body through which waste flows into a discreetly positioned bag. Women who undergo a mastectomy are faced with living without a breast or, if they choose, with a prosthesis or reconstructed breast. Similarly, someone who loses an arm or leg must adjust to functioning without that limb or learn to use an artificial one (see Chapters 20 and 22).

Complications

Although many side effects of cancer surgery are predictable, unexpected problems sometimes arise. The most common complication is impairment of lung function, and it usually results from previous lung disease, a smoking habit, or failure to move about adequately after surgery. The ultimate risk, operative mortality, refers to a death occurring within thirty days of an operation. This may be due to complications of the surgery, or it may be directly related to the cancer.

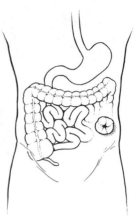

A colostomy is the removal of a portion of the colon and creation of an opening through which waste material is excreted. A bag with an opening that fits over the ostomy collects the waste.

The Emotional Impact of Surgery

Although surgery offers hope of substantial relief, in the short term it is a stressful experience. Apprehension about being in the hospital and being operated on, plus the fear of pain, side effects, and temporary or permanent changes in how the body functions, can intensify the fear associated with having cancer. However, managing as much of that anxiety as possible before surgery will help you achieve peace of mind and improve your chances of a smooth recovery. Research shows that people who are extremely fearful and anxious before an operation tend to experience more complications afterward.

The best way to quell fear is to voice your concerns about the operation and its aftermath to your doctor and other medical personnel. Try to get specific answers to your questions. If you ask when you can go back to work following surgery and are told, "As soon as you feel comfortable," press for a time frame. Likewise, if your doctor prescribes "plenty of bedrest" after you go home, get him or her to explain what "plenty" means. Does it mean that you will need to spend several hours a day in bed or that after a day or so, you will just curtail your normal activities for a while? Details such as these will give you a clear picture of what your life immediately following surgery will be like, and you'll be better able to prepare for it. Often your doctor can also arrange a visit with a person who has undergone similar surgery.

If your operation involves changes in how you look or how your body works, again, get as many details as you can. If you are having a mastectomy, discuss the pros and cons of a breast prosthesis versus breast reconstruction with your doctor, and if you opt for reconstruction, find out when you can undergo that procedure. Ostomies can be especially traumatic if you don't know what to expect afterward. Find out what the stoma (opening) will look like, and get specific information from an enterostomal therapist about caring for it before you leave the hospital. You will be assured that the ostomy will not be noticeable to other people and will not limit the amount of time you can spend away from home, which are two of the biggest fears of people with ostomies.

Equally important are the support of others and learning to relax. A support network of family, friends, and medical personnel can help relieve your fear and anxiety. You may also find it helpful to join an established support group of people who also are cancer surgery patients. They can share with you some of the coping strategies they've found useful. There are a variety of mind-body techniques you can use to relieve pre- and postsurgery anxiety and manage pain and discomfort (see Chapter 27). These techniques can prove just as important to you as making the necessary physical preparations.

Surgery is an essential element of cancer treatment, and in many cases it is a positive step toward cure. Even so, the prospect of staying in the hospital, undergoing anesthesia, being "opened up," and facing possible postsurgical consequences such as pain or disfigurement is distressing. Asking questions and carefully weighing the benefits and risks of surgery should lessen your apprehension and give you a more positive outlook.

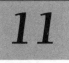
Radiation Therapy

At least half of all people who have cancer receive radiation therapy (also known as radiotherapy, x-ray therapy, cobalt therapy, and irradiation), a treatment that uses x-ray waves or a stream of energy particles to destroy cancer cells or damage them so much they cannot multiply.

Radiation only damages cells directly in the radiation field. Not only can it be used as the primary treatment to cure or control cancer, it can be combined with other therapies such as surgery, chemotherapy, or both. Vulnerable areas of the body can also be shielded during treatment so they are not exposed to radiation. Radiation is also used for palliation. This means that treatment can be directed to a tumor that is causing symptoms such as pain or blocking an important passageway in the body. By destroying this local tumor, the radiation will relieve the pain or blockage.

Harnessing Energy to Fight Cancer

Waves of radiation energy, from short to long waves, permeate the atmosphere. This background radiation is, for the most part, quite harmless. In the form of x-rays, radiation is used to diagnose broken bones and visualize internal organs.

Radiation therapy relies on high-energy x-rays, electron beams, or radioactive isotopes (from sources such as cobalt and cesium, or created in a machine called a linear accelerator) to shrink or destroy malignant growths. Radiation does this through a process that destroys living cells called ionization. Ionizing means removing electrons from atoms to create ions. The higher the energy of ionizing radiation, the deeper it penetrates. The radiation oncologist determines what specific type of ionizing radiation should be administered for each individual patient. Sometimes the cells are destroyed immediately; more often, however, certain components of the cells are injured, such as their genetic material or DNA. Because this injury interferes with the cells' ability to reproduce, they eventually die.

Electron beams don't penetrate deeply and are useful for treating superficial tumors like skin cancer. When cancer cells involve organs deep within the body, a new form of radiation therapy available at a few medical centers uses protons, which cause little injury to tissues they pass through but kill cells at the end of their path. This makes proton therapy useful for treating tumors that are very near vital structures. Another type of radiation therapy that is still being tested relies on neutrons. Neutrons are very damaging to tissues. Because of this, it has been thought they could treat cancers more effectively. So far the results have been mixed and more work is needed to perfect this approach. Neutron radiation therapy is sometimes used to treat cancer of the head, neck, and prostate.

INFORM

YOURSELF

Informed Consent for Radiation Therapy

Informed consent is your written permission to receive radiotherapy and the tests that may be necessary to plan the treatment and assess its results. Although the specifics of the form may vary from one state to another, an informed consent form usually attests to the fact that your doctor has explained your condition to you and how radiation therapy will affect it.

Before signing the informed consent form, you should have discussed with your doctor the potential benefits, side effects, and complications of radiation therapy in general and those associated with the particular type of therapy being recommended to you specifically. You should understand how the treatment will be administered. You should also be informed of the pros and cons of the alternative therapies, if there are other options. Finally, when you sign the form, you are acknowledging that you understand there is no guarantee that the treatment will achieve its purpose.

What Radiation Does to Malignant Cells

The life cycle of any cell, malignant or healthy, has five phases, one of which is the dividing or mitotic stage. During this process the cell must produce a copy of its DNA for the new cell. Because radiation damages DNA, the cell will be unable to reproduce its DNA and form new cells. This makes rapidly growing tumors very sensitive to radiation (see the box *Words You Will Hear*, page 174). Examples of highly radiosensitive cancers include lymphoma (cancer of the lymph nodes), leukemias, and testicular cancers. Although cancers in other organs such as the prostate or breast are less sensitive, they are still treatable by radiation. It is important to remember that cancer cells can often repair their DNA damage. That is why the radiation must be given repeatedly.

Cells' sensitivity to radiation also depends on the amount of oxygen in their environment. The more oxygenated the cells are, the more susceptible they are to radiation. Conversely, cells that are hypoxic (that is, their environment contains little, if any, oxygen) are not very radiosensitive. It takes two to three times more radiation to kill hypoxic cells than well-oxygenated ones. One of the hopes for neutron therapy is that because it is so potent, it would still be effective if the tumor was poorly oxygenated.

Tumors become hypoxic when they grow very large and their blood supply is diminished. In that case, radiation may first shrink the tumor, which brings the hypoxic cells closer to blood vessels. As the oxygen supply to the cancer cells increases, so does their vulnerability to additional radiation treatments.

Effects on Healthy Tissue

Normal tissues vary in their degree of radiosensitivity. Bone marrow, reproductive glands, skin, mucous membranes, and the organs of the lymph system, such as the tonsils and the lymph nodes, are all highly radiosensitive. Mature bone and cartilage, the brain, and the spinal cord are not very radiosensitive, but high doses can still cause severe side effects in these tissues.

Radiation does not distinguish between tumor cells and healthy tissue, but normal tissue usually is able to recover with little or no permanent damage. Nevertheless, great care is taken to shield healthy body parts during treatment, although certain predictable side effects may occur.

Radiation as Cancer Therapy

Radiation is the primary treatment for certain types of cancer, which are especially vulnerable to it. These include certain head and neck malignancies (such as early-stage cancer of the larynx), early-stage Hodgkin's disease and non-Hodgkin's lymphomas, and certain cancers of the lung, cervix, prostate, bladder, thyroid, and brain.

In the early stage of disease, radiation therapy can cure or control the cancer. It can shrink a tumor to facilitate surgery or relieve pain. When cancer cells have spread beyond the tumor, radiation therapy to the surrounding area can prevent the cells from gaining a foothold and halt their growth.

CANCER

BASICS

Radiation Therapy Alone

Unlike chemotherapy, which requires exposing the entire body to cancer-fighting chemicals, radiation therapy and surgery are considered local treatments, affecting only the tumor and the area surrounding it. Radiation and surgery have similar cure rates for some types of cancer, but radiation therapy may be preferred to surgery if there is a pre-existing condition that makes surgery impossible or if surgery would require removing part or all of a limb or organ. Radiation therapy, therefore, is often chosen to preserve normal organs, to keep the body functioning fully, and sometimes to avoid disfiguring surgery. For example, radiation therapy may be used to treat cancer of the larynx in order to preserve the voice.

Combined Treatment

Radiation therapy is frequently combined with other treatments to enhance the chances of curing or controlling the cancer. For instance, radiation may be used to shrink the tumor so that it can be more easily removed by surgery or to limit the extent of the operation and preserve more normal tissue.

Radiation therapy is also recommended after surgery to prevent the cancer from coming back by killing cells that may have been left behind. For example, radiation may be used after removal of a malignant breast tumor (lumpectomy) to prevent a recurrence. How soon the radiation therapy begins after an operation depends on the extent of the surgery and how well you are recuperating. In some cases, radiation therapy begins only a few days after surgery; most times, it's best to wait until the surgical wound has healed.

Chemotherapy can also be a helpful addition to radiation therapy; often these two modes of treatment follow surgery to rid the body of any remaining malignant cells. Chemicals may work by rendering cancer cells more radiosensitive, by independently killing cells, or by enhancing the effects of radiation therapy by preventing the cancer cells from repairing their radiation-damaged DNA (see Chapter 15).

When combination therapy is a consideration, the proposed treatment plan is discussed by the surgeon, the medical oncologist, the radiation oncologist, and the person receiving treatment.

Questions to Ask Your Doctor About Radiation Therapy

QUESTIONS

TO ASK

Part of deciding on a particular treatment is determining whether the benefits of the treatment are worth its costs, side effects, and risks. These vary according to the area being treated, the type of radiation given, and its dose and frequency. Therefore, you should understand the goals of the treatment and what your doctor predicts the benefits will be. Some people never have any side effects, and a very small percentage have severe ones. For the most part, side effects are mild and temporary, subsiding completely within days or weeks after treatment ends. Some cases, however, (especially when large doses of radiation are necessary) produce chronic problems and permanent interruption of body functions.

Considering the range of possibilities, it's important to ask your doctor about all the risks and weigh them against the hoped-for benefits. The following questions are general ones, regardless of the type of radiation recommended.

- What is the purpose of radiation treatment for my cancer? For example, will my therapy totally destroy the tumor or merely shrink it? Will it prevent the spread of cancer?

- How will the radiation affect the surrounding area?

- If radiation therapy is to follow surgery, its purpose may be slightly different, and you might ask, "Is this treatment designed to destroy any remaining cancer cells? Could radiation alone be used instead of surgery?"

- If the cancer has recurred or spread to other organs and radiation is being suggested, you might ask, "Why is radiation therapy being suggested? Will it destroy the spreading cancer cells? Will it control further spread? Is it being recommended primarily to relieve symptoms such as pain or bleeding?"

- Whatever the purpose is, what are the chances that the radiation therapy will work?

- Are there other ways to achieve the same goals?

- What problems typically result from treatment?

- Which, if any, of these effects will interfere with my functioning? My ability to eat or drink? My physical activity? My ability to work? My sexual activity? My reproductive capability?

- Will any of the effects temporarily or permanently change my appearance?

- How long will the side effect(s) last? Is it likely that any will become chronic?

- What is the probability that the cancer will worsen, spread, and/or recur if I don't receive radiation therapy?

- Is there an alternative treatment that could spare me the risk of a particular side effect? If so, what are the risks and benefits of altering the treatment you have recommended?

Types of Radiation Therapy

There are two main types of radiation treatment: external beam radiation, or teletherapy, which directs radiation from an outside source into the body; and internal therapy, or brachytherapy, in which a radioactive source is placed inside the body, near the cancerous growth.

INFORM

YOURSELF

Team Members

It takes a number of medical professionals to plan and administer radiation therapy, as well as to care for you during the treatment. These people must work together, sharing information about your particular illness. They include the following:

- The *radiation oncologist*, a doctor who specializes in treating cancer with radiation. He or she will make many of the decisions affecting your radiation therapy, starting with the recommendation that you should receive radiation in the first place and deciding what kind and approximately how much radiation you should get. The radiation oncologist will evaluate you frequently during the course of treatment and at intervals afterward.

- The *medical* or *radiation physicist*, an expert in medical physics who is trained in planning radiation treatment. He or she helps determine the treatment plan and makes sure the equipment is working properly to deliver the appropriate dose of radiation.

- The *dosimetrist*, a technician who assists the physicist in planning and calculating the dosage of radiation and in deciding how long each treatment will last, often using a computer.

- The *radiation technologist* or *therapist*, a specially trained technician who operates the radiation equipment and positions the patient for treatment.

- The *radiation therapy nurse*, a registered nurse who has trained extensively in oncology and the care of people receiving radiation therapy. For instance, he or she is familiar with the side effects of radiation therapy and will be able to give you information about coping with fatigue, appetite loss, and skin reactions.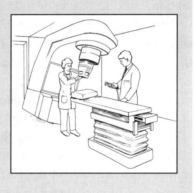

External Beam Radiation Therapy

External beam radiation therapy is used for many different tumors, including cancers in the head and neck area, breast, lung, rectum, and prostate. A machine positioned several feet from the person being treated strikes the target area with radiation.

Low-energy, or orthovoltage, radiation does not penetrate very deeply into the body and is used mainly to treat surface tumors, such as skin cancer.

High-energy, or megavoltage, x-ray radiation is used to treat most other cancers. Megavoltage is able to penetrate the skin. It is strong enough to penetrate the skin as well as most internal organs and structures; and it is able to strike deep tumors. Equally important, megavoltage radiation doesn't attain its full strength until it has reached some depth in the body. This means that the skin and tissues close to the skin receive only mild radiation, which usually causes only minor and temporary side effects. Moreover, the radiation beam is often directed from more than one location so that the radiation is focused on the tumor, sparing all but a small margin of surrounding normal tissue.

Typically, external beam radiation is given in a daily dose or fraction, Monday through Friday, for several weeks. (Doses given twice a day are called hyperfractionated. This altered fractionation is sometimes necessary for tumors that are not very responsive to radiation.)

Planning External Beam Radiation Treatment. Before the therapy begins, a team of specialists plans how the treatment will be carried out. This treatment planning procedure uses a simulator and treatment planning computer to create images of the areas to be treated and to plan the procedure.

A special diagnostic x-ray machine, called a radiation simulator, maps the treatment area. In fact, the simulator does everything the treatment machine does except deliver the radiation beam. Ultrasound or a computerized tomography (CT) scan may also be used to help pinpoint the location of the tumor.

While undergoing radiation simulation in what may be called a marking session, you must lie very still on a table or special chair in the position you will assume for the treatment. For the next thirty minutes to two hours, the simulator and/or other devices are used to make careful measurements, locate the tumor, and delineate the areas on your body through which the radiation will be directed. Then the port will be drawn on your body and a small number of tattoos placed in strategic places so the beam can always be directed at the same place on your body. The rest of the markings are then washed off.

Finally, using the images that precisely locate the tumor, the planning team—which includes a radiologist, a physicist, and a dosimetrist—determines, with the aid of a treatment-planning computer, the best plan for treating the tumor. They will consider the size of the tumor and how sensitive it is to radiation as well as the ability of the normal healthy tissue to tolerate the therapy. The dose is measured in grays or rads: 1 gray = 100 rads.

The ultimate success of treatment depends in part on how successfully the cancer cells continue to multiply between fractions. Allowing too much time to pass between fractions gives cells an opportunity to double; and the more cells there are, the less likely it is that a dose of radiation will destroy them all. Therefore, the interval between treatments must be reasonably short for the radiation to kill the greatest number of cancer cells.

Body Supports and Shields. Before the treatment begins, foam, plaster, or plastic devices may be custom-made to conform to the body. During the treatment, these will help you remain comfortably in the proper position.

The radiation team often produces customized "blocks." These blocks, which are made of either lead or "Cerrobend," a lead-like material that is easy to mold, are designed to protect normal tissues and organs. During treatment, these are attached to a transparent plate located between you and the radiation source. During radiation therapy for Hodgkin's disease, for instance, the blocks may be arranged to protect the lungs and larynx. Newer linear accelerators can actually shape the field properly without the use of blocks.

Treatment Intervals. External beam radiation therapy is usually given five days a week for five to eight weeks or more, though this schedule may vary. (This schedule prevents the skin and normal tissue from receiving too much radiation at one time.) For instance, radiotherapy may last for two to three weeks when given mainly to treat symptoms. For a slow-growing skin cancer, radiation may be administered only two to three times a week for three to five weeks. Split-course therapy allows several weeks off in the middle of a radiation treatment to allow the body time to recover from minor side effects while the tumor regresses. For treatments that are not responsive to radiation, patients may be treated twice a day, in what's called a hyperfractionated schedule. This sometimes seems to enhance the effect of radiation.

Intraoperative Radiation Therapy (IORT). Radiation is sometimes used to treat the tumor or adjacent tissue during surgery. This technique, which utilizes external radiation beam equipment and a special adapter, makes it possible to deliver a large dose of radiation to the tumor without harming healthy tissue in the path of the beam. IORT is often used as a preventive measure, to destroy stray cancer cells that may proliferate, even though the initial tumor has just been removed. It's most commonly used in abdominal or pelvic cancer.

Stereotactic Radiation Therapy. Currently, this type of radiotherapy is used to treat brain cancers, but as the technology evolves, this technique may one day be used to treat tumors in other sites. Stereotactic radiation therapy involves targeting a tumor from many different directions so a large, precise radiation dose converges on a small tumor. In that way, the amount of radiation needed to destroy tumor cells is delivered directly to the growth, but the amount of exposure to the area surrounding the tumor is minimal.

During the procedure, the person's head is held perfectly still by a temporary frame surgically attached to the skull. Then, using a map based on images of the tumor and the brain obtained from computerized tomography (CT) scans, magnetic resonance imaging (MRI), and/or arteriography, a movable, robot-like arm of the x-ray machine is guided by a computer around the head, delivering hundreds of beams of radiation to the brain during a typical forty-minute session.

Special immobilization devices that allow stereotactic treatment without requiring surgery are now available at a number of institutions.

Conformal Radiation Therapy. In this method, computers map the location of the cancer and then the beam targets the cancer from several directions. Long-term advantages of this technique over the usual method of external beam

INFORM

YOURSELF

What to Expect During External Beam Therapy

Typically, external beam therapy is given on an outpatient basis, although sometimes it is begun in the hospital and completed at a clinic. In any case, you may have to undress at least partly, depending on what part of your body is being treated. So it is wise to wear loose-fitting clothing that is easily removed.

The actual treatment takes only a few minutes, though you may spend as many as fifteen to thirty minutes in the treatment room "setting up." This room is designed to contain the radiation.

First, you are asked to lie on a cushioned table, which is then positioned beneath the radiation machine. The technicians focus the machine according to the parameters determined during the simulation. Any pads, casts, or other immobilizing devices designed for you are put in place to ensure that you are in precisely the right position. Lead blocks or shields may be suspended from the machine to protect areas of your body further. These blocks shape the beam so that it is exactly on target.

Once you are positioned correctly, the technicians go into an adjacent room where they can monitor you on closed-circuit TV and talk to you over an intercom.

The machine is then turned on. Radiation equipment is large and often noisy. It may whir, click, or sound something like a vacuum cleaner as it moves around to aim at the cancer from different angles.

Radiation therapy does not hurt, though some people have a sensation of warmth or mild tingling, which is normal. Once the machine delivers the prescribed dose to your body, usually in less than a minute, it is turned off and the therapist returns to help you out of the immobilization devices. You can then dress and leave. Depending on the size of the radiation field and the part of the body being treated, you may not need to be accompanied to your radiation treatment and may be able to drive yourself home. In fact, many people continue to work and engage in their normal activities while receiving courses of radiation therapy.

radiation are not yet known, but it is being used increasingly, particularly to treat prostate cancer. The theoretical advantage of this approach is that the radiation is concentrated on the tumor and spares the surrounding tissue.

Internal Radiation Therapy

Internal radiation therapy, also called brachytherapy, places radioactive material inside the body to deliver radiation to the tumor at point-blank range. Sometimes the radioactive material is inserted into a body cavity, or it may be injected or swallowed in a special solution. Most often, however, internal therapy involves implanting a radioactive substance in or near the tumor.

The most common radiation sources are iridium, cesium, iodine, phosphorus, and gold, all of which give off low-energy radiation, which makes it easier to spare healthy tissue. The advantage of this method is that more radiation can be delivered to the target within a shorter time than with external radiation. Also, the source of radiation is close to the cancer cells so that less healthy tissue is exposed, and higher doses can be used than those in external beam radiation.

Internal radiation therapy is often used as an adjunct to external treatment to avoid the side effects of using full doses of either. For instance, it is used in combination with external beam radiation to treat prostate cancer. This can help avoid damage to the rectum caused by the external beam. There are several ways of placing radiation inside the body. These procedures usually require hospitalization.

Interstitial Radiation Therapy. Using local or general anesthesia, a radiation oncologist places an implant that will contain radioactive material directly into the tumor and the surrounding tissues. Later it is filled with ribbons of radioactive seeds, which are smaller than grains of rice.

When the ribbons are added after the tubes are in place, the procedure is known as afterloading. Afterloading takes place in the person's hospital room following surgery.

Implants typically remain in place for three to five days while the radioactive source decays, giving off radiation that the tumor absorbs. Like the batteries in a flashlight that gradually lose their power, the radioactive material inside the body gives off less and less energy over time. Most interstitial implants are removed once the prescribed dose has been delivered, but some are left in the body permanently.

Interstitial radiation therapy is a common treatment for cancers of the mouth, tongue, lip, neck, and prostate.

Intracavitary Radiation Therapy. A radiation oncologist places a container into a body space, most commonly the vagina or uterus. Usually the radioactive source is afterloaded into the container. When the specified dose of radiation has been delivered to the tumor (over forty-eight to seventy-two hours), the doctor removes the container containing the isotope.

Intraluminal Radiation Therapy. Intraluminal radiation therapy delivers radiation to hollow organs. In esophageal cancer, for instance, a surgeon or a radiation oncologist inserts a specially designed tube or container into the lumen, or opening, of the esophagus. A special imaging technique allows insertion of small radioactive sources into the tube near the tumor so it receives a specified dose of radiation.

High-Dose Rate Remote Afterloading. This method of brachytherapy uses containers similar to those used for intracavitary or intraluminal radiation therapy, but does not require manual loading of a radioactive source. Instead, the radiation is delivered remotely from a machine into the container through a special conduit or catheter. The same radiation dose that may take days to deliver using other implant methods can be given as an outpatient treatment.

Radiopharmaceuticals. Radioactive materials can be administered by mouth, injected intravenously, or inserted into a body cavity. For example, radioactive strontium (Metastron) is one of the radiopharmaceuticals sometimes used to kill cancer cells that have spread to the bones. Sometimes a radiopharmaceutical is used in combination with external beam radiation.

Radioactive iodine is sometimes given by intravenous injection to destroy thyroid gland tissue—and the thyroid cancer that absorbs the iodine—that is not removed surgically. It is not used to treat anaplastic and medullary thyroid cancers, and there is disagreement on its usefulness for those with small tumors that have not spread to surrounding tissue.

Radioactive phosphorus 32 can be injected into the abdominal cavity or linings around the lungs.

INFORM

YOURSELF

What to Expect During Implant Radiation

Most implants are done in a hospital, where you will need to stay for several days. Depending on the type of implant you receive, you may undergo minor surgery—with either local or general anesthesia—to enable placement of the empty container into your body. You will then be taken to your room so that the radioactive material can be afterloaded, or placed inside the container.

While the radioactive source is in place, you will remain in your room. Often you must sit or lie very still in bed so that the implant does not shift. You may undergo certain procedures to ensure that you're comfortable and that the treatment will be as effective as possible. For instance, for implants in the vagina or uterus, an enema is given the night before surgery, and a catheter is inserted into the bladder so that you won't have to use a bedpan or move about. The bladder and rectum may be packed with gauze to protect them from the radioactive implant. These procedures are generally done at the same time the container is put in place.

Likewise, if implants are placed in your head or neck, a tube may be inserted in your nose so you can receive liquid nourishment in case you cannot chew or swallow.

During the days that the radiation is active, you will be cared for by nurses trained to deal with radiation. They will be able to provide everything you need, but to protect themselves they will work quickly and may often speak to you from the door of your room or behind a lead shield. You may be able to have visitors for short periods of time, although some hospitals do not allow them. Pregnant women should not visit, since the fetus could be harmed by even small amounts of radiation.

Once the treatment is over, the implants are usually removed (although some are left in permanently and are harmless). You will then be able to check out of the hospital.

New Therapies

Besides these fairly conventional methods of radiation therapy, a few other promising techniques are currently being studied.

Radiosensitizers or Chemical Modifiers. Drugs called chemical or clinical sensitizers are being studied to see if they enhance the effects of radiation. For instance, some drugs, such as Etanidazole, take the place of oxygen in hypoxic cells (cells that don't receive enough oxygen); others transport oxygen to hypoxic cells; and still others are taken up by the DNA in a cell, inhibiting its ability to repair itself after being damaged by radiation. Some drugs such as Flusol DA both transport oxygen and make cellular repair difficult. None of these drugs has yet been shown to improve the results of radiation therapy.

Will I Be Radioactive?

SPECIAL

CONCERNS

Because of the powerful effects of radiation, people often are afraid that even when it is used therapeutically, they will become permanently radioactive. They won't. In fact, with external radiation therapy, even the cells targeted by the high-energy waves are affected only for a moment.

When radioactive particles are injected into the body or swallowed, a very small and harmless amount of radiation may be emitted from the body. If the source of radiation is contained in a closed implant, the radioactive material cannot escape, although precautions are taken nevertheless. For these reasons, you are hospitalized and your visitors are limited. A pregnant woman, whose fetus is vulnerable to even small doses of radiation, is not allowed to visit. In fact, some hospitals do not allow visitors at all. Being touched and cared for poses no risk to anyone, provided the exposure time is limited. The health professionals assigned to your care will be able to tell you and your visitors what a safe exposure time is.

If you are given a permanent implant (such as sometimes used to treat prostate cancer) and discharged from the hospital, the amount of radiation you receive and others are exposed to is safe.

People who receive radioactive iodine are kept in isolation until their bodies no longer contain enough radioactivity to be a radiation hazard. They are instructed to drink a lot of fluid to flush the iodine from the body. Kissing and sexual contact must be avoided for a time and contact with children and pregnant women should be brief. Talk to your doctor about how long contact should be restricted.

Hyperthermia. It has been known for some time that tumor cells are sensitive to heat. Heating body tissues to more than 43 degrees centigrade (105 to 110 degrees Fahrenheit) kills cancer cells directly and enhances the effects of radiation.

Tumors are exposed to heat either before or after radiation therapy. Hyperthermia has become an increasingly refined technique, so it is now possible to heat the whole body, specific areas, or just the tumor with ultrasound, microwaves, immersion in a heated bath, or a heat probe inserted into the tumor.

Boron Neutron Capture Therapy. This experimental therapy is sometimes used to treat brain tumors. When a boron compound is injected, the boron is absorbed by the brain tumor. When the brain is irradiated with neutrons and the boron is bombarded, a type of high-energy radiation is released to destroy the tumor cells, but it does not penetrate far into normal brain tissue. The value of this approach is still undetermined.

Side Effects

Although enormous efforts are made to prevent the radiation beam from striking normal tissue, some contact is unavoidable and side effects often occur. Some of these affect the area being treated; others are more general. But most of them are temporary, and there are ways to cope with them.

If side effects are severe and debilitating, the type of treatment or the schedule may be adjusted. Although a break in treatment may be prescribed, this is a last resort since it may delay the effectiveness of radiation therapy.

When Should I Call the Doctor?

If you have any of these problems, tell your doctor at once:

- A pain that doesn't go away, especially if it's in the same place.

- Lumps, bumps, or swelling.

- Nausea, vomiting, diarrhea, loss of appetite, or difficulty swallowing.

- Unexplained weight loss.

- A fever or cough that doesn't go away.

- Unusual rashes, bruises, or bleeding.

- Any other signs mentioned by your doctor or nurse.

Fatigue

Tiredness and lethargy are among the most common reactions to radiation therapy, especially among people who are receiving radiation to large areas, such as the abdomen. Fatigue is likely to begin early and increase during the course of treatment, peaking between the third and fifth weeks.

Why the body reacts to radiation in this way isn't exactly understood, although there are a number of plausible explanations. It may be that the healing process drains the body's energy. Another reason may be the buildup of toxic wastes resulting from cell destruction. An increase in the body's metabolism may play a role, too. Furthermore, daily trips to a radiation center disrupt the normal activities of life and may cut into rest time. (For more information about fatigue and cancer, see Chapter 24.)

Poor Appetite

Many people receiving radiation lose their appetite. This may happen because changes in the body's cells affect hunger signals or because the perception of taste is altered. The stress of being sick also takes a toll on the desire to eat. It is important not to give in, however, because the energy that food provides is vital to the damaged tissues that are trying to repair themselves. It's important to communicate appetite and nutrition problems to the doctor as soon as they occur so that they can be attended to promptly (see Chapter 18).

A simple multivitamin may be advised to help ensure adequate nutrients, but it's best to avoid high doses of supplements. For instance the antioxidant vitamins A, E, and C may interfere with radiation therapy. Antioxidants prevent the formation of DNA-damaging ions, but radiation therapy works by producing ions that damage the DNA of cancer cells. Before taking any vitamin, mineral, herb, or other nutritional supplement, check with your doctor.

Perking Up Your Appetite

While you're receiving radiation, you may have digestive problems and not feel like eating, but it is very important to overcome this temporary loss of appetite. Your body is being bombarded with radiation and is using extra energy, therefore it needs more than the usual amount of calories and nutrients. The trick is to note when during the day you feel most like eating and then to take advantage of that time.

Eat when you're hungry, even if it's not a regular mealtime and even if it means eating several small meals each day, rather than three big ones. Be sure to have healthy snacks, such as low-fat frozen yogurt, fruits, and fruit juices. If you are losing weight, you may need to choose high-calorie snacks or nutritional supplements. Take the time to make your meals as pleasant as possible: play your favorite music, watch television, read, or dine with friends—whatever makes eating enjoyable for you. And if friends offer to cook for you, don't hesitate to tell them the foods you like. See Chapter 18 for more information about nutrition and appetite during treatment.

Skin Problems

The skin surrounding the area receiving radiation therapy undergoes some temporary changes, reacting much as it would to a long day at the beach without sunscreen. About two weeks after the therapy begins, the skin begins to redden and becomes very dry and itchy. Occasionally, it may peel as the cells in the top layer of skin shed. Rarely, a reaction called moist desquamation may occur, in which skin folds (under the breasts and buttocks, for example) become wet and often very sore. Most skin reactions go away a few weeks after treatment is completed. When hair loss occurs, it's important to care for the skin that was covered by hair the same as skin in any area affected by radiation.

Caring for Your Skin

Technical improvements have greatly reduced the amount of radiation absorbed by the skin, but local, temporary reactions do occur. You may continue your usual bathing routine. The only skin that will be affected is in the area receiving the radiation. Here are some ways to minimize and treat these problems:

- Wash the skin in the treatment area gently with warm water, and pat it dry; don't rub it. If you must use soap, use a mild, unscented one. Take care not to wash away the skin markings.

- Do not use lotions, creams, perfumes, deodorant, powder, pre-shave or aftershave lotions, hair removal products, makeup, or other scented or alcohol-containing skin preparations on the affected area unless approved by your doctor.

- You may be able to relieve dryness with moisturizing creams and lotions such as Eucerin, Aquaphor, lanolin, or gels containing aloe vera (check with your doctor or nurse). Avoid petroleum jelly, since it is insoluble and hard to remove.

- Do not use adhesive tape or rub or scrub treated skin.

- Wear loose-fitting, cotton clothing over the skin exposed to radiation, and avoid tight girdles, hose, bras, and close-fitting collars.

- Do not use hot water bottles, heating pads, heat lamps, or cold packs on the area.

- Wear protective clothing in cold weather, and avoid sunlight on the treatment area, particularly while you are receiving treatment. Apply a broad-spectrum sunscreen with an SPF of 15 or higher, and/or cover the area to provide additional protection. After the radiotherapy has been completed, the treated area will likely remain more sensitive to sunlight and cold, so you need to take similar precautions for at least a year.

Hair Loss

Radiation therapy will cause hair loss in the area being treated. The amount that grows back and the texture and density of the hair will vary according to the type and dose of radiation administered.

Local Reactions

Some symptoms are responses of the organ or structure receiving radiation. They usually are temporary and are experienced differently by different people.

Effects on the Mouth. When the radiation is directed to the head and neck, the mucous membranes of the mouth may become red. You may have difficulty swallowing and suffer from xerostomia, extreme dryness of the mouth and lips. Your sense of taste may be impaired, particularly if your tongue is in range of the radiation beam, and your salivary glands may be unable to produce a normal amount of saliva, thereby contributing to the dryness. Drinking a lot of fluids and sucking on hard candy should provide some relief.

Moisten foods with gravy or sauces. Do not use alcohol-containing mouthwash; it can intensify the radiation reaction. Do not smoke or drink alcohol during your treatment. Avoid sugary snacks, spices, and coarse foods, such as raw vegetables, nuts, and dry crackers. Don't eat very hot or cold foods.

Meticulous mouth care can help you avoid complications affecting your mouth and teeth. Special, gentle care is needed because of mouth soreness. Use a very soft brush and a fluoride toothpaste to clean teeth and gums after meals and at least once more each day. Rinse after brushing with cool water or a solution of one teaspoon baking soda to a quart of water. Gently floss between teeth once a day with unwaxed dental tape. And, if a dentist prescribes it, apply fluoride regularly.

It may be necessary to remove dentures for a while if the gums are sore. Mouth dryness that isn't relieved with sipping cool drinks throughout the day may be helped by artificial saliva.

Effects on the Stomach and Bowel. Radiation therapy directed to the abdominal or pelvic area may cause nausea and vomiting. Antinausea drugs taken before therapy and as needed afterward may prevent or relieve these reactions. Diarrhea, along with cramping, gassiness, and bloating, may occur in the third or fourth week of treatment. Radiation affects the function of the bowel, and food slips through the body without being properly absorbed. A clear liquid diet as soon as the diarrhea begins is recommended. When the diarrhea improves, eat small, frequent meals and avoid high-fiber foods. Avoid milk and milk products, too, if they are irritating. Since potassium is lost when you have diarrhea, include dietary sources such as bananas, potatoes, and apricots in your meals and snacks. Over-the-counter preparations for diarrhea, such as Kaopectate, Immodium, or prescription medications such as Lomotil help. Some people complain of queasiness immediately after being treated. It may be helpful to eat a bland snack before the treatment or not to eat at all for a few hours before and an hour or two after the treatment. Antinausea medication is also helpful.

Effects on the Bladder. Radiation to the pelvis can also cause temporary bladder irritation, causing discomfort and frequent urination. A drug called pyridium can help alleviate these symptoms. Women may have vaginal itching, burning, and dryness. Intercourse may be painful for women, and some may notice slight bleeding afterward even if they don't have pain.

A long-term side effect of pelvic irradiation is scarring which can shorten or narrow the vagina. To prevent this from happening, it will help to have intercourse three or four times a week during treatment and about two to three weeks afterward. Or a woman may use a rubber or plastic dilator similar to a large tampon to stretch the vagina for a few minutes each day until about two to three weeks after the radiation is complete.

Effects on the Lungs. Radiation to the chest may cause difficulty swallowing, a cough, and even shortness of breath. Any of these side effects should be reported to the doctor. Some medications, such as steroids, may relieve the inflammation that keeps the lungs from expanding fully.

Effects on the Breasts. People who receive radiation therapy as part of breast cancer treatment may notice that their breasts are sore and may swell. The breasts may feel more sensitive, and skin changes that last a month or two after treatment may be annoying. If you must wear a bra, choose one that is made of soft cotton with no underwires. Shoulder stiffness may be relieved with flexibility exercises and stretching. Long-term changes include a change in skin color, skin pore size, breast firmness, and perhaps breast size. If any changes are noticed more than a year after therapy, they should be reported to your doctor.

Long-Term Effects

Whereas physical responses such as fatigue and tissue damage become apparent during the course of treatment, some side effects do not appear until after the treatment has been completed. Chronic side effects or reactions can occur months or years later and affect the body part that was treated.

Effects on Reproductive Organs. For some people receiving radiation treatment in the pelvic area, the most feared irreversible side effect is diminished fertility. Women may have difficulty becoming pregnant, sometimes stop menstruating, and experience symptoms of menopause. The infertility may be permanent in some cases; however, it's sometimes possible to prevent sterility by shielding the ovaries during treatment so they are not damaged. Nevertheless, women of childbearing age are urged to practice careful birth control to avoid conceiving while undergoing radiation therapy.

For men, radiation to the testicles can reduce both the number of sperm and their ability to fertilize an egg. Many men have their sperm stored in a sperm bank before beginning radiation therapy. Some men may become impotent after radiation to the prostate gland, and men who have had radiation to the pelvis may also have erection problems (see Chapter 21).

Risk of Developing Another Cancer. It is rare, but radiation therapy may cause the very disease it is treating. Evidence suggests that low doses of radiation increase cancer incidence. This means in a few cases, it may eventually lead to a second primary cancer. The most common radiation-induced cancer is leukemia, which usually shows up from five to nine years after therapy. Thyroid cancer, breast cancer, lung cancer, and sarcomas can appear fifteen years or more after treatment if these areas of the body were subjected to the radiation beam.

The incidence of radiation-induced cancer is quite low, however, and depends on several factors. The younger a person is when he or she receives radiation treatment, the greater the risk will be of developing cancer later. Also, the risk is greater with certain types of cancer, namely Hodgkin's disease and non-Hodgkin's lymphoma. Experts believe that not treating a cancer with radiation is a greater risk than the chance that a secondary cancer will occur as a result of the treatment. Some radiation-induced cancers can be prevented. For example, lung cancer is much less likely to occur after radiation to the chest for Hodgkin's disease if you don't smoke.

Emotional Effects

Having a life-threatening illness is enough to evoke fear, anger, depression, anxiety, a sense of helplessness, and other strong feelings, and the fatigue that accompanies radiation therapy only makes these feelings worse. Having to schedule daily radiation appointments—and get to them—also adds to the emotional mix, as does coping with uncomfortable side effects.

It is important to keep in mind that most of the unpleasantness that may develop with radiation therapy will, in all likelihood, last only as long as the treatment continues or for only a limited time afterward. Once the course of therapy is over, a significant step will have been taken in treating the cancer. A support group or therapy group can be helpful in easing emotional symptoms and even some physical ones. See Chapters 8, 26, and 27 for more information on coping, getting support, and help with managing your feelings.

Follow-up Care

Sometimes the tumor shows measurable changes in size during treatment, but more likely it will take weeks or months after therapy for a tumor to shrink significantly. Some people return to their primary oncologist for follow-up care immediately after their radiation therapy is completed, and others continue to see their radiation oncologist frequently for a while after treatment. During the follow-up visits, blood tests and x-rays are taken to determine the response to treatment and whether further therapy is needed. If it proves necessary, these tests help in the decision about the type of treatment to use next.

The lingering effects of radiation therapy may require some additional care. For instance, some skin reactions take a while to heal, and fatigue continues as tissues regenerate. If you experience these persistent symptoms, continue caring for yourself as you did during treatment—being gentle with the skin and taking naps. As your energy levels increase, you can ease back into a normal daily routine, including work, exercise, and sexual activity.

12

Chemotherapy

A t some point in their treatment, most people with cancer receive one or more of over 100 anticancer drugs. These drugs are used to destroy cancer and often represent the only method capable of treating widespread disease. Surgery and radiation therapy are local therapies that treat a malignant tumor and the area directly surrounding it. Chemotherapy destroys cancer cells that have metastasized to parts of the body far from the primary tumor. This bodywide, or systemic, capability is due to the fact that medications enter the bloodstream and are distributed throughout the body to kill cancer cells wherever they are.

Chemotherapy may either cure the cancer or lead to its remission. It may control the disease by slowing the tumor's growth, if not stopping it, or preventing its spread. It also may be used to relieve symptoms and improve quality of life.

All the tissues and organs of the body are subject to an anticancer drug's action, which is to destroy rapidly dividing cells or prevent them from reproducing. Cancer cells, which continuously divide and replace themselves, are obvious targets. But some healthy cells that are also continuously dividing— such as those in the bone marrow, hair follicles, and lining the mouth, stomach, and intestines—are vulnerable to the drugs as well. Consequently, low blood cell counts, temporary hair loss, mouth sores, nausea, and diarrhea are common side effects.

The side effects have given chemotherapy such a bad reputation, that it has become the most anxiety-provoking treatment that people with cancer face. Fortunately, being educated about chemotherapy and more clearly understanding its benefits helps people manage their anxiety and tolerate the treatments much more easily than in the past (see Chapter 27). The challenge for the oncologist is to balance the cancer-destroying benefits of a particular drug or combination of drugs against their toxic effects. It is sometimes quite a delicate balance, but with good emotional and physical care and support, the side effects can be managed in most cases and, if not fully controlled, at least made tolerable.

How Chemotherapy Destroys Cancer Cells

All cells, healthy and malignant, pass through distinct phases in their life cycle: the stage during which the cell replicates genetic material (DNA); the mitotic stage, during which the cell is dividing; and the resting stage. Chemotherapy drugs are designed to disrupt a cell's function at one or all of these stages. Cell cycle dependent agents kill only cells actively undergoing DNA replication or division; cell cycle independent drugs kill both resting and dividing cells. Often, combinations of these drugs are used.

Most cancer drugs belong to one of several classes of drugs used in chemotherapy. They are categorized by how they affect chemicals in cancer cells, how they interfere with the cell's function, and what phases of the cell's cycle they affect.

- *Alkylating agents* are cell cycle nonspecific, meaning they work in all phases of the cell cycle. They bind with DNA, preventing the cell from dividing. These were the first anticancer drugs. Examples are cyclophosphamide (Cytoxan), melphalan (Alkeran), busulfan (Myleran), dacarbazine (DTIC-Dome), ifosfamide (IFEX), mechlorethamine (Mustargen), and mitomycin C (Mutamycin). Nitrosoureas are also called alkylating agents. Examples include carmustine (BiCNU) and lomustine (CCNU).

- *Antimetabolites* are cell cycle specific because they prevent the cell from making DNA or ribonucleic acid (RNA). Sometimes they do this by making it hard for the cell to make the nucleic acids that are the building blocks of DNA or RNA. Examples of this are fluorouracil (5-FU) and methotrexate. Other antimetabolites mimic the nucleotides needed for producing DNA or RNA and interfere with their production. Examples are gemcitabine (Gemzar), cytarabine (Ara-C), and fludarabine (Fludara). If the cell cannot make DNA, it cannot enter its S-phase (when DNA is being replicated) and divide. Without RNA, the cancer cell cannot make the proteins it needs for its growth.

- *Platinum drugs* are chemicals that contain platinum. They bind to DNA and block it from functioning. They are cell cycle nonspecific and work mostly in the growth phase of cancer cells. The most commonly used platinum compounds are cisplatin (Platinol) and carboplatin (Paraplatin).

- *Mitotic inhibitors* are plant alkaloids that are cell cycle specific and work during the mitosis phase when the cell actually divides to form two cells. They inhibit enzymes necessary for cell division. Examples are vincristine (Oncovin), vinblastine (Velban), VP-16, VM-26, paclitaxel (Taxol), docetaxel (Taxotere), etoposide (VePesid), and vinorelbine (Navelbine).

- *Antitumor antibiotics* are cell cycle nonspecific. They are called antibiotics because they were originally isolated from growing microorganisms just like the antibiotics used to treat bacterial infections, but they are much more toxic. These drugs mainly work by interfering with DNA and sometimes RNA. Examples are mitomycin C (Mutamycin), doxorubicin (Adriamycin), bleomycin (Blenoxane), dactinomycin (Cosmegen), daunorubicin (Cerubidine), and idarubicin (Idamycin).

- *Topoisomerase inhibitors* are a new class of drugs called campothecins. These also interfere with DNA and RNA formation. The two drugs in use today are called topotecan (Hycamtin) and irinotecan (Camptosar, Camptothecan-11, CPT-11).

- *Sex hormones* occur naturally in the body and support the growth of tissues such as the breast and prostate. Tumors in these organs also often depend on hormones to grow. Because of this, one strategy to treat cancers in these organs has been to block the action of the appropriate hormone. For example, the antiestrogen drug tamoxifen (Nolvadex) is given to women with breast cancer when estrogen receptors are present in tumor cells. Examples of hormonal therapy for breast cancer are antiestrogens, progestins, aromatase inhibitors, which block estrogen production in the adrenal glands, and occasionally androgens (male hormones). For prostate cancer, antiandrogens such as flutamide (Eulexin), bicalutamide (Casodex), and nilutamide (Nilandron), luteinizing hormone–releasing hormones (LHRH), agonists such as leuprolide acetate (Lupron) and goserelin acetate (Zoladex), which block testosterone production, and occasionally estrogens are used.

- *Corticosteroid hormones* have many medical uses, but when they are used to kill cancer cells, they are considered chemotherapy drugs. They are often used with other types of chemotherapy drugs to increase their effectiveness. Examples include prednisone and dexamethasone.

New Therapies

New drugs, new combinations of chemotherapy drugs, and new delivery techniques hold significant promise for curing or controlling cancer and improving the quality of life of people with cancer, including:

- New chemotherapy drugs that are directed against new targets in the cancer cells, such as Gleevec, which blocks an enzyme needed for the growth of some types of leukemia cells, and arsenic trioxide (Trisenox), which makes another type of leukemia cells transform into normal cells.

- Novel approaches to targeting drugs more specifically at the cancer cells (like attaching drugs to monoclonal antibodies or packaging them inside liposomes) to produce fewer side effects.

- Drugs to reduce side effects include chemoprotective agents such as mesna, dexrazoxane, and amifostine (amifostine prevents cisplatin toxicity to kidneys and dry mouth from radiation).

- Antiangiogenesis drugs, which stop the development of the blood vessels necessary for a tumor's growth and cause few side effects.

New Chemotherapy Drugs

Every year, many chemotherapy agents are tested in phase I and II clinical trials. Clinical trials determine optimum doses of these drugs and whether the drugs are effective in treating the cancers (see Chapter 16). Some drugs transform cancer cells into normal cells; others are new formulations of existing drugs that are hoped to be more effective; and still others activate or inhibit proteins in order to control cancer growth.

Two chemotherapy drugs that have recently proven successful in these trials are Gleevec and arsenic trioxide. Gleevec is very effective in treating chronic myelogenous leukemia. It works by interfering with a novel protein in the leukemia cells that seems to be responsible for the growth of the cells. Arsenic trioxide (Trisenox) causes the leukemia cells in people with a rare type of leukemia (acute promyelocyitic leukemia) to transform into normal cells.

Another drug that has been successful is capecitabine (Xeloda), a form of the 5-FU chemotherapy drug that can be given orally. Although it is not a new kind of drug, its new formulation may make it more effective than standard 5-FU treatment. Another agent used mostly for brain tumors is temozolamide (Temodar). This drug can cause modest shrinkage of some brain tumors.

Several new agents that are chemically similar to older drugs are being tested in these phase I and II studies. Only a few examples are listed here because although many drugs exist, most will not be more effective than the drugs that are used now. One drug being tested is rebeccamycin, which is an antibiotic. Another is nearabine, which acts to prevent DNA synthesis. Several drugs are being tested that are similar to existing drugs like paclitaxel (Taxol) or irinotecan (Camptosar) or etoposide (VePesid) but may be more powerful.

The most exciting area of new drug discovery is in drugs that block specific proteins in the cancer cell. For example, a drug called SCH 66336 blocks farnesyl transferase, an enzyme that causes a special cell protein called

Ras to become activated, which then causes the cell to grow out of control. There are several drugs being studied that inhibit other proteins that seem to be important in the development of cancer cells. None of these are ready to be used on patients except in clinical trials.

Liposomal Therapies

New research has also included new agents such as liposomal therapies, which reduce the severity of side effects. Liposomal therapy is a new technique that uses chemotherapy drugs that have been packaged inside liposomes (synthetic fat globules). These liposomes, or fatty coatings, help the drugs penetrate the cancer cells more selectively and decrease possible side effects (such as hair loss and nausea and vomiting). Examples of liposomal medications are Doxil (the encapsulated form of doxorubicin) and Daunoxome (the encapsulated form of daunorubicin).

See Chapter 13 for information about monoclonal antibodies, which can be designed to guide chemotherapy medications to tumors, but are also used without chemotherapy, as immunotherapy drugs.

Chemoprotective Agents

Some drugs are given to protect people from the side effects of chemotherapy or in one case, radiation therapy. Mesna (Mesnex) is a drug given with alkylating agents such as ifosfamide or cyclophosphamide to protect the bladder from the toxic effects of these drugs since they are excreted from the body through the kidneys. A second drug, dexraxoxane (Zinecard), is helpful in reducing heart damage by drugs such as the antitumor antibiotic doxorubicin (Adriamycin). Another drug that can protect against chemotherapy damage and radiation damage is amifostine (Ethyol). This drug can help prevent kidney damage in patients receiving the platinum drug cisplatin (Platinol) and is also useful in preventing mouth dryness in patients who have received radiation therapy to their mouth and throat.

Antiangiogenesis

For tumors to be able to grow, new blood vessels must develop (through a process called angiogenesis) to nourish cancer cells. Antiangiogenesis therapy is the use of drugs or other compounds that interfere with the development of new blood vessels that feed the tumor. This can "starve" tumors by cutting off their blood supply.

Angiogenesis shows promise for treating tumors effectively with few side effects. Unlike chemotherapy or radiation, both of which can damage normal cells in addition to cancer cells, antiangiogenesis therapy would simply turn off the growth of new blood vessels without affecting normal cells, whose blood vessels are already established.

Initially, antiangiogenesis substances are most likely to be used in conjunction with conventional chemotherapies. Animal research has shown that combinations of antiangiogenesis substances and chemotherapy drugs or radiation are more effective than chemotherapy or radiation alone.

The potential for antiangiogenesis therapy is enormous. New antiangiogenesis drugs, including angiostatin, endostatin, SU 5416, VEGF inhibitor (anti-VEGF compound), and TNP-470 (AGM-1470) are under development and testing in clinical trials.

What Chemotherapy Can Do

Chemotherapy can cure cancer, particularly if it is given in the early stages of the cancer. When cure can't be achieved, chemotherapy is used shrink cancers or at least to stop the cancer from growing. In advanced cancer, when neither cure nor control can be achieved, it can relieve symptoms by shrinking tumors and is used for palliation—that is, to relieve cancer symptoms even when life cannot be prolonged.

Anticancer, or cytotoxic, chemotherapy can be given before other treatments such as radiation or surgery. In these cases it is called neoadjuvant or primary therapy (see Chapter 15). An advantage of neoadjuvant therapy is that the cancer cells are especially vulnerable because they have not been exposed to other drugs. A disadvantage is that its toxic effects may weaken the body and leave it more susceptible to the side effects of the treatments that follow, such as radiation therapy.

Adjuvant therapy means the chemotherapy is given after other treatments. In this case, the anticancer drugs target stray cancer cells that remain after local therapy with surgery, radiation therapy, or both.

QUESTIONS

TO ASK

What Will Chemotherapy Do for Me?

Before you elect to have chemotherapy you should understand the expected benefits, side effects, and risks. You can get this information from your doctor. Answers to the following questions will give you important facts about your treatment and will help you make a decision about treatment and have realistic expectations about its outcome.

- What is the purpose of chemotherapy for my cancer? Is it likely to kill all the malignant cells in my body so that my disease will be cured or only kill some of them and put my cancer into temporary remission? Or is it designed to relieve the symptoms I'm experiencing, without curing the disease?

- If the chemotherapy is to follow surgery and/or radiation, you might ask: Is this treatment designed to destroy stray cancer cells that may have been missed by the initial treatment? What are the chances that my cancer will recur if I don't have chemotherapy? Will it improve my chances of cure?

- When chemotherapy is suggested before surgery or radiation, you might ask: Why is this approach being recommended? Will it make it easier to remove or irradiate the tumor? What are the chances that the tumor will respond to the drugs?

- What are the potential risks and side effects of the anticancer drug(s) I will be taking? How do they compare with other treatments or with not receiving any treatment at all? Will the quality of my life be better or worse with chemotherapy?

- How will I be taking my medication, how often, and for how long? Will I be given the drugs in the hospital or my doctor's office?

- Are there ways you will help me prepare for the treatment and to lessen the side effects?

- Will my diet be restricted? My activity? Will I have to take a leave of absence from work or curtail my hours? Will I feel like exercising or pursuing hobbies?

- How much will my therapy cost? Will this cost be covered by my insurance or health plan?

Designing a Treatment Plan

Every cancer is unique, and therefore every chemotherapy plan or regimen must be individually tailored by an oncologist. The doctor must choose the drug—or, more commonly, combination of drugs—and determine the dosage, the best way to administer the drugs, how often to give them, and how long the treatment should last.

One of the most important decisions is how much medication to prescribe. Large doses kill more cells. But the greater the dose of chemotherapy, the more likely that it will produce side effects. Still, lowering the dosage to minimize side effects also reduces the chances of success. When the chemotherapy is being given to cure your cancer, the doctor will try to give you the full dose of the drugs. However, since side effects can be so severe and potentially damaging to certain organs, if cure is not possible, oncologists will moderate the dose according to the side effects you experience. There are exceptions, however, and in some cases full drug doses may be the most effective way to kill cancer cells and help you in the long run.

Before Treatment Begins

Because many anticancer drugs are harmful to certain organs, a number of preliminary tests are necessary. For instance, because the bone marrow, where blood cells are formed, is especially susceptible to cytotoxic drugs, a blood sample is obtained to determine that a person with cancer has a healthy number of red and white blood cells and platelets.

Other important tests include an assessment of the health of certain organs, such as the liver, kidney, and heart. All these tests help determine dosages and whether you will be able to tolerate the chemotherapy. For example, a lower-than-normal white blood cell count can indicate a lowered resistance to infection; therefore, drugs known to suppress the immune system will be too risky to use until the person's white blood cell count returns to normal.

Testing also provides baseline information that the treatment team uses throughout chemotherapy to determine how well the drugs are working or if they are causing damage.

Combination Chemotherapy

The current practice is generally to combine two to five or more drugs to treat cancer. This strategy serves several purposes. Anticancer drugs often are more powerful when used in combination (see Chapter 15). Also, if each drug causes different side effects, then a combination that allows the doctor to use lower doses of each drug and still give a higher total dose of drugs can avoid severe side effects. And because malignant cells that are exposed to a particular drug eventually develop a resistance to it, mixing several drugs increases the chances that a cancer will be vulnerable to their anticancer effects.

In order to avoid potentially harmful combinations, the oncologist will also consider other medications the person is taking when determining which drugs to use. It's important to inform your doctor of any medications you are taking, including supplements and over-the-counter drugs. For example, high doses of antioxidants can interfere with the effectiveness of chemotherapy. Other drugs may make side effects worse. Some bodybuilding drugs, for example, contain male hormones, which will make prostate cancer worse. Certain teas increase nausea and perhaps vomiting.

The dosage of drugs prescribed is very individualized. The first factors considered are body weight and height, which can be converted to body surface area. Most cancer drugs are dosed based on body surface area. The dosage is likely to be adjusted for the elderly or the very young, and for those who are not well nourished, who have had radiation therapy, who have low blood cell counts or liver or kidney disease, and/or who are taking other medications.

Treatment Cycles

Chemotherapy is often given in several phases, called cycles. Each cycle consists of administering the drugs, waiting for them to work, and then allowing the body to recover before beginning the next cycle. A woman being treated for breast cancer, for example, might receive chemotherapy in four three-week cycles in order to maximize the benefits of chemotherapy while optimizing her recovery.

During a cycle of therapy, a percentage of cancer cells throughout the body die. Between cycles, the remaining cancer cells continue to divide, but before they can reach their original number, the next onslaught of anticancer drugs begins. These cycles continue until there are sufficiently few cancer cells that the body can handle them on its own. Theoretically, for instance, if one cycle kills 75 out of 100 cancer cells, 25 cells will be left. During the rest interval, these cells might multiply to 27, but then the next cycle of treatment will kill 75 percent of these remaining cells, and so on, until the cells are virtually or completely eliminated. The time between treatments is just long enough to allow healthy body tissues that are sensitive to chemotherapy to recover but not so long that the remaining cancer cells have time to regain their original numbers.

INFORM

YOURSELF

Informed Consent for Chemotherapy

Informed consent is your permission to receive chemotherapy, based on your understanding of the drugs the oncologist recommends, how they will be administered, how often and for how long, what their side effects are, and how likely it is that the therapy will be successful. Although many people think of having to sign an informed consent form only before surgery or an invasive test, it is also sometimes done before chemotherapy. More often, your informed consent is verbal. Generally your doctor will tell you the benefits and side effects of your chemotherapy and you can then accept or reject the treatment. If you are being treated as part of a clinical trial, however, you must be asked to sign an informed consent form.

Understanding these details should make chemotherapy less daunting, so make sure you and your immediate support team understand what you are agreeing to. If you know what to expect, you can prepare for the side effects. Knowing that the treatment may help you get better should also make it easier to take pills on schedule and keep chemotherapy appointments.

How Chemotherapy Is Administered

Chemotherapy drugs are administered in a variety of ways. They can be given by mouth (orally) or applied to the skin (topically). They may also be injected: into a muscle (intramuscularly), under the skin (subcutaneously), into a vein (intravenously), into an artery (intra-arterially), into the cerebrospinal fluid (intrathecally), into the chest cavity (intrapleurally), into the abdominal cavity (intraperitoneally), into the bladder (intravesically), or directly into the tumor (intralesionally).

The method of administration depends on the type of cancer and the particular drug or drug combination. For example, drugs that are not well absorbed by the gastrointestinal tract are injected directly into the bloodstream. Drugs that are in pill, capsule, or liquid form can be taken at home, accompanied by regular visits to the doctor's office to evaluate how well the treatment is working. Injections are usually given in a hospital or doctor's office. Sometimes drugs given intravenously or into a body cavity require a short hospital stay.

Systemic Delivery

When the goal of treatment is to attack metastatic cells, the drugs must enter the bloodstream for delivery throughout the body.

Oral Chemotherapy. Taking anticancer drugs by mouth is more convenient and sometimes less costly than other methods, in large part because you take them at home. The disadvantage is that there are usually a lot of instructions to follow—some drugs require drinking lots of water, some must be taken on an empty stomach, and others should be swallowed with food. Therefore, for oral chemotherapy to be successful, you must keep careful records of which drugs

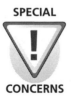

SPECIAL

CONCERNS

Caring for a Catheter

In many ways, having a catheter in place makes the chemotherapy easier, mainly because it avoids multiple injections. But the catheter and the skin around it need special attention. To prevent infection, you must clean the area where the catheter enters the skin and regularly change the bandages covering it. Then a nurse must periodically inject heparin, a drug that prevents blood from clotting and blocking the tube. A nurse will instruct you on how to care for the catheter and practice with you until you feel comfortable doing it yourself.

If you develop a fever while you have a catheter in place, you should notify your doctor. It might be caused by a catheter infection. If an infection does develop around the catheter, you may receive antibiotics, or your doctor may decide to remove the catheter.

are taken and when. Since accidental overdosing could cause serious problems, doctors often prescribe just enough medication for one treatment at a time.

Intramuscular or Subcutaneous Injection. Chemotherapy drugs are occasionally injected into the muscle or under the skin. Although this method does allow for slow absorption, it is not often used because some drugs can damage tissues.

Intravenous (IV) Chemotherapy. The quickest way to get the medication into the bloodstream and to all parts of the body—except perhaps the central nervous system—is by injecting it directly into a vein (IV). There are several ways this can be done.

Push or continuous infusion is one method. A needle or a tiny plastic tube called a catheter is inserted into a vein in the forearm or hand. The oncologist or nurse then either "pushes" the drugs from a syringe directly into the vein or mixes the drug in a solution and allows it to flow slowly into the tube from a bag containing the mixture. This "drip" may take from a few minutes to several hours to complete, depending on the drug. Afterward, the IV catheter is removed.

A drawback to this method is that some people have very small veins and thus it becomes difficult to insert an IV needle or catheter repeatedly for subsequent treatments. Although veins in the hand are easier to see, those in the lower arm have more protective tissue surrounding them and may better withstand repeated needle sticks. Even so, veins can become scarred or collapse after several chemotherapy sessions. Also, some chemotherapy drugs, known as vesicants, can leak out of veins and seriously damage nearby tissue. Even if they don't leak, they can still damage veins.

Extravasation Signs and Symptoms

SPECIAL

CONCERNS

One small risk of chemotherapy is the leakage of drugs from a vein into nearby healthy tissue. Some drugs that are capable of causing serious damage are doxorubicin (Adriamycin), mitomycin (Mutamycin), and vinblastine (Velban). The early signs of leakage may be subtle. Later there may be pain, stinging, burning, or swelling around the area where the drug was injected. After three to five days, the area may become inflamed and painful to the touch, and within about two weeks, ulceration and other damage can develop that affects the function of tendons and nerves in the area.

Fortunately, serious injury is rare, but any unusual symptoms should be promptly reported to your doctor. Usually only a small amount of drug leaks out, and applying ice to the area and changing the injection site are all the treatment necessary.

An alternative to a catheter or needle is a vascular access device (VAD). This is a catheter that can remain painlessly in place in the skin to provide access to a large vein in the chest, neck, or arm. Chemotherapy drugs can be injected directly into a VAD or can be administered through an IV tube connected to the VAD.

There are several types of VADs. In one type, the thin catheter is inserted in the large arm vein and remains there for several weeks. Another type is inserted into a large vein that runs under the collarbone or in the neck. Part of it remains outside the body and is taped to the skin. It can have several openings so that not only can chemotherapy be given through the VAD, but blood can also be sampled from it. Another type is attached to a small metal or plastic port. After the catheter is inserted into the large vessel of the neck or below the collarbone, it is attached to a quarter-sized shallow cup-like structure that is surgically implanted beneath the skin of the chest. Drugs are injected into the port via a needle through the skin that punctures a rubber diaphragm covering the port "cup." The advantage of an implanted port is that it requires no special care, since it is completely under the skin. On the other hand, there is a slight risk that the drug can leak or that the port can shift out of position. It can also be difficult to draw blood out of a port.

All these devices carry the risk of a clot developing in the large vein in which they sit. This clot can interfere with blood returning to your heart from your face and arms and cause them to swell. If you have one of these devices in your vein and your face begins to swell, you should contact your doctor right away.

Vascular Access Systems

A port through which medication can be infused directly into the bloodstream can be implanted beneath the skin. It's usually placed in an inconspicuous place such as just below the collarbone. Medication is injected through a needle into a round chamber about an inch in diameter. The person usually feels a mild prick as the needle enters the covering over the chamber, which is a major advantage over having to have repeated intravenous injections. Once in the chamber, the medication will flow through a flexible tube into the bloodstream. The port can also be used to obtain blood samples.

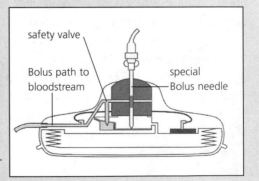

Vascular access system by Arrow International

Regional Chemotherapy

Although chemotherapy is almost always a systemic treatment, sometimes an anticancer drug is delivered directly into the area of the body where the tumor is located, bathing it in larger than usual doses of the drug without affecting healthy cells throughout the body. This increases the chances of destroying localized cancer cells and decreases the risks of the treatment.

Intra-Arterial Chemotherapy. Administering the drug to a tumor via the artery supplying blood to the area where the cancer is located is called intra-arterial chemotherapy. This is done in a hospital, using a special pump that can override the pressure of the blood flow in the artery and allow the drug to travel to the targeted spot. The area of the body most commonly treated this way is the liver.

Intraperitoneal Chemotherapy. Delivering drugs into the abdominal cavity, or peritoneum, is called intraperitoneal chemotherapy. The doctor will place a catheter in the abdomen using local anesthesia in order to deliver the chemotherapy into the abdominal cavity. Intraperitoneal chemotherapy is sometimes used to treat ovarian cancer and can be administered either in the hospital or doctor's office. If the treatment is to be repeated several times, sometimes the catheter will be attached to a port that is surgically implanted in the abdominal wall.

Intravesical Chemotherapy. Bladder cancer is treated by chemotherapy administered directly into the bladder, called intravesical therapy. The drugs flow through a catheter inserted into the bladder for one to three hours. The person being treated shifts position every fifteen minutes so that the drug reaches all areas of the bladder. This therapy is commonly used for early bladder cancer and is usually done in a urologist's office.

Intraventricular and Intrathecal Chemotherapy. Administering drugs directly into the spinal fluid is most often done in treating leukemia and cancers that have spread to the spinal fluid and the tissues surrounding the spinal fluid space. The drugs can be injected directly into the lower spinal canal (which is safe because lower down, the spinal cord has broken into smaller nerve fibers and there is little chance of injuring nerves) by means of a spinal tap (intra-thecal chemotherapy). If these injections are to be repeated often, a surgeon can implant a device like a port under the scalp and threads the small catheter into the fluid-filled center of the brain (called the ventricle). The drug is placed into the Omaya reservoir, which is connected to a catheter that has been placed into the ventricle (intraventricular chemotherapy). Chemotherapy drugs can then be injected directly into the reservoir, avoiding the repeated injections that would be necessary to deliver the drug to the spinal fluid that continuously flows through and around the brain.

Side Effects

Healthy cells that reproduce rapidly and often—such as those in the bone marrow, mouth, stomach, intestines, and hair follicles—are especially susceptible to temporary damage from chemotherapy. Since chemotherapy also may cause serious toxic effects—such as damage to the bone marrow—that can be life-threatening, anyone undergoing treatment must be monitored carefully and the treatment plan changed if the problems become severe. Some examples of toxic effects are a lowered resistance to infection or damage to vital organs.

No two people experience chemotherapy and its side effects in the same way. This is partly because people have inherent differences and responses and partly because their health varies. In addition, each chemotherapy drug differs in its side effects. Many are notorious for inducing nausea, others for causing hair loss, and still others for affecting bone marrow. Most have more than one potential side effect. The side effects also may change as the treatment progresses; some get worse as more and more normal cells succumb to the constant bombardment of drugs. In any case, most are temporary, and there are ways of relieving them.

Nausea and Vomiting

Nausea and vomiting are two of the most common and most dreaded side effects of chemotherapy. Some drugs cause queasiness or are only mildly nauseating; and sometimes a drug induces nausea only when given in large doses. In any case, vomiting occurs because the drug stimulates an area of the brain called the chemoreceptor trigger zone, which then sends a message to the vomiting center. Irritation of the gastrointestinal tract, overeating, motion sickness, or nervousness can also activate this zone. Fortunately, new drugs have been developed that interfere with the activation of the chemoreceptor trigger zone. These are most effective if they are given before chemotherapy treatment.

If nausea, retching, and/or vomiting are going to occur, the side effect usually starts a few hours after treatment (acute onset) and lasts a very short time, but any of these problems may not begin until the day after the treatment. For some people, even the thought of chemotherapy causes nausea and vomiting (anticipatory nausea).

According to one survey, many people receiving chemotherapy have anticipatory nausea, and some vomit before receiving any drugs at all. No one knows why this phenomenon occurs. One theory is that after you have undergone a chemotherapy session that made you sick, you associate the treatment room, the smell of the hospital or clinic, or even the sight of the hospital with nausea. The worse your experience with these side effects, the more likely you will develop anticipatory nausea. Those who are prone to motion sickness or are generally anxious or nervous may be more apt to have this problem.

Most oncologists try to prevent anticipatory nausea by using powerful antiemesis drugs before the first treatment so that chemotherapy is never associated with severe nausea and vomiting. If this did not work, the best way to handle anticipatory nausea is through simple relaxation techniques. For instance, imagining a very pleasant scene can be helpful. You might picture yourself on a beach, feeling the sun on your back and hearing the crash of the waves. Focusing on the detail of this image can distract you from the treatment (see Chapter 27).

Severe nausea and vomiting can last from twelve to twenty-four hours and sometimes a day or two, or you may experience a vague, sick feeling that doesn't let up.

Persistent vomiting can cause dehydration and loss of appetite. Attempts are made to overcome or prevent both nausea and vomiting with medication and/or other measures such as ginger ale or guided imagery so that the body gets the fuel it needs to recover from the drugs' effects.

Coping with Nausea and Vomiting

TIPS AND

ADVICE

Besides taking antinausea medications and practicing relaxation and self-hypnosis techniques (see Chapter 27), there are some simple steps you can take to curb queasiness and curtail vomiting:

- Eat small meals throughout the day. Avoid sweet, fried, or fatty foods, which tend to stimulate the stomach and intestinal tract. Foods that are cold or at room temperature are less likely to have strong aromas that may trigger nausea.

- Eat and drink slowly, chewing the food thoroughly so that you can digest it easily. Small amounts of food are less stimulating.

- Wear loose-fitting clothes to avoid pressure on the abdomen.

- Keep air moving by running a fan or leaving a window open. Patients who are nauseated often perspire and feel as if they might faint. Moving air helps decrease this sensation.

- Drink liquids at least an hour before and after meals, and restrict fluids with meals. Clear unsweetened fruit juices and "flat" ginger ale or other light-colored sodas are often best. (Carbonated beverages produce gas bubbles in the stomach, which can increase the likelihood of vomiting when nauseated.)

- Ginger in tablets or tea may be helpful because of ginger's soothing effect on the lining of the stomach.

- Eat only small amounts for at least a few hours before treatment if you tend to become nauseated during chemotherapy.

- Steer clear of your favorite food while you are sick so you don't begin to associate it with the side effects. Save it for a day when you're feeling good. On your good days, make an attempt to eat regular healthy meals and snacks.

- Try to avoid any sights, sounds, or smells that you associate with nausea and vomiting.

- If morning nausea is a problem, have some dry cereal, toast, or crackers by the bed to eat before you get up. These substances are the least likely to cause nausea. They absorb some of the stomach acids that can cause irritation of the lining of the stomach that could lead to vomiting.

- Rest in a chair after eating, but do not lie down for at least two hours. This helps prevent someone who is nauseated from regurgitating food.

- Relaxation exercises, guided imagery, and soothing music may help you relax.

- Call your doctor or nurse if the antinausea medicine is not reducing the episodes of vomiting, if you cannot keep any liquids down, or if you become faint.

Nausea-Curbing Drugs. Antinausea medications are selected by the oncologist according to how much nausea and vomiting the chemotherapeutic drugs are expected to cause. The most important drugs for treating severe nausea caused by chemotherapy are ondansetron (Zofran) or granisetron (Kytril). These can be given either intravenously or in pill form and are very effective in preventing nausea and vomiting for the first day or two of treatment. They are less effective in treating delayed nausea (nausea that occurs twenty-four hours after treatment).

Other commonly prescribed medications are dexamethasone (Decadron), often given with ondansetron or granisetron, and metoclopramide. These can be used for less severe nausea. Another drug is prochlorperazine (Compazine). This can be given by pill or suppository.

Diarrhea

Diarrhea means having loose or watery bowel movements three or more times a day, and it usually occurs because chemotherapy drugs are affecting the lining of the intestines. This troublesome side effect can last briefly or for some time, usually depending on the drug and the dose given.

There are several drugs that may offer relief, and if one is not effective, another might be. Most drugs are available without a prescription.

Call your doctor if diarrhea persists for more than twenty-four hours. It's very important to avoid dehydration.

SPECIAL

CONCERNS

Should an Elderly Person Choose Chemotherapy?

It was once assumed that the elderly could not tolerate chemotherapy simply because their organs do not function as well as a younger person's, and therefore they are more vulnerable to side effects. As a result, even though cancer is more common in older people, treatment was often withheld or not provided aggressively enough to do much good.

Scientists now know that older people are usually just as able to tolerate chemotherapy as the young, and treatment can be just as successful for the elderly. For instance, one study of women who had been treated for breast cancer found that those over age 70 live just as long after treatment as younger women do. Therefore, a person's health is a better criterion than age when deciding if chemotherapy is an option.

Mouth Sores

The inside of your mouth can be injured by chemotherapy—the lining may bleed and sores may develop, making the mouth susceptible to infection. The throat and esophagus can also become sore. Good oral hygiene is the key to protecting your mouth from the adverse effects of chemotherapy.

TIPS AND

ADVICE

Soothing a Sore Mouth

A sore mouth can make eating difficult and is, of course, just plain uncomfortable. The following are some suggestions for relief:

- Use a cotton swab to apply Maalox or milk of magnesia to soothe and dry out sores in the mouth.

- Eat foods cold or at room temperature, and choose soft foods such as ice cream, mashed potatoes, cooked cereals, macaroni and cheese, custards, and gelatin.

- Avoid acidic foods, such as tomatoes and citrus fruits and juices, and spicy, salty, and rough-textured foods.

- If all else fails, ask your doctor to prescribe a pain-easing medication.

Hair Loss

Nausea may be one of the most dreaded chemotherapy side effects, but hair loss (alopecia) can be devastating because it seems like such a gross violation of a healthy appearance. Not all chemotherapy drugs cause hair loss, however, and some people experience only mild thinning that is obvious only to them. Some people lose only the hair from their heads, but others also lose eyebrows, eyelashes, and pubic, leg, and underarm hair.

Hair loss doesn't happen immediately. Your scalp may feel tingly and tender for a few weeks after treatment. Your hair may begin to fall out from the roots gradually at first and then in large clumps. Distressing as this is, there are many ways to cope with it. For instance, women with long hair often have their hair cut very short when they begin chemotherapy.

Remember that hair almost always grows back once the chemotherapy is completed; it may even start growing again before treatment is over. The good

TIPS AND

ADVICE

Coping with Hair Loss

If you know that the drugs you will be taking typically cause hair loss, the following are some useful steps for making the transition easier:

- Before beginning chemotherapy get a stylish, short haircut. This change will prepare you for the effect that the hair loss will have on your appearance. It will also cut down on the amount of hair you find on your pillow or in the shower.

- Once your treatment has begun, handle your hair gently: wash it with a mild shampoo, pat it dry, and comb it through carefully without pulling or tugging. Use low heat if you must use a dryer. Don't use harsh chemicals such as hair dyes or permanent waving products. Temporary hair rinses are not thought to cause problems, but beauticians are often hesitant to take the chance.

- Sleep on a satin pillowcase to reduce the friction between hair and scalp.

- Some people find the daily handfuls of hair falling out difficult to deal with and so feel more in control if they shave their heads.

- Once all your hair has come out, you may either bare your bald head (many people do) or cover it with a hat, scarf, or wig.

- If you plan to wear a wig, buy it before you begin losing your hair. That way you can match your natural hair color and style more exactly. Some shops specialize in wigs for people undergoing chemotherapy. For recommendations look in the yellow pages or ask your doctor, local chapter of the American Cancer Society, or support group (see Chapter 20).

news for some people whose hair is naturally straight is that their "new" hair often is thicker and even curly and stays that way for as long as two years.

Weight Gain and Loss

Some people (usually women undergoing adjuvant chemotherapy for breast cancer) put on weight during chemotherapy. It is unclear why this happens. It may have to do with the intense food cravings that develop, despite the nausea. These cravings may be for foods that you once disliked. Generally, you should eat whatever you want as long as your diet contains enough nutritious foods to fuel your body's energy and repair processes. The average weight gain for women is six to eight pounds, although greater gains are not unusual. Most people prefer to wait until their chemotherapy is completed before dieting to shed the added pounds (see Chapters 18 and 20).

Loss of appetite (anorexia) and weight loss is more easily understood. It may be caused by the nausea and vomiting that are side effects of certain drugs, or the changes in taste sensations that sometimes occur. It can also be due to the metabolic changes that result from the cancer itself. Anorexia usually resolves itself when chemotherapy is complete. If it doesn't, certain drugs can be prescribed to resolve the problem. Large doses of a female hormone called megace as well as cortisone-like drugs can improve appetite and help you gain weight. Most oncologists avoid using these unless absolutely necessary, however, because they cause side effects.

Fatigue

Tiredness is one of the most common side effects of chemotherapy (see Chapter 24). It can range from mild lethargy to feeling completely wiped out. It may occur because the body is working especially hard to recover from the effects of the drugs and is using lots of energy to dispose of dead cells and build new ones. Tiredness also results from anemia, a dearth of the red blood cells that carry oxygen to body tissues.

Fatigue tends to be most severe at the beginning of a treatment cycle, tapering off toward the end, but it may get progressively worse after a number of cycles. When the chemotherapy is completed, the fatigue will gradually disappear.

Should you push yourself? The key to coping with fatigue is listening to your body: if you don't feel like doing something, don't do it. Of course, this advice isn't always practical. Enlist the help of friends and family for the unavoidable tasks of day-to-day life, and pace yourself in regard to other activities. Note when you feel most energetic, and schedule exercise or work for that time. Take rest breaks and naps throughout the day if you can (see Chapter 19). Keep in mind that a little daily exercise, even walking, can help you maintain your fitness and keep weight off if you are gaining weight on chemotherapy.

You can also plan your treatment session with fatigue in mind. For example, you may feel especially tired the day after intravenous chemotherapy. If so, try to schedule the treatment sessions for a Friday so that you will have the weekend to rest. This way, you may feel more energetic for work by Monday morning.

Effects on Bone Marrow

Chemotherapy's effects on bone marrow are often the most severe side effects experienced by people with cancer. The bone marrow produces several types of blood cells essential to health. Because these cells are constantly dividing to produce new blood cells, they are vulnerable to the effects of chemotherapy. The term used to describe impaired bone marrow function is bone marrow suppression or myelosuppression.

The bone marrow produces three important blood components: red blood cells, which carry oxygen to cells throughout the body; white blood cells, which fight infection; and platelets, which seal damaged blood vessels so they don't bleed. A drop in the levels of any of these cells results in specific side effects. Some drops in cell levels can be serious, so blood cells are monitored carefully throughout the chemotherapy, even daily if necessary.

The treatment team performs a blood test to count the blood cells at the beginning of each treatment cycle and again a week to ten days later. This phase of the cycle, known as the nadir, is when white blood cells and the longer-lived platelets reach their lowest levels, leaving the body most vulnerable to infection. (Various drugs have different nadirs; most but not all of them arrive between seven and fourteen days.)

Anemia. Anemia means there are not enough red blood cells. A measurement called hematocrit is the percentage of the blood that is red blood cells. The normal range is 36 to 45 percent. The other measure is hemoglobin, which is the oxygen-carrying red pigment of red blood cells. Normal range is 12 to 16 grams per deciliter (g/dl).

The symptoms of anemia are fatigue, dizziness, paleness of the skin, and a tendency to feel cold. There may be shortness of breath and an increase in heart rate. Mild anemia usually is not serious and can be handled with more rest, but sometimes when anemia becomes severe, it interferes with daily living, and a transfusion of red blood cells or treatment with red cell growth factor (Procrit, Epoietin) may be necessary.

Leukopenia or Neutropenia. Leukopenia refers to a lowered number of white blood cells. This condition can make it difficult for the body to fight infection in the mouth, skin, lungs, and urinary tract.

Normally there are 4,000 to 10,000 white blood cells per cubic millimeter in the blood. There are granulocytes—which are the infection-fighting neutrophils, eosinophils, and basophils—and agranulocytes, including lymphocytes, monocytes, and macrophages.

When the number of neutrophils drops below 1,000 (the normal range is 2,500 to 6,000 cells per cubic millimeter of blood), the person is said to have neutropenia and is at risk of developing a serious infection in the blood or pneumonia. Should an infection take hold, the symptoms are typically chills, high fever, and malaise.

Preventive antibiotics are sometimes prescribed when white blood cell counts are low. There are also growth factors that stimulate production of white blood cells (see Chapter 13). Granulocyte-macrophage colony stimulating factor (GM-CSF, sargramostim, Leukine) and granulocyte colony stimulating factor (G-CSF, filgrastim, Neupogen) may be given the day after a chemotherapy treatment or as long as two weeks afterward. When the blood cell count is very low, chemotherapy may be delayed until it returns to a healthier level.

Very high doses of chemotherapy or radiation therapy may require stem cell transplantation to replenish the bone marrow (see Chapter 14). Common signs of a serious infection are high fever, sore throat, coughing, and chills or sweating. Always tell your doctor if any of these symptoms develop.

Thrombocytopenia. Thrombocytopenia is an inadequate number of platelets, which are the cells necessary for blood sealing damaged blood vessels. Normally there are 150,000 to 450,000 platelets per cubic millimeter. A deficiency can cause nosebleeds and bleeding gums, blood in the urine or stool, unusually heavy menstrual flow, or bleeding under the skin, which shows up as bruises. Internal bleeding is a serious symptom. A low platelet count usually resolves itself, but if it is very low a platelet transfusion may be given.

When to Call the Doctor

TIPS AND

ADVICE

Even when chemotherapy side effects are fleeting and minor, they may not feel so inconsequential at the time, and some symptoms do signal potentially serious problems. Call your doctor immediately if you experience any of the following:

- a fever of more than 100.5 degrees

- bleeding or unexplained bruising

- a rash or allergic reaction such as swelling of the hands or feet

- violent chills

- pain or soreness at the chemotherapy injection site

- unusual pain, including intense headaches

- shortness of breath

- diarrhea or prolonged vomiting

- bloody urine

Organ Damage

Some chemotherapy drugs have the potential to damage organs such as the heart (e.g., daunorubicin and doxorubicin); lungs (e.g., bleomycin); nerves, including numbness and some weakness (e.g., vincristine); urinary system, including the kidney (e.g., cisplatin); liver (e.g., methotrexate); and the ovaries and testicles (e.g., alkylating agents).

The symptoms vary according to the organ involved, and the doctor caring for you will be alert to any indication of toxicity. Periodic testing for expected toxicities may also be done. In some cases the problems are temporary, but they can be permanent. The doctor should discuss the potential for organ damage with you as part of the informed consent process.

Nerve and Muscle Side Effects

When chemotherapy drugs affect the nervous system, a condition called peripheral neuropathy results. The symptoms include tingling, burning, weakness, or numbness in the hands or feet or both. When the nerves are affected, you may experience a loss of balance and clumsiness, jaw pain, hearing loss, stomach pain, constipation, and difficulty walking or picking things up. Your muscles may be affected as well, and you may feel weak, tired, and sore. Even when such symptoms are mild, you should always report them to your doctor.

Effects on Sex and Fertility

Chemotherapy has direct and indirect effects on sexual function and fertility. Fatigue and nausea can lower libido, and changes in appearance (particularly hair loss) make some people feel they are less attractive to their partners. In addition, the rapidly dividing cells of the reproductive tract are prime targets for anticancer drugs, resulting in a number of side effects for both men and women (see Chapter 21).

Men. Chemotherapy does not cause erection problems or inhibit sexual intercourse, but the drugs may reduce and/or damage sperm cells, resulting in infertility. Men undergoing combination chemotherapy that includes alkylating drugs are particularly at risk. Once treatment is complete, fertility may be restored, but perhaps not for two to four years. Some men never regain their fertility. Since it is impossible to predict the extent of damage to sperm production that will result from chemotherapy, it makes sense for men who know they want to become fathers to bank healthy sperm before undergoing treatment.

Women. The ovaries are highly sensitive to chemotherapy drugs, especially alkylating agents. Menstrual periods may become irregular. Or menstruation may stop altogether during therapy, accompanied by menopause-like symptoms, such as hot flashes, night sweats, and vaginal dryness. Usually, menstruation starts up again after the chemotherapy is completed, although the periods may be irregular for a while. Women who are close to menopause may not resume menstruating. Damage to the ovaries can result in either temporary or permanent infertility.

Because the mucous membranes may be irritated, the lining of the vagina can become dry and inflamed, and intercourse may be painful. Yeast infections may arise and worsen the inflammation. (To prevent this, a vaginal cream or suppository may be prescribed, and women are encouraged to wear loose clothing and cotton underwear.) Genital herpes or genital wart infections may flare up again since the immune system has been compromised.

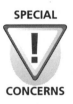

SPECIAL

CONCERNS

Pregnancy and Chemotherapy

Although chemotherapy often makes both men and women infertile, it is possible to become pregnant during treatment, which may be risky for both the woman and the fetus. Furthermore, the physical changes of pregnancy only compound the unpleasant side effects of chemotherapy. More seriously, the drugs can cause severe birth defects, although current studies are finding that many women who had chemotherapy have healthy babies afterward, even if they were exposed to the drugs early in their pregnancy, when the fetus was most susceptible to damage.

If a woman is already pregnant when she is diagnosed with cancer, it is sometimes possible to postpone chemotherapy until after the baby is born. If not, doctors may recommend delaying treatment until after at least the twelfth week of pregnancy, when the fetus is at less risk of being affected by the drugs. Sometimes, however, the safest approach for the woman's health is terminating the pregnancy. Obviously, you must discuss these issues with your treatment team, family, and others who provide your emotional support.

Effects on Emotions, Mood, and Thinking
The strain of being sick, coupled with the side effects and disruptions brought about by chemotherapy, can take a toll on mental well being. Chemotherapy can make you feel angry, depressed, anxious, and afraid. It's emotionally wearing to feel queasy all the time, to have to reschedule work around treatment appointments, and miss out on enjoyable activities because of fatigue. Also, the drugs can cause mood swings. Chemotherapy has also been known to cause confusion, memory loss, agitation, and even periods of unconsciousness. Older people are particularly vulnerable to these side effects, and anyone taking tranquilizers or painkillers may notice these changes.

It helps to remember that the emotional and cognitive side effects of chemotherapy are temporary and that once the treatment is over, the mood swings will probably end, your thinking will become clearer, and recovery will begin. Meanwhile, talking about your fears, anxiety, anger, and confusion with doctors, friends, family, or support group members can help ease the emotional burden (see Chapters 8 and 27).

Drug Resistance

Sometimes cancer cells do not respond at all to chemotherapy, or the drugs work well for some time but then the cancer cells begin to flourish again despite continued treatment. Some cells do not respond because they are in areas of the body that anticancer drugs cannot easily reach, such as the central nervous system. Other types of cells are inherently resistant to drugs, and some cells develop resistance in ways that are not entirely clear.

Cancer cells that are easily destroyed with chemotherapy at the start of treatment can develop multidrug resistance, meaning that the cells are resistant not only to the drugs they have been exposed to, but also new ones. It seems that when cells are bombarded with anticancer drugs, a defense mechanism is activated that is effective against many anticancer drugs.

Life After Chemotherapy

Once the chemotherapy has ended, the body usually returns to normal, often bouncing back from most side effects in a relatively short time. Lost hair grows in and energy levels rise. But some consequences may linger, such as infertility, menstrual changes, and damage to organs. Similarly, anxiety and fear may continue, especially regarding the possible recurrence of your cancer. Many cancer survivors are helped greatly by joining support groups, where they can share their feelings with others who are going through a similar experience. After treatment ends, family members may not understand why you are not acting like everything is all right again. But cancer survivors know full well about the emotional course of the illness (see Chapters 26 and 28).

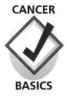

CANCER

BASICS

Defining Remission

Cancers are often described as being in "remission," meaning a complete or partial disappearance of signs and symptoms and a good sign that the chemotherapy is working. Partial remission means that the tumor has diminished to less than half its original size. Complete remission means that no cancer can be found. Because stray cancer cells are difficult to detect, however, doctors may continue chemotherapy for some time even after they remove the tumor and/or they believe complete remission has been achieved.

13

Biological Therapies

For many years, the three main methods of treating cancer have been surgery, chemotherapy, and radiation. Recently, excitement has grown about a fourth approach, one that stimulates the body to recognize, attack, and destroy cancer cells or protect the body against the damaging side-effects of chemotherapy and radiation therapy. It's known by several terms: biological therapy, biotherapy, biological response modifier therapy, immunotherapy, and cytokine therapy. All of the agents used in this approach—such as growth factors, interferon, monoclonal antibodies, and vaccines—are made from living cells.

One aspect of biological therapy, immunotherapy, began with the discovery of immunization more than 200 years ago. In modern times, research has centered on isolating specific cells of the immune system and their chemical products and manipulating them in the laboratory in order to target their activity and control their effects.

Research in humans is underway throughout the world in hopes of identifying which biological approaches work best for which types of cancer and in which kinds of people. Also, because the side effects can be serious, even life-threatening, and may alter the person's quality of life, studies to determine how the agents can be used safely is an active area of scientific endeavor.

With few exceptions, biological therapy is not considered a frontline approach. In other words, although it is most often used in conjunction with surgery, radiation, or chemotherapy, it does not replace these other methods, nor is it usually the first treatment tried. Also, in many instances, biological therapy is considered an investigational treatment (see Chapter 16).

Currently, some biological agents have been approved by the U.S. Food and Drug Administration (FDA) for use in particular types of cancer. Interferon alpha, for example, is approved for a rare type of cancer called hairy-cell leukemia, the more common chronic myeloid leukemia, melanoma, and AIDs-related Kaposi's sarcoma. Interleukin-2 (Aldesleukin and Proleukin) is approved for treating advanced renal cancer and advanced melanoma. However, clinical trials—a step toward FDA approval—of these agents for other cancers as well as new agents are being conducted in medical centers nationwide.

Defending the Body

To understand immunologic therapy, it helps to know a few basics about the immune system, the network of organs and cells that recognizes foreign materials and attempts to rid the body of them.

The body's first line of defense against foreign invaders is the skin, mucous membranes, lining of the respiratory tract, and so on. Like the moat surrounding a castle, this first line of defense is a physical barrier that works regardless of the invader (a nonspecific response).

If that defense fails, the immune response is set in motion. First the body must recognize the invaders—such as bacteria, viruses, parasites, or cancer cells—as being foreign. Then it musters the specific weapons needed to fight the detected invader and sends those weapons to the site of the battle. Anything the immune system recognizes as foreign is called an antigen. Antigens are small molecules that are part of the invader and that the immune system can detect. After achieving victory over the invader or anything the antigen is attached to, it must be able to remember what the invader looked like so the next time its response will be even swifter.

This military imagery—invaders, weapons, battles—is appropriate, since the immune cells circulating throughout the body are very much like a well-organized, well-trained army. As in any army, success in the battle against the cancer, or any foreign invader, depends on the ability of these various parts of the system to communicate.

Understanding how cells exchange messages and finding ways to make these messages clear and strong are the goals of research. The following section briefly describes the key components of the immune system. The main point to keep in mind is that each of these components, indeed each step in the immune response, represents a potential avenue for the development of a cancer therapy.

Immune System Cells

The most important cells of the immune system are certain white blood cells known as lymphocytes. Lymphocytes come in two main varieties, T cells and B cells.

T Cells. These lymphocytes are created in the bone marrow, but their name—T cells—derives from the fact that they mature in the thymus, a small gland in the chest between the breastbone and the heart. T cells accumulate in lymph nodes and the spleen along with other immune cells. There are three types of T cells that may be called into action: killer T cells (cytotoxic T lymphocytes), which are poisonous to cells and destroy the invader directly; helper T cells, which boost the activity of the B cells; and cytotoxic T cells, which do not directly destroy invaders.

B Cells. B cells are so-named because they develop within the bone marrow. Attracted by signals from helper T cells, B cells link up with these T cells. The T cells program the B cells to produce the appropriate antibody. The B cells quickly mature and become factories for producing antibodies against the specific invaders. Millions of antibodies released from the B cells then circulate in the blood and lymphatic system to seek out other invaders of the same type.

Tumor-Infiltrating Lymphocytes (TIL). TILs are immune system cells within tumor tissue. These are removed from the tumor and treated in the laboratory with IL-2 (see page 222 on interleukins), then injected into the person from whom the tumor was removed. TILs are being tested in people with melanoma, ovarian cancer, and other cancers.

Other Immune Cells. Natural killer (NK) cells are a third kind of lymphocyte. NK cells get their name because they function naturally; that is, they can attack invaders without having to be "switched on" by messages from other immune cells. But they can be activated by interleukins. When this happens, they become much more potent and are called lymphokine-activated killer (LAK) cells.

Antigen-presenting cells are a special class of cells that are very important in starting the immune process. These cells can be macrophages, monocytes, or dendritic cells. These cells are produced in the bone marrow. Their major role is to process the antigens attached to invading organisms and "present" the processed antigen fragments in order to attract and activate the T cells, beginning an immune response.

Therapy from Within

There are three categories of immunotherapy: active, passive, and nonspecific or adjuvant.

Active Immunotherapy

Every cell in your body contains an identical copy of your unique DNA, the molecule that serves as a blueprint for making more cells. In a sense, DNA is like a cellular identity card proving that a particular cell belongs to you. Accordingly, cells that do not carry the same DNA look foreign to your immune system. The surfaces of these cells are studded with antigens that reveal the invader to be "non-self."

Certain cancer cells contain antigens that appear foreign to your immune system. In some cases, it is possible to remove cancer cells, analyze them in the lab, and identify their antigens. Theoretically, once the antigens are known, a treatment can be designed that stimulates a specific immune response against them. This is called specific active immunotherapy. This method has been effective in treating certain lymphomas. However, it is very difficult and time-consuming because a new antigen needs to be found for each person's cancer.

Tumor Cell Vaccines. These are killed tumor cells that retain antigens on their surface. When injected into a patient, his or her immune system responds and attempts to destroy them. These are sometimes mixed with other substances (nonspecific adjuvants) that help stimulate the immune system. Sometimes these are just foreign proteins. Other times biological therapy is used, such as interleukin-2 or GM-CSF (see pages 222–223, 226).

The tumor cells may come from the person who will receive the vaccine (an autologous tumor cell vaccine) or from another person (an allogeneic tumor cell vaccine). Currently, tumor cell vaccines are not routinely used to treat cancer, but some are available in clinical trials. Melanoma vaccines have been used for several years in people who have a high risk of recurrence. One such vaccine is made from several melanoma cell lines that have been killed with radiation.

Antigen Vaccines. Instead of using the whole killed tumor cell and its large number of antigens, an antigen vaccine is created by genetic engineering techniques that mass produce specific antigens. These antigens may be used alone or several may be combined. These are now being evaluated as a treatment for breast, colorectal, ovarian, and pancreatic cancers and melanoma.

Anti-Idiotype Vaccines. A particular antibody (called an idiotype) will attach to an antigen like a lock and key. However, antibodies are antigens, and an antibody can be made that attaches to another antibody. On a molecular level, they will appear very much like the original antigens that produced the first antibodies.

Now that these anti-idiotype antibodies can be mass produced, they can be injected into a person, causing the immune system to produce antibodies that react with the injected antibody. Because the injected antibody resembles the antigen on the cancer cell surface, the newly formed antibodies will also react with the cancer cell. Subsequently, there is an immune response against those cancers. The antibody produced in this way is more potent than if an antibody were produced against the original antigen, although it is not known exactly why.

Anti-idiotype vaccines are being evaluated as a treatment for melanoma, lymphoma, and other types of cancer.

Dendritic Cell Vaccines. Dendritic cells are a type of antigen-presenting cell, meaning they help lymphocytes recognize antigens on cancer cells. Dendritic cells, in particular, are found in the blood, lymph nodes, skin, and some internal organs, and they present antigens from cancer cell surfaces to T cells.

Dendritic cells are taken from a person, isolated and exposed in the laboratory to antigens from that person's cancer cells, then returned to the person. Then the dendritic cells will be better able to present the cancer antigens to the T cells, which will then seek out and destroy cancer cells that have the recognizable antigen.

Clinical trials are in progress to study the effectiveness of dendritic cell vaccines in treating prostate, colorectal, and lung cancers and melanoma.

DNA Vaccines. Scientists use genetic engineering techniques to sort out bits of DNA that, when injected into a person, stimulate the production of particular antigens, which in turn stimulate an immune response. Another method of using DNA vaccines is by treating (in the laboratory) cells removed from a person with those antigen-producing bits of DNA and then injecting the cells into the person. The altered cell continues producing the antigen and stimulating the person's immune system. One trial, which used a DNA specific vaccine for a melanoma antigen, was unsuccessful in patients with melanoma. No immune response could be detected.

Nonspecific Immunotherapy

This approach uses agents that set a generalized immune response in motion, activating a wide range of immune cells in hopes that cancer cells will be attacked. *Bacillus* (or *bacille*) *Calmette-Guérin* (BCG), the organism that causes tuberculosis, is one example. The immune response to tuberculosis can also cause certain cancers to regress. These agents are sometimes called adjuvants and are used to improve another therapy's effectiveness. BCG, for example, and interleukin-2 have been used in experimental cancer vaccines. Another treatment using BCG involves instilling it into the bladder after surgery to treat superficial bladder cancer. The solution remains in the bladder for about two hours if possible before the person has to urinate. The treatment may be repeated once a week for six weeks.

Another adjuvant, levamisole, is sometimes used along with chemotherapy after surgery for advanced colon cancer.

Cytokines. The immune cells produce chemical messengers called cytokines that regulate the blood and immune cell activity and reproduction. As nonspecific immunotherapy agents, they have been used both to provide a general boost to immunity and as adjuvants given with other therapies such as vaccines. Clinical trials are underway to evaluate the use of cytokines for melanoma, leukemia, lymphoma, neuroblastoma, AIDS-related Kaposi's sarcoma, mesothelioma, and cancer of the brain, kidney, cervix, and other organs.

Cytokines have other therapeutic uses as well. For example, hematopoietic growth factors help the bone marrow recover after chemotherapy. Other growth factors are named for the type of blood cell they stimulate, such as granulocyte colony stimulating factor (G-CSF, filgrastim, or Neupogen), which stimulates granulocyte production. (See page 226, *Colony Stimulating Factors*.)

Interferons. Interferons are a family of cytokines that normally function in our bodies to interfere with a virus' ability to reproduce and proliferate, but they can also inhibit the growth of cancer cells. There are several types of interferon, and they affect cancer cell growth in different ways. They also enhance the effectiveness of natural killer cells and other immune system cells.

There are three main types of interferon, and it is possible that more will be discovered. So far, only interferon alpha has been approved as a cancer treatment, but interferon beta and gamma are being studied as well. Interferon alpha has been approved by the FDA for the treatment of hairy-cell leukemia, chronic myeloid leukemia (CML), melanoma, and AIDS-related Kaposi's sarcoma.

Interferon is also indicated for the treatment of genital warts known as condylomata acuminata, which have been linked to cervical cancer. Studies have shown that interferon alpha may be effective for metastatic kidney cancer and non-Hodgkin's lymphoma.

As a rule, interferon appears to be most active when used in cancers of the blood and is not as effective against solid tumors. However, interferon alpha appears to enhance the effectiveness of other treatments. For example, it may be combined with the chemotherapy drug fluorouracil in treating colorectal cancer.

In laboratory studies, interferon beta seems to enhance the effects of radiation therapy; whether similar results will be seen in humans is not yet clear. This approach may have particular value in treating cancer of the bronchial tubes of the lung. Interferon beta also suppresses cell growth and differentiation, especially when used in combination with other interferons, tumor necrosis factor (see box on page 223), or interleukins. Interferon is usually administered on an outpatient basis. Initially, close monitoring of side effects is essential. Often, though, injections can be provided at home if the people responsible have been given careful instruction. A typical course of treatment involves three to seven doses of interferon each week for a period of time from a month to a year.

The injection site can become red and sore. When the agent is given intra-venously, possibly serious phlebitis (vein inflammation) can result. Flu-like symptoms—fever, chills, and muscle aches—are the most typical side effects, affecting nine out of ten people taking interferon. The chills usually begin between two and six hours after administration and are marked by teeth chattering, shivers, and a pale complexion. The shivers can cause the body temperature and pulse rate to rise.

The day after the interferon is administered, the fever usually abates, but it is often replaced by malaise and achy muscles. Some people feel so fatigued that they can barely drag themselves out of bed. They may eat poorly and neglect their personal hygiene. Skin rashes and thinning hair may occur. Sometimes just knowing what to expect will lessen the impact of these side effects. Also, a kind of tolerance develops that helps in enduring the treatment.

Long-term side effects may be distressing and can have a serious impact on a person's quality of life. For instance, the fatigue can become chronic. About 70 percent of people taking interferon experience confusion, disorientation, and depression. They may have trouble concentrating, performing simple calculations, or remembering appointments. Not surprisingly, these difficulties may interfere with their ability to work.

Many people stop taking interferon because of the chronic fatigue and/or the cognitive problems, feeling that the benefits are not worth the costs. But others find effective ways to manage the problems.

Some side effects stem from high doses of interferon. These reactions, which are usually temporary and reversible, include nausea, vomiting, diarrhea, low blood pressure, burning or prickling sensations, sleepiness, and a general "slowing down" of the body. Tests of liver and kidney functions may be abnormal, indicating that these organs are temporarily compromised. Heart function can also be affected. Low blood pressure is common and in rare cases, there is danger of an irregular heartbeat, loss of blood flow to the heart, and acute cardiac failure.

Managing the Side Effects of Interferon Therapy

TIPS AND

ADVICE

The severity of the flu-like side effects often depends on the dose. Unfortunately, at this time, high doses appear to be most effective. However, there are ways to manage the side effects.

Acetaminophen relieves the aches and fever. (Aspirin can interfere with immune function, so it is not recommended.) Ask your nurse or doctor how much acetaminophen you should take and how often. Your doctor may offer to prescribe acetaminophen with codeine if the over-the-counter medication doesn't adequately control your discomfort.

Commonsense remedies such as blankets and warm beverages can provide relief for the chills and shaking, which occur for up to six hours after an interferon injection. In severe cases, morphine may be needed to relieve muscle contractions.

Ask your doctor about taking the interferon injection in the evening, so that you're able to sleep through the worst of the adverse reactions.

You may experience a change in your taste for food. Old favorites may lose their appeal, or you may have no appetite at all. A dietitian can help with planning meals so you get the most nutritive value from the foods you do eat and you don't lose too much weight. Sometimes sipping high-protein, high-calorie liquid meals can get you through days when you just don't feel like eating anything (see Chapter 18).

Inflammation at the site of injection is common. Alternating sites minimizes the risk of serious infection, and corticosteroid medication can help relieve inflammation, redness, and pain.

Low blood pressure can often be managed through drinking more fluids and by avoiding sudden changes in position, such as quickly standing up from a chair or a bed. If you are taking a medication for high blood pressure, your doctor may lower the dosage or take you off the medication while you're taking interferon.

Since interferon can lead to trouble concentrating, you may want to ask your family or a close friend to check with you often during therapy about the medicines you're taking and to be certain you keep your doctor's appointments. It may be necessary to take time off from work, and it may help to delegate such responsibilities as paying bills to someone else for a while.

Fatigue is the most distressing side effect and one that can dramatically affect your quality of life. You might need to cut back on activities, allow plenty of time for rest, and take naps frequently. Don't hesitate to ask others for help, even for small things like getting dressed or helping you wash your hair. You need to conserve your strength so the treatment has the best chance of working.

Interleukins. Treatment with the cytokine interleukin-2 (IL-2 or aldesleukin) has become a standard therapy for advanced renal cancer and melanoma. Several different interleukins have been identified, but IL-2 is the only one being used in clinical practice. It can be mass produced using genetic technology.

IL-2 may also be combined with lymphokine-activated killer (LAK) cells and tumor-infiltrating lymphocytes (TILs) vaccines. IL-2 helps these cells reproduce after injection into the body.

Treatment with IL-2 is complicated and expensive. It has been given intravenously in high doses, but this was complicated by serious side effects. It seems to be just as effective given in lower doses subcutaneously. In a typical protocol for renal cell cancer, for example, IL-2 is given subcutaneously for five days. Then, a week later, a second IL-2 cycle begins at lower doses.

Most people receiving IL-2 gain weight and about one-third experience nausea and vomiting or diarrhea. Other flu-like symptoms include chills, fever, fatigue, and disorientation. Treatment with high doses of IL-2 carries considerable risk of serious side effects; therefore, it is typically given in intensive care units (ICUs) or at least in hospitals that have an ICU and emergency doctors available. Blood pressure, urine output, and breathing must be monitored closely for a few days.

Of great concern is capillary leak syndrome, in which fluids escape from small blood vessels, resulting in swollen tissues. Symptoms include rapid weight gain, a drop in blood pressure, and difficulty breathing. Left untreated, the syndrome can cause kidney failure or respiratory arrest. For these reasons, it should only be given at major cancer centers by doctors who are experienced at using IL-2.

Tumor Necrosis Factor (TNF)

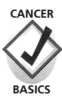

CANCER

BASICS

TNF, a protein secreted by macrophages and other cells, kills tumor cells directly. It appears to enhance the effectiveness of some anticancer drugs and gives a boost to the interleukins and interferons. There is evidence that injecting TNF directly into AIDS-related Kaposi's sarcoma lesions provides some benefit. Unfortunately, the side effects of TNF are very severe and patients cannot tolerate large enough doses to kill tumors.

As a way of avoiding needing large doses, TNF is being tested in low doses combined with chemotherapy or other treatments. So far, these trials haven't been successful. Another use of TNF that has been more successful is using it for regional therapy. In this form of treatment, the TNF is infused directly into the tumor or part of the body carrying the tumor. This approach is still experimental.

Passive Immunotherapy

Passive immunotherapy uses antibodies and other agents that have been made in the lab and given to the person with cancer. With the developments of production techniques for monoclonal antibodies, passive immunotherapy has recently become an important biological therapy. This approach is sometimes called adoptive immunotherapy because the person adopts an immune response that has been developed in a test tube.

As with active immunotherapy, the passive approach can be specific (aimed at certain targets) or nonspecific (aimed at a range of targets). Specific treatments include monoclonal antibodies (MAbs), the so-called magic bullets that can be designed to target certain cancer cells.

Monoclonal Antibodies (MAbs). When monoclonal antibodies (also known as MAbs, MOABs, or MoABs) were developed in 1978, the idea of a single agent that could target and destroy cancer cells became possible. These laboratory-made antibodies are manufactured or cloned from the same living parent cell (hence the word monoclonal) and are designed to link up with matching antigens on the surface of particular cancer cells. The cells usually come from an animal that has been immunized against the cancer and then "humanized" (made to resemble human antibodies so they are not rejected as foreign) by genetic engineering. These designer antibodies can be made either to react directly against cancer cells or to carry radioactive molecules or anticancer drugs to them (conjugated antibodies).

Naked MAbs work in one of two ways: 1) they attach to antigens on cancer cells and destroy them, or they enable them to be recognized and destroyed by immune cells, or 2) they attach to growth-stimulating molecules on cancer cells and block the cells' growth. Monoclonal antibodies are also used by pathologists in the laboratory to test blood and tissue samples, and experimentally by radiologists to highlight sites of metastasis so they will be noticeable on x-rays. MAbs with substances attached are said to be labeled or loaded. An MAb with a radioactive particle attached is called radiolabeled.

Two naked MAbs have been approved by the FDA: trastuzumab (Herceptin), used to treat advanced breast cancer in those who have tumors that produce excessive amounts of a protein called HER-2, and rituximab (Rituxan), used to treat B cell non-Hodgkin's lymphoma that has returned or no longer responds to chemotherapy. A third, Campath, which would be used to treat chronic lymphocytic leukemia, is under consideration by the FDA.

Clinical trials are in progress that use various types of MAbs to treat people with leukemia, lymphoma, multiple myeloma, neuroblastoma, and breast, prostate, colorectal, ovarian, lung, brain, thyroid, and other cancers.

Monoclonal antibodies can play a key role in bone marrow transplantation. For example, cells harvested from donated marrow are mixed with antibodies in the lab and prepared to seek out and disable T-lymphocytes that would normally lead to rejection of the marrow. The marrow, now free of the T cells, can then be infused into the host. Other antibodies can be used to remove malignant cells, a process called purging.

Cancer cells are wily opponents, defending themselves in a variety of ways against MAbs. The cells sometimes shed their antigens, thereby leaving the MAbs without a docking site. Or the cells may secrete a blocking factor that coats their antigens, disguising their appearance.

Monoclonal antibodies, like other biological therapies, have side effects. There is often pain or inflammation at the injection site. Many people experience flu-like symptoms of fever, fatigue, chills, headache, nausea, and vomiting. There may be a drop in blood pressure, weight gain, and shifts in body fluids, resulting in mild swelling. To some extent, the side effects depend on the target of the antibodies. For example, MAbs aimed at colon cancer may cause diarrhea, and those used against a blood disorder may cause the number of white blood cells to decrease. In general, all of the side effects are mild and rarely cause patients to abandon the treatment.

Some people experience allergic reactions, including cough, wheezing, and skin rash. In severe cases, there is an extreme, potentially fatal allergic reaction, called anaphylaxis, which produces a drop in blood pressure, swelling, severe rash, and difficulty in breathing. Although these are rare, the risk of allergic reactions increases with each injection because the body eventually forms antibodies against the monoclonal antibody itself, since it is made from mouse cells. Although the antibody has been "humanized," it can still carry some mouse antigen that the body recognizes as foreign.

People receiving monoclonal treatments need to be in a facility equipped with resuscitation equipment in case of a rare serious allergic reaction. Close observation for at least an hour after the injection is important. Heart and lung functions are checked frequently. In the weeks following the injection, various blood tests, scans, and tumor measurements routinely monitor the person's response to treatment. The problems and side effects associated with MAb therapy are the subject of several areas of research. For example, scientists are using genetic engineering techniques to eliminate the mouse antigens given with human antigens and thus reduce the risk of allergic reaction. Figuring out ways to prevent tumor cells from changing their antigens would facilitate the MAbs' ability to bind to their targets. It is likely that combinations of treatments using MAbs and other biological agents such as IL-2 or interferon will increase the success of this approach.

Conjugated Antibodies. Monoclonal antibodies can be produced to bear poisonous toxins or radioactive molecules that will destroy cancer cells. These conjugated antibodies have been in clinical testing and are slowly working their way into practice. So far, the radioactive conjugates appear to be more successful, because the toxins can be taken up by normal cells.

Clinical trials using conjugated antibodies are underway in people with many different types of cancers.

Other Biological Therapies

Growth factors and hormones help normal cells grow. Growth factors are also known as colony stimulating factors or hematopoietic growth factors. Two

FDA-approved types of growth factors are used in cancer treatment: those that stimulate bone marrow to make normal cells and those that act as anti-cancer agents.

Erythropoietin

Called epo for short, erythropoietin is one of the first growth factors to be synthesized and is perhaps the best known. It was approved in 1989 for use in chronic kidney disease. This hormone, partially produced by the kidneys, stimulates the production of red blood cells and their release from the bone marrow (see Chapter 12).

People with advanced kidney failure often cannot make enough epo, and so in addition to dialysis, they may require many blood transfusions. Injections of epo, however, maintain a healthy level of red blood cells and can eliminate the need for dialysis and transfusions altogether.

This treatment does not address the cause of kidney failure directly, but it does offer a valuable form of support that enhances the quality of life. Epo replacement also helps reverse the anemia that often results from certain chemotherapy drugs. People receiving epo report a sense of well-being and higher levels of energy that allow them to live more normally.

Colony Stimulating Factors

Colony stimulating factors (CSFs) are proteins that induce granulocyte cells to multiply. Granulocytes are the major circulating blood cells that directly fight infections. That means they actually seek and destroy invading organisms by ingesting them. They are named granulocytes (other names are neutrophils, or polymorphonuclear leukocytes—"polys" for short) because they contain tiny granules, or particles, essential to various cellular functions.

Given by injection to people with small-cell lung cancer, granulocyte colony stimulating factor (G-CSF) increases the number of certain granulo-cytes that can destroy microorganisms. It can be given before chemotherapy to prevent the granulocyte level from dropping too low. Granulocyte-macrophage colony stimulating factor (GM-CSF) is another growth factor that works in much the same way. These agents usually cause few serious side effects, although some people experience mild fever, nausea, vomiting, and diarrhea. Perhaps the major side effect is bone pain, which can be very disturbing for some patients.

Megakaryocyte-Stimulating Factors

As discussed in other chapters, one of the side effects of chemotherapy is that it often lowers the platelet count just as it lowers the white blood cell count. Platelets, which are made in the bone marrow by large cells called megakary-ocytes, are small cell fragments (they are not complete cells because they don't have a nucleus) that seal damaged small blood vessels. Without them, people would bruise easily and bleed excessively from the mouth, gums, and any small cuts or scrapes.

Doctors have been trying to develop megakaryocyte-stimulating factors for many years and have partly succeeded. The only one available to date is an interleukin, IL-11 (Neumega). This can raise platelet counts in people undergoing chemotherapy, but it is associated with some side effects, such as fatigue and muscle aches. A new agent, called thrombopoietin, is in the development stage and not yet available for general use in patients.

Tumor Necrosis Factor (TNF)

TNF, secreted by macrophages and other cells, kills tumor cells directly. It appears to enhance the effectiveness of some anticancer drugs and gives a boost to the interleukins and interferons. There is evidence that injecting TNF directly into AIDS-related Kaposi's sarcoma lesions provides some benefit. Many researchers believe the role of this factor will be to shrink tumors, enabling other treatments that activate the immune system to destroy malignant cells more effectively.

The side effects with TNF resemble those of other biological treatments: flu-like symptoms of shivers, fever, and headache, and inflammation at the injection site. People with abdominal disease may experience nausea and vomiting. Less common side effects include a change in blood pressure, rapid heartbeat, mild chest discomfort, and fatigue.

The route of administration is determined by the type and severity of adverse reactions. Intravenous infusion produces longer-lasting and more severe shivering and fevers, but after injection under the skin, fatigue is more common and severe, and skin rash more likely. Fortunately, people who are given daily doses of TNF often find they become able to tolerate the side effects fairly well.

Questions to Ask Your Doctor About Biological Therapy

QUESTIONS

TO ASK

Weighing the physical, emotional, and financial costs of biological therapies and the serious nature of their side effects against the potential benefit is difficult. One reason is that the risks and benefits are hard to pin down, particularly with the newest agents, since experience with them is so limited. Therefore, try to discuss the state of the research with more than one doctor. It may also help to talk about the option being suggested to you with a person who has undergone the treatment.

The following are some suggested questions to ask your doctor:

- Is biological treatment an option for my kind of cancer?

- What agent will be used and why?

- Has the agent been proved effective?

- If not, why do you believe it will help me?

- At what point in my illness will biological treatment be used?

- What experience do you have with this particular agent?

- What are the chances of success?

- What are the risks? The complications?

- How much will it cost? Is this treatment covered by my insurance or health plan?

- Will I be part of a research protocol?

- What are the immediate side effects? Long-term effects?

- Will I have to be in the hospital during my treatment?

- Will I be in an intensive care unit?

- What will happen if I stop the treatment?

The Future

Each day, the immune system gives up more of its secrets. Researchers are learning more about how cells multiply and mature, and how they exchange messages. Just as important, they are learning about the relationship between the host and the disease, how tumor cells and immune cells interact, and how they try to outwit each other in the battle for survival. The results of the Human Genome Project will provide countless opportunities for developing gene therapy aimed at improving the body's ability to fend off disease.

For researchers, health care providers, and people with cancer, the promise of biological therapy has been a roller coaster ride. The hope that biological therapy would produce a cure, or at least a vaccine, has been scaled back to a more reasonable understanding that biological treatments have clear value in certain cancers when given in certain ways. There is no doubt that the role of biological treatment will continue to grow in the years ahead.

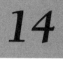

14

Stem Cell Transplants

In the 1950s, scientists discovered that bone marrow taken from one person could be infused into the bloodstream of another person and that the immature cells (called stem cells) it contained would shortly begin to produce normal blood cells. In this way, stem cells in the bone marrow that had been destroyed by high doses of anticancer drugs and/or radiation could be replaced. The replacement cells would begin turning out oxygen-bearing red blood cells; infection-fighting white blood cells; and platelets, which assist blood clotting.

In the late 1960s, when techniques were developed that allowed precise genetic matching of bone marrow recipients and donors, this procedure, known as bone marrow transplant (BMT), became a viable tool in the treatment of leukemia, a cancer of the blood-manufacturing cells in the bone marrow.

Today, stem cell transplant (SCT) is a therapy for leukemia and other cancers of the bone marrow as well as some noncancerous conditions. When the stem cells come directly from the bone marrow, the spongy tissue from the center of bones where the cells are formed and where most of them mature, the procedure is called a bone marrow transplant. When the stem cells are collected from the circulating blood, the procedure is called a peripheral blood stem cell transplant.

Techniques that enhance the recovery process—for example, using new drugs to boost cell production—are making transplants safer and shortening hospital stays. Studies are underway that allow for outpatient care for part of the procedure. More than 500 specialized transplant centers throughout the world perform BMT on a daily basis. Despite their widespread use, stem cell transplants are very demanding treatments. The decision to have a transplant is not an easy one to make. SCT requires a tremendous investment of time, energy, patience, and bravery, because of the toxicity of the high-dose chemotherapy that precedes it, the risks of rejection, and the long-term consequences.

When is SCT an Option?

Most stem cell transplants are done in people with cancer. Sometimes, however, SCT is a rescue procedure, replacing diseased or damaged stem cells with healthy new ones. Certain types of anemia and immune conditions can also directly affect blood cell production, and new indications continue to be added to the list. The following are some cancers for which blood and marrow transplants are most often used. The transplants are usually, but not always, done if standard treatment has failed.

- several types of leukemia: acute myelogenous, acute lymphocytic, chronic myelogenous, and chronic lymphocytic leukemias

- myelodysplastic syndromes

- multiple myeloma

- non-Hodgkin's lymphoma and Hodgkin's disease

Even though SCT was considered experimental for breast cancer, this was the most frequent use in recent years. However, several recent trials have had disappointing results. They should only be done as part of a clinical trial as researchers study how to improve the results.

Types of Transplants

Transplants are categorized according to how closely the recipient and the donor of the stem cells are matched. The closer the match, the less likely the cells will be rejected.

Syngeneic Transplant

The most compatible cells are from an identical twin because his or her tissue type is the same as the recipient. Less than one percent of STCs are syngeneic.

Allogeneic Transplant

An allogeneic transplant is donated by a person chosen through a tissue typing process (see the *Testing the Donor* section on page 234). The more similar the donor's tissue is to the recipient's tissue, the lower the risk of rejection will be. The first choice is always a sibling. Siblings are always likely to be a closer match than either parent or other relatives. If there is not a donor in the immediate family, the patient may consult a national registry for donors in the general population. The best matches of non-family members come from someone of the same ancestry. Currently, it is more difficult to find a match for people belonging to minority populations, such as those of African or Asian descent, because fewer minorities are in the donor pool at this time. An effort is being made to encourage members of minority groups to become donors, so this scarcity may be overcome in the future.

Non-Myeloablative Transplant. One of the most promising new types of stem cell transplants is the non-myeloablative transplant, or minitransplant. Instead of destroying the recipient's immune system with high doses of chemotherapy drugs or total body irradiation, these allogeneic transplants use lower, far less toxic doses of the chemotherapy used in BMTs. Also, some of the drugs used—for example, fludarabine—specifically suppress the immune system. Consequently, the conditioning treatment is more easily tolerated than traditional treatments. In fact, the procedure is sometimes called an outpatient allogeneic transplant, because hospitalization isn't necessary.

This investigative approach to transplantation is based on a phenomenon called graft-versus-malignancy (GVM) effect or graft-versus-leukemia effect, since it was noted to improve long-term survival in people with leukemia and lymphoma. GVM is what happens when donated cells target and destroy cancer cells that have managed to survive the conditioning treatment. GVM occurs after all types of transplants.

A minitransplant takes advantage of this phenomenon. Although the lower doses of chemotherapy drugs and/or radiation leave some of the recipient's own blood and marrow intact for a while, they are eventually driven out by the new cells from the donor. Any cancer cells that remain after the conditioning treatment, or that develop soon after, are under attack from donor cells. In some cases, when a person has a relapse after a minitransplant, a donation of the donor's white blood cells, called a donor leukocyte infusion, will put the recipient back in remission.

A minitransplant can only be done as an allogeneic transplant from a donor that is not an identical twin, because restored cells from the person with cancer cannot recognize—and therefore cannot destroy—his or her own cancer cells.

Since the conditioning treatment used for a minitransplant is not toxic, this procedure may be useful to elderly people who might not otherwise be transplant candidates, as well as people who have organ damage and are unable to tolerate STC. Also, non-myeloablative transplants do not cause major liver damage, a serious complication common after high-dose conditioning treatments.

The procedure is so new—it was first done in humans in the late 1990s—that long-term studies have not established its risks and benefits, nor are there any statistics yet available on long-term survival. Clinical trials are underway to evaluate non-myeloablative transplants for leukemia, lymphoma, multiple myeloma, melanoma, and kidney cancer, among others. It may also be useful for people with inherited blood disorders or immunodeficiency disease.

Autologous Transplant

An autologous transplant is the removal of stem cells from the person with cancer before treatment with high doses of chemotherapy and/or radiation and returning the stem cells to him or her after treatment. During the days that the chemotherapy and/or radiation therapy are given, the stem cells are frozen.

This is a frequently used type of transplant, particularly for cancers that are not leukemia. Although there is no risk of rejection because the stem cells used are the person's own, there is a chance of reintroducing cancer cells that may be in the marrow. To minimize this risk, some laboratories treat the marrow with chemotherapy or antibodies in a procedure called purging before reinfusing it.

Cord Blood Cell Transplant

A recent development is the banking of frozen umbilical cord blood, which is obtained from the placenta when a baby is born. These contain a high number of stem cells that seem to be less likely to cause graft versus host disease (see pages 241–243) and may be more potent at repopulating the bone marrow. They are being used for allogeneic transplants for recipients who have no sibling donor. Because the volume of stem cells is low, cord blood transplants are usually done in children who don't require as many stem cells as adults because of their smaller size.

Candidates for Stem Cell Transplants

Your body must be strong enough to withstand a variety of potential complications as well as endure the aggressive treatment with radiation and chemotherapy. For example, you have absolutely no bone marrow for some time during the transplant procedure and the circulating blood cells take a while to mature after the transplantation is done. With these challenges in mind, doctors at stem cell centers carefully screen each candidate.

Age

The risk of complications generally increases with age. Stem cell transplantation is commonly performed in people up to age 50, provided they meet certain health criteria. This maximum age has been increasing in recent years, and it is not unreasonable to expect the age limit to climb as techniques become better and success rates improve. People over age 50 now account for 10 percent of allogeneic transplants and 28 percent of autologous transplants.

Still, it seems that the older you get, the more trouble you will have with stem cell transplantation, particularly allogeneic transplants. Children tolerate the procedure better than adults.

General Health

People who undergo SCT must be in reasonably good health aside from their cancer and should not have had infections recently that may have weakened their bodies.

Intestinal difficulties are one reason that a person may not be accepted for SCT, because the high doses of anticancer drugs or radiation can damage tissue in the intestinal tract, making existing intestinal problems worse.

Pneumonia usually rules out or postpones SCT, even if the patient is under age 30, because the lungs are especially vulnerable to complications after a transplant.

Therapy Trial

Chemotherapy and/or radiation precedes SCT. The cancer must be responsive to chemotherapy for the transplant to be successful. A course of treatment with standard (not high) doses of chemotherapy will reveal whether a person's cancer is responsive to that therapy. This is given before the transplant until the cancer has shrunk as much as possible.

Emotional Resilience

Blood and marrow centers differ in how they evaluate a potential recipient's ability to cope with the psychological stress of the procedure. Some insist on psychiatric interviews. Some ask a potential recipient to complete a questionnaire that assesses whether he or she is emotionally capable of enduring the procedure and its potential side effects and can cope with the uncertainty of the outcome. At many centers a social worker evaluates the candidate and decides whether a consultation with a psychiatrist would be helpful.

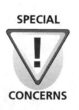

SPECIAL

CONCERNS

How Much Does SCT Cost?

Typically, a SCT procedure requires about four to six weeks in the hospital and can cost upward of $100,000. Whether or not a transplant is covered by insurance—especially for cancers in which its use is considered investigational—varies widely from one health care plan to another. And even when the cost of the transplant is reimbursed by insurance, there still can be staggering out-of-pocket, uncovered expenses such as return visits to the transplant center and travel and housing for family members who want to be nearby during the procedure.

Finding a Donor

A sibling is an ideal donor candidate, but if he or she is not a good match—and 60 to 70 percent are not—a parent is considered as a donor possibility. Other family members—aunts, uncles, and cousins—are next to be considered. A final option is an unrelated donor. But even though more than a million volunteer donors are registered, it is extremely difficult to find a donor whose bone marrow is genetically similar to that of the individual in need.

Finding a family member whose stem cells match those of the patient can be difficult. Family members from around the country or even abroad must be contacted and have their blood tested. If a good match is found, it may be necessary to arrange and pay for travel. If the recipient was adopted, it can be even more challenging to find relatives who are potential donors.

Other difficulties may arise as well. Sometimes the patient is not emotionally close to the family member whose stem cells match. A person in need of stem cells might feel guilty asking an estranged relative to provide stem cells. Or a relative may decide not to be a donor, which can create resentment and anger.

In the early years of BMT, a person without a relative who could be a donor would have to search on his or her own for a volunteer whose bone marrow closely matched. This process was haphazard and draining. Now, with computers and large marrow banks, it is increasingly possible to find a stem cell donor. Some communities even host "matching" parties, inviting people to come to a barbecue or pancake breakfast for testing to see whether they might be potential donors.

Testing the Donor

The technique for matching is called HLA (human leukocyte antigens) tissue typing. This is a kind of fingerprinting for tissues. HLAs are proteins produced by HLA genes on white blood cells that help the cell recognize foreign substances. They thus play a key role in the immune response and in the acceptance of the transplant. The better the match of the donor's and recipient's HLA antigens, the less likely the stem cells will be rejected and the fewer complications there will be. Once a match is made, the donor is tested for human immunodeficiency virus (HIV), hepatitis infection, and other diseases that might be spread by the transplanted cells.

The Donor's Responsibility

Aside from the actual discomfort of the procedure, the donor must be available to have his or her stem cells removed (a procedure called extraction) when the recipient's blood count is favorable and he or she is in good general health. The donor will also be subjected to a complete medical exam and a series of blood tests, including screening for viruses like hepatitis, cyto-megalovirus, and HIV. In some cases they will have a pint or two of blood taken for transfusion back to them later.

Most donors are happy that they can help, but some worry that their marrow won't be "good enough" to cure the recipient. Some people feel responsible for the success or failure of the treatment, as if it were under their control. Although some donors are hesitant to mention it, they may also feel ignored, as most of the concern and attention are focused on the recipient.

QUESTIONS

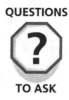

TO ASK

Finding a Stem Cell Transplant Center

Your doctor will refer you to a stem cell transplant center, but you may prefer to evaluate others as well. A directory of centers is available from marrow donor programs (see *Resources*). Some centers have more experience with specific cancers. It's helpful to visit the center(s) you are considering. (Most of them will request a "transplant interview" before accepting you.) Speak with the doctors and other staff members there. If your donor is able to visit as well, you'll know that both of you understand the process. You may want to ask the following questions:

- Does the center have extensive experience in treating the type of cancer I have?

- Has the doctor likely to treat me had experience with similar cases?

- Does the center meet the minimal criteria set up by the American Society of Clinical Oncology and the American Society of Hematology, which have jointly recommended standards for transplant centers? (There is no accreditation of stem cell transplant centers, although the hospitals that house them or are associated with them must meet the general accreditation standards of the Joint Commission on Accreditation of Health Care Organizations.)

- Does the center sponsor support or discussion groups for patients and their families? If not, is there a referral service to connect me to such groups or help?

- Is there a waiting list?

The Procedure

For the recipient, allogeneic SCT begins with a pretreatment or conditioning treatment. The high-dose chemotherapy, radiation therapy, or both that are given to kill the cancer cells also destroy the bone marrow. Pretreatment also temporarily suppresses the immune system, which will allow the body to accept the transplanted cells. In the case of an autologous SCT, the conditioning treatment will be preceded by harvesting or retrieving blood or marrow cells.

QUESTIONS

?

TO ASK

Questions to Ask Your Doctor About Stem Cell Transplants

Part of deciding on a particular treatment is determining whether the benefits of the treatment are worth its costs, side effects, and risks. Weighing the physical, emotional, and financial costs of stem cell transplants against the potential benefit is difficult. Therefore, try to discuss the state of the research with more than one doctor. When considering a transplant, it's important to ask your doctor about all the risks and weigh them against the hoped-for benefits. It may also help to talk about the procedure with a person who has undergone the treatment. The following are some suggested questions to ask your doctor:

- Is SCT the best option for me? Why?

- Can my cancer be treated by any other method besides high-dose radiation or chemotherapy?

- What are the chances of success in my case?

- Is SCT considered experimental for my disease or my type of cancer? Why?

- What are the risks of the SCT?

- What type of conditioning treatment will I receive?

- What is the estimated cost? What costs, if any, will be covered by my insurance or health plan?

- What side effects might I expect? How severe are they likely to be? How long will they last? Can they be controlled by medicine or other means?

- When will I be able to visit with people? Participate in social functions? Return to work?

- What type of monitoring will be required after SCT? How often? What are the chances that my cancer will recur even after SCT?

The Conditioning Treatment

The conditioning treatment usually takes three to five days, during which time the recipient is hospitalized. If the anticancer drug cyclophosphamide is given, electrocardiograms will be done periodically because the drug can be toxic to the heart (see Chapter 12).

Such side effects as nausea, vomiting, severe mouth sores, and diarrhea are nearly universal; however, medications are available to ease the distress. The large doses prescribed have a sedative effect. Intravenous fluids are often given to prevent dehydration and to provide nutrients. Bladder inflammation and bleeding may occur.

Total body irradiation (TBI)—the use of high-energy x-rays to kill cancer cells throughout the body—may be given in combination with chemotherapy in one session or over several days. Although the side effects are less severe than those following chemotherapy, nausea and vomiting are not unusual (see Chapter 11).

QUESTIONS

TO ASK

Questions to Ask Yourself About Treatment

Deciding whether to undergo SCT can seem like an overwhelming decision. Here are some questions to consider:

- Am I strong enough, or can I get strong enough, for the procedure?

- Is a good donor match likely?

- Does my family understand the length of time, the expense, and the effort involved with this treatment?

- Do I have a strong support system in place to help with the physical and emotional side effects?

Donor Preparation and Procedures

As noted earlier, once someone has consented to be a donor, he or she is given a complete medical examination and a series of blood tests to ensure that he or she is in good health. Sometimes the donor may have one or two pints of blood removed in advance, stored, and given back on the day of removing the bone marrow cells. The procedure for collecting stem cells from the bone marrow (usually from the iliac crest bones in the pelvis) is the same whether the source is the recipient or a donor.

Preparation for BMT. Cells "harvested" from marrow for a bone marrow transplant are retrieved through a large needle placed into the marrow, usually of the hipbone. Since a spinal or general anesthetic is used, this is not painful. However, the area remains quite tender for several days afterward. The donor stays in the hospital for a few hours or a day while he or she is monitored closely. Antibiotics may be given to prevent infection, and pain medication is administered if necessary. There are few risks involved in this harvesting procedure, and side effects, if any, are usually related to the anesthesia.

About 10 percent of the donor's marrow is removed. It will gradually replenish itself within a few weeks. Some doctors recommend that donors take iron supplements until their red blood cell count returns to normal.

Preparation for Allogeneic or Syngeneic Transplant. Cells harvested for an allogeneic or syngeneic transplant are processed and filtered and given back to the recipient within several hours, but those harvested from marrow for an autologous transplant are filtered to remove any fat or bits of bone that may be in the sample. The stem cells are cleansed or treated with anticancer drugs to purge any cancer cells that may be present. The stem cells are then frozen so they may be reinfused later.

When stem cells are retrieved from the bloodstream, a technique called apheresis separates the different types of cells. The red blood cells and platelets and the fluid portion (plasma) are reinfused to the donor or patient. Some centers also purge stem cells retrieved from the bloodstream.

Colony stimulating factors may be given before apheresis so that more stem cells than usual are released by the bone marrow into the bloodstream. Even so, stem cells in the blood are ten to one hundred times less concentrated than in the bone marrow. Each apheresis session may take as long as four hours and usually several sessions over days to weeks are needed to gather enough stem cells for transplanting. Although this is inconvenient and time-consuming, it can be done on an outpatient basis and no anesthetic is necessary.

The donor or patient may feel lightheaded during the apheresis session and experience some tingling and chills, but side effects are usually limited to the procedure itself—that is, placement of the catheter, blood clots and other blockages in the tubing, and possibly infection at the site of the catheter.

The Transplant

A few days after the conditioning treatment, the stem cells are infused into the recipient's vein through a catheter much like a blood transfusion. No anesthesia is needed for this procedure, which takes a few hours. When peripheral blood stem cells (PBSCs) are infused, a great volume of them—as many as thirty-two bags—are needed. So much fluid can cause a temporary accumulation in the lungs—a major side effect—and kidney problems. Marrow-derived stem cells are more concentrated and two to eight bags are typically infused. Even though the cells are infused into the blood, they find their way to the bone marrow where they settle and begin to divide and repopulate the marrow.

Recovery

Immediate side effects are unusual, and if they do occur, they are generally mild. They include nausea and vomiting, fever and chills, shortness of breath, chest tightness or pain, a drop in blood pressure, decreased urine output, and malaise. A preserving agent, dimethylsulfoxide (DMSO), that is used when autologous stem cells are frozen causes some patients to have a strange taste in their mouths (similar to that of garlic or creamed corn) that can last a day or so and may cause nausea. Sucking on hard candy or sipping flavored beverages during and after the infusion may combat this unusual sensation.

It takes several weeks for the number of red and white blood cells and platelets in the blood to return to normal and resume their functions. It is during this period that dangerous complications, mainly infections and bleeding, are most likely to occur.

For several weeks following the transfusion, the focus of nursing and medical care is on maintaining the recipient's health until the transplanted cells begin to function. Although most people survive the procedure, no one should consider SCT without recognizing that complications—some of them life-threatening—may occur.

Infection. The most serious early danger of SCT is infection, because most of the recipient's infection-fighting white blood cells are destroyed. While waiting for the white blood cells to return, stem cell recipients may spend up to four weeks (usually much less with autologous transplants) in a laminar airflow room. This is a special sealed-off hospital room in which an air filter continuously removes bacteria and other impurities. Because of the risk of infection, visitors are limited, and those who are permitted must carefully wash their hands and wear sterile gowns and masks. Flowers and plants are not permitted during this early high-risk period and all food is cooked thoroughly to eliminate bacteria. The recipient is closely monitored for fever and other signs of infection and receives antibiotics as well as red blood cells and platelets. Blood-forming growth factors may shorten the length of time a recipient is very susceptible to infection, but the recipient's immune system will not completely recover for at least six months to a year.

Nausea and Vomiting. These side effects of the conditioning treatment can be severe. Mucositis, an inflammation of the membranes lining the mouth, causes intense pain and is another common side effect (see Chapters 11 and 12). It is often treated with morphine infusions.

TIPS AND

ADVICE

Nutrition and SCT

Because of appetite loss, nausea, vomiting, diarrhea, and other side effects of aggressive treatment, nutritional monitoring and counseling are vital before, during, and after SCT. Taking into account individual differences, experts offer the following tips:

- Meal replacement products are not well tolerated immediately after SCT. Within a few weeks, though, such supplements may be helpful (see Chapter 18).

- Total parenteral nutrition (TPN) or intravenous feeding may be necessary to ensure an adequate intake of fluid and nutrients.

- Because nausea and vomiting can make eating difficult, try clear liquids, salty foods, and fruits such as watermelon, and avoid very sweet and greasy foods. Drink and eat slowly and avoid sudden movements, which can precipitate vomiting (see pages 205, 301).

- A dry mouth can make it difficult to chew and swallow foods such as meat and bread (see pages 187–188, 300). Gravies, broths, or sauces make these foods easier to swallow. Citric acid from lemonade or sugarless lemon drops increases saliva production. Also try eating crackers, plain meat, and bananas.

- Thick saliva makes swallowing difficult. Try an all-liquid diet. Hot tea with lemon or sour lemon drops can help break up the thick saliva.

- Changes in the way foods taste are widespread and may last as long as two months after SCT, but changing taste sensation interferes most with eating during the first twenty-five days. (Adults suffer changes in taste perception more often than children do.) Interestingly, smell perception isn't affected, so foods with an attractive aroma may stimulate your appetite. As long as there is no inflammation in your mouth, strongly flavored foods are the most appealing. Avoid bland, unsalted, and overcooked foods. Eventually, taste perception returns to normal. Sweet taste comes back first, followed by bitter, sour, and salty tastes.

- If possible, work with a dietitian to ensure an adequate intake of food and liquids.

Bleeding. Platelets which enable blood clotting are destroyed by the conditioning treatment and don't fully recover for several weeks, making this a particularly vulnerable time for nosebleeds, bleeding gums, bruising, and bleeding at other sites. Usually the stem cell recipient will be given regular transfusions of platelets and red blood cells (white blood cells cannot be easily transfused).

Veno-Occlusive Disease. Veno-occlusive disease (VOD) of the liver is a complication of conditioning treatments, particularly those that contain cyclophosphamide or higher than usual doses of radiation. It is most often seen with allogeneic transplants and not autologous transplants. The blood vessels of the liver become swollen and obstructed, which interferes with the organ's ability to perform its normal functioning, such as removing toxins and waste products from the blood. The liver swells and becomes tender and fluid builds up within it. The kidneys may become involved and retain fluid and sodium and cause water retention in the legs, arms, and abdomen.

Some people appear to be at higher risk for developing VOD than others. These include recipients with chronic hepatitis, cirrhosis of the liver, or a persistent fever at the beginning of the conditioning treatment. Those who have undergone a previous transplant are at increased risk. Those who are having SCT because of cancer are at greater risk for VOD than those having a transplant for other reasons.

The symptoms of liver problems are weight gain and pain in the upper right side. There is no specific treatment for VOD, but anything that diminishes stress on the liver—such as discontinuing drugs that affect liver function—is helpful. Over 80 percent of people who develop this complication recover completely, but it can be fatal, especially when the disease is severe.

Rejection. One of the major risks of allogeneic SCT (never autologous SCT) is that the recipient's T cells will reject the transplanted "foreign" stem cells. If the donors are unrelated, which is increasingly common, the likelihood is greater that the new marrow will be rejected. Although the cells initially appear to function, the blood counts may not return to normal; or if they do, the number suddenly drops. Graft rejection is frequently fatal.

To avoid rejection, immunity-suppressing drugs and/or total body radiation therapy may curtail the body's ability to fight the donor cells.

Acute Graft Versus Host Disease (GVHD). About 30 to 50 percent of allogeneic transplant recipients (never autologous transplant recipients) develop a condition in which rejection occurs in reverse; that is, the white blood cells (T-lymphocytes) in the newly transplanted cells (the graft) recognize the recipient (the host) as foreign and launch an attack against the host's cells. Acute GVHD can occur ten to seventy days after the transplant; the average time of onset is around day twenty-five.

Often the skin, liver, and gastrointestinal tract are affected, and symptoms range from a mild skin rash (affecting 25 percent of the body) and severe diarrhea to blistering, peeling skin, liver damage, and stomach and intestinal problems.

Initially, GVHD may be difficult to diagnose because the symptoms so closely resemble other complications or side effects of the chemotherapy and radiation therapy. Most people survive acute GVHD and the disease disappears, although some recipients die of GVHD.

The risk increases in those over the age of 30. Generally, the older both the recipient and the donor are, the greater the risk. Risk of developing GVHD is also higher among those whose donors are of the opposite sex. For unexplained reasons, female recipients whose female donors previously were pregnant have a higher risk. The less well matched the donor and recipient are, the greater the risk of GVHD.

The incidence and severity of GVHD may be reduced by immunosuppressive drugs or removing T cells from the donor's marrow. Removing T cells reduces the chance that the graft will take and so is not done regularly. Treatment involves suppressing the immune system—specifically the T cells—and avoiding infection.

Pneumonia. Adult respiratory distress syndrome (ARDS), a kind of pneumonia, is a grave danger for allogeneic transplant recipients (not autologous transplant recipients). The symptoms are similar to those of other types of pneumonia—although ARDS usually comes on more rapidly—such as a dry cough and difficult, rapid breathing. ARDS may occur approximately two months after the transplant, after the recipient has been discharged from the hospital. It is usually treated with steroid drugs. ARDS is the most common cause of death during the one hundred day window after a transplant.

The most frequent cause of pneumonia is infection by the cytomegalovirus (CMV). Since CMV is such a grave danger, some doctors suggest screening potential donors to make sure they do not have the virus. Another approach is to prophylactically treat the recipient with anti-CMV drugs.

Long-Term Complications

Complications may occur months or years after a transplant. After a year, the complication rate drops to about 5 to 10 percent, and after two years, it declines to less than 5 percent. The following are common long-term complications:

Chronic Graft Versus Host Disease. If chronic GVHD develops, it usually does so three months or more after an allogeneic transplant (it never occurs with autologous transplants). About 70 to 80 percent of people who develop chronic GVHD have experienced the acute form. Symptoms affecting the skin are common, such as temporary hardening and darkening (a kind of mottled appearance), as well as an itchy dry rash that begins on the hands or soles of the feet. Other typical symptoms include fever, infections, and weight loss. Problems also may arise in the intestinal tract, the esophagus, and the liver. Abdominal cramping and bloating, pain in the upper right abdomen, and jaundice are symptoms of chronic GVHD. Mucus-secreting glands are affected by chronic GVHD, so eye dryness and stinging, dry mouth, difficulty swallowing, and burning in the mouth can be problems. Hair may thin and/or become gray. The joints may tighten, making moving difficult. Lung problems can be serious, even life threatening.

There is no convincingly effective therapy for chronic GVHD. Treatment with drugs that suppress the immune system, such as steroids or methotrexate, may be given for as long as two years, but using them involves a delicate balancing act between the benefits of the drugs and their side effects. Antibiotics help prevent infection.

Some experts believe the key to preventing chronic GVHD is in effective pretreatment, which involves removing or inactivating the T-lymphocytes, a component of the immune system, so they won't attack the transplanted marrow.

Most people do not have long-lasting effects, but when they do, problems include chronic diarrhea, failure to absorb nutrients in the stomach, persistent liver and lung problems, skin sensitivity, and contractures.

Cataracts. Very high doses of radiation can cause cataracts (a clouding of the eye's natural lens) as much as five years after treatment. This condition can usually be corrected surgically.

Fertility Problems. High doses of radiation and chemotherapy can make people sterile. Men about to undergo SCT may consider banking their sperm before the pretreatment. For women, the issue of maintaining fertility is more difficult. Retrieving eggs requires surgery and is not generally recommended for female transplant candidates. And even if a woman successfully stored her eggs, it would be questionable whether her uterus could later support a pregnancy after such aggressive cancer treatment. Women under age 25, however, often maintain their fertility if they do not receive high doses of radiation to the pelvis. In children, SCT may delay or arrest puberty.

Learning Problems. Experts notice a tendency among children to develop permanent learning disabilities after SCT, especially if they have received high doses of radiation to the brain or if they have taken high doses of the chemotherapy drug methotrexate. Since the children often have undergone intensive therapy for acute leukemia, which may also cause mild learning disabilities, it is difficult to identify the cause.

Emotional Problems. People undergoing SCT face the challenge of isolation both immediately—in the hospital—and after the procedure, because they can wait six months or more to go out into public, where germs proliferate.

Feelings of isolation can be extremely stressful for even the most emotionally stable person, but the combination of isolation and physical discomfort is particularly distressing. After SCT, many of the recipients who are placed in laminar airflow rooms feel especially isolated. There, in the sterile calm, the recipient begins to realize, perhaps for the first time, the seriousness of his or her condition and the demands of the treatment.

Although a few recipients sail through with few psychological repercussions, many become quite depressed and anxious. Some experts believe that being informed about what emotional upheaval to expect before the procedure helps people cope more effectively. If recipients are informed, they won't be surprised by certain physical and emotional reactions and will be better prepared to accept feelings that otherwise might be misconstrued as abnormal. People who develop GVHD may also have emotional reactions to the drugs that relieve the problem. Depression, confusion, mood swings, and exaggerated responses are temporary side effects.

Long-term emotional challenges can seriously hamper quality of life. Studies of transplant recipients have concluded that sexual problems, occupational disability, and mood disturbances are not unusual. In general, older people have a harder time returning to a normal life.

Most blood and marrow centers have a social worker available to help recipients and their family and friends cope during the hospital stay. In addition, the center's staff members are usually trained to deal with the unique issues surrounding SCT.

Memory Lapses. Recipients experience memory problems, poor concentration, and a shortened attention span after SCT. Although such problems as slowed reaction time and difficulties in problem solving and reasoning are rarely severe, they can last for several years.

Recurrence

The main reason for SCT failure is recurrence of the original cancer. New cancers at other sites also occasionally occur after SCT. Some experts believe that the treatments designed to destroy the original cancer—radiation, chemotherapy, and immunosuppression—may predispose a person to develop another cancer. But it's important to remember that the initial treatments were often the only hope for treating the original cancer.

Getting and Giving Support

The recovery period following SCT is quite prolonged, taking from six months to a year. Even then, returning to work may be delayed another six months or longer. During this time, a support group can be extremely valuable (see Chapter 8).

Today, experts in SCT recognize that the family members or friends involved in a recipient's care are under enormous pressure and have serious emotional needs as well. They often feel exhausted in their roles as supporters and caregivers, and sometimes, as stand-in breadwinners. Many frequently believe they must keep a stiff upper lip. These factors can take a toll on their health and emotional well being (see Chapter 28).

Support groups can give family and friends an opportunity to talk about their experiences and learn how others have dealt with similar issues. A good transplant center is likely to offer support groups for transplant recipients and to provide outreach programs for family members. Or, they may be able to refer them to counseling services, which many recipients take advantage of for many months.

It is important to remember, however, that ongoing support groups are not helpful for everyone. Some transplant recipients remain friends with fellow patients, drawing strength from them. Others, however, want to cut off such relationships once they leave the hospital, feeling that being around others who have undergone SCT only reminds them of all the unpleasant possibilities.

Others draw strength from each other. Frequently, people who "graduate" from BMT centers volunteer to help other SCT recipients. They enjoy the feeling of repaying the center that saved their lives.

Quality of Life

Because the side effects of SCT can be seriously debilitating for some people, the difficulties raise questions about the quality of life afterward. It is especially important for those contemplating the procedure to be aware that their life may not return to normal following their recovery from the actual procedure. Nausea, vomiting, poor appetite, and changes in taste may be nagging side effects, as can itching skin, mottling, sleep problems, diarrhea or constipation, mouth sores, and dizzy spells. Joints can be stiff. Headaches, blurred vision, and shortness of breath may be problems.

But not everyone has these complications, and many transplant recipients do report a return to normal. As researchers clarify areas of unresolved psychological needs for those with SCT, social workers and others can concentrate on those needs and improve the overall quality of life for more and more people who choose this often life-saving procedure.

How One Woman Coped

Jean was 25 years old when she was diagnosed with leukemia. When her doctor suggested aggressive chemotherapy followed by SCT, she set to work finding a donor. Fortunately, her sister was a good match.

Jean's goal was to survive so that she could care for her 4-year-old twins, one of whom had undergone heart surgery the year before. She decided to "go for the cure" as soon as possible so that other complications wouldn't weaken her.

She asked question after question, including how to best help her husband care for their sons when she had to be hospitalized. Jean made good use of the social worker at the blood and marrow center at her hospital, conferring with her frequently.

A combination of humor and grit helped Jean get through the ordeal. She joked about windy days, because her wig wouldn't stay on. She had to learn to deal with adults who made cruel comments about her mottled skin. Nonetheless, everything went well for about eight months after the transplant, and then she developed chronic GVHD. She was fatigued and unable to do things for her children, such as drive them to kindergarten and take part in social functions. She felt she was not contributing to the family, even though she spent many hours with them. The goal then became how to control the GVHD. Jean now accepts the fact that she often cannot do everything she could before SCT. But she hopes that her strength will return or at least improve.

She credits her very close-knit family, especially her husband, with helping her keep a grip on reality. He has taken over many of the child care tasks and keeps the atmosphere as upbeat and cooperative as possible.

Her bottom line: Even though she has a chronic disease, Jean firmly believes the SCT was worth doing. She can still take part in many aspects of her family's life. And she values being with them every day.

15

Combination Treatments

Today, cancer is typically treated with two or more types of treatments—such as surgery, radiation, chemotherapy, and immunotherapy. Also, under certain conditions combination or multimodal therapy may also cause less damage to vital organs and tissues than a single approach.

A dramatic example of the success of combining therapies is the treatment of osteosarcoma, a cancer of the bone that occurs most often in young people. Not long ago, amputation of the affected limb was the only treatment. Today, radiation therapy directed to the tumor and chemotherapy delivered through the bloodstream may destroy the cancer without loss of the limb. Another example is the change in treatment of early-stage breast cancer from mastectomy (removal of the entire breast) to lumpectomy (removal of the lump) followed by radiation therapy. This is often combined with treatment such as tamoxifen, chemotherapy, or both. This has allowed many women to retain their natural contour without compromising the possibility of cure.

Why Treatments Are Combined

Doctors prescribe combined treatments in situations where:

- one treatment alone may not treat all the cancer at a certain stage.
- one may enhance the effectiveness of another.
- one may reduce the extent or intensity of another.
- one alone may not affect the tumor.

Multimodal therapy requires a well-planned strategy designed to exploit the unique qualities of each of the component treatments. It should balance their strengths and weaknesses, increasing the likelihood of success.

Depending on the stage of a person's cancer, the oncologist chooses a primary or definitive therapy, the one that might have the greatest impact on the cancer. Then one or more other therapies may be selected to increase the possibility of cure. The secondary treatments may come before, after, or at the same time as the primary one.

Often the therapies are equally important, so it is hard to say which one should be called primary. In certain breast cancers, for example, combined surgery, radiation, and drug therapy with tamoxifen (Nolvadex) and chemotherapy are all essential; omitting any one diminishes the possibility of cure.

Multimodal approaches can be designed to work in various ways. One treatment can fill in the gaps of another. For example, radiation therapy is generally most effective at the edges, or margins, of a tumor, where the bulk of the tumor is small and the cells are well supplied with blood vessels. (Blood brings in the oxygen required for radiation to work.) However, radiation therapy may not be as effective in the center, or core, of a tumor, where there is a dense collection of cells with a poor oxygen supply (see Chapter 11). Surgery, on the other hand, can remove the tumor, but it does not eliminate undetected cancer cells in surrounding tissues. Therefore, the two treatments can cover for each other's weaknesses. Adding chemotherapy can eliminate small numbers of cancer cells that have spread to other parts of the body.

Combining therapies may enhance the immediate and long-term effects of both. For example, the chemotherapy drugs fluorouracil (5-FU) and mitomycin C (Mutamycin) can make certain kinds of cancer cells more susceptible to radiation and are often given along with radiation therapy.

Combining two therapies may also allow for a less intense treatment than would be required if one were given alone.

The mixture and sequence of therapies depend chiefly on the risk of spread and on whether the cancer cells are dividing rapidly or slowly—along with such factors as your age, general health, and ability to tolerate the therapy. The various modalities may interact in ways that vary with the kind of cancer and its stage. Because there are so many aspects to consider, doctors caution patients against comparing their treatment plan with that of another person even if he or she has the same kind of cancer.

Of greatest importance is that the doctor discuss the whole treatment plan and any options with you in advance. Of course, some changes may be necessary during treatment. For example, if you seem to be responding unusually well to a certain drug, the doctor may alter the dose and schedule to take advantage of it. Of course, the regimen will change as well if you experience excessive side effects or unexpected toxicity. For these reasons, the primary doctor or oncologist must carefully monitor your response and adjust the treatment strategy as needed.

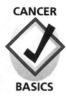

Terms You May Hear

The following terms are used to describe how several therapies may be used together.

- The words *combination* and *multimodal* are often used interchangeably, although they may have somewhat different meanings. *Combination* sometimes describes a single treatment that incorporates more than one variety of the same therapy. For example, chemotherapy may include two or more different drugs, or radiation may be delivered from an external source and an implant.

- *Multimodal* refers only to the use of two or more kinds of therapy (for example, surgery and chemotherapy). It may consist of a sequence of treatments, such as surgery followed by radiation therapy; simultaneous treatments, such as radiation and chemotherapy given during the same time period; and various combinations of treatment type and timing, such as alternating courses of radiation therapy and chemotherapy.

- *Adjuvant therapy* refers to giving a secondary treatment *after* the primary treatment, such as radiation after surgery.

- *Neoadjuvant therapy* is sometimes referred to as up-front treatment, because it is given *before* the primary therapy. Sometimes both neoadjuvant and adjuvant therapies are used. One recent approach for treating advanced lung cancer is surgery "surrounded" or "sandwiched" by chemotherapy.

Multimodal therapy calls for a team approach using the expertise of several doctors to ensure the most effective type and timing of treatments with the least risk. The primary doctor, radiologist, pathologist, surgeon, oncologist, and other specialists confer to tailor therapy for each individual with cancer. Among the issues they discuss is how to integrate conflicting treatments. For example, radiation therapy before surgery may help to shrink a tumor, making it easier to remove surgically, but it also can permanently affect other vital organs or slow the healing process or both. The surgeon and the radiologist work together to assess these possibilities. Sometimes it is best to give chemotherapy and radiation together; other times they work best when used sequentially.

In the ideal situation, members of the team don't simply manage their part and then turn the treatment over to the next specialist in line. Nor do they administer one therapy and then try to decide what to do next. Preferably, all the specialists will express their views and recommendations at the beginning, reach agreement with the person being treated on the plan and its details, and continue to consult with each other and the patient throughout the administration of therapy. This is why assessing a doctor's willingness to work with others is important when choosing the primary doctor (see Chapter 6).

How Combinations Evolved

Cancer does not always move directly and progressively outward from its primary site (see Chapter 30). Instead, cancer cells may travel from the local site to a distant area through the blood and lymphatic systems. And they may do so before the primary tumor is discovered or produces symptoms. Neither surgery nor radiation therapy addresses the problem of tumor cells that escape surgery or that have already established themselves elsewhere. Something more is needed.

That something was found in the 1960s. Research showed that certain drugs could kill cancer cells throughout the body. Doctors began combining chemotherapy with surgery for certain stages of breast cancer, and the outlook for people with this disease improved.

These results quickly led to combining surgery and chemotherapy for other cancers. The greatest success came with colorectal cancer, where chemotherapy was able to reduce the recurrence rate and save lives. Combination therapy was also used for cancers of the head and neck. Such tumors had continued to have a high relapse rate even after doctors began treating them aggressively with surgery and radiation. A combination of chemotherapy with surgery proved successful in shrinking tumors and helping to avoid mutilating surgery. This also helped to lower the recurrence rate of these cancers in other parts of the body.

Although multimodal treatment is now the most common approach, some cancers and certain circumstances call for a single type of treatment. For example, early-stage skin cancer is curable with surgery alone. Similarly, certain types of leukemia and lymphoma can be cured using chemotherapy or radiation therapy alone. In these situations, multimodal therapy would be unnecessary and could be detrimental. One example is Hodgkin's disease. Treatment is so successful with either chemotherapy or radiation that doctors are reluctant to combine the two, because the combination increases the long-term complication rate.

What Lies Ahead?

Cancer specialists are constantly adjusting, refining, and investigating ways to improve treatment planning, primarily through the use of clinical trials (see

Chapter 16). One of the newest developments is to add immunotherapy to boost the body's natural immune defenses (see Chapter 13).

Hormones or hormone suppressants are being added to enhance chemotherapy in some multimodal plans for cancers that are influenced by their hormonal environment, such as cancers of the breast, uterus, prostate, and thyroid. Another treatment being used is high-dose chemotherapy followed by stem cell transplantation after surgery or standard-dose chemotherapy (see Chapter 14).

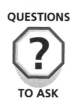

QUESTIONS

TO ASK

Questions to Ask Your Doctor About Combination Treatments

Multimodal therapy is not a standard recipe for treatment but a strategy that must be tailored to your unique situation. The answers to the following questions will help you understand your treatment plan. You will also want assurance that you are getting the teamwork that combination treatments require. The following are some suggested questions to ask your doctor:

- Why is multimodal therapy being recommended for me? Does this mean my cancer has spread or is likely to recur?

- What is the evidence that multimodal treatment is best for my kind of cancer?

- What are the major side effects? How long will they last? Are any permanent?

- Who are the people on my treatment team? Did they agree on the details of the proposed plan? Will they all be involved throughout? Who will monitor the different types of treatment?

- If I get better after the first kind of treatment, can I skip the next one?

- Will the first treatment have side effects that may affect the second treatment? If I get radiation or chemotherapy first, will I have to delay surgery? For how long? How will it affect my recovery?

- What if I choose not to have additional treatment?

- What is the timetable for treatments? How long do I wait in between? How long will the whole plan take? Will I have to be hospitalized? Can any of the treatment be done on an outpatient basis? Will I be able to continue working? Will I be able to travel?

- How much will it cost? Is my treatment plan covered by my health care plan?

- Is there a clinical research trial available for my type of cancer?

Neoadjuvant Therapy

Because surgery was the only treatment for cancer for so long, most people still assume that it is always the doctor's first and most important weapon. This is not always the case.

If there is a suspicion that your cancer has spread, your doctor may advise neoadjuvant therapy. For example, he or she may want to attempt to eliminate distant colonies of cancer cells by ordering chemotherapy before surgery. Radiation therapy or chemotherapy may also be used before surgery to reduce the size of a very large tumor so that less drastic surgery is required.

Neoadjuvant therapy has several advantages:

- People may tolerate radiation therapy or chemotherapy better before surgery, when they are usually stronger and in a better nutritional state.

- The blood supply hasn't been interrupted by surgery, so high concentrations of chemotherapy can reach the tumor. A good oxygen supply via the bloodstream also makes cancer cells more susceptible to radiation.

- Large numbers of rapidly growing cells can be destroyed.

- Neoadjuvant therapy provides a guide for later treatment. For example, a good response to chemotherapy before surgery usually means a good response to chemotherapy afterward.

Neoadjuvant therapy does have disadvantages:

- It can mask the true extent of the disease. Reduction of the tumor makes it harder for the surgeon and the pathologist to determine its original margins; thus, the operation may not be extensive enough.

- When radiation therapy is provided first, it may make proper staging impossible.

- Other treatment may be delayed or limited, sometimes seriously. This is a minor disadvantage if the first treatment produces no complications and the second treatment is postponed only for the normal time needed to administer the first.

- Immune defenses may be weakened just when they are especially needed to promote recovery from surgery.

Radiation Therapy

Doctors may prescribe neoadjuvant radiation therapy when they are concerned that cancer cells may become dislodged during surgery and spread elsewhere in the body. The radiation not only prevents these cells from reproducing if they are displaced, but also can shrink tumors so they are easier to remove.

Chemotherapy

Chemotherapy before surgery or radiation can be useful in shrinking cancers that would otherwise require drastic or extensive surgery. Sometimes combining chemotherapy and radiation can eliminate the need for surgery. Neoadjuvant chemotherapy is also being evaluated in cancers that are not expected to respond well to other therapies.

Timing Treatments

Treatment schedules vary widely, depending on the type of cancer, the extent of spread, and the person's physical condition. The timing of any combination of treatment depends on how each therapy works and how it relates to the others. Radiation treatment may precede surgery by only a few days or even hours. On the other hand, several months of chemotherapy may precede radiation therapy (in breast cancer and some lymphomas, for example) or surgery (for instance, for large breast tumors).

Neoadjuvant radiation is usually given in the smallest possible doses over the shortest time period, to destroy cancer cells with minimal side effects and the least delay before surgery. A typical schedule might consist of radiation therapy five days a week for two weeks, followed by a two-week recovery period before surgery.

Risks and Complications

All cancer therapies have some side effects and can cause complications, but combining them doesn't necessarily pose greater risks. However, where a certain therapy is more toxic when used with another, the doctor chooses it only if the benefits outweigh the added burden of side effects.

Radiation therapy or chemotherapy given first in the treatment plan may exaggerate some of the potential long-term and permanent side effects of surgery. These include such complications as adhesions of tissues, fibrosis, abscesses, and fistulas.

Radiation therapy may trigger side effects from subsequent chemotherapy. For example, doxorubicin (Adriamycin) given weeks after radiation therapy may be followed by a sunburn-like reaction in the skin of the irradiated area.

One of the greatest risks of neoadjuvant therapy is that it will be ineffective or produce intolerable side effects. These possibilities are considered as part of the treatment planning.

Knowledgeable doctors, careful monitoring during treatment, use of the safest and most effective doses, and continuous teamwork are the keys to preventing or managing most complications.

Adjuvant Therapy

Adjuvant therapy usually refers to hormonal therapy, chemotherapy, radiation therapy, or immunotherapy added after surgery to increase the chances of curing the disease or keeping it in check. It is a kind of one-two punch. First, definitive primary treatment removes the tumor, or as much of it as possible. Then either a supplemental local treatment kills any cancer cells remaining in the immediate area and/or a systemic treatment destroys cancer cells in other parts of the body. A common sequence is surgery followed by radiation, chemotherapy, or both. The choices depend on the type of tumor, whether there is a danger of recurrence, if it is largely local or systemic, and how rapidly the cancer cells are growing.

Timing

Chemotherapy usually begins as soon as possible after surgery, allowing time for a necessary degree of recovery. Postsurgical radiation therapy, however, must be delayed until the wound has healed. Chemotherapy is usually given before radiation to make sure cells distant from the tumor don't start growing while the tumor is being treated with the radiation. Also, body tissues seem to best tolerate the chemotherapy followed by radiation.

Combining Radiation Therapy and Chemotherapy

When there is a known likelihood of recurrence or clear evidence that cancer has spread, doctors may combine radiation and chemotherapy to treat both the primary cancer and any potential disease. Depending on the extent of the cancer, these treatments may even be used without surgery.

In some cancers both radiation therapy and chemotherapy are advantageous because each attacks different "volumes" of cells—that is, large tumor masses versus microscopic scattered cells. Chemotherapy given first can shrink a tumor to make it more susceptible to radiation therapy, which tends to work best against smaller tumors.

The effects of chemotherapy and radiation therapy also supplement each other, depending on the cancer cells' rate of growth. Radiation therapy works better against older and slower-growing cells; chemotherapy is best against the younger, more rapidly growing ones.

In some cases the two therapies are used because one makes the other possible. In head and neck cancer, for example, chemotherapy may be given for a few months before radiation therapy begins. Or chemotherapy may be given simultaneously with radiation therapy to make the cells more vulnerable to the radiation. For instance, rectal cancer may be treated simultaneously with fluorouracil (5-FU), mitomycin C (Mutamycin), and radiation. Here chemotherapy and radiation are combined because the total effect seems to be greater than the sum of the parts.

Intraoperative Radiation Therapy (IORT)

Radiation is sometimes used during an operation to treat the tumor and the surrounding area directly (see Chapter 11). Sometimes this intraoperative therapy is given in addition to postoperative external radiation therapy. Intraoperative radiation therapy is being used in cancers of the breast, colon, rectum, stomach, brain, pancreas, and female reproductive organs.

Advantages and Disadvantages

Performing surgery first allows the surgeon, pathologist, radiologist, and oncologist to review the results of surgery, looking at the size and type of the tumor that was removed and examining cells from the surrounding area. This direct analysis helps them to determine whether postoperative therapy will be helpful. If radiation is indicated, the precise target area is defined. The team can also identify those who won't benefit from radiation therapy and who should therefore be spared the exposure.

The disadvantages of having initial surgery depend on the situation. For instance, certain kinds of abdominal surgery may make the small intestine more susceptible to damage from radiation therapy.

Risks and Complications

Combining chemotherapy with radiation therapy may produce the same side effects as either treatment given alone and will not necessarily create any additional ones when combined. Nor will this combination aggravate the consequences of previous surgery, as long as adequate time is allowed for postoperative recovery. Conversely, the acute and long-term effects of surgery don't seem to increase or change the side effects of chemotherapy or radiation therapy.

Sticking with the Plan

Occasionally, people stop their cancer treatment or fail to keep their medical appointments. Those undergoing multimodal therapy are especially vulnerable to this kind of noncompliance, because the treatments are often long term, inconvenient, and expensive—not just in medical costs but in out-of-pocket costs, such as transportation to the doctor's office.

Unfortunately, some people who respond dramatically to the first part of a treatment plan may think they are cured and don't need to proceed with adjuvant therapy, especially if the next treatment is expected to have unpleasant side effects. Multimodal therapy, however, is an overall strategy that must include all of its interlocking parts to be successful.

16

Investigational Treatments

Scientific studies involving humans are crucial to conquering cancer. Over the last forty years, such investigations, called clinical trials, have led to the development of more precise methods of detecting and diagnosing cancer as well as highly effective prevention and treatment strategies.

Clinical trials are designed to follow the principles of ethical medical practice and to provide nothing less than the current standard of treatment—that is, the therapy that oncologists, the National Cancer Institute (NCI), the U.S. Food and Drug Administration (FDA), and the American Cancer Society (ACS) agree is the most effective and safe. In fact, since new drugs are approved and regimens are altered continuously, many people enter a trial to ensure they will receive the most current therapy available.

The potential benefit to a person volunteering for a clinical trial varies considerably, depending on the stage of the research. In the earliest phases, direct benefits are limited, because the purpose of these trials is to establish whether the treatment or drug should be evaluated at all. In the last phase, where the prospects of the treatment or drug's usefulness are good, the potential for benefit is much greater. Some people enter clinical trials in the last phase, because they want to be among the first to benefit if the new treatment being studied does prove superior to the current standard of care.

Some people also volunteer for altruistic reasons. They have the satisfaction of knowing they are helping to solve the mysteries of the disease. And even if the treatment fails to cure their illness, they have contributed to future, more successful therapies.

Only 2 to 3 percent of adults with cancer participate in clinical trials, yet many experts believe that if more people volunteered, cancer treatment would be improved significantly. About half of those with cancer today are cured, but that rate could climb considerably if more people would join research studies. Considering that the large number of children in trials has been accompanied by steadily higher survival rates for some childhood cancers, this prediction seems plausible. Nearly 75 percent of children with cancer are enrolled in clinical trials today. However, participation of teenagers is much lower, causing an "adolescent gap." Only 5 to 10 percent of 15 to 21 year olds participate in clinical trials.

Researchers are investigating basic biology to learn what causes cancer, testing current diagnostic methods, and evaluating new ones to determine how best to detect and define the disease. Epidemiologists are studying the impact of suspected risk factors such as diet on the incidence of cancer, and researchers are conducting prevention trials to learn what might help people avoid developing cancer. Some studies focus on rehabilitation methods after treatment, and some aim to devise better ways of controlling some of cancer's most devastating effects, such as pain. But most clinical trials are designed to determine how to safely and effectively administer a new treatment and whether the new treatment is better than the older treatments. The type of treatments studied may include:

- new chemotherapy drugs or different combinations of standard ones

- innovative types of radiation therapy

- ways of combining standard radiation therapy techniques with surgery and/or chemotherapy

- different surgical approaches

- various biological therapies—either alone or in combination with standard treatments.

Besides looking at how a particular treatment may improve chances for cure, researchers often examine how it may enhance a person's quality of life—perhaps by relieving pain, psychological stress, or other symptoms—thus allowing more people to continue working and enjoying life as long as possible. Clinical trials also allow comparison between treatments and are essential to learning whether or not one therapy is more effective than another.

From the Laboratory to Real Life

The NCI currently sponsors approximately two-thirds of clinical trials and studies over 250 anticancer agents. Other institutes at the National Institutes of Health sponsor or conduct clinical trials related to cancer, as do the Department of Defense and the Department of Veterans Affairs. Voluntary organizations like ACS, Susan G. Komen Foundation, and CaP CURE also sponsor or support clinical trials. Pharmaceutical companies often join forces with universities and cancer centers to conduct these trials. The main thrust of these studies is to see if a new drug or combination of drugs or therapies is ultimately more effective than the interventions currently in use. Clinical trials are part of the long, slow, and often expensive process that improves standard treatments. Typically, it takes six to eight years for an anticancer drug to complete human testing in clinical trials and become a standard treatment.

Before human testing of a drug begins, researchers conduct rigorous preliminary experiments in the test tube (in vitro) and in animals (in vivo) to determine which drugs are most likely to affect the cancer and make educated guesses about how best to administer them. Finally, if the laboratory research is promising and the FDA approves the drug for investigation, scientists begin human studies in three phases, each of which has a different purpose. Each phase builds on information gleaned from the phase that preceded it.

INFORM

YOURSELF

Informed Consent for Clinical Trials

An informed consent agreement that details the potential benefits and risks is essential for many treatments (see Chapter 9). But it is especially important in the case of clinical trials, since the outcome of the proposed intervention is unknown to some degree or may have some risk.

The details of an informed consent form for clinical trials include the expected benefits of the study, other treatment options, assurance that your personal records will be kept confidential, provisions for compensation for injury, and a statement that your participation is voluntary and that you are free to withdraw without penalty at any time.

To cover all of this information, consent forms are often lengthy and riddled with medical terminology with which you may not be familiar. For that reason you should ask your doctor, nurse, or other health care professional to go over the form with you before you sign it and to help you fully understand every aspect of the study you are considering. In fact, most people are given informed consent forms to read on their own, and then make appointments soon after to discuss their questions and concerns with the doctors and nurses involved with the trial.

Even though you sign the form, you are not legally bound to complete the trial. The informed consent form will state that you will be regularly updated regarding any new results coming from the trial, including unexpected risks or toxicity. Similarly, you or your doctor may determine that the problems you are experiencing do not warrant your staying in the trial. In either case, you can leave the trial at any time if you or others determine it is wise to do so.

Phase I Clinical Trials

During a phase I trial—the initial investigation of a treatment's safety and effectiveness in humans—a promising new therapy is tested to learn the best way to administer a new treatment and the dosage that can safely be administered. This is when researchers learn about a new drug's effects by gradually increasing the dosage in a stepwise fashion and carefully analyzing the responses among the participants.

This is a preliminary trial in which the researchers learn, for example, how well the drug is absorbed by the body, how much of it reaches the bloodstream, and how it is metabolized and eliminated from the body. The results let the scientists know if a larger study is possible that will reveal the drug's potential effectiveness.

Because participants in a phase I study can experience toxic and other undesirable side effects, only a few people—usually no more than fifty—are recruited. Most participants in a phase I study have advanced cancer that is no longer responding to conventional therapies. Typically, the person who enters this early phase of a clinical trial has no other treatment possibilities, and the study offers some hope of a response.

SPECIAL

CONCERNS

Compassionate Need

In some instances a promising anticancer drug may have been proven effective before all the trials have been completed and it becomes approved for use by the FDA. In this case, an argument can be made for compassionate need, which is a process that has been developed to allow cancer patients who have exhausted most available standard therapies to receive the experimental drug. The use of the drug is called off protocol, meaning that even if the person is eligible, he or she is not part of a clinical trial.

Phase II Clinical Trials

Once researchers determine the safe dosage and other specifics of administering a treatment, they focus on how effective the treatment is on people with one or more types of cancer. Phase II studies are often slightly larger than phase I studies and may involve groups of twenty to forty people. The larger numbers of participants allow researchers to note less common side effects.

In some ways, a phase II trial is a preview of a new treatment. The results may not indicate for certain that a treatment is an improvement on current therapy; instead researchers may learn whether it has the potential to be better.

Participants in a phase II trial often have been treated with a standard therapy before but have had a relapse or recurrence of their cancer. Although they are no longer responding to the standard treatment, their doctors believe the new approach being evaluated may be of benefit.

To gather information about how well people are responding, researchers will measure the size of tumors for shrinkage or, in the case of a systemic blood disease such as leukemia, they will analyze blood samples for changes in the circulating blood cells. The study may also involve monitoring the patient's blood for substances called tumor markers that often indicate whether their cancers are growing or shrinking. Subjective experiences, such as relief of certain symptoms, are noted, but objective measures that allow for accurate analysis and comparison of treatment results are important. If enough people show a response to the treatment, it goes to phase III testing.

Phase III Clinical Trials

A phase III trial is the final and definitive round of study before FDA approval. A phase III trial is designed to determine if the new intervention is better than, as good as, or inferior to the accepted standard treatment. Often many hundreds of people who have the same type of cancer at the same stage are involved in these studies. Phase III trials require a large number of participants for several reasons. For one, the levels of improvement may be small, and so many subjects are needed to determine by reliable statistical methods how the benefit compares to that achieved with standard treatment.

As a general rule, participants in a phase III trial are receiving the drug or therapy being studied as their initial treatment—that is, they have not received any prior interventions for their cancer. In this way, any changes in the subjects' condition are due to the treatment being studied and not to the delayed effects of any other therapy. Other factors may also make some patients ineligible for the trial, such as the presence of another disease with the potential to affect the person's health. The study design usually provides one group of people with the treatment currently thought to be the best available. This is the control group. Another group receives the new treatment being studied, which may be a modification of the standard one. For example, in the case of a chemotherapy trial, the promising treatment may be an entirely different medication, or it may be the standard drug plus a second one that scientists believe may boost the effectiveness of the first.

If at some point during the study the new treatment is found to be more effective than the standard one, the trial is stopped, and all the participants receive the more successful intervention. The trial is also stopped if there is any evidence that the intervention is inferior, unduly toxic, or otherwise harmful.

The trial may be completed, or closed, when enough people have been treated to satisfy the statistical requirements for answering the experimental question. Once a drug is found to be safe and effective, the FDA is likely to approve it for commercial use. At this point it is available to anyone who might benefit. However, the researchers will continue their observations. They may want to know that the new treatment offers better results in terms of preventing a recurrence or of lengthening survival time and to observe the patients for long-term side effects. Or they may want to confirm other advantages, such as improved function and fewer undesirable effects.

From Phase I to Phase III

Although most experimental cancer treatments go through all three trial phases, there are exceptions, such as studies designed to assess a prevention strategy. Usually, evidence from population studies has already indicated that the intervention, such as a dietary change, may be beneficial, so a phase II trial to determine the potential efficacy of a particular change is unnecessary. What remains to be tested is whether the new intervention or strategy can be implemented and whether it is truly beneficial. For example, a phase I trial, which is sometimes referred to as a pilot study, may determine that it's possible to get people to modify their diets in a particular way. It will then be compared to other prevention strategies or to no specific preventive measures in a phase III trial to establish the effectiveness of the intervention.

Terms You Will Hear

CANCER

BASICS

These are terms commonly used in discussing clinical trials:

- *Protocol* is a formal outline or plan of a clinical study. You are not likely to receive a copy of the protocol, which spells out, among other things, the objectives of the trial, how it will be carried out—what treatment a person will receive and when—and a list of scientists involved in the study. However, you will receive an abbreviated form that is written in language you can understand, called the informed consent document. If you request it, you can review the actual protocol.

- *Standard treatment* refers to the therapy for a particular cancer that is accepted by the medical community and has FDA approval, if it is a drug. This standard treatment for cancer is promoted by both the NCI and the ACS in most instances and is used for comparison with the "new" treatment. (The investigational treatment is usually a variation of the "standard" treatment. The researchers hope the variation will yield better results, but it may not.)

- *Placebos* are rarely used in clinical trials of cancer patients except in adjuvant trials where it is not certain that the cancer is present. A placebo is a harmless inactive substance given to members of the control group when the study is attempting to evaluate the benefits of a new drug. It is usually a pill, capsule, or injection indistinguishable from the active drug being tested. For some situations, such as in adjuvant trials where doctors are trying to learn if treatment can prevent recurrence, a placebo is sometimes necessary as a standard of comparison. But all patients with known cancer entered into a clinical trial generally receive active anticancer treatment.

- *Control group* refers to those people in a clinical trial not receiving the investigational treatment but undergoing the standard treatment approach.

- *Randomization* is a distribution process. Participants are randomly assigned to a control group or to one or more other groups receiving the new or modified treatment. Chance determines who goes into which group.

- *Double blind* describes a randomized trial in which neither doctors nor participants know which treatments are being administered to whom until the study is over.

- *Study arm* is the group in a study to which a participant is assigned: Each arm receives a different treatment.

Myths and Misunderstandings

You may be hesitant to participate in clinical trials because you have heard that there's no guarantee you will receive appropriate treatment, or that you will be lost in some scientific shuffle. If you are considering joining a clinical trial, it's important to know what's myth and what's reality.

Fear of Being Treated Like a "Guinea Pig"

Trial participants commonly worry that they will no longer be treated as individuals, that they will become just a "face in the crowd" and their care will be compromised in the name of science. In fact, study participants typically receive the best care available. Rather than being treated by only one or two doctors, they are monitored carefully by a number of specialists who are aware of privacy concerns and care about the subjects' well being. If anything, clinical study participants in phase III trials have a better chance of gaining benefits from treatment than nonparticipants, because they will receive either the best standard treatment known or an experimental therapy with the potential to be even more effective. (The likelihood for benefit with phase I and phase II trials is considerably less than that with phase III trials.) Most doctors in clinical trials are very sensitive to patients' experiences, the demands of participating in a clinical trial, and the need for individualized care. It is a general rule among doctors working with experimental therapies that these needs are considered and supersede those of the trial. The patient comes first.

Fear of Side Effects

It is true that, depending on which phase a trial is in, an experimental treatment may have unknown side effects. Most side effects in drug trials are similar to those brought about by standard drug therapies, such as hair loss, diminished blood counts (increasing the chance of infection), and nausea, and they are usually temporary. Although there is considerable information about side effects from animal studies that precede phase I trials, as a general rule more is known about how people will tolerate a drug during a phase III trial than in a phase I trial.

Of course, it is always possible that a treatment under investigation will cause serious, even life-threatening problems. These may be permanent, or they may not appear for a long time after the treatment is completed (e.g., problems affecting the kidney or heart, or the later appearance of a second cancer). Some of these problems are also associated with standard treatments. Consequently, all possible risks are carefully discussed with potential participants during the informed consent process described earlier in this chapter.

The decision to participate should not be made impulsively; it may require several discussions with your primary doctor or oncologist and other members of the treatment team. A family member or close friend may also join you when you discuss this with the doctor responsible for the trial and help you weigh the risks and benefits of volunteering.

Fear of Receiving a Placebo

The use of the term placebo when discussing clinical trials is often misleading. Clinical trials of anticancer drugs are never designed so that any participant will receive a placebo as the sole treatment unless, of course, the current standard is no treatment. For instance, in a clinical trial evaluating the effects of a new drug given with radiation therapy on a particular type and stage of cancer, radiation therapy alone may be the recommended treatment. Therefore, all study participants will receive radiation therapy; but some will also receive the drug being tested. Those in the control group will take a placebo in addition to the radiation therapy. No one in such a study will go without treatment. If during the course of the research the new drug is found to boost the effectiveness of the radiation therapy, all participants will immediately get the additional drug and the trial will end.

Fear of Missing Out on a Promising Treatment

Some experimental treatments are available outside of the clinical trial arena, and some doctors, encouraged by reports of promising results early in the investigation phase, may offer unapproved treatments as standard care. You may be tempted to seek treatment in this way rather than via a clinical trial. Some people do this because they fear that if they enter a study, they will be part of the control group that does not receive the new and potentially beneficial experimental treatment. This perception is unfortunate on two counts: if a treatment is still being investigated, it has not been proven to be better than standard care; also, its risks and side effects may not be clear.

Whatever you choose to do about an investigational treatment, it's important to understand that until all phases of the trial are completed, there is no proof that it is superior to any other option.

Financial Fears

Extra follow-up office visits and frequent monitoring with laboratory tests are part of participating in a clinical trial. The extent to which insurance and health plans cover these additional costs varies. Some do pay for the cost of phase III trial treatments. Indeed, there is much pressure being put on managed care organizations to include clinical trials as treatment options. However, if your plan doesn't cover the costs of experimental treatments, be sure the researchers in charge of the study you are considering are aware of it. Most doctors who plan clinical trials know the status of coverage and are careful to keep the number of office visits, laboratory tests, hospital stays, and other potentially costly conditions of clinical investigations to a minimum. In fact, clinical trials are sometimes less expensive to patients than receiving standard treatment, since many of the charges may be borne by those funding the study.

As for travel costs, as more and more trials are conducted in community hospitals rather than in major cancer centers, participants travel no farther for treatment and checkups than if they were receiving standard care.

Safeguards

Although there are no guarantees about the outcome of a clinical trial, safeguards are built in. One of the most important is the Institutional Review Board (IRB), a group of doctors, knowledgeable lay people, and other experts such as nurses, scientists, and clergy based at the facility where trials are carried out. IRBs are specifically responsible for protecting the welfare of trial participants in their institution. Members examine all aspects of each study before it is initiated to make sure that the risks are reasonable compared to the potential benefits to the patients. These groups also periodically monitor the data from the trial at their institution while it is underway. Studies funded by the federal government and under its jurisdiction are also reviewed by the NCI.

How to Find a Clinical Trial

Most cancer studies are funded by the NCI through cancer centers or cooperative networks made up of research institutions, university and community hospitals, and clinics associated with them.

Currently, the NCI is sponsoring hundreds of experimental treatment programs. Many of these studies take place at community hospitals as part of the Community Clinical Oncology Program (CCOP). This links community oncologists and primary doctors with NCI-funded researchers at medical centers, so that people can participate in cancer treatment trials without having to leave their area (see *Resources*).

Most pilot or exploratory studies (phases I and II) are carried out by single institutions such as universities and/or cancer centers. Even pharmaceutical companies that have a vested interest in proving that a medication works must adhere strictly to the scientific rules of research outlined earlier. Often they join forces with university medical centers to fund the necessary studies of drug efficacy, and any reputable company will scrupulously avoid potential conflict of interest.

There are many ways to find out about a clinical study that may benefit you. The most obvious place to start is the office of your own oncologist. You can also contact an NCI-designated clinical cancer center. The Cancer Information Service (CIS; 800-4-CANCER), a program supported by the NCI, can provide you with the names and numbers of centers near you (see *Resources*).

When contacting the CIS, you can also request a Physician's Data Query (PDQ) search. PDQ is a computerized database system supported by the NCI. It contains information about the latest nationwide cancer treatments for each type and stage of cancer. It lists more than 1,500 ongoing clinical trials and is updated monthly.

You can also access the PDQ (www.cancer.gov) on line with your own computer. In addition, the NCI has begun to collaborate with patient advocacy groups (starting with NABCO, the National Alliance of Breast Cancer Organizations) to offer information about relevant clinical trials through their own Internet sites. Patient advocacy organizations can be excellent sources of information about experimental treatments generally (see *Resources* for contact information).

Another valuable source of cancer research information is the ACS (800-ACS-2345).

QUESTIONS

?

TO ASK

Questions to Ask About Clinical Trials

If you are considering entering a clinical trial, you will want to gather as much information about the study as you can before you make a decision to participate. The following questions are a good start:

- What is the study trying to find out? Is the purpose to determine the safest dosage of a new drug or to determine the most effective treatment for my type of cancer?

- Who is sponsoring the study? Has it been reviewed by a bona fide national group, such as the NCI? Has it been approved by an institutional review board?

- How is my cancer most likely to progress or change if I join this study? What will happen regarding treatment if I don't?

- What are the other alternatives to the treatment proposed in this study? Are there standard options that may be just as beneficial as those in the study? What are the risks and advantages of these alternatives?

- What kinds of additional tests, such as blood tests or biopsies, will I undergo for the specific purpose of the study? Do any of these have side effects or risks that are of particular concern to me?

- How will being in the study affect my daily life? Will I be able to continue work? Will I feel like pursuing social activities?

- Will I have to be hospitalized? How often and for how long?

- How long will my active participation in the study last?

- Where will I be treated and evaluated? Will I have to travel? How frequently? Will much of my time be taken up by visits to the doctor or place where the trial is being coordinated, or can much of the treatment be given at my local cancer treatment center?

- What are the potential short-term and long-term side effects of the treatment alternatives? Are any of them likely to be permanent or life-threatening? Will I be allowed to take medications to relieve side effects such as nausea? Will I be able to continue other medicines?

- How will I know if the treatment is working properly or if I am responding? How will I know whether I should receive a different treatment plan from the one being studied?

- What if I seem to be harmed during the research program? Will I be entitled to care for problems related to the treatment?

- Will the treatment involve additional expense? Will any or all of the costs be covered? If not, are there other sources I can turn to for financial help? Do you know of any organizations that can help me convince my insurance company or health plan to cover the costs?

- What type of long-term follow-up care will I receive after the study is completed?

- How much will my personal doctor be involved?

- Who will be professionally responsible for my health care while I am in the trial?

Complementary and Alternative Therapies

Health care consumers in America are turning to complementary and alternative medicine in record numbers, despite little or no evidence to support their use in many cases. According to a 1998 study published in the *Journal of the American Medical Association (JAMA)*, an estimated 42 percent of adult Americans—about 83 million people—used at least one complementary or alternative therapy the previous year, spending about $34 billion. These therapies are being used for a variety of illnesses, ailments, and diseases, such as cancer. It has been reported that up to 50 percent of people with cancer use complementary and alternative medicine.

A *Consumer Reports* survey of 46,000 people conducted in the year 2000 found that 35 percent used complementary and alternative therapies. Although such methods have become popular, the survey reported that conventional medicine is still the treatment of choice. For example, prescription drugs were rated as being more effective than herbal remedies. They recommended that consumers consult a medical doctor for diagnosis and advice before seeking help from any alternative practitioner.

This trend of using complementary and alternative treatments is predicted to grow even more in the twenty-first century. The *JAMA* study showed that Americans now visit alternative practitioners more often than they see primary care doctors. In addition, herbal remedies and megavitamins are selling fast in health food stores and pharmacies, making promises of relief from common complaints and long-term illnesses, despite being virtually unregulated for safety, effectiveness, quality, and actual content.

How Complementary and Alternative Therapies Are Defined

The words complementary and alternative are often used interchangeably. However, there are important distinctions between the two terms. Complementary therapies are those that are used along with conventional medicine. Some of these therapies can help relieve symptoms and improve the quality of life by lessening the side effects of conventional treatments or by providing psychological benefits.

Alternative therapies are unproven treatments that are used instead of conventional therapy to attempt to prevent, lessen, or cure disease. Alternative therapies may be harmful in and of themselves or because they are used instead of conventional medicine, and thereby delay treatments that are proven to be helpful. Until the late 1990s, the term alternative was generally used to describe most of the therapies that are not part of conventional medicine.

What Does Alternative Mean?

INFORM

YOURSELF

There is often confusion surrounding the use of different terms in the field. Here are some definitions of commonly used terms.

- *Proven* treatments refer to evidence-based, conventional, mainstream, or standard medical treatments that have been tested following a strict set of guidelines and found to be safe and effective. The results of such clinical studies have been published in peer-reviewed journals— meaning that other doctors or scientists in the field evaluate the quality of the research and decide whether the article will be published. These treatments have been approved by the U.S. Food and Drug Administration (FDA).

- *Research* or *investigational* treatments are therapies being studied in a clinical trial. Clinical trials are controlled research projects that determine whether a new treatment is effective and safe for patients. Before a drug or other treatment can be used regularly to treat patients, it is studied and tested carefully, first in laboratory test tubes and then in animals. After these studies are completed and the therapy is found safe and promising, it is tested to see if it helps patients. After careful testing among patients shows the drug or other treatment is safe and effective, the FDA may approve it for regular use. Only then does the treatment become part of the standard, conventional collection of proven therapies used to treat disease in human beings.

- *Complementary* refers to supportive methods that are used to comple- ment, or add to, conventional treatments. Complementary therapies may lessen the side effects of standard treatments or provide mental and physical benefits to the person with cancer. Examples of complementary methods include meditation (to reduce stress), peppermint tea (to relieve nausea), and acupuncture (to relieve chronic back pain). Methods now called complementary, such as massage therapy, yoga, and meditation, have actually been referred to as *supportive therapies* in the past.

- *Integrative therapy* refers to the combined use of evidence-based proven therapies and complementary therapies. This is the term that many people in the field are using more frequently. In fact, integrative medicine services are becoming part of cancer centers and hospitals across the country.

- The terms *unproven* or *untested* can be confusing because they are sometimes used to refer to treatments with little basis in scientific fact, while they may also refer to treatments or tests that are under investigation. In general, adequate scientific evidence is not available to support the use of unproven or untested treatments.

- *Alternative* treatments are unproven because they have not been scientifically tested, or they were tested and found to be ineffective. Alternative treatments are used *instead of* conventional treatment. They may cause the patient to suffer, either from lack of helpful treatment, delay in treatment, or because the alternative treatment is actually harmful.

- *Quackery* refers to the promotion of methods that claim to prevent, diagnose, or cure cancers that are known to be false or that are unproven. These methods are often based on the use of patient testimonials as evidence of their effectiveness and safety. Many times the treatment is claimed to be effective against other diseases as well as cancer.

- *Unconventional* is a term used to cover all types of complementary and alternative treatments that fall outside the definition of proven, conventional therapies.

- *Nontraditional* is used in the same way as unconventional to describe complementary and alternative therapies. However, some therapies that seem nontraditional to modern American or European doctors may have been used in certain cultures for thousands of years, such as traditional Chinese medicine or traditional Native American medicine. These traditional native medicines are often used in complementary or alternative therapies.

- *Questionable* treatments are those that are unproven or untested therapies.

The Appeal of Alternatives

What is fueling this enormous appetite for the unregulated and largely unproven variety of treatments, practices, and products that make up alternative medicine? Ironically, the boom in complementary and alternative medicine may be based on the successes of conventional medicine. Primarily through the efforts of scientific medicine in the twentieth century, the average life expectancy rose from 48 years in 1900 to 76 years by 2000. As more and more people live longer lives, chronic diseases and disorders, including cancer, have become more common. While conventional medicine can extend the lives of people with chronic illnesses, it cannot cure all chronic illness. Therefore many health care consumers with long-term complaints are turning to alternative medicine with the hope of a better chance for effective treatment.

Advances in modern technological medicine may also play a role. Many Americans see high-tech medicine as impersonal and expensive. With increasing pressure on doctors to provide cost-effective care, they tend to spend less time with patients in an effort to see more people. On the other hand, many alternative practitioners spend an average of thirty minutes with their patients, or about four times the amount of time that doctors now spend with patients.

Several large surveys have reported that the holistic approach to medicine, which focuses on the whole body rather than on just the illness, is one of the main reasons Americans seek complementary and alternative therapies. Holistic medicine has roots in the centuries-old customs of traditional Chinese medicine, Ayurveda (traditional medicine from India), European folk medicine, and Native American medicinal traditions in North America. Proponents argue that modern scientific medicine tends to overlook the ancient healing traditions and their gentle methods of care.

Undoubtedly, the attitudes of those in conventional medicine toward alternative and complementary medicine are changing, but most still insist on objective, scientific evidence as the basis for judging complementary and alternative treatments.

Evaluating Claims

Promoters of alternative medicine may make claims about the effectiveness of these therapies ranging from the reasonable to the extraordinary. The most outlandish claim is that any alternative therapy can actually cure people with cancer. Even conventional cancer therapies, such as surgery, chemotherapy, and radiation therapy, cannot guarantee a cure. If certain cancers are diagnosed early enough in their development, conventional therapies may completely remove or destroy the cancer. Many cancer specialists do not even like to use the term cure, but prefer to say that a cancer is in remission. Alternative therapies cannot cure cancer, and any claims for a cure should be treated with skepticism.

The promise of a cure is often the main allure of alternative cancer therapies. Another appeal is the claim that the alternative therapy not only cures cancer or prolongs the survival time of a person living with cancer but also has no objectionable side effects. People should also be skeptical of these claims. Promoters usually have no evidence to back up these claims, except, perhaps, testimonials from some people who have used the therapies. The reality is that some alternative therapies can actually cause serious side effects, including allergic reactions, liver toxicity, heart problems, nutritional deficiencies, and harmful interactions with medications, including cancer drugs (see pages 275–276 and 278–279).

Supporters of some alternative cancer therapies may claim that the treatments can reduce a person's risk of developing cancer, stop the progression of cancer once it has occurred, or stop cancer recurrences. All of these claims should be evaluated on the basis of the evidence presented to back them up. Is there solid scientific evidence based on clinical trials to support the claim or is the claim based solely on the word of the manufacturer, promoter, or certain people who have tried the therapy? Controlled human clinical trials of complementary and alternative cancer therapies are needed to evaluate the therapies. Animal and laboratory studies may show that a certain therapy holds promise as a beneficial treatment, but further studies are necessary to determine if the results apply to humans.

Because laws prohibit manufacturers and marketers of dietary supplements, such as vitamins, minerals, and herbal medicines, from claiming that their products can cure or prevent disease, many claim that the products "boost the immune system" to help the body fight disease naturally. This commonly used phrase leads one to believe that the product will increase the function of the immune system. Yet, these claims are often made without any evidence to back them up. All claims should be evaluated on the basis of available scientific evidence to support them. The same standard of proof should be held for claims that an herbal product or other type of complementary or alternative cancer therapy can inhibit the growth or spread of

SPECIAL

!

CONCERNS

Signs of Possible Fraudulent Products Include:

- Claims that promote the supplement with such terms as *miracle cure, breakthrough,* or *new discovery*.

- Claims that the supplement has benefits but no side effects.

- Claims that the supplement can be used for a wide variety of unrelated illnesses.

- Claims that the treatment is safe and effective based solely on testimonials.

- Claims that the treatment is based on a secret ingredient or method.

tumors or actually destroy cancer cells. In some cases, these claims may be based on solid evidence; in many other instances, they are not.

Dietary Supplements

Dietary supplements have received a tremendous amount of attention over the past decade. What exactly is a dietary supplement? If you take a vitamin pill regularly, you are taking a dietary supplement. That is, you are adding something to your diet of foods, most likely in an attempt to make up for a less-than-perfect diet, to promote good health, or to help speed healing when illness strikes.

The term dietary supplement includes vitamins, minerals, herbs, amino acids, and other products that are not already approved as drugs. Dietary supplements are sold in grocery stores, health food shops, drugstores, national discount chain stores, mail-order catalogs, television programs, the Internet, and direct sales. Vitamins are the supplements most often purchased in this country.

Dietary ingredients used in dietary supplements are not subject to the premarket safety evaluations required of other new food ingredients, such as "food additives." It is up to the manufacturer to ensure that the dietary supplement is safe and properly labeled before marketing. Dietary supplements can make claims regarding effects on nutrition (e.g., works as an antioxidant), body function (e.g., maintains a healthy circulatory system), and well being (e.g., helps you relax). Because these statements are not reviewed by the FDA prior to being sold to the public, manufacturers are required to include a disclaimer on the label: "This statement has not been evaluated by the Food and Drug Administration. This product is not intended to diagnose, treat, cure, or prevent any disease." However, claims regarding effects on treating or preventing disease (e.g., vitamin C prevents scurvy) require testing and approval by the FDA.

Guidelines for the Safe Use of Dietary Supplements

INFORM

YOURSELF

Rule One: Investigate before you buy or use. There are many resources in libraries and on the Internet. However, much of this information is produced by promoters and it contains biased or incorrect information. Rely on materials by reputable organizations, a recognized expert, or government agencies with which you are familiar.

Rule Two: Check with your doctor before you try a dietary supplement. He or she may or may not be thoroughly versed in all of the product areas, but hopefully your doctor will prevent you from making a dangerous mistake.

Rule Three: Do not take any self-prescribed remedy instead of the medicine prescribed by your doctor without discussing it first.

Rule Four: Introduce one product at a time. Be alert to any negative effects you experience while taking the product. Any product that produces a rash, or a feeling of sleeplessness, restlessness, anxiety, GI disturbance (nausea, vomiting, diarrhea, or constipation), or severe headache, should immediately be stopped and the reaction should be reported to your doctor.

Rule Five: Avoid any dietary supplements not prescribed by a licensed doctor during pregnancy or if you are breast-feeding. Few, if any, of these products have been studied for safety, and their effects on the growing fetus are largely unknown.

Rule Six: Don't depend on any non prescription product to cure cancer or any other serious disease. Regardless of the claims you might hear, "if it sounds too good to be true, it probably is."

Rule Seven: Never give a product to a baby or child under 18 years old, without consulting your doctor first. Their bodies metabolize nutrients and drugs differently from an adult's body, and the effects of many of these products in children are not known.

Rule Eight: Always follow the dosage recommendations on the label. Overdosage could be deadly. Do not take a dietary supplement any longer than experts recommend.

Rule Nine: Try to avoid mixtures. The more ingredients, the greater the possibility for harmful effects.

Making Informed Choices

There is a great need for public protection in this area. We are in a "let the buyer beware" mode when it comes to nutritional dietary supplements and herbal medicines. To this day, there is no requirement for proof of safety, accurate labeling, or proof of a health benefit for dietary supplements sold in the United States. Congress has seen the need to protect the public against harmful prescription medications, but this protection is not extended to dietary supplements sold directly to consumers. The FDA has permission to stop production of a product only when the FDA proves that the product is dangerous to the health of Americans. Manufacturers still are not required to show that their products are safe or effective prior to marketing. The public still has limited protection against the marketing of products that often promise much and produce little if any benefit. Indeed, some products marketed in health food stores have recently been removed from shelves only after serious harm and even death from those products were reported.

The challenge to consumers is to determine which products are safe and which are not. Consumers should read the product label to be sure they are purchasing what they think they are. Some botanicals contain ingredients that can interact with conventional products or treatments, or may interact with other dietary supplements or food products. If a label on a dietary supplement makes a claim that the product can diagnose, treat, cure, or prevent disease, such as "cures cancer," the product is being sold illegally as a drug.

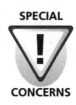

SPECIAL

CONCERNS

Buyer Be Aware

Consumers should be aware of the ingredients in the herbal medicines and other dietary supplements they take and be wary of false claims. To help protect consumers, the FDA recommends that consumers:

- Look for products with the USP notation, indicating that the manufacturer of the product followed standards set by the *US Pharmacopoeia* in formulating the product.

- Realize that the use of the term natural on an herbal product is no guarantee that the product is safe. Poisonous mushrooms are natural but not safe, for example.

- Take into account the name and reputation of the manufacturer or distributor. Herbal products and other dietary supplements made by nationally known food or drug manufacturers are more likely to have been made under tight quality controls because these companies have a reputation to uphold.

- Write to the manufacturer for more information than what is on the label of the supplement. Ask about the company's manufacturing practices and the quality-control conditions under which the product was made.

The Possible Dangers

Although some complementary and alternative treatments are harmless and inexpensive and can renew a person's feelings of hopefulness, not all are benign. It is possible that some treatments can interfere with the effectiveness of a conventional medical therapy; there are very few scientific studies to guide us. More information is needed on the safety of these therapies. Some diet therapies actually cause nutritional deficiencies that interfere with the body's ability to heal and withstand the side effects of conventional treatment. Others may involve procedures that can lead to serious injury or infection. Many botanicals

INFORM

YOURSELF

Supplements and Surgery

A number of ingredients sold in supplements can produce severe swings in blood pressure and other dangerous interactions with anesthetics and, therefore, should not be taken before surgery. In fact, the American Society of Anesthesiologists advises that patients stop taking herbal medications at least two to three weeks before surgery to allow enough time for the herbals to clear from the body. If the patient does not have enough time to stop taking herbal medicines before surgery, he or she should bring the product to the hospital and show the anesthesiologist what it is.

contain ingredients that can cause side effects, hazardous drug interactions, and allergic reactions. The possibility of drug supplement interactions is so high that cancer experts recommend that patients undergoing chemotherapy or radiation therapy avoid taking dietary supplements at the same time.

It is extremely difficult for the public to determine which of the many proliferating alternatives are safe or provide any benefits at all. Just because a practice is legal or natural does not mean it is harmless. Laws and regulations protecting people from unsafe practices are sometimes vague, and few attempts are made to enforce those that do exist. Certainly, there is no law against traveling to another country for a treatment that is illegal or not available in the United States. Indeed, several treatments that are not considered effective by American doctors are used in conventional practice in European countries, which only increases the confusion for someone with cancer.

It also is unfortunate when those with very advanced disease turn to an unconventional therapy simply because they believe they have "nothing to lose." This decision to pursue an alternative treatment as a last resort, without careful consideration of what the real costs are, may lead to unnecessary grief and pain. People have been known to spend their remaining weeks receiving ineffective and expensive treatments overseas, for instance, rather than enjoying the company of loved ones, receiving care that keeps them comfortable, and seeing to their financial affairs. Even when an alternative therapy is less costly than conventional medicine, the fees paid for it may still be wasted.

At the very least, the promises made by the proponents of some of these treatments create false hope and can cost a significant amount of money. What often causes so much dismay among conventional practitioners is that alternative therapies sometimes steer people away from treatment that would have been effective if they had not delayed it. The greatest danger in alternative medicine for people with cancer lies in losing the best opportunity to help treat cancer and prolong survival by avoiding conventional therapy. *Unnecessary delays and interruptions in conventional therapies are dangerous.*

QUESTIONS

TO ASK

Guidelines for Using Complementary and Alternative Methods of Cancer Management

Many people with cancer use one or more kinds of alternative or complementary therapies. They are often reluctant to tell their doctors or nurses about their decision. The best approach is to look carefully at your choices. When evaluating any complementary or alternative method, ask yourself the following questions.

- What claims are made for the treatment: To cure the cancer? To enable the conventional treatment to work better? To relieve symptoms or side effects?

- What are the credentials of those supporting the treatment? Are they recognized experts in cancer treatment? Have they published their findings in trustworthy medical journals?

- How is the method promoted? Is it promoted only in the mass media (books, magazines, TV, and radio talk shows) rather than in scientific journals?

- What are the costs of the therapy?

- Is the method widely available for use within the health care community, or is it controlled with limited access to its use?

- If used in place of conventional therapies or clinical trials, will the ensuing delay in conventional treatment affect any chances for cure or advance the cancer stage?.

In addition, use the checklist below to spot those approaches that might be open to question. If you are not sure, talk to your doctor or nurse before moving ahead.

- Is the treatment based on an unproven theory?

- Does the treatment promise a cure for all cancers?

- Are you told not to use conventional medical treatment?

- Is the treatment or drug a secret that only certain people can give?

- Is the treatment or drug offered by only one individual?

- Does the treatment require you to travel to another country?

- Do the promoters attack the medical or scientific establishment?

Talking with Your Doctor

About 60 percent of all people trying complementary or alternative therapies do not tell their doctors they are trying these treatments. Many people feel uncomfortable asking their doctor or nurse about complementary or alternative treatments. But most health care professionals understand that patients and caregivers want to do all they can to improve their quality of life or improve the quality of life for their loved ones. Although people may be reluctant to share their complementary or alternative therapy interests with their health care team, it could be dangerous to the health of the person with cancer to withhold information.

The best approach is to look carefully at your choices. Talk to your health care team about any methods you are considering. Consider the risks and benefits of using any complementary or alternative methods and make an informed decision in an atmosphere of shared decision-making. There are many *complementary* methods you can safely use along with conventional treatment to help relieve symptoms or side effects, to ease pain, and to help you enjoy life more.

If you are considering using complementary or alternative therapies, here are some tips for your discussion with your doctor and other members of your health care team:

- Educate yourself first. Before beginning a conversation with your doctor, research the proven conventional treatment for your disease. It is important to be as informed as possible before the office visit. Then, find out as much as you can about the alternative method that you wish to discuss. Some questions for patients to ask the doctor are: What do you know about this alternative? Can you give me additional sources of information? Do you know someone who tried the alternative method? What was their experience?

    When looking at information, particularly on the Internet, try to determine whether or not the information is provided by someone selling a product. If a product is being promoted for sale, then information will likely be slanted toward helping to sell the product. The objectivity and accuracy of the information may not be reliable.

- Let your doctor know before beginning an alternative. Tell your doctor that you are thinking about taking an alternative therapy but that you want to make sure it does not interfere with the treatment he or she prescribes. Once the treatment is recorded in your medical record, your doctor will be able to watch for potential drug interactions and/or harmful effects.

- Ask questions. It can be helpful to write down a list of questions for the doctor and bring in any literature you want to discuss. Let your doctor know you are an educated consumer; even though you may be apprehensive about what you are facing, you are seeking as much information as you can. Let your doctor know you want him or her to be a supportive partner in your education and treatment process.

- Bring someone with you to the doctor's office. A friend or relative can help you retain information, ask questions, and remain more objective than you may be able to alone. Support from your loved ones will not only help you communicate but can also help lessen the stress of making decisions alone.

- Understand your doctor's perspective. If you take herbs or megadoses of vitamins or start on a special diet, the doctor needs to know. Some therapies are considered alternative because they have not been proven to be safe and effective in controlled scientific studies. People with cancer who rely on alternative therapies may run the risk of jeopardizing their primary treatment because of possible drug interactions or they may harm themselves with unsafe methods. If your doctor has not heard of the particular therapy, don't become discouraged. Ask your doctor to help you find out more about it.

- Don't delay or forgo conventional therapy. If you are considering stopping or not taking current conventional treatment, discuss the implications of this decision with your doctor. You may be giving up the only proven treatment for your cancer.

- If you're taking dietary supplements, review your usage. Whenever you receive new medication or there is a change in medication or medical history, review the list of supplements you are taking with your doctor or nurse. Also, let your health care team know if you change or add any dietary supplements. By telling your health care providers about supplement use, the medical record can be used to analyze the risks, benefits, and interactions with medications.

- Ask about the use of alternative therapies if you are pregnant or breast-feeding. Most herbalists advise not using alternative medicines if you are. Do not give alternative medicine to children.

- Ask your doctor or nurse to help you identify possible fraudulent products.

- Follow up with your doctor. On your next office visit, be sure to continue your conversation about your use of any alternative therapies. Discuss any decision you have reached about using an alternative method. Your doctor may or may not agree with your decision, but it's important that your doctor know if you're planning to use alternative therapies so that he or she can provide you with the best possible care.

- Be open to change. Realize that new studies may yield new information about complementary and alternative methods of managing cancer that may change your treatment plan.

Where the American Cancer Society (ACS) Stands

The ACS believes that all cancer interventions must withstand the scrutiny of scientific evaluation before they can be recommended for the prevention, diagnosis, or treatment of cancer. The following are questions that researchers, doctors, and other health care professionals use when evaluating treatment:

- Has the method been objectively demonstrated in peer-reviewed scientific literature to be more effective than doing nothing?

- Has the method shown a potential for benefit that clearly exceeds the potential for harm?

- Have objective studies been conducted properly, appropriately evaluated by other qualified scientists, and approved by responsible human studies committees to answer these questions?

The ACS urges individuals with cancer to remain in the care of doctors who use standard, conventional therapies for cancer and approved clinical trials of promising new treatments. The ACS also encourages patients to talk openly with their health care providers about any other therapy they are considering, and to seek information from unbiased and reliable sources. Open, trusting, noncritical communication is essential in making health care decisions. In this way, patients will be able to make informed decisions by selecting methods most likely to be safe and effective in relieving symptoms and improving their well being. They will also be able to avoid methods that are dangerous, likely to interfere with conventional treatments, and known to be ineffective. For more information about specific methods, contact the ACS at 800-ACS-2345 (www.cancer.org) or read the *American Cancer Society's Guide to Complementary and Alternative Cancer Methods*.

Categories of Methods

The list of complementary and alternative methods changes continually. Most of the methods can be grouped within the five major areas that follow. They are classified within categories based on similar characteristics and how the treatment is administered or performed.

Mind, Body, and Spirit Methods

These methods focus on the connections between the mind, body, and spirit, and their power for healing. Many of the methods in this category are considered complementary methods you can safely use along with conventional treatment to help relieve symptoms or side effects, to ease pain, and to help you enjoy life more. Some of these methods include aromatherapy, art therapy, biofeedback, meditation, music therapy, prayer, spiritual practices, tai chi, and yoga. (For more information about coping methods such as these, see Chapter 27).

Meditation. One example of a mind-body process is meditation, which uses concentration or reflection to relax the body and calm the mind in order to create a sense of well being. It is a relaxation method approved by an independent panel convened by the National Institutes of Health as a useful complementary therapy for treating chronic pain and insomnia. It may help people with cancer control pain, decrease stress, and improve quality of life.

There are many ways to practice meditation, such as sitting quietly and concentrating on breathing in a regulated way, focusing on a repeated word, or concentrating on an object such as a lighted candle. Some practitioners recommend two fifteen- to twenty-minute sessions a day. Meditation can be self-directed, or guided by doctors, psychiatrists, other mental health professionals, and yoga masters. The ultimate goal of meditation is to separate oneself mentally from the outside world.

Diet and Nutrition Methods

Many complementary and alternative therapies designed to prevent cancer involve nutrition. There is a growing body of scientific evidence available to suggest that a diet high in fiber, fruits, and vegetables can help protect the human body against some types of cancer. These foods contain vitamins and minerals necessary for normal growth and development and overall health and well being. The ACS and many conventional doctors recommend that people get these essential vitamins and minerals from foods rather than from supplements. Supplements have not been proven to have the same cancer-protective effects as foods rich in vitamins, minerals, and other nutrients. Furthermore, foods provide nutrients in a complete package that may allow the vitamins and minerals to work together to help prevent cancer.

Gerson Therapy. Gerson therapy was developed by Max Gerson, M.D., a German doctor who immigrated to the United States in the late 1930s. The therapy is based on the theory that disease is caused by the body's accumulation of toxic substances. Practitioners believe that chemical fertilizers, insecticides, and herbicides contaminate food, and that food processing and cooking adds sodium to food which changes the metabolism of cells in the body, eventually causing cancer.

Gerson therapy involves coffee enemas and a special diet with supplements claiming to cleanse the body and stimulate metabolism. This therapy can be very harmful to the body. Coffee enemas have been associated with serious infections, dehydration, constipation, colitis (inflammation of the colon), electrolyte (salt and mineral) imbalances, and even death. According to a critique in a major peer-reviewed journal, the explanation for how the method is supposed to work does not follow the established scientific principles of basic nutrition, biology, and cancer immunology. There is no scientific evidence that Gerson therapy is effective in treating cancer.

Herbs, Vitamins, and Minerals

It is estimated that 4 billion people, 80 percent of the world's population, currently use herbals as medicine for some aspect of their health care. They have a long history of use in virtually every ancient culture. About one in four drugs prescribed today came from plants. Although many chemotherapy drugs, such as paclitaxel (Taxol), are derived from plant sources, no raw herbal medicine has yet been approved by the FDA for use as a drug to treat cancer.

Herbals are made up of many chemicals, some helpful and others dangerous. Because they have an impact on a variety of systems in the human body, they present a potential danger by affecting the way drugs exert their activity on the body, either by increasing the drug's activity or by blocking it. Drug companies have been slow to conduct research on such supplement-drug interactions, and herb manufacturers generally do not have the resources or the desire to do that type of research. So consumers are left to search out information about possibly dangerous interactions on their own.

Essiac Tea. Essiac is a mixture of herbs that are combined to make a tea. The original formula included burdock root, slippery elm inner bark, sheep sorrel, and Turkish rhubarb. Watercress, blessed thistle, red clover, and kelp were added to later recipes.

Promoters claim that Essiac strengthens the immune system, improves well being, relieves pain, reduces tumor size, and extends survival. It was originally claimed that Essiac changed tumors into normal tissue. Proponents claimed that after a few doses of Essiac, a tumor would grow larger and harder, then soften, shrink, and be discharged by the body.

There is no scientific evidence to support these claims in humans. One study found reduced tumor growth after giving oral and intravenous doses of Essiac to mice injected with human cancer cells. Also, some laboratory research found anticancer effects related to the specific herbs studied separately. Animal and laboratory studies may show that a certain compound holds promise as a beneficial treatment, but further studies are necessary to determine if the results apply to humans.

There have been no clinical trials (trials with humans) proving the effectiveness of Essiac. In 1983, NCI tested Essiac and found that no anticancer activity occurred. Canadian health officials at that time found that there was no evidence that Essiac slowed the progression of cancer, but that there were few serious side effects, and that people may have benefited psychologically from the treatment.

Hoxsey Herbal Treatment. In the 1920s, Harry Hoxsey, who had no medical training, marketed a mixture of herbs that he believed would effectively treat cancer. Over the next few decades he opened clinics in the United States and at one point operated clinics in seventeen states. By 1960, after battling with Hoxsey for over a decade, the FDA banned the sale of the Hoxsey herbal treatment in the United States. In 1963 Hoxsey opened a clinic in Tijuana, Mexico, which still operates today. Hoxsey developed prostate cancer in 1967. When he did not respond to his own treatment, he underwent conventional surgery. He died seven years later.

The Hoxsey herbal treatment is an herbal mixture taken internally or applied externally. The pastes or salves that are applied externally contain antimony trisulfide, zinc chloride, and bloodroot, and a yellow powder consisting of arsenic sulfide, sulfur, and talc. Both the paste and powder are escharotics, which means they can burn the skin.

Proponents of the treatment claim that the mixture eliminates toxins from the body, strengthens the immune system, and enhances its ability to slowly absorb and excrete tumors. The external treatment is used to treat skin cancer by allegedly keeping cancer from spreading and helping to destroy cancer cells. There is no scientific evidence to support these claims.

Manual Healing/Physical Touch

The methods in this category involve touching, manipulation, or movement of the body. These techniques are based on the idea that problems in one part of the body often affect other parts of the body. Examples of this include electromagnetic therapy, massage, hydrotherapy, chiropractic, acupuncture, and transcutaneous electrical nerve stimulation.

Electromagnetic Therapy. Electromagnetic therapy involves the use of electrical and magnetic energy to diagnose or treat disease. Practitioners claim that when electromagnetic frequencies or fields of energy within the body go out of balance, disease and illness occur. Practitioners claim they can correct the imbalances in the body by applying electrical energy from outside the body, usually with electronic devices.

Electromagnetic therapy, which encompasses several different kinds of therapy, uses an energy field—electrical, magnetic, microwave, or infrared—to diagnose or treat an illness by detecting imbalances in the body's energy fields and then correcting them. Electronic devices, which emit some form of low-voltage electrical current or radio frequency, are often involved.

Dozens of unconventional and unproven electronic devices have been marketed over the years. One electronic device that has been promoted to cure cancer is the Zapping Machine. Based on the claim that cancer is related to parasites, promoters say it kills the parasites that cause cancer; however, there is no evidence for this claim. Other devices promoted for electromagnetic therapy include the BioResonance Tumor Therapy Device, the Cell Com System, and the Rife Machine. There is no scientific evidence to support any of the claims made for these devices. The FDA has not approved any of the alternative machines or products connected to electrical sources (electronic devices) used to cure illness and does not recognize any frequency generator as a legitimate medical device.

Untested, unproven electrical devices may pose some risk. There have been reports of injuries due to faulty electrical wiring, power surges during lightning storms, and misuse of equipment. Relying on this type of treatment alone, and avoiding conventional medical care, may have serious health consequences.

Pharmacological and Biological Treatment Methods

The methods in this category include substances that are synthesized and produced from chemicals or concentrated from plants and other living things. Some of these methods are highlighted below.

Antineoplaston Therapy. Antineoplaston therapy is an alternative form of cancer treatment that involves using a group of synthetic chemicals called antineoplastons to protect the body from disease. Antineoplastons are made up mostly of peptides and amino acids originally taken from human blood and urine.

Supporters claim that antineoplastons are a part of something called the body's natural biochemical defense system. This system is said to operate independently from the body's immune system and protect against diseases like cancer, which involve a breakdown in the chemistry of the body's cells. Proponents claim that people with cancer have a deficiency of naturally occurring antineoplastons, and that this therapy replenishes the body's supply, allowing the body's biochemical defense system to convert cancer cells into normal cells.

Proponents claim that antineoplaston therapy is nontoxic. Side effects may include stomach gas, slight rashes, chills, fever, change in blood pressure, and unpleasant body odor during treatment. High levels of blood sodium can also be a significant problem with this therapy.

Due to a lack of scientific evidence regarding antineoplaston therapy and the popularity of this therapy among some people with cancer, the FDA has recently granted the developer of the therapy (Stanislaw Burzynski, M.D., Ph.D.) permission to conduct clinical trials of antineoplaston therapy at his clinic.

There is not yet any scientific evidence that antineoplaston therapy is effective in treating cancer or any other disease. Relying on this type of treatment alone, and avoiding conventional medical care, may have serious health consequences.

Dimethylsulfoxide (DMSO). DMSO is an industrial solvent, produced as a byproduct of paper manufacturing, that has been promoted as an alternative cancer treatment since the 1960s. There is no scientific evidence that DMSO is effective in treating cancer. It is currently under study as a drug carrier used to increase the effectiveness of some chemotherapy agents for the treatment of bladder cancer. If administered in high concentrations, DMSO can cause death.

Proponents say that DMSO can cause malignant cells to become benign and slow or halt the progress of cancers in the bladder, colon, ovary, breast, and skin. Some claim that it is effective in treating leukemia, and it has also been used as a component of some metabolic cancer therapies. Some people claim that DMSO works as a cancer preventive agent by "cleaning" the cell membrane and decreasing the effect of cancer-causing substances. DMSO is also promoted to reduce the side effects of chemotherapy and radiation treatments in people with cancer. This activity is supposedly due to the ability of DMSO to stimulate the immune system and neutralize free radicals that are produced by these treatments and are a main cause of the side effects. These claims have not been proven.

Research has shown that DMSO does appear to have some effect in reducing swelling and inflammation. Dimethylsulfoxide is approved by the FDA to treat a single type of bladder disorder (interstitial cystitis) in humans and as veterinary therapy to reduce swelling in horses and dogs.

Laetrile. Laetrile is a compound produced from amygdalin, a naturally occurring substance found primarily in the kernels of apricots, peaches, and almonds. Promoters claim that Laetrile can prevent cancer from occurring and can help patients stay in remission. It is also promoted to provide pain relief to people with cancer. One of the proponents' theories is that cancer cells trigger the release of the cyanide found in Laetrile, causing cyanide poisoning and the death of the cancer cells. The second theory is that cancer is really a "vitamin deficiency" and that Laetrile is the missing "vitamin B-17."

There is no scientific evidence to support these claims. Studies have been done to determine Laetrile's effectiveness and none has been demonstrated. Laetrile contains a small percentage of cyanide, and several cases of cyanide poisoning and death have been linked to its use. The FDA has not issued approval for Laetrile as a medical treatment and its use is illegal in the United States. This treatment should be avoided, especially by women who are pregnant or breast-feeding. Relying on this type of treatment alone and avoiding conventional medical care may have serious health consequences.

Shark Cartilage. Shark cartilage is extracted from the heads and fins of sharks. Cartilage is a type of elastic tissue that is found in the skeletal systems of many animals, including humans. Sharks have no bones, so cartilage is the primary component of their skeletal system. The major compounds in shark cartilage are glycoproteins and calcium salts.

Proponents believe that shark cartilage contains a protein that slows or stops the growth of cancer through preventing angiogenesis, the process of blood vessel development. Tumors require a network of blood vessels to survive and grow, so cutting off the tumor's blood supply starves it of nutrients it needs to live, causing it to shrink or disappear. Finding drugs that halt the spread of cancer by inhibiting the growth of blood vessels has been the subject of many serious research studies in recent years. A number of antiangiogenesis drugs have been developed and are currently under investigation. However, the most promising antiangiogenic substances now in existence are those that have been purified from sources other than cartilage or have been synthesized in laboratories.

Shark cartilage is available as a capsule, powder, or liquid extract. It can be applied directly to the skin or injected by needle into the bloodstream, under the skin, into the lining of the abdomen, or directly into the muscle. It is also sometimes used as an enema.

Interest in shark cartilage increased after a television newsmagazine aired a segment in 1993 that showed a study of patients with advanced cancer in Cuba that had gone into remission after being treated with shark cartilage. The National Cancer Institute later concluded that the results of the Cuban study were "incomplete and unimpressive." In June 2000, the Federal Trade Commission ordered shark cartilage manufacturers to stop making unsubstantiated claims that their products have cancer-fighting abilities, and fined them $1 million for false advertising.

There is no scientific evidence that shark cartilage, sold as a food supplement, is an effective treatment for cancer, osteoporosis, or any other disease. Although some laboratory and animal studies have shown that components isolated from shark cartilage possess a modest ability to inhibit the growth of new blood vessels, these effects have not been proven in humans. No well-controlled clinical studies have been published; however, clinical trials are currently underway.

Shark cartilage is not thought to be toxic, although it has been known to cause nausea, indigestion, fatigue, fever, and dizziness in some people. It may also slow down the healing process for people recovering from surgery. People with a low white blood cell count should not take shark cartilage enemas, because there is a risk of life-threatening infection. Children should not take shark cartilage because it could interfere with body growth and development. Women who are pregnant or breast-feeding should also avoid these supplements. Relying on this type of treatment alone, and avoiding conventional medical care, may have serious health consequences.

Living
with Cancer

Food and Nutrition

The importance of good nutrition for people with cancer is well documented, whether for people who are undergoing active therapy, recovering from cancer treatment, or currently cancer-free.

The goals of optimal nutrition intake (healthy eating) during cancer care include:

- preventing or reversing nutrition-related nutrient deficiencies
- preserving lean body mass (muscle)
- minimizing nutrition-related side effects
- maximizing energy level and quality of life

At a time where people with cancer and health care professionals alike are inundated with nutrition-related complementary and alternative therapy choices, seeking sound nutrition information and guidance for informed decision-making is vital.

Nutrition Basics

A healthy diet helps maintain strength and resistance to infection, prevents body tissues from breaking down, and helps rebuild tissues that have been affected by therapy. Those who eat well and maintain their weight are in better shape to withstand the side effects of therapy and may even be able to handle more aggressive treatments and, therefore, increase their chances for survival.

Eating well for people who have cancer means eating the same healthy diet generally recommended for all Americans: one that is high in complex carbohydrates and low in fat while ensuring an adequate intake of protein.

SPECIAL

CONCERNS

A Nutritional Cure for Cancer?

Eating a balanced, healthy diet during cancer treatment and recovery is important to promote strength and healing. Many people immediately change their diets when they learn they have cancer. For example, according to one survey of women recently diagnosed with breast cancer, 80 percent altered their food intake in some way as a result, and 85 percent started taking vitamins.

But nutrition is no panacea. Despite the increased interest in and research on the relationship of nutrition to health and healing, no unimpeachable evidence yet exists that a particular diet or combination of nutrients can bring remission or cure. The interrelationship of nutrients and cancer is extraordinarily complex and not yet well understood. Thus far, more light has been shed on the role of diet in prevention than in treatment or cure.

When supplementing a conventional cancer treatment with an unconventional nutritional intervention, beware of any practitioner who claims to have a dietary cure for cancer (see Chapter 17).

Carbohydrates

The most efficient source of energy that the body receives from the diet is carbohydrates, which should account for 55 to 60 percent of the calories eaten each day. Most of the calories should come from starches (also called complex carbohydrates) rather than sugars (also called simple carbohydrates).

Starches are found in grains (cereals, pastas, rice, flour, and bran), legumes (beans, lentils, and peas), potatoes, and other vegetables. Sugars are found in fruit, milk, honey, table sugar, jams, jellies, syrups, and other sweets.

The body needs the energy from carbohydrates to breathe, move, and handle extra stress posed by cancer and its treatment. If the diet doesn't contain enough carbohydrates, the body will turn to its protein stores for energy, thereby risking the loss of lean body mass.

Fat

Most Americans eat too much fat. Even though numerous health authorities suggest limiting fat calories to 30 percent of daily intake, the average American's diet is 35 percent fat. The links between fat and cardiovascular disease are well known. Less well defined but under careful study are possible links between fat and cancer, especially colon, breast, and prostate cancer. The amount of fat in the diet can be reduced simply by eating only lean meats; removing the skin from chicken and turkey before eating the meat (and preferably before cooking it); avoiding fried foods, spreads like butter and mayonnaise, and fat-filled fast foods and snacks; and substituting skim milk for whole milk. When oils are needed for cooking, monounsaturated fats like olive oil or canola oil should be used instead of butter or lard. If you are trying not to lose weight, small amounts of fat can help increase your calorie intake for weight gain. The use of foods containing fat—such as a pat of margarine or butter or a spoonful of peanut butter or sour cream—can add flavor and may help to improve your appetite as well. If you're experiencing stomach upset, avoid foods that are high in fat, deep-fried, or greasy. These foods are more slowly digested and absorbed by the body and can make you feel full for a longer period of time.

Protein

Protein is vital to the life of every cell, as it continuously builds, maintains, and repairs cells. During treatment and recovery, protein requirements increase as the body repairs and rebuilds damaged tissue and works toward maintaining a healthy immune system. (In order for your body to use protein in the most effective way, you must also consume adequate calories.)

Protein should account for about 15 to 25 percent of a person's total daily calories, depending on age and nutritional status. The normal requirement is about 50 to 75 grams per day. If you are experiencing weight loss, it may be helpful to increase protein to 80 to 90 grams a day. Counting grams of protein is not necessary, but to estimate grams consumed use the following examples:

1 cup of milk = 8 grams of protein
1 ounce of meat, poultry, or fish = 7 grams of protein
1 serving ($\frac{1}{2}$ cup) of dry beans, lentils, or peas = 6 grams of protein
1 ounce of cheese = 6 grams of protein
1 serving ($\frac{1}{2}$ cup) of pasta or rice = 2 grams of protein
1 serving (1 slice) of bread = 2 grams of protein

Quality sources of protein are found in animal products as well as in vegetable sources. Examples of quality protein foods are non-fat dairy foods (such as skim milk and cheeses made of skim or low-fat milk), grains, legumes, fish, lean meat, and poultry.

Counting Calories

Most people only think about calories when they want to lose weight, but those with cancer may need to count calories in order to maintain or gain weight.

The easiest way to determine your daily caloric needs is to multiply your current weight in kilograms (divide your weight in pounds by 2.2 to determine your weight in kilograms) by the recommended caloric needs for your sex and metabolic needs. Caloric needs for women are 20 to 30 calories per kilogram of current body weight, and for men, 25 to 35 calories per kilogram. When your body needs extra energy and more calories, such as before and after surgery or when you are running a fever, boost your intake to 40 to 50 calories per kilogram.

If you are experiencing weight loss, here is another quick method to figure out how many calories you need for weight gain. One pound of body weight is equal to 3,500 calories. If you want to gain one pound a week, try adding 500 calories a day. A quick calculation shows that if you eat 500 more calories a day for a week (seven days), you will be taking in 3,500 calories and that should result in a one-pound weight gain. If eating 500 calories a day seems too much, you can gain a half-pound each week by adding 250 calories per day.

INFORM

YOURSELF

Calculating Your Caloric Needs

To determine the range of your daily caloric needs, first weigh yourself and convert your weight in pounds to your metric weight in kilograms (divide your weight in pounds by 2.2 to determine your weight in kilograms). Then men should multiply their current weight in kilograms by 25 and then multiply their weight in kilograms by 35. The lower number is the low end of the range, while the higher number is the upper end of the range. Women would multiply by 20 and then 30.

Let us use as an example a woman weighing 140 pounds, which is 63 kilograms. If we multiply her metric weight first by 20 and then again by 30, we will get an estimated daily need of 1,260 to 1,890 calories to maintain weight. For a man of 190 pounds, or 85.5 kilograms, the recommended range for weight maintenance comes to about 2,138 to 2,993 calories.

Vitamin and Mineral Supplements

Although essential micronutrients are necessary for optimal health, research studies have not shown that vitamin and mineral supplements, even at high doses, are useful in promoting cancer remission or improving cancer-related symptoms. Large doses of some vitamin and mineral supplements may actually cause adverse side effects such as gastrointestinal distress and discomfort after eating. Large amounts of antioxidants, especially single nutrients, just before and during therapy may actually interfere with the action of prescribed anticancer treatment regimens. The use of vitamin and mineral supplements should never replace the consumption of regular foods and the goal of eating a healthy diet.

When cancer or its treatment interferes with the body's absorption of certain nutrients, especially the B vitamins, supplements are sometimes recommended. Further, recent research suggests that certain vitamins—called antioxidant vitamins because they help prevent the oxidative destruction of cells—may help lower the risk of cancer. However, these same nutrients may interfere with therapy in a person who has cancer.

The antioxidants are vitamin C, vitamin E, and beta carotene (which is converted to vitamin A in the body). Antioxidant vitamins are in plentiful supply in colorful foods. Dark green, yellow, and orange foods such as cantaloupe, carrots, spinach, and sweet potatoes are good sources of beta

What to Eat Every Day

INFORM

YOURSELF

Eating a wide variety of foods is the best way to ensure getting the nutrients you need. The following are recommendations adapted from the U.S. Department of Agriculture's Dietary Guidelines:

Food Group	Servings Daily	Sample Servings
Breads, cereals, grains	6–11	1 slice bread; small roll or muffin; ½ cup cooked cereal, rice, or pasta; 1 ounce cold breakfast cereal; 3–4 small crackers
Vegetables	3–5, including dark green leafy vegetables several times a day	½ cup cooked vegetables; ½ cup raw vegetables; 1 cup leafy raw vegetables such as lettuce or spinach; 1 medium potato; ¾ cup vegetable juice
Fruits	2–4	1 whole medium fresh fruit, such as an orange, apple, or banana; a grapefruit half; a melon wedge; ½ cup berries; ¾ cup fruit juice; ½ cup cooked or canned fruit; ¼ cup dried fruit
Lean meat, poultry, dry beans, fish, eggs, nuts	2–3	2–3 ounces lean meat, fish, or poultry; 1 egg; ½ cup nuts; ½ cup cooked beans or tofu; 2 tablespoons reduced-fat peanut butter (equal to 1 ounce meat); 2½ ounce soyburger
Milk, cheese, yogurt	2	1 cup skim milk; 8 ounces low-fat yogurt; 1½ ounces low-fat cheese

carotene. Citrus and other fruits and dark green vegetables such as broccoli and green peppers are rich in vitamin C. Green leafy vegetables, dried beans, and whole-grain cereals and breads contain vitamin E.

The use of a multivitamin and mineral supplement that provides no more than 100 percent of the U.S. Recommended Dietary Allowances is generally considered safe. Because cancer and its treatment can affect the body's metabolism in many ways, however, you should discuss taking any supplements, particularly antioxidants, with your doctor before taking them.

Planning Daily Meals

It may be useful to schedule an appointment with a registered dietitian who is familiar with the nutritional demands of cancer. He or she can help determine, for example, how many calories you need daily and how to select foods that will provide those calories and be healthful.

In health care settings where the services of a registered dietitian are unavailable, you need to be assertive and persistent in order to have your diet and nutrition questions addressed by other members of the health care team. You can also call the American Dietetic Association, your own state's Dietetic Association, or the local American Cancer Society for assistance in locating a qualified registered dietitian in your area.

The Mechanics of Digestion

A malfunction or alteration anywhere in the alimentary tract (from the mouth to the colon) can affect your nutritional status. Obviously, if a tumor is pressing on an area of the alimentary tract or affecting one of the digestive organs, it can impair the normal movement of food, nutrient absorption, or both. For example, tumors in the mouth or throat can interfere with chewing and swallowing. Tumors in the stomach or intestines can cause obstructions, blocking the passage of food or decreasing the flow of fluids and interfering with their absorption. Tumors in the liver or pancreas can cause changes in the production of digestive enzymes and hormones. Mechanical difficulties may also cause early satiety, a feeling of fullness that occurs shortly after you begin to eat. This can happen when a tumor decreases the size of the stomach or causes changes that slow the movement of food through the intestinal tract. Early satiety is apt to worsen during the day; that is, it may be absent at breakfast, mild at lunch, and severe at dinner. Reversing the typical order of meals can help; you could eat the main meal for breakfast or have many small meals throughout the day.

Nutritional Effects of Cancer Treatment

As described in earlier chapters, conventional methods of cancer treatment include surgery, radiation therapy, chemotherapy, and biological therapy. In many instances, individuals receive a combination of therapies (multi-modality) to most effectively treat their cancer (see Chapter 15). Cancer treatments can have temporary or sometimes permanent side effects that can impact nutritional needs and the ability to eat. People receiving multimodality therapy may experience side effects sooner and with greater intensity.

Surgery

Immediately after any type of surgery, nutritional needs increase for wound healing and recovery. After surgery many people also experience tiredness, pain, loss of appetite, and are unable to consume their regular diet. Most people benefit from some type of diet progression (clear liquids, then easy-to-digest foods, and then a regular diet) for a few days after the surgery. Unfortunately, most people don't feel much like eating at this time. Furthermore, if the surgery has involved the alimentary tract, eating may be uncomfortable, and the digestion and absorption of nutrients from food may be compromised. Most side effects are temporary and go away within a few days of the surgical procedure; however, some surgeries cause long-lasting nutrition-related changes. For example, the surgical removal of all or part of the stomach or small intestine may mean that food moves through the system and reaches the colon too quickly, leading to a condition known as dumping syndrome, which can cause nausea, diarrhea, rapid heartbeat, weakness, and dizziness.

Radiation Therapy

Radiation therapy uses photons or electrons to treat cancer in a specific area of the body. Side effects experienced are usually limited to the area being treated. People receiving radiation therapy generally begin to notice the effects of therapy after eight to ten days of treatment, and side effects usually resolve after two to four weeks after treatment has been completed.

Regardless of which area is being treated, the most commonly experienced side effects are tiredness, loss of appetite, and skin changes, as well as hair loss in the treated area. Irradiation to cells anywhere along the alimentary tract can affect a person's ability to eat and his or her nutritional status. For example, radiation to the head and neck can: inhibit the activity of the salivary glands, leading to dry mouth (xerostomia); cause a sore throat and/or mouth; and lead to dental problems that inhibit chewing or change the taste of food. Radiation to the stomach or intestines may cause nausea, vomiting, or diarrhea (see Chapter 11).

Chemotherapy

Chemotherapy uses chemical agents and medications to treat cancer. It is a "systemic" therapy that can affect the whole body. The action of chemotherapy can be harmful to healthy cells as well as cancer cells. The type of cells most sensitive to chemotherapy are those that are rapidly growing, such as hair cells, blood cells, and cells that line the alimentary tract. Commonly experienced side effects include tiredness, loss of appetite, nausea, vomiting, changes in taste and smell, sore or tender mouth and throat, dry mouth, and changes in normal bowel function. The severity of side effects experienced is related to the amount of chemotherapy prescribed, its frequency, whether single or multiple agents are used, individual response, and current health status. In contrast to the appetite and weight loss associated with most cancer treatments, hormonal therapy (for instance, tamoxifen or steroid drugs) can stimulate the appetite and cause weight gain. In this case, you may be advised not to eat too much, particularly high-fat foods, to avoid becoming overweight (see Chapter 12).

The new generation of antinausea medications currently available make extreme, hard-to-control nausea and vomiting less common today.

Biological Therapy

Individuals receiving biologicals for the treatment of their cancer often experience side effects somewhat similar to those seen in chemotherapy. Commonly experienced side effects include flu-like symptoms, nausea and vomiting, diarrhea, sore mouth, dry month, and changes in the taste of food. Moreover, loss of appetite and weight loss may be severe.

Loss of Appetite

In early or localized cancer, poor appetite may be due to depression or being emotionally upset (such as coping with a cancer diagnosis), or loss of appetite may be a side effect of the treatment. Those affected in this way are encouraged to do whatever they can to stimulate their appetite and eat healthy meals—that is, meals low in fat; containing whole-grain foods, fruits, and vegetables; and containing adequate protein.

Mind, Body, and Appetite

The impact of stress, anxiety, fear, and depression on appetite varies from person to person. Some people eat more when they're stressed, whereas others can't stand the thought of food. Indeed, a change in appetite is one of the diagnostic hallmarks of depression. Because a diagnosis of cancer can be frightening and its treatment can bring discomfort and disruption to daily life, anxiety and appetite loss are not uncommon.

Other aspects of the daily life of a person with cancer can also impair appetite. For example, someone who has done most of the cooking at home but is no longer able to do so may miss its appetite-stimulating effects. Or perhaps the meals prepared by others are not as appealing because the seasoning is different or because the foods are unfamiliar. The appetite of someone accustomed to sharing meals with others may suffer if he or she is no longer able to socialize.

Pain interferes with appetite, too. If the brain is focused on dealing with discomfort, responses to other stimuli, even pleasant ones such as the aroma and taste of a delicious meal, may diminish.

Coping with Loss of Appetite

In most cases, it's not difficult to explain the loss of appetite and to understand the ways of dealing with it. For example, consider when it occurs. If you began to lose weight when your cancer was first diagnosed or in anticipation of a doctor's visit or chemotherapy or radiation therapy, the cause is probably related to depression or anxiety. Appetite loss during or after chemotherapy or radiation therapy is probably due to the treatment.

Your doctor can help assess your situation and help you respond to the loss of appetite at any stage of treatment.

TIPS AND

ADVICE

Appetite Boosters

Sometimes simple changes in daily habits boost appetite, especially if psychological factors appear to be the underlying problem. Here are some suggestions:

- Ask those preparing your meals to follow your recipes or preferences.

- If you usually cooked your own food and are not feeling nauseated, stay in the kitchen to participate in its preparation even if you are not physically able to do the cooking.

- Ask friends and family to bring food from home to the hospital, if it is permitted.

- Arrange to eat meals with others.

- Disregard the "rules" of specific mealtimes. Instead, eat when you're hungry.

- Have small, frequent meals—six or more times per day—rather than three large ones.

- Foods that are visually appealing can stimulate the appetite. For example, brightly colored foods can accent pale ones. Fruits could be served over cereal or cottage cheese. Green and yellow vegetables and other garnishes could decorate pale sauces and casseroles. Contrasting texture and temperature also enhance the appeal of food. For example, soups could be seasoned with crunchy croutons; raw vegetable curls could top a soft casserole.

Medications to Stimulate Appetite. Some individuals may experience a lack of appetite that can lead to poor intake and weight loss. These people may benefit from the use of medications to boost their appetites so that muscles can be rebuilt (lean body mass). A variety of medications have been used to stimulate appetite. Examples of these medications include corticoidsteriods, dronabinol (Marinol), metoclopramide (Reglan), and megestrol acetate (Megace). These medications are most effective when used in combination with nutritional counseling and support and encouragement for increased physical activity.

Coping with Treatment Side Effects at Mealtimes

When treatment side effects cannot be avoided, dietitians offer a variety of techniques to ease problems while still ensuring adequate nutrition.

- *Mouth inflammation, difficulty chewing or swallowing:* Avoid spicy, salty, and acidic foods. Instead of hot food, try eating room-temperature or chilled foods. Also try soft foods such as milkshakes, bananas, applesauce, cottage cheese, mashed potatoes, macaroni and cheese, cooked cereals, pureed vegetables, and scrambled eggs. Careful attention to daily mouth care (regular brushing, flossing, and rinsing with a mix of baking soda and water or a saline rinse) will help keep the mouth clean and can enhance the healing of a tender, inflamed mouth.

- *Dry mouth:* Try to drink plenty of fluids throughout the day to keep a dry mouth more moist. The use of extra fluids at meal and snack time can also help to moisten foods for ease in chewing and swallowing. Eat soups and foods in sauces or gravies. Liquefy foods in a blender, or drink liquids in between bites of food. Very sweet or tart foods and beverages may help you produce more saliva. Use caution with especially sticky or overly sweet foods, as these foods can stay in contact with the teeth for a longer period of time and increase the likelihood of dental decay in a dry mouth.

- *Altered taste and smell perception:* Many people receiving chemotherapy commonly experience changes in taste and smell. These alterations in normal taste and smell are often described to as "off" smells and metallic tastes. A cleaner mouth can definitely help. Many people state that eating foods with a cool or room temperature has less taste and aroma. If sweet foods don't seem sweet enough, add a little extra sugar, such as honey, molasses, marmalade, syrup, apple butter, or jam. If your sour or bitter threshold is decreased, you may find that beef and pork taste bad. The addition of extra herbs and seasonings may remedy the problem. Or simply avoid the offensive foods and choose other sources of protein, such as poultry, fish, beans, peanut butter, nuts, and seeds. In particular, tart foods such as oranges or lemonade, or foods seasoned with citrus, may be appealing.

- *Diarrhea:* For four to eight hours after diarrhea subsides, try to limit your intake to only clear liquids such as weak tea, juices, broth, or sport drinks. Then add foods such as bananas and rice dishes, and low-fiber foods such as farina, scrambled eggs, pureed vegetables, canned fruit, and skinned poultry. Eat small amounts frequently throughout the day rather than three large meals, and include plenty of fluids. Foods and beverages should be at room temperature. Avoid foods and beverages that produce gas: greasy, fatty, spicy, or fried foods as well as raw vegetables and fruits and high-fiber vegetables. Medication may be needed to stop diarrhea.

- *Constipation:* Increase your consumption of fluids and fiber-containing foods, such as salads, colorful vegetables, bran, and other whole grains. Some fiber-containing foods may cause bloating, cramping, and gas and can add to constipation discomfort. Use caution with the following foods: dry beans and peas, melons, vegetables from the cabbage family, and carbonated beverages. If possible, get some exercise, such as walking, every day. If this regimen is not well tolerated, try a daily dose of psyllium seeds in products such as Metamucil. Medication to relieve constipation may be necessary.

- *Nausea:* If possible, stay out of the kitchen to avoid cooking aromas that may trigger nausea. If you must do the cooking, avoid aromatic foods (such as cabbage) and keep foods covered during cooking to minimize odors. Try to eat slowly in a relaxed atmosphere, avoiding a room that is stuffy or too warm. Eat dry, bland foods such as crackers or toast before meals. Eat your largest meal in the morning, when you may be less apt to be nauseated. Or eat small meals throughout the day, stopping when the nausea hits. Avoid any food that seems to trigger or aggravate the nausea, such as fatty, spicy, or other strongly flavored foods. You may be better able to tolerate foods that are chilled or at room temperature than hot foods. When nausea hits, take deep breaths to relax and sip small quantities of a carbonated beverage or warm tea, or chew ice chips until the nausea passes. Rest for a half-hour after eating, preferably sitting in an upright position, as reclining may trigger reflux, nausea, and vomiting. If nausea is persistent or treatment-related, ask your doctor about medications that may help.

- *Vomiting:* Do not try to eat or drink until the vomiting has stopped. Then try drinking a teaspoon of cool or room temperature clear liquids every ten minutes. Gradually increase the quantity until you can hold down two tablespoons every thirty minutes. Other liquids can be gradually introduced. If you know when nausea and vomiting are likely to occur, such as shortly after a treatment, eat a bland, easy-to-digest meal several hours beforehand, making sure to avoid milk products. If home remedies are not sufficient to control nausea and vomiting, ask your doctor about medication.

Understanding Weight Loss

The presence of cancer and the effects of cancer therapy put extra demands on your body and can alter your nutritional status. More than half of all people with cancer lose weight. Poor nutritional intake can lead to weight loss and can be caused by loss of appetite, or it may be the result of the effects of the cancer, cancer-related symptoms, or treatment. For some people, severe weight loss that results from or is aggravated by a treatment's side effects may require stopping the treatment until their nutritional status can be improved.

Weight loss and poor nutritional status can affect your strength and energy level, which can affect your quality of life by not allowing you to do the activities that you normally do. Not surprisingly, the prognosis for those who lose too much weight is not as good as for those who are able to maintain their weight. However, it is still not clear whether survival time is affected directly by weight loss. It may be that weight loss is a symptom of an aggressive form of cancer and that it is the disease—not the body wasting itself—that is responsible for the shortened survival time.

Maintaining body weight requires eating enough calories to replace those being burned and being able to digest food and absorb the nutrients. Any impairment of digestion and metabolism can lead to malnutrition, and in advanced cancer, weight loss may not be preventable.

How Cancer Affects Loss of Appetite and Weight

The relationship between the presence of a tumor in the body and loss of appetite and weight loss despite caloric intake continues to mystify researchers. There are two theories to explain the phenomenon. One is that the tumor secretes a substance that suppresses the appetite or affects the body's use of energy or both. The other theory is that the body secretes substances that have an anorexic effect, which enables it to defend itself against the tumor. Although the research is not conclusive, it may be that the loss of appetite starves the tumor. Many scientists believe that multiple mechanisms may be at work.

Clues to these phenomena have been found in many research studies. For example, a brain chemical called tryptophan is elevated in animals with tumors. Tryptophan is used by the body to make a neurotransmitter called serotonin, which plays a key role in controlling the appetite. Although it is not known why or how the tryptophan level rises in people with cancer, the finding supports the theory that the body's chemistry changes and leads to loss of appetite. People with cancer may metabolize carbohydrates, fats, and proteins differently, which helps support such theories.

In addition, certain types of cancer cause specific metabolic abnormalities that contribute to loss of appetite. For instance, a cancer that begins in or spreads to the liver produces high levels of lactic acid, a chemical that can cause both loss of appetite and nausea.

Beyond overall appetite loss, many people—especially those with metastatic cancer—report changes in their taste and smell sensations and say they develop aversions to certain foods. Meat and meat products, for instance, can become quite distasteful. Such people may have increased tolerance for sweet substances and decreased tolerance for sour and salty foods. Although such changes may occur as a side effect of treatment, they may also stem from the body's response to the tumor.

Although people with loss of appetite do eat—albeit far less food than is usual for them—they may lose weight (both lean body mass and fatty tissue) far out of proportion to their caloric intake. This type of weight loss seems to indicate a wide range of metabolic abnormalities, including aberrations in energy expenditure and in the body's use of sugar, fat, and protein.

A condition called cancer cachexia, which involves a loss of body weight and muscle mass, can occur in people with advanced stages of cancer. Its cause is not clearly understood, but people with cachexia experience weakness, involuntary weight loss, and hormonal imbalances, and they are malnourished (unable to eat enough calories and protein to meet their bodies' needs). Cachexia also compromises the body's immune system because the white blood cells that battle disease do not function properly and thus lower the person's resistance to even minor infections. Furthermore, once malnutrition is underway, changes occur in the gastrointestinal tract that worsen the situation. For example, cells lining the small intestine may be shed, thereby reducing the absorption of food. So even though the person may eat, the food's nutrients are not put to use.

Today, cancer experts and nutritionists are rethinking their advice that even people with advanced cancer *must* eat. Now doctors are concluding that loss of appetite and weight in the presence of cancer should not necessarily prompt efforts to force-feed or give supplements. Eating a few bites a day may make people feel independent and give them some strength and energy. Still, food is not necessarily what the body needs as it does battle with advanced or metastatic cancer.

It is important to remember that tumor cells require nutrients to grow, just as normal cells do. And when a tumor cell uses large quantities of nutrients, healthy cells may be deprived of their essential nutrients. Such body wasting is very disturbing, yet the body's response may be the best one.

Methods of Nutrition Support and Care

If at all possible, the preferred route for meeting nutritional needs is the consumption of regular meals and snacks by mouth (orally). Due to the effects of cancer or treatment-related side effects, some individuals may be unable to take in enough calories and protein to maintain their weight and optimal nutrition status. Three different approaches of nutrition support to consider are: the use of oral liquid nutrition supplements to boost calories and protein; enteral nutrition, also known as tube feedings; and parenteral nutrition, or intravenous feedings.

TIPS AND

ADVICE

A Word to Family Members: Food Is Not Necessarily Love

We grew up learning that "food is love" and "food is good medicine," so it's hard to accept that the opposite may be the case in advanced or metastatic cancer.

"He's becoming a skeleton," many a wife has lamented. How can she resist heading to the kitchen to whip up her husband's favorite high-calorie—and probably high-fat—dessert when cooking has been one of the ways she has expressed her love throughout their marriage? How can a partner resist taking his or her mate to a favorite restaurant to offer cheer and "put a little meat on your bones?" How can one not provide the nourishment to a parent that he or she never withheld?

If it is clear that the appetite and weight loss are related to the cancer rather than the result of emotions or treatment side effects, resist the urge. Your desire to see your loved one gain weight is well intentioned, but ill founded. Avoid hounding him or her to eat.

Liquid Nutritional Supplements

In circumstances when enough nutrition cannot be obtained from a regular diet and snacks, consider liquid nutritional supplements. The majority of these products are available in ready-to-drink boxes or cans, or are powders that can be easily mixed with liquids to reconstitute. The products' nutritional contents vary widely. Some are classified as complete mixtures of nutrients; some are modular, providing sources of protein, carbohydrates, or fatty acids alone or with a carbohydrate; some are designed specifically for those with liver, kidney, or lung failure; and some address various needs, such as lactose intolerance. The doctor's choice of a supplement is based on the person's specific nutritional needs. Most are available in drugstores and supermarkets. Examples include Ensure and Instant Breakfast.

Enteral Nutrition

When individuals are unable to meet their needs by mouth, other routes of nutrition support need to be considered. Enteral nutrition should be used when individuals cannot eat due to obstruction, prolonged anorexia, or if they are unable to consume adequate oral intake due to treatment-related side effects. For example, this may happen if your mouth, throat, or esophagus is severely inflamed because of radiation therapy. Or it may be needed when neurologic or psychiatric disorders, including severe depression, prevent normal eating.

The most common method of enteral nutrition involves a nasogastric tube, a flexible plastic tube that is passed through the nose into the stomach. A specific formula is delivered directly to the stomach through the tube, which remains in place continuously. Less commonly, an orogastric tube is used, entering through the mouth rather than the nose. If you cannot tolerate a tube in the nose or mouth, a surgical opening can be made in the abdomen, and a gastrostomy tube can be placed directly into the stomach or, if the stomach must be bypassed, a jejunostomy tube is inserted directly into the small intestine. Another option is a Percutaneous Endoscopic Gastrostomy (PEG). PEG feeding tubes can be placed on an outpatient basis and can be placed endoscopically (through hollow, tube-like instruments used for viewing the interior of the body).

The nutrients delivered through a tube are usually in a liquid formula such as those provided in commercial meal replacements. With surgically placed tubes to the stomach or intestine, sometimes normal food pureed in a blender can be used. Enteral nutrition may be delivered to the stomach at specified meal times every three or four hours (called bolus feeding), intermittently, or continuously by a special pump.

Once the tube is in place, enteral nutrition can be provided in the hospital or by a trained family member or health care worker at home. This has become a relatively common and safe practice that permits you to be sent home earlier, where you may recuperate more rapidly and in your own environment. In any case, when you are receiving enteral nutrition, you must be monitored for such side effects as nausea, vomiting, diarrhea, and constipation. A change of formula can usually relieve these problems.

Parenteral Nutrition

Parenteral nutrition delivers nutrients directly into the bloodstream on a short-term or long-term basis depending on the needs of the person. It may be recommended when the intestinal tract is not functioning; for example, when surgery has caused a temporary but severe gastrointestinal malfunction. It is also used when radiation therapy has caused severe inflammation to the gastrointestinal tract. These people may need parenteral nutrition indefinitely.

For short-term nutrition of less than ten days, a catheter is inserted into a vein in the arm, peripherally delivering a solution of amino acids, simple sugars, electrolytes, and vitamins. This is called peripheral parenteral nutrition.

For longer-term nutritional support, a large needle is inserted into a large vein in the chest, and a tiny catheter is threaded through it. This is called central parenteral nutrition. Fluid and nutrients flow through the catheter directly into the heart, where it enters the bloodstream and circulates throughout the body.

As with tube feeding, once the catheter for central parenteral nutrition is in place, fluid and essential nutrients can be provided either in the hospital or at home by home health workers or trained family members. Hyperalimentation, or intravenous feeding, need not be continuous but can often be done while you sleep at night. During the day, the catheter can be disconnected from the intravenous tube and discreetly concealed.

Central parenteral nutrition is the least preferable route for providing nutrition because of the high risk of mechanical difficulties, infection, and other complications. Moreover, central parenteral nutrition is very expensive.

When Extra Nutrition Is Necessary

Although oncologists do not routinely use nutritional support with liquid-food supplements or tube or intravenous feeding for extra nutrition, regardless of the stage of cancer, there are some exceptions.

Extra energy is needed to cope with the stress of recovery from an operation and to promote healing. The American College of Physicians found that nutritional support is useful for certain high-risk patients. For example, a number of studies have shown that seven to ten days of aggressive pre- and postoperative nutritional support in cancer patients reduces the morbidity and mortality associated with surgery.

Supplementation also is recommended, even for those who are well nourished, for people about to undergo operations (such as removal of part of the stomach) that will result in a postoperative period of ten days or more when they will not be able to eat. It is advised as well for those who develop postoperative complications that similarly impair the ability to eat. People who have mechanical difficulties that interfere with their ability to eat and digest food may not obtain adequate nutrition from meals. Furthermore, radiation therapy to the gastrointestinal system can cause side effects that damage the ability to eat, digest, and/or absorb food. In such cases, a period of tube or intravenous feeding, depending on the site of gastrointestinal impairment, can help maintain body weight until the person is again able to eat.

Physical Activity

The evidence in favor of the health benefits of physical activity (including for people with cancer) continues to accumulate. Research shows that exercise may help prevent some cancers, particularly cancer of the colon, rectum, prostate, testicles, ovary, endometrium, kidney, and breast. Exercise also seems to help counter some aspects of cancer and to relieve some treatment side effects. Although the effects of physical activity on people with cancer have not yet been studied extensively, physical activity is known to enhance self-esteem and provide a sense of autonomy. A recent study suggests that regular physical activity helped women with breast cancer avoid a general decline that often occurs after surgery, and both men and women report that exercise helps them feel better.

Of course, the ability to exercise depends on your general health and physical condition, including the stage and type of cancer you have as well as the treatment and its side effects. For instance, a fitness regimen that might be beneficial to a woman recovering from a mastectomy could be counterproductive for a man in the late stages of lung cancer.

Why Exercise?

Although it is not known whether physical activity can prevent a recurrence of cancer or slow the progress of metastasis (spread), it has many positive emotional and physical benefits. People with cancer should be encouraged to accumulate thirty minutes of activity each day (see the *Limitations on Physical Activity* section of this chapter and consult your doctor about physical activity that is appropriate for your individual circumstances).

Physical Benefits

Physical activity builds muscle tissue, strengthens the heart, increases the capacity of the lungs to take in oxygen, and improves circulation. It may even help healthy tissue compensate for compromised tissues and organs. For example, walking or swimming twice a day for fifteen minutes may increase the efficiency of the healthy areas of the lungs and enable a person with lung cancer to breathe more easily.

CANCER

BASICS

Physical Activity and Cancer Prevention

Some intriguing findings have emerged from studies of the role of physical inactivity in the development of cancer. It's now known, for instance, that physically fit people tend to have a lower incidence of cancer. According to one large study of people at various levels of fitness, the least fit men died from cancer at a rate that was more than four times higher than that of the most fit men, and the least fit women had fully sixteen times the cancer death rate of the most fit women. Studies have linked inactivity to colon cancer and breast cancer. Physical activity may also influence the risk for cancer of the endometrium, ovary, testicles, and prostate, but the research is either too limited or too inconsistent to support any definite conclusions. Unfortunately, finding a correlation is not the same as identifying a cause, but researchers are exploring several theories that may explain the link between inactivity and cancer. People who exercise tend to be leaner than those who do not, and excessive body fat is a risk factor for some cancers (see Chapter 2). Obesity is linked to higher risks of several cancers, and regular exercise can help people maintain a healthy weight, particularly as they age and their metabolism slows.

Another theory is that because exercise such as walking or jogging helps speed food through the digestive tract, carcinogens (including certain bile acids that help digest fat) interact with the intestinal wall for a shorter time. Girls who exercise vigorously begin menstruating later, which appears to reduce their chances of getting breast or reproductive cancers in the future. This finding has led some scientists to speculate that exercise might help prevent certain forms of cancer by affecting hormone levels.

Stimulating Appetite. Moderate activity stimulates appetite when worry and the physical effects of the disease or the side effects of treatment interfere with the desire for food.

Boosting Energy. Men and women who have survived cancer and exercise regularly say the main reason they keep active is that they feel more energetic.

This probably occurs for two reasons: first, exercise increases stamina that has been diminished by bed rest or depression; second, activity increases muscle strength, so movement requires less effort.

Improving Immunity. Aerobic exercise is any activity that increases the blood flow to the heart and the amount of oxygen the lungs take in. Fast walking and running are common examples. Aerobic exercise is believed to improve the immune function by enhancing the production of interferon and inter-leukin-2, normal body proteins that also are used to treat cancer (see Chapter 13). This may explain why physical activity seems to help the body fight infection. Remember, though, that moderation is the key. Some evidence suggests that overtraining—that is, repeatedly working out to the point of exhaustion—can depress immunity.

Preventing Complications. Poor physical condition invites a worsening of problems that arise from confinement to bed or restricted movement. These can range from minor annoyances, such as skin sores, generalized aches or localized muscle spasms, and constipation to serious health problems such as breathing problems, pneumonia, and poor circulation. Regular movement of the entire body will help avoid these effects of immobility.

If you were very active before treatment, you may find that you have to resume a lower level of activity after surgery or chemotherapy and then gradually build up your stamina again. You may not achieve your pre-treatment level of conditioning, but by working with a doctor who can help monitor your progress and physical capability, a program can be designed that works for you.

If your lifestyle hasn't included much physical activity until now, slowly and gradually increase your level of exertion so that it challenges but does not exhaust you.

Fighting Fatigue. Traditionally, the only medical treatment for fatigue has been rest, yet this can create a dangerous fatigue spiral: the more you rest, the weaker your muscles become and the more your circulation is compromised, which increases your tiredness. In fact, to regain the lean muscle mass lost during one week of bed rest, it's necessary to exercise regularly for two to three weeks.

A program of moderate exercise combats the fatigue syndrome by keeping muscles in good condition and elevating your mood (see Chapter 24).

Maintaining Range of Motion. Studies show that increasing physical activity improves the range of motion of the body's joints, which often diminishes as the cancer progresses or whenever bed rest or general inactivity is prolonged. (Range of motion is the degree to which a joint can be moved in a circle.) Maintaining and restoring flexibility and range of motion are essential to preserving general strength. (See *Exercises to Do in Bed* on pages 362–363.)

Preserving Lean Tissue. Muscle fibers, which give your body strength and allow you to move freely, consist of lean tissue. If you lose too much weight or lose weight too quickly, you lose lean tissue, or lean body mass. Activity can help counter that loss. As you build strength and endurance through exercise, you increase the amount of lean tissue in your body.

If your prognosis is good and you can tolerate a 1,500-calorie diet, it's usually safe to do some form of aerobic exercise four or five times a week, along with some strength training to build muscle. Always discuss your exercise program with your doctor before starting your activity.

Weight Gain. Exercise can also counter some weight gain because it raises the body's metabolic rate so that calories burn faster. During cancer treatment, however, your doctor may be less concerned about weight gain than assuring that you are getting the nutrition you need.

Weight Loss. The interrelationship between cancer, physical activity, and appetite becomes complicated when the disease is advanced. Since exercise helps preserve lean muscle tissue, it may slow the wasting process that accompanies advanced disease. However, this benefit has not been confirmed by research. Most doctors believe that if you feel up to it, moderate exercise is probably not harmful.

Emotional Benefits

Exercise enhances emotional well being in a variety of ways. Immediately after cancer is diagnosed, people may feel depressed, lethargic, hopeless, anxious, angry, or a combination of all these emotions. Exercise can go a long way to counteract these feelings by inducing feelings of relaxation and optimism.

Decreasing Depression. Activities that are pleasurable and constructive appear to decrease feelings of apathy, inadequacy, and helplessness. Physical activity provides a sense of accomplishment, control, and independence. Some scientists speculate that aerobic exercise may have a direct effect on the brain's chemistry, increasing those natural agents that enhance pleasurable sensations and reducing those associated with stress.

Reducing Anxiety. Exercise also has a temporary calming effect on angry or anxious people. Muscle tension is especially troublesome, because when the muscles are tense, their blood supply is constricted, which contributes to a generalized weakness. Fatigue may follow, which often contributes to depression.

Improving Self-Esteem. Physical activity can prompt a feeling of control in a situation in which constant tests, visits to the doctor, and treatments make it easy to feel helpless. Therefore, exercise is a worthwhile activity, if only through encouraging a sense of autonomy and personal power. It also provides goals to work toward and accomplish, which can be quite satisfying.

A Prescription for Physical Activity

Physical activity falls into two categories: aerobic and anaerobic. Walking, jogging, cycling, and swimming are examples of aerobic exercise. Any of these activities can increase the heart rate and, as a result, increase the lungs' capacity to take in oxygen. Thus more oxygen is delivered to the muscles.

Aerobic exercise also increases metabolism, lowers blood cholesterol, strengthens bones, and increases endurance.

Anaerobic exercise is characterized by short bursts of intense activity. Weight lifting or sprinting, for example, helps develop muscles and strength, speed, and power.

- *Walking.* Walking is an excellent exercise for people with cancer, because it increases lung function, stimulates bone growth, and strengthens leg and back muscles. Although a metastasis to the leg, back, or pelvic bone rules out running, it may not preclude walking, because walking does not jar the joints as much as running. (If you have metastatic disease in your bones, consult your doctor before starting any exercise program.) Walking in a swimming pool is especially gentle to joints and bones, yet stimulates the heart and lungs, building endurance.

- *Swimming.* When walking is painful, swimming can be a good aerobic substitute. It is not stressful to joints, and swimming far and fast enough increases a person's aerobic capacity. Swimming's major advantage is that it stretches the muscles, including those of the ribcage, which increases the amount of air you can inhale and exhale. Swimming also strengthens your muscles without jarring as your body moves against the water's resistance.

- *Resistance or strength training.* Anaerobic exercise, such as lifting weights or working out with weight resistance machines, helps build muscle. However, because you burn more calories if you have more lean muscle mass, it's important to be closely supervised and have your weight monitored to make sure your increased caloric needs don't exceed the number of calories you are able to eat.

    Some experts feel that weight resistance machines are safer than free weights because they are more easily controlled. If you have never done strength training before, work with an experienced trainer who understands the needs and limitations of a person with cancer.

- *Stretching and yoga.* Both stretching the major muscle and tendon groups and doing yoga promote flexibility and relieve muscle tension. Well-stretched muscles are less vulnerable to injury than tight muscles, and they require less energy and effort to move. Stretching and yoga are gentle anaerobic movements designed to extend and tone muscles that have become shortened as a result of lengthy periods of inactivity, such as prolonged bed rest after surgery. Stretching also produces a feeling of well being and increases blood circulation.

In addition, yoga and the deep breathing it requires can help you relax and gain a feeling of serenity. Some experts say it helps restore emotional equilibrium.

There are many varieties of yoga available today, and some of them are quite strenuous or done in quite warm environments. When selecting a yoga class, be careful to select one that is appropriate for your abilities. In addition to consulting with your doctor, it's also wise to let the instructor know of your condition, since some postures may not be safe for you to do.

Getting Started, Keeping Going

There are no rules in regard to maintaining your current level of activity, but if you have been sidelined for a while or want to begin an exercise program or take a new class, it's important to first consult a doctor. He or she may need to run tests on your heart and lung function before making a safe recommendation. For example, a runner or a person with a previously diagnosed heart condition may need to have an exercise stress test to be certain that his or her heart can handle the increased workload. A physical exam that includes an evaluation of joint and muscle function is important to forestall such problems as stiffness of the hips or unstable knees. If the cancer has metastasized, x-rays of the legs, pelvis, spine, and other areas may be needed.

People who have never exercised before or active people who have been confined to bed for a while need to start slowly, perhaps walking only five to ten minutes several times a day initially. With daily effort, endurance will increase. The key is to have a willing, positive attitude; to set reasonable goals; and to stick to a program. Avoid competitive activities if they make you feel tense; exercise should promote relaxation. As your endurance increases, be sure to take a rest day or two each week to avoid overtraining.

The Right Combination

If you enjoyed physical activity before your diagnosis, you will probably be able to continue the activities that gave you pleasure. Your safe level of activity depends in part on the location of your cancer and which treatment you have received. If you are a runner or a golfer, for example, you should still be able to run and play after a prostatectomy, a mastectomy, partial removal of the large bowel, or even removal of one kidney. Many who have had a portion of a lung removed return to their original level of activity. But you must avoid intense exertion that produces exhaustion and muscle strain and that lowers the body's resistance to infection. People with cancer also frequently have anemia,

Moderate Physical Activity Examples*

- Washing and waxing a car for 45–60 minutes

- Washing windows or floors for 45–60 minutes

- Playing volleyball for 45 minutes

- Playing touch football for 30–45 minutes

- Gardening for 30–45 minutes

- Wheeling self in wheelchair for 30–40 minutes

- Walking 1¾ miles in 35 minutes (20 minutes/mile)

- Basketball (shooting baskets) for 30 minutes

- Bicycling 5 miles in 30 minutes

- Pushing a stroller 1½ miles in 30 minutes

- Raking leaves for 30 minutes

- Walking 2 miles in 30 minutes (15 minutes/mile)

- Water aerobics for 30 minutes

- Swimming laps for 20 minutes

- Wheelchair basketball for 20 mintues

- Basketball (playing a game) for 15–20 minutes

- Bicycling 4 miles in 15 minutes

- Jumping rope for 15 minutes

- Running 1½ miles in 15 minutes (10 minutes/mile)

- Shoveling snow for 15 minutes

- Stairwalking for 15 minutes

Less Vigorous, More Time

↑

↓

More Vigorous, Less Time

* A moderate amount of physical activity is roughly equivalent to physical activity that uses approximately 150 calories (kcal) of energy per day or 1,000 calories per week. Because amount of activity is a function of duration, intensity, and frequency, the same amount of activity can be obtained in longer sessions of moderately intense activities (such as brisk walking) as in shorter sessions of more strenuous activites (such as running).

Adapted from: *Chronic Disease Notes & Reports*, a publication of the Centers for Disease Control and Prevention.

which makes them tired and susceptible to cold. Never exercise so vigorously that you feel unable to do your normal activities. For instance, don't walk so long in the afternoon that you are too tired to eat dinner that evening.

An ideal exercise program combines aerobic and anaerobic exercises such as strength training with stretching components as part of the warm-up and cool-down. It's a good idea to alternate aerobic and strength-training exercises. If you enjoy a half-hour walk every day, you might add a strength-training session two or three times a week. A day of rest and/or easy activity will give muscles time to recover.

Warming up for five to ten minutes before exercising will help you avoid injuries. To warm up, start the activity slowly, then briefly limber up muscles in the arms, legs, and trunk through stretching movements. As circulation to the muscle increases, pick up the pace. Do the last few minutes of the activity at a slower pace. This cool-down allows the muscles to relax and prevent cramping. Each episode of exercise should begin and end with some gentle stretches.

Where to Get the Right Supervision and Help

Your doctor or the physical therapy department at the hospital where you're being treated should be able to recommend an exercise professional to you. For help with all types of exercise, you can check with your local American Heart Association for cardiac rehabilitation classes, which are designed for people who need to be careful about how much they stress their system. The YMCA and YWCA may have programs for people with cancer, and the American Lung Association offers special programs in some areas. Road runner clubs, local hiking groups, and cycling groups also may have programs for people with chronic diseases and/or cancer. Yoga and stretching classes are offered at health clubs throughout the country. In any class or program, stop if you feel pressured to push yourself to the point of discomfort or if you feel any pain or unusual twinges.

Limitations on Physical Activity

Despite the obvious benefits of exercise, people with cancer need to take into account their special circumstances. Each person is the best judge of how much activity is tolerable. There is nothing to be gained from attempting to "work through" symptoms or the side effects of treatment with excessive exercise. Also, even if physical activity was your way of coping with stress and tension before you became ill, pushing yourself too hard now may be discouraging and end up making you feel worse.

Chemotherapy can adversely affect the capacity to exercise by inducing nausea and decreasing the number of red and white blood cells and platelets, which not only reduces the body's ability to deliver oxygen to the muscles but raises the risk of infection and bleeding. However, during chemotherapy,

Why Walk?

Walking is the perfect exercise. It can be done in nearly any type of weather and is not jarring to the joints. Moreover, a five-year longitudinal study showed no significant difference in the improvement of aerobic capacity between joggers and walkers who kept to a brisk pace. In addition, walking provides a feeling of well being, relaxation, and emotional uplift.

Begin by walking for ten minutes three times a week, and then build to twenty minutes four times a week. Depending on your condition, your goal may be to walk four to five times a week for thirty minutes or longer.

Keep in mind that the rate at which you walk and the difficulty of the terrain you're able to safely cover depend entirely on your condition. Your doctor can give you specific recommendations.

walking and stretching or gentle yoga, which incorporate deep breathing, can be helpful. Remember that some medications you are taking may cause drowsiness. Do not attempt to exercise while you are feeling drowsy.

Conditions Aggravated by Exercise

Although it is important to resist the impulse to stop exercising altogether when you're not feeling energetic, there are times when it's wise to give yourself a break. Some of the following situations or conditions may alter your ability to exercise.

Dehydration. Some cancers can cause electrolyte imbalances and deplete the body of fluids. Dehydration in these cases can have severe consequences. Never exercise in extreme heat, and always drink plenty of fluids. If you perspire a lot, you may feel better drinking a sport drink that is fortified with electrolytes such as salt and potassium.

Bone Stress. Many people with cancer are at risk for bone fractures, especially in the long bones, spine, pelvis, and ribs. If the cancer has spread to the bone, strength training is not recommended. Activities such as basketball or tennis that involve jumping or twisting the hips are not advised if there is bone loss or metastatic disease in the bones.

Anemia. If the cancer has metastasized to the bones or treatment has affected the bone marrow, anemia and a low platelet count, which causes bruising or bleeding into the joints and elsewhere, can make you vulnerable to injury. Accordingly, activities that exert a force on the bones, such as running or step classes and dance, may be restricted. Until the condition is corrected, your activities may be limited to walking and stretching or gentle yoga.

My Life as a Runner with Cancer, by Fred Lebow

Fred Lebow, a member of the national Track Hall of Fame and founder of the New York City Marathon, died of brain cancer—a recurrence of lymphoma—four years after his condition was diagnosed. In 1992, while his cancer was in remission, Lebow completed the 26-mile marathon he created—in five hours, 32 minutes, and 34 seconds. In the introduction to *The New York Road Runners Club Complete Book of Running*, Lebow described how important exercise was during his illness:

My physical fitness was critical. I used it to make sure I didn't stagnate. You can be sick in bed, unable to do almost anything, but you can still wiggle your fingers and toes. I found this out through experience. Over the months in and out of hospitals, I believed that if I let myself be ruled by the disease, I could succumb to my own laziness. I fought that tendency with exercise.

On the journey to save my life, I started chemotherapy, a horrible odyssey of nausea, weakness, weight and hair loss. I felt like Methuselah in his nine hundredth year—yet I continued to proclaim myself the healthiest cancer patient on earth.

The first day back in my own apartment, I decided to walk in Central Park. I was tired before I started. But I was spurred on by greetings from the doorman I used to pass on my daily runs during my pre-disease days. Every day I went walking, starting with one mile, and by the third day I walked 2³/₄ miles in one hour. After about three weeks of walking, I was able to insert short bursts of running, 10- to 15-yard jogs, into my walking routine. I never thought running could be so difficult! I was amazed how I could be jogging and every walker in the park could still pass me. But with each day I improved, inserting more and longer intervals of jogging. One minute of running became ten, and eventually, I worked my way up to post levels of training.

Then I began a 37-day cycle of radiation at Memorial Sloan-Kettering Cancer Center. Because the hospital is within blocks of my apartment, it was convenient to walk there for treatments. This was the only convenience, however.

With chemotherapy, I lost my hair. With radiation, I lost my trademark beard. Initially, I became bloated, then I lost weight. Eventually I was down to 124 pounds from my running weight of 144. I had no hair, and very little meat on my bones. But I had made great progress in my recovery. One day I managed an entire lower loop of the park running, it took me 30 minutes to cover the 1.7 miles. Pills, operations, doctor's guidance, and the love of family and friends all aid recovery. But there is something more, something crucial to overcoming the failure of the body, and that is physical fitness.

When I look back over my experience with cancer, I am struck by how little other patients exercise. At Mount Sinai [Hospital], younger, fitter patients than I didn't move a muscle. Only one other patient—a 2:48 marathoner—ever seemed to join me in activity. When I became ill, I got the best doctors, treatment, and advice. And then I did more. I moved my hands, my legs. I made my blood pump. Other patients at Mount Sinai would ask me, "Why do you do this?" I'd respond, "The question isn't why I'm doing this, but why you aren't."

I know it's sometimes hard to get motivated to run even in the best of health and under the best conditions. Part of my desire to run is to stay in shape to race. Even after cancer therapy, I walked, then ran, with the goal of getting back into racing. However, I was no longer racing to break a 7-minute per mile pace. I'm delighted now to break 10 minutes per mile.

Since my illness, I have been taking my life back, slowly but confidently. My body has changed. I'm not as strong as I was before, but I can manage more and more each day. I'm thinner, but I've always been fairly "runner thin." But the real change is inside me, a change I understand best through my running. I'm glad to be alive and I live with that feeling every day. It's like being a beginner again, in love with the idea of my body moving along, content with the weather, the seasons, and the sound of each footfall.

Hypercalcemia. Too much calcium in the blood, or hypercalcemia, may occur in patients who have bone metastasis. This condition causes muscle weakness and leaches calcium out of bones, making them vulnerable to fractures. Acute hypercalcemia can even cause cardiac arrhythmia and kidney failure, therefore aerobic exercise that stresses the heart is not recommended until the condition is corrected.

Nerve Damage. If your brain or nerves are affected and you are unsteady, exercising by yourself is not advised. Plan walks with a friend. You could also consult with a physiatrist, a specialist in rehabilitation medicine, to learn compensatory training methods to help you overcome some problems such as unsteadiness in walking (see Chapter 22).

Physical Activity During Advanced Illness

Exercise counteracts feelings of listlessness and can slow the fatigue spiral and tissue loss, so some form of physical activity is beneficial at an advanced stage of cancer, even when generalized weakness is present.

Activity for those confined to bed may consist of passive range-of-motion exercises (where someone else moves your extremities) and general stretching. You can do active range-of-motion movements of your joints by yourself, or a physical therapist can show you and a friend or family member a passive exercise routine.

Even if you are confined to bed most of the time, you still may be able to sit in a chair by the bed or sit at the edge of the bed. Doing as much self-care as possible will help avoid immobility.

Physical activity will help you maintain some mobility and relieve muscle tension, providing a temporary psychological boost. In fact, pain medication combined with stretching exercises is one of the best solutions for keeping comfortable when confined to bed.

It's important to listen to your body. If a physical activity causes you pain, stop the activity.

The Gift of Physical Activity

Besides all the good reasons for exercising, remember that physical activity can also be pleasurable. It can add to your quality of life by making you feel better mentally and physically. The bonus can be a sense of pure joy that improves your quality of life.

Many of the people with cancer who engage in physical activity revel in meeting personal challenges. Some walk the length of their street, while others run marathons or climb mountains. These people thrill at seeing their own capabilities increase and take pride in their successive accomplishments. They are champions.

Body Image
and Self-Esteem

A diagnosis of cancer can feel like a betrayal of your body, inside and out. It may feel as though the body you had always counted on is now unpredictably out of control, especially if you have never been seriously ill before.

Cancer and its treatment may result in physical changes that are obvious to everyone, or they may only be noticeable to you and those closest to you. They may be temporary, such as hair loss, or permanent, such as an amputation. Whatever the nature of these changes, cancer draws inordinate attention to you and your body.

Although most people worry about survival and recovery early in the diagnostic and treatment stages, some are just as concerned about how the diagnosis will affect their appearance and how they feel about themselves. How you feel about those changes and how well you are able to accept them as part of yourself will influence the quality of your life from now on.

Recognizing body-image problems and their relation to self-esteem generally, and understanding how to resolve them helps men and women of all ages accept themselves during and after cancer treatment. This chapter addresses these concerns by focusing on the following questions:

- What is body image and how does cancer alter it?

- What is the relationship between body image and self-esteem?

- What are the signs of problems with body image and self-esteem?

- How can body image and self-esteem be strengthened?

- What can be done to improve your appearance while being treated for cancer or recovering from it?

- Who can help?

Body Image and Cancer

Body image has two major components: your feelings about how your body looks and your feelings about how it functions. Cancer and its treatment can drastically affect both, and in turn can challenge your self-esteem—your entire sense of identity and value as a human being.

Appearance

The loss of a limb or other body part, hair loss, cracking and peeling skin, and facial disfigurement, among other things, can dramatically change outward appearance. In a society that emphasizes physical attractiveness, youth, and fitness, people who don't look "normal" can be stigmatized. When the alteration is to the face, which others study first when meeting and communicating with you, reactions can be especially difficult.

Sometimes the permanent physical change is not so obvious to others—such as a small scar or the indelible marks left after radiation therapy—but serves as a lifelong reminder to you that you have had cancer.

Body Functioning

The need for an ostomy and alterations in sexual functioning are just two of the many ways that cancer treatment can affect the way the body works. It can be traumatizing and upsetting to your self-concept if your body does not function the way it used to (and if you are not able to take care of your body by yourself anymore). Although physical changes may not be noticed by strangers, coworkers, or friends, the reaction of more intimate friends and family is an issue, since those who do see the altered parts are the very people whose acceptance matters most.

Common Reactions

It is not unusual to feel angry or outraged, depressed, anxious, or hostile toward health care professionals or family members, at least initially. Those to whom appearance is especially important will have a difficult time if their looks are altered, whether by illness or age. Since women are under greater cultural pressure to be attractive, they are more vulnerable to the emotional consequences of looking sick or different. Men may be somewhat more concerned about changes in the way their bodies function.

People who fear they are being judged according to their altered appearance may well feel reluctant to leave the house or to interact with others. And although it is possible to conceal a mastectomy scar or ostomy bag, for example, it is common to feel extremely self-conscious, at least for a while, and to wonder whether observers can see the change.

The Process of Adjustment

Most people eventually come to terms with a new body image, but learning to accept the differences takes time and work. Those who cannot handle the changes right away need to respect their own timetable and work on self-acceptance when the time is right for them. Most people successfully accept and integrate body changes within one to two years following treatment.

There are no predictable stages in coming to terms with such changes, however, because each person copes in a different way. For some people, any perceived defect in their physical appearance is embarrassing and shameful. Others may initially refuse to accept that anything has changed at all. Still others grieve and cry so much that they seem as if they'll never deal with it, yet they eventually are able to look on the bright side. For example, an athletic, fit, and extremely attractive woman in her 50s underwent surgery on her face. For months she grieved over the loss of her looks. Over time, however, she was able to see another side to her situation. She told her family, "Well, at least the surgery didn't make me fat. I couldn't deal with that."

As with the diagnosis of the cancer itself, the process of coming to terms with an altered body may include shock and dismay, denial, fear and anxiety, depression, and eventual acceptance. Ultimately, how you handle such body image issues depends on your general coping skills, family dynamics, social support systems in place before the diagnosis, and the sum total of your self-esteem (see Chapter 26). These adjustment factors combine with the nature of the change itself—how much of your appearance and/or functioning is lost—and how diminished the alteration makes you feel.

People who are used to feeling good about themselves and who have a solid support network of family and friends generally manage to incorporate these changes into a positive image of themselves. This doesn't mean that they don't struggle with difficult feelings, of course, or that they don't miss their former appearance or abilities.

People who are more likely to find the adjustment difficult are those who have:

- problems with self-esteem

- a history of depression

- negative feelings about their body beyond the part affected by the illness

- no support systems or shaky relationships before treatment

People who experience one or more of these factors generally have fewer resources in dealing with crisis. But it can be done, perhaps with professional guidance.

What Your Body Really Means to You

Chapter 26 will help you understand your usual style of coping with crisis and stress. In addition, it may be helpful to think about the personal significance of the changed body part or function. For example, some women see their breasts as signifying their sexuality and/or motherhood, and so losing one or both may mean to them that they are "no longer women." Others, perhaps those who have already experienced a loss of bodily functions or aesthetics through illness or aging, may adapt to surgery without damage to their identity as women.

Understanding the highly individual meaning of the change in what your body looks like or what it can no longer do will help you understand the degree of distress you are experiencing. Men with testicular cancer (which usually occurs in young men), for example, commonly hear from well-meaning friends and relatives that they don't need that "extra" testicle, since they still have one that works. But having their manhood altered in any way may be devastating, despite their continued ability to function.

Building Up Other Components of Self-Esteem

Body image is only one component of self-esteem. Other aspects include what you do, what you value and believe in, and your relationships with other people. As this chapter explains, working to strengthen all these aspects of identity will help you weather not only challenges to your bodily self-image but also the many other ways that cancer can threaten self-esteem.

Although it may be difficult to believe if you are just beginning to face the crisis of cancer, coping with this disease offers an opportunity to gain self-esteem. After enduring the trauma of cancer treatment, many men, women, and children realize their own strengths for the first time. They now have a new sense of what is and is not important in life and they feel empowered by capabilities they never knew they had.

Body Image and Self-Esteem

The key to recovering from assaults on body image is caring for all parts of yourself. Self-esteem has four components:

- The *body self* (or *body image*): how your body looks and functions. In addition to specific physical appearance and functioning, the body self can be viewed more broadly. For example, some people (such as models and performers) emphasize how they look, and others are more concerned with what their bodies do (such as machine operators, police, athletes, artists).

- The *interpersonal self:* how you respond to others (coworkers, friends, lovers, and family members) and how they respond to you. Those who are happy with their family relationships, get along easily with others, and have people they can count on usually feel an important sense of connection.

- The *achieving self:* your goals and aspirations. How you perform at anything you do—from work, to hobbies, to providing for and taking care of your family—contributes to your achieving self.

- The *identification self:* your spiritual or ethical beliefs, values, and behaviors. People who gain strength from spiritual or ethical beliefs usually have a sense of meaning and a sense of fulfillment in their lives.

How Cancer Threatens Self-Esteem

Cancer and its treatment can disrupt self-esteem by undermining any or all of these selves in several ways:

- As discussed in the first part of this chapter, cancer affects your body self by altering your looks and your physical ability to function.

- The illness often disrupts important relationships. For example, feeling that a mate, lover, child, friend, or a coworker is avoiding you because of your illness can shatter your sense of connection to others.

- A missed promotion at work because of time off for treatment, a role change at home, or the necessity of giving up a favorite sport because of a physical change can make you feel less of a person.

- Cancer can challenge your faith in the fairness of life. If you feel angry at God or at life for allowing such a terrible thing to happen, you may feel spiritually adrift.

Maintaining the Balance

To safeguard your self-esteem during cancer treatment, it is essential to maintain a balance among these four components of yourself, so that if one aspect of self-esteem is diminished, another will be enhanced. For example, when body image is affected, you can concentrate on how important your friends or family are to you. If treatment has interrupted your work or other important activities, you can pay more attention to your loved ones, spiritual life, or other interests.

The following are two examples of ways in which people who lost a limb balanced their resources and regained their self-esteem:

- A teacher nearing retirement lost a leg to cancer. During his recovery, as two generations of students came forward to show their love and concern for him, he realized what a great teacher he had been. The more he thought about his professional competence and what he had yet to accomplish, the better he felt about himself, despite his difficulty dealing with his amputation. Although he was single, the realization of how important he was to others helped strengthen his faith in people and reassured him that life really had been good to him after all.

- A woman in her 40s who had often said she "lived for tennis" lost her right arm, putting an end to her game. While recovering, she spent much more time around the house. At first she was extremely depressed by her amputation and inactivity. She felt she no longer had an outlet for her energy. Then, out of sheer boredom, she started cooking more adventurously than she had before. She found that having one arm did not limit her as much as she had thought it would, and her family was delighted with the food and her newfound culinary creativity. Spending more time with her teenagers helped her realize just how important she was to them and they to her. Once she was fitted for a prosthesis, she became less self-conscious about her appearance. Jogging eventually replaced the tennis. When she ran her first marathon, she realized she had never in her life felt more vital.

Strengthening Your Body Image and Self-Esteem

The following are suggestions for preventing body-image problems and strengthening self-esteem and relationships with others, both of which may be challenged during cancer treatment.

Learn as much as you can about your body change and how to manage it. For example, learn how to care for an ostomy or how to identify an infection. Information and knowledge enable most people to feel less frightened or intimidated by physical changes and restore their sense of control over their body and their life.

Begin to touch and look at the altered body site. This is the new you, and you'll need to get used to your new body as it is now. If you can't touch or look at it right away, don't worry about it. You may need to try many times to get comfortable with the change.

Work on becoming more comfortable showing your body to other people like health care professionals, a spouse, or significant other. When you feel comfortable and relaxed about how you look, the people around you generally will feel more comfortable too.

Restore your physical fitness, or start exercising for the first time. People who are committed to fitness as a way of life often have greater mastery over their bodies. As the previous chapter explains, trainers and physical therapists can devise fitness strategies for all levels of activity, even for the bedridden. Even

Charting Self-Esteem

Everybody has a characteristic way of relating in the world—as strong, smart, beautiful, caring, hardworking, and so on. Changes or losses of abilities, looks, roles, or independence resulting from cancer can alter your usual way of obtaining the self-enhancing feedback or "strokes" that you've always counted on.

This chart can help you identify how you felt about yourself in the four self-esteem areas before cancer and how you feel about yourself now. If you discover that your self-worth before cancer rested heavily on one of the four components now being threatened, try to locate strengths in other aspects of yourself to which you can shift your attention. By recognizing your remaining strengths or where you can turn to renew your sources of self-esteem, you can still maintain a positive balance of self-esteem.

Circle how much good feeling you had about yourself both before your cancer and now in each of the four components, with 1 indicating very little and 5 quite a lot:

	Before					Now				
Body self	1	2	3	4	5	1	2	3	4	5
Interpersonal self	1	2	3	4	5	1	2	3	4	5
Achieving self	1	2	3	4	5	1	2	3	4	5
Identification self	1	2	3	4	5	1	2	3	4	5

Compare the *Before* and *Now* columns for each aspect of self-esteem and notice where there has been a change. Think about the possible reasons for any low scores and whether you can do anything to improve the scores. Suggestions for building up your feelings about yourself and enhancing your appearance are offered throughout this chapter.

if you cannot return to your previous activities, you'll appreciate what you still can do to restore your strength and muscle tone. It can also be helpful to focus on what your body can do, rather than on what it can't.

Shift your emphasis to another attractive part of your body. A woman with a mastectomy, for example, might decide to wear skirts or tights to show her nice legs.

Do something new and different. Another way of taking your mind off a changed body is to find a way to do something that makes you feel capable and valued. Take up golf or pottery, start a journal, do volunteer work—anything that makes you feel competent and worthwhile.

Shift your values. If you cannot continue your career or household responsibilities, turn your attention to something else (another kind of job, gardening, painting). A former carpenter might turn to wood carving, a former secretary might find a new joy in writing poetry, and a woman who can no longer do the physical cleaning for her family might become a fabulous cook. A one-time executive might turn to teaching.

Learn to value your body as a whole. Just because one part of your body has changed in some way does not mean you are an unattractive person. Wearing an ostomy bag, for example, does not mean you've become worthless. Even if others have a hard time at first looking at your surgically changed face, this does not mean that you are no longer a sensuous, sexual, athletic, physically vital, or interesting person—the characteristics you value in yourself are not erased by changes to your body.

To distract yourself and others from the problem, create a "healthy illusion." A man who has lost his hair during chemotherapy might have some fun with baseball caps or hats. Many women decide to wear wigs or scarves. (Not everyone feels the need to cover up a cancer-related alteration or to create the illusion of health, however, as we will discuss later in this chapter.)

Try to find some value in what has happened. This may take some real work and growth to accomplish, but a positive attitude can dramatically improve your quality of life. For example, instead of perceiving a stoma as unnatural or embarrassing, think of it as a way of having the freedom to go out in public and interact with others without having to worry about incontinence or frequent trips to the bathroom. If you have a reconstructed breast, instead of thinking of it as asymmetrical, tighter, or harder than your real one, think of it as a way of gaining new freedom in clothes.

In your relationships, how you look and control your own physical functions can affect even your closest ties to other people. In addition, changes to your body may threaten an already poor relationship with an intimate partner. To determine whether body-image problems are causing or contributing to relationship difficulties, see the box on page 331.

Talk about it. Open communication can help alleviate stress and clear up any misconceptions about what the cancer has and has not changed about you.

It is not unusual to discover that your partner is less upset about the changes than you imagined. A husband, for example, may be grateful his wife is alive and not be concerned at all about her mastectomy scar. Furthermore, he may be avoiding his wife not because he is turned off by her body but because he is afraid of causing pain when he hugs or makes love to her. But when partners are afraid of or repulsed by the changes and cannot resolve these feelings on their own, this is even more reason for them to talk and seek help. Frank discussion is equally important with children, whose fears about a parent need to be explored (see Chapter 28).

Look the best you can. Physical appearance can reveal not only how ill you are but also your attitude about yourself. Exercise or dieting can tone and firm your body and make you look healthier and more attractive to others and to yourself. A new hairstyle, clothes, jewelry, perfume or aftershave, although seemingly insignificant, suggest that you are interested in yourself and others again (for more ideas, see *Appearance Tips* below).

Start to value new activities with other people. If because of a cancer-related change you can no longer do something you used to do with a friend, try sharing something else. If you can no longer go bowling with friends or ballroom dancing with a spouse, for example, find other activities that are fun or meaningful in order to maintain the relationship. Volunteer with a friend at the senior center or in a literacy program. Take up cards or join a book discussion group—anything that keeps you enjoying your time together. This advice is equally valid for relationships with children and grandchildren.

Appearance Tips

Whether or not it is possible to restore your body to what it was before treatment, you can regain control over your appearance. Feeling attractive and looking like yourself again are important to both men and women as they return to their careers and day-to-day lives. For most people, feeling good about their appearance restores self-confidence and improves interactions with others.

Restoring appearance does not, however, necessarily mean hiding all the physical changes brought on by cancer treatment. Rather, it means expressing positive feelings about yourself through your appearance in whatever feels like "you."

The Option of Not Covering Up

There is a new freedom in today's more accepting social climate that gives women and men the option of being seen in public without covering up a hair loss or a disfigurement. For some people, the cancer experience even enables them to discover and demonstrate their acceptance of who they are. For example, some women may choose not to conform to societal expectations and go without breast prostheses or reconstructive surgery. Art photographs of nude women without breasts that have been shown in some magazines and exhibitions prove that sensuality comes from within a person's whole body, not from one particular body part.

In addition, some people are refusing to hide their bald heads or create the illusion that no change has taken place. For some women with breast cancer, the decision is political: they want to call a disinterested public's attention to the desperate need for research to cure the disease.

If you feel more comfortable covering up, however, there are many options available, including the following.

Hair and Complexion. Even though treatment-related baldness is temporary, hair loss can be as devastating for men as it is for women. Although some people are proud of a bald head, others feel more comfortable and self-confident with a wig or some other covering.

If you choose to wear a wig, select one before you lose your hair so that the hairdresser or wig salon can match your color and style. Your local American Cancer Society (ACS) may have a list of stores experienced in working with cancer patients. Since hair usually falls out in clumps rather abruptly during treatment, it's a good idea to have a wig available when you need it.

There are several other options besides wigs. Women may feel attractive in stylish hats, turbans, or scarves; men can wear baseball caps or hats.

Even for those who feel comfortable with no hair, be aware that family and friends may view the baldness as a constant reminder of your illness and feel more comfortable when you're covered up. Discuss it with them and then decide what to do.

Some people like to wear a wig or head covering during lovemaking, whereas others don't. Talk it over as a couple and decide on whatever makes you both comfortable.

The ACS, in partnership with the National Cosmetology Association and the Cosmetic, Toiletry, and Fragrance Association (CTFA) Foundation, offers a free national public service program dedicated to teaching women with cancer how to restore a healthy appearance and self-image during and after chemotherapy and radiation therapy. *Look Good…Feel Better* teaches women who have undergone cancer treatment how to improve their appearance using cosmetics, wigs, turbans, and scarves. Pampering yourself can improve your attitude, so don't feel embarrassed or vain about attending such a group. For further information, contact your local ACS, look for posters in your hospital or clinic, call 800-395-LOOK (see also the *Resources* section in the back of the book or visit the LGFB web site at www.lookgoodfeelbetter.org).

Clothing. Clothing says a lot about personality. It still is possible to be fashionable and look your usual self even if you've lost a body part or gained an appliance.

Although you may need to make some adjustments after cancer treatment, you can still dress to look your best. Catheters can be hidden beneath high-neck blouses or shirts or under long sleeves; pleated slacks can hide an ostomy; and breast forms can camouflage a mastectomy. Choose fabrics that are soft and flowing, and select styles that draw the eye away from the changed body part.

If you've lost or gained a lot of weight because of chemotherapy, buy a few new clothes that fit well. Loose or tight clothing draws attention.

Metamorphosis, by Judith Hooper

About two or three weeks into chemotherapy, I began to wake up to a tangled wad of hair on my pillow. Hair fell into my plate as I ate. It fell on my clothes, on the floor, on my son's bed when I read him a bedtime story, prompting him to call, Mommy, you forgot your hair! It clogged the vacuum cleaner, filled the plastic, handle-tie garbage bags. When the part in my hair become an inch wide, I knew it was time to visit Audrey's Wigs.

Audrey was in her late 50s, I estimated, and sported a lemon-yellow cascade of hair resembling the hair on a doll I had as a little girl. She confided that the bulk of her clients were chemotherapy patients or country and western singers. I could tell that she disapproved of me, perhaps because I was not wearing makeup or perhaps because my head was too small for most of her wigs. She produced a longish light-brown wig with a shag cut. When I put it on, I looked like a failed cocktail-lounge act. "Do you have anything else?" I asked. Finally we settled on a short, curly wig that didn't look anything like me, but did look vaguely natural. I bought a couple of terry cloth turbans, too. I never wore the wig. I did wear the turbans day in and day out, often coordinating them with my outfits....

My chemotherapy ended in mid-January...by mid-February I had eye-brows and eyelashes, and my skin had returned to normal earthling color. I was even pleased to see tiny hairs appear on my arms and legs. During the late turban-early-hair phase, which happened to coincide with late winter-early spring, I felt that I was a creature undergoing a profound metamorphosis. I was cocooning, molting, transforming. The new being that would emerge from this process, I visualized, would be beautiful, tran-scendent. Even while ignorant observers saw an unresplendent woman with sallow skin and an unbecoming hairstyle, I knew I was incubating my reborn self. About the time that blossoms and new pole-green leaves appeared on the trees, I was growing my new foliage.

Reconstructive Surgery. Reconstructive surgeries—such as breast reconstruction or plastic surgery to correct face or head deformities—are common and are no longer considered vain or purely cosmetic.

When considering reconstruction, you must decide for yourself whether the benefits of the surgery outweigh the risks. Although reconstructive surgery improves the quality of life for many people, many of these procedures are considered elective and thus may not be covered by insurance. Be sure to discuss this fully with your insurance company or health plan before you agree to any kind of surgery.

Many people feel reconstruction helps them feel whole again and happier about their body image. Some even find that they feel healthier.

Signs of Body-Image Problems

People who are concerned about their body image often feel self-conscious, embarrassed, and/or inadequate. They may spend a disproportionate amount of time and energy feeling bitter about their bodies, leaving little time or inclination for more productive activities.

Other indications include no longer wanting to hug or be hugged and avoiding touching or looking at what's different. Switching to unflattering styles of clothing is often a giveaway that someone is struggling with a body-image problem. So is giving up exercising in front of others for fear of being seen in revealing workout clothes or undressing in a locker room.

Avoiding discussing the body changes, continually displacing anger toward health care professionals or family members, refusing to talk about distressing changes, and denying that anything unfortunate has happened are other signs of problems (see Chapter 26).

Body-image difficulties are almost always revealed in sexual avoidance or outright problems with sexual functioning. Fear of rejection or abandonment can make people retreat from intimacy for fear that loved ones have the same negative reactions to their bodies as they do. Sexual difficulties resulting from cancer treatment, such as anxiety about erections or painful intercourse due to vaginal dryness, can also change people's image of themselves as sexual beings (see the next chapter for a further discussion of sexuality and cancer).

Failing to accept a changed body can lead to problems that extend far beyond the bedroom. People who withdraw from others because of their appearance or because they are depressed about their looks have a substantially reduced quality of life, not because their looks have changed, but because they no longer have vital human companionship. These reactions can become life threatening for those who become so overwhelmed and depressed that they choose not to continue treatment.

Where to Go for Help

When your self-esteem is low, it feels like everyone is staring at, criticizing, or judging you, which can make you feel isolated and alone just when you need other people the most.

People who also have cancer or have the same type of cancer can often identify best with your problems and can offer the most practical advice, not to mention crucial companionship. Support groups give people with cancer a chance to see that their feelings are normal and shared by others. Exchanging information and ways of coping helps them regain their sense of control and gives them a more positive outlook toward life (see Chapter 8).

Is a Poor Body Image Causing Relationship Problems?

If you answer yes to two or more of these questions, you may wish to talk to someone who can help you to work through these concerns:

- Do you feel self-conscious when your children, friends, or colleagues look at you or hug you?

- Do your children, friends, or colleagues feel self-conscious when they look at you or hug you?

- Are there subtle signs of negative changes in your relationships with others? Do you argue more or laugh less when you are together?

- Do you feel uncomfortable when your spouse or significant other touches, kisses, or fondles you?

- Does your partner feel uncomfortable when he or she touches, kisses, or fondles you?

- Are you spending less time with your spouse, children, friends, colleagues?

- Are you avoiding sex?

Several professional mental health resources are available to make the adjustment process smoother or to provide essential help for those who can't cope. All reputable cancer centers can put you in touch with a sensitive, trained counselor with expertise in the issues that people with cancer face.

Body Image and Self-Esteem in the Hospital

Almost everyone would agree that staying in a hospital can be a dehumanizing experience. You have to wear awful gowns that never tie right in the back. Strangers keep coming in and out of the room to poke and prod your body and to discuss private bodily functions. There is a lack of personalization and a lack of sensitivity. You feel more like an object than a human being.

What to do? Make your part of the hospital room your own personal environment. Bring in things from home that make you feel happy—your own night clothes (if appropriate and allowed), framed photographs, your own pillowcase and blanket (that can handle occasional spills), a tape recorder, and your favorite music or meditation tapes.

Establish a relationship with the hospital staff so they know your name and not just your room and bed number. Don't be afraid to ask questions of your doctors and nurses. You have a right to know what they're doing to you and why.

Set up visits and/or phone calls from people you love. The support of friends and family can make you feel better.

The aim is to bring you as an individual to the hospital with you, with as many loves, tastes, and quirks as you can fit into the room. In the hospital or at home, at work, or anywhere else, it's the sum total of who you are, not what you look like, that shines through.

Loving Yourself

You've just finished what may have been several months of grueling cancer treatment. You know you should feel happy to be alive, but instead you feel unhappy about the way you look. There is no reason to feel guilty or vain about feeling that way. Your looks have changed, either temporarily or permanently, and you need to grieve for the loss of your old body image—and it may be an enormous loss—before you can accept the new one.

The most important thing you can do for yourself is to grow comfortable with your new body, both with how it looks and how it functions. You need to accept your body as it is now so you can get on with your life.

One way to do that is to look at yourself in the mirror and become accustomed to your new body. Try it at first with your clothes on, and if you normally wear certain clothing or accessories to disguise the changes occurring from treatment, wear those too. Find at least three positive things about your looks that you like.

Now take off your clothes and face yourself in the mirror. How you look to yourself is more important than how you look (or think you look) to strangers. Examine your scar, appliance, or other body change. Get used to touching it. Try thinking of the change as a life-saving change—without it, you wouldn't be here. Some people consider it a badge of courage—they had the strength to go through a difficult ordeal and come out the other side. Think about yourself as a whole person, not just a body part. Try to put things into perspective. You have changed, but you still have positive traits and personal attributes that you and others value. Indeed, you may find that the way you are handling the cancer experience has enhanced your personality and made you a better person. The people who truly loved and cared for you before your treatment still love and care for you now, maybe even more than before.

Whether or not to conceal a body change is up to you. Do whatever makes you feel comfortable and makes you feel good about yourself.

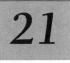

Sexuality

Sexuality is an important quality-of-life issue in surviving cancer, whether you are young or old, single, or have a partner. Even during advanced illness, the physical expression of caring—a touch, a kiss—can help you feel connected and loved.

The effects of cancer on sexuality receive more attention today than they have in the past. It is now widely accepted that, whether directly or indirectly, cancer and its treatment can affect sexual desire, pleasure, and function in virtually everyone. Nonetheless, according to experts on sexual health, pleasurable feelings and sexual performance can continue in some way for almost everyone. Partners may have to change positions, habits, or notions about how sex "should" be or otherwise adapt to new ways of expressing caring in order to meet each other's need for intimacy. Part of sexuality is learning to deal with feelings about one's body and the effects of these changes on self-esteem, which is the subject of the preceding chapter. Open discussion about cancer and sexuality among those with cancer, their partners, and their treatment team is crucial. Equally important is getting an accurate diagnosis of any sexual problems that occur.

How Cancer Affects Sexuality

Sexual response depends on a finely tuned balance of physical and emotional factors. Your nerves, blood vessels, muscles, hormones, sex organs, senses, and brain centers that control sexual response all must function harmoniously. Moreover, you must be able to clear your mind of other concerns (worries, fears, depression, pain, anger) in order to engage yourself in sexual intimacy. Even in the best of circumstances—in a good relationship with a caring and attractive partner—smooth sexual functioning can be difficult to achieve. For people with cancer, it can seem impossible (at least temporarily) for a number of physical and emotional reasons.

The Sexual Response Cycle

Sexual functioning consists of a four-phase cycle including desire, excitement, orgasm, and resolution. Desire is having an interest in sex; excitement is becoming physically aroused; orgasm is the climax; and resolution is the body's returning to its unexcited state. Desire and arousal—waiting to have sex and getting mentally and physically "turned on" by it—are the phases most often affected by cancer.

Physical Disruptions

Physically, cancer can disrupt sexual function directly through the disease process itself or, more commonly, through the side effects of treatments. For example, the cancer can damage the blood vessels, organs, glands, or nerves necessary for sexual arousal. Some surgical procedures cut nerves or remove the organs involved in sexual response. Chemotherapy and pelvic radiation can affect a variety of body systems, including hormone levels, vessels that carry blood to the genital areas, and nerves involved in sexual function. Hormone therapy may directly alter the balance of body chemicals necessary to achieve a smooth sexual response. Nausea, fatigue, or pain in the genital areas or in other parts of the body can dampen any interest in sex. Many drugs taken to counteract side effects or symptoms also can interfere with sexual desire or response.

Emotional Factors

Emotional concerns are probably the most common causes of sexual problems in people with cancer. But this is good news, since sexual anxieties can be successfully treated if properly diagnosed.

Cancer produces no end of psychological stresses, or so it often seems. Learning that one has cancer, for example, can be so emotionally overwhelming that sex is the last thought to come to mind. Anxiety about sexual performance after treatment, worry about changing roles at home or at work, or fear of no longer being attractive can diminish sexual interest. Depression is also a factor. One of the classic symptoms of depression is loss of interest in sex.

In addition to leaving physical scars, cancer treatment can alter body or self-image. A man who loses a testicle, a woman who loses a breast, or a person with a facial disfigurement might feel undesirable or embarrassed by the changes in his or her body, causing great reluctance to engage in sexual intimacy. As the preceding chapter explains more fully, a negative self-image or the fear of appearing unattractive because of hair loss or weight changes can change your self-perception and how others see you.

Of course, partners are also powerfully affected by the cancer. They may feel frightened about initiating sex, perhaps for fear of causing pain, or they may find the changes in their loved one's body hard to accept, at least at first. In a troubled relationship, the cancer may worsen an already threatened level of intimacy (see Chapter 28). Or a partner's sadness over a loved one's illness may affect his or her own ability to respond sexually.

The Importance of Diagnosis

Many problems in sexual functioning after cancer can be improved with medical treatment or counseling. Treatment is keyed to an accurate diagnosis of the problem and its causes. Ideally, you should be able to discuss your sexual problems with a doctor, but in reality, not all professionals are comfortable with the subject or are aware of the impact of cancer on sexuality. And not all people have the courage to bring it up.

If you are having some of the problems discussed in this chapter, the suggestions here about dealing with them may be helpful. Just understanding what is causing the sexual difficulties may help you feel better about what is happening. But if difficulties persist and the members of your health care team can offer no solutions, take advantage of the specialists available to diagnose and treat the problem.

Effects of Chemotherapy on Sexuality

The side effects of chemotherapy, including upset stomach and weakness, reduce both the physical energy and the emotional desire for sex. But most people find that their sexual desire returns after the side effects go away. It can be frustrating, however, that you may not feel in the mood until it's just about time for the next treatment. Sexual desire ordinarily returns after the entire course of chemotherapy is over.

For both men and women, the temporary changes that chemotherapy causes in appearance can also interfere with feeling sexy or sexual. Not only is hair loss from the head and face upsetting, but it may also be hard to get used to losing pubic hair or, for men, chest hair. Weight gain, weight loss, or extremely pale skin also commonly interfere with a person's sexual self-image, even if these side effects do not directly affect the ability to engage in intimate behavior.

For Men

Some chemotherapy drugs, such as cisplatin (Platinol) or vincristine (Oncovin), may interfere with the nerves that control erection. Most men continue to have normal erections during chemotherapy, although their desire may decrease temporarily because of the physical effects of and emotional responses to chemotherapy. Erection problems that do occur are usually resolved a week or two after chemotherapy ends. Sexual desire is likely to recover soon, too.

Some chemotherapy drugs, including Oncovin, can also damage nerves controlling the emission of semen and produce what is known as a dry orgasm, that is, having the feeling of pleasure but no semen (retrograde ejaculation or complete failure of emission, as explained on pages 348–349). This effect, however, is rare. Once in a while, chemotherapy dampens sexual desire and causes erection difficulties by slowing down the production of testosterone, a male hormone. The areas in the testicles that produce testosterone are not as easily damaged as those that make sperm cells, however.

For Women

Although many women lose interest in sex because of the side effects of chemotherapy, understanding that the change may not be permanent usually eases the concern.

Premature Menopause. For women of childbearing age, the critical issue affecting sexuality and reproductive capability is premature menopause brought on by chemotherapy drugs that temporarily compromise or permanently destroy the functioning of the ovaries. For example, women over 35 years old who are treated with combination chemotherapy for breast cancer may stop menstruating permanently. Those under age 35 may recover their menstrual periods but begin menopause sooner than they would have without the chemotherapy. The extent to which the ovaries are damaged depends on the type of drugs used and the size of the doses. Therefore, women who wish to have children should discuss the possible effects of chemotherapy on their reproductive capacity with their doctors before undergoing treatment (see box on pages 350–351).

When the ovaries stop functioning, they no longer produce the hormones estrogen and progesterone, which control the menstrual cycle. Women thus lose their ability to produce ripe eggs and become pregnant. Symptoms of premature menopause can appear quite suddenly and be more severe than those occurring with natural menopause, which takes place gradually over several years. Hot flashes, vaginal dryness, partial loss of the vagina's capacity to expand, and the absence of menstrual periods are the usual symptoms caused by a lack of estrogen. Vaginal dryness and loss of elasticity can make intercourse painful and are a chief cause of sexual difficulties for women who have undergone chemotherapy. It is not unusual to have a light spotting of

Premature Menopause: Some Solutions

Premature menopause can be caused by chemotherapy, radiation treatments to the pelvic area, or surgical removal of the ovaries. After what are often months of treatment, vaginal dryness and hot flashes may seem like the last thing you need, but don't despair. Understanding that these side effects are to be expected is the first step in planning how to cope with them.

Is estrogen replacement for you? Many women who naturally enter menopause decide to take replacement hormones (usually estrogen is taken in combination with progesterone if the woman has her uterus) to ease the symptoms and to prevent the long-term risks of osteoporosis and heart disease. This may be an option for you, too—unless you have a cancer that is sensitive to estrogen such as breast or endometrial cancer or melanoma.

Vaginal Dryness

Vaginal dryness is the most common cause of sexual difficulties. It causes not only physical problems (tightness and pain during intercourse), but also emotional ones (you know the intercourse is going to hurt, so you lose interest). Vaginal lubricants can sometimes provide enough extra lubrication to make intercourse comfortable. Look for over-the-counter, water-based gels rather than other oil-based lubricants such as petroleum jelly that may contribute to yeast infections.

For severe dryness, a vaginal moisturizer such as Replens can be used several times a week to keep the vagina moist at all times. Since the moisturizer is used on a regular basis and not just during intercourse, you don't have to stop in the middle of lovemaking to apply a lubricant. If you still have pain, continue using the moisturizer, but try using a gel lubricant during intercourse.

The lining of the vagina thins during chemotherapy. Light bleeding after intercourse is not unusual and is no cause for alarm. However, a burning sensation during intercourse may indicate that the vagina is inflamed because of a yeast infection, in which case medication will be required to treat it.

Self-Help for Symptoms of Menopause

Many self-help books on menopause suggest that exercise and relaxation techniques such as meditation or yoga may help ease the symptoms. (Relaxation techniques are detailed in Chapter 27.) The most important thing to do is to talk to your doctor about any symptoms you may be having and then decide what treatment is right for you. If your doctor offers no solutions, ask for a referral to a specialist.

blood after intercourse because of small tears in the vaginal lining, which is not in itself serious but can be frightening if you do not expect it.

Finally, a lack of testosterone (a male hormone that is also present, albeit in lower levels, in women) can result in a loss of desire for sex (see page 343).

Women who have already gone through menopause may not notice so much change after chemotherapy, although those whose cancers are sensitive to estrogen (breast or endometrial cancers) may have to stop taking replacement hormones. The lack of estrogen may then become more obvious.

There is much that can be done to make intercourse more comfortable following chemotherapy, as described on pages 352–354. For tips on coping with premature menopause, see *Premature Menopause: Some Solutions* (page 337).

Pregnancy. Although many chemotherapy drugs interrupt the menstrual cycle, the ovaries do not necessarily stop functioning altogether. A woman therefore may occasionally ovulate and have a period even if she has not menstruated for several months. Thus, it still may be possible to get pregnant while undergoing chemotherapy. Since many chemotherapy drugs can damage the fetus, a woman should discuss methods of birth control with her doctor.

Infection. Since chemotherapy weakens the immune system, women undergoing chemotherapy are vulnerable to yeast infections. Symptoms such as vaginal itching, a whitish discharge, or a burning sensation during intercourse can make a woman less interested in sex. Yeast infections can be easily treated with medication.

For the same reason, genital herpes or warts can flare up if a woman had them before treatment. Any infection can become a problem, so it is important to contact a doctor as soon as symptoms appear. Some chemotherapy drugs can also cause thinning of the vaginal lining that may lead to painful inflammation.

Chemotherapy for Bladder Cancer. Chemotherapy drugs are sometimes placed directly into the bladder through a catheter in the urethra. Because the drugs do not circulate to the ovaries, the treatment does not cause menopause, but intercourse can be painful soon after treatment while the bladder and urethra are still irritated.

Effects of Radiation Therapy on Sexuality

Radiation therapy can cause fatigue and weakness toward the end of the course of treatment, leaving little or no energy for sexual activity. In addition, radiation that includes the pelvic area (e.g., for prostate, bladder, colon, and cervical cancers) causes physical changes that result in sexual problems for both men and women.

For Men

Although radiation to the pelvic area is one of the most common causes of erection difficulties in men with cancer, the majority of men do not have permanent sexual problems after they undergo radiation.

Problems with Erections. The higher the total dose of radiation is and the wider the pelvic area that is being treated, the greater the chance of developing erection difficulties. Some men have a normal erection initially, but cannot sustain it to the point of climax. Others don't have firm erections at all.

The problem is caused by a loss of elasticity in the arteries that carry blood to the penis and the result: a narrowing of these blood vessels. The pelvic arteries can also be damaged, which contributes to the problem. Men whose arteries may already be damaged by high blood pressure or heavy smoking are at increased risk of erection problems.

Testosterone production may also slow after pelvic radiation, because the testicles may be affected, but hormone levels usually recover within six months.

Of those men who had good erections before the radiation, about one-quarter to one-third will have difficulties that often develop slowly after a year or so after radiation therapy. Those most at risk are men who already had a decline in erections as a result of inadequate blood flow before radiation.

TIPS AND

ADVICE

Coping with Lost Erections

Erection problems can have either emotional or physical causes, or a combination of both. Stress from the diagnosis or treatment, fear of not being able to get an erection or satisfy your partner, or pain and side effects of cancer treatments may be responsible for erection problems.

- The first step is to get a proper diagnosis to determine whether the cause is physical, psychological, or a combination of both. If you find that your erection difficulties occur all the time in all situations, the problem may be largely physical and perhaps permanent. But if you sometimes awake with an erection, can stimulate your own penis, have an erection and orgasm during sex with your partner, or become sexually aroused unexpectedly, your problem is probably psychological and temporary.

- Erection problems do not make you less masculine, and you shouldn't feel embarrassed to seek help; sex therapy has been very successful in treating sexual problems caused by anxiety and stress. Even if the problem is physical, a sex therapist can explain things you might not even realize about your own body. For example, many men do not know they can still have an orgasm with a flaccid penis, with manual or oral caressing.

- If your problem is physical, several effective treatments can restore firm erections. Men can learn to inject several types of medications into the penis to make it firm. Although the erections feel and look natural, injection therapy can cause scarring inside the soft tissue of the penis. A less risky option is a plastic vacuum erection pump. A man places a cylinder over his penis and uses a hand- or battery-powered pump to produce a vacuum that draws blood into the penis and makes it firm. A medical doctor (urologist or family practitioner) can prescribe a vacuum erection device if you and your partner would like to try it, and one model is also available over-the-counter.

- Although there are also some experimental surgical procedures to correct erection problems due to blockage of the arteries, only a small number of men have realized any long-term improvements. Far more successful are penile prostheses, or implants. The two most common types are a semirigid prosthesis that stays about 80 percent erect all the time or an inflatable penile prosthesis that gives a man the option of having his penis hard or soft, as he chooses. The implant is placed surgically inside the body.

- Be sure to discuss the benefits and risks of any medications, devices, or implants with your own doctor to find which is best. Each of these treatment options can provide firm erections, but none can restore sexual desire or improve skin sensation. Sexual counseling can help you cope with permanent changes in your ability to experience sexual pleasure.

- It's a good idea to include your partner in these talks, so that she or he can understand what's happening to you and how it affects your sex life together.

- It's important to also talk to your partner about what's happening to your body and find new ways of giving you both pleasure. Sex therapy can help you both in this regard.

Ejaculation Difficulties. After radiation to the prostate, some men find that the amount of semen they ejaculate has decreased to only a few drops. Since the urethra has been irritated during radiation, it is not unusual, toward the end of treatment, to feel a sharp pain during ejaculation. Although the semen may not return to previous levels, the pain will fade, and sexual desire will return within several weeks after the treatment has been completed.

Loss of Desire. Once in a while, scattered radiation can affect a man's testicles, decreasing testosterone production, which causes temporary erection problems and a loss of desire. These problems usually improve within a few months, however, as hormone levels recover (see pages 342–343, *Lost Sexual Desire: Is Androgen Replacement for You?*).

For Women

Radiation to a woman's pelvic area affects all organs in the region (but not those outside the target area) and thus can influence her sex and reproductive life in several ways. Radiation can make the lining of the vagina thin and fragile. As a result, some women experience light bleeding after intercourse. This is not unusual and can often be prevented by using lubricants and more gentle sexual stimulation. If the ovaries are within the area being treated, reproduction may be affected.

Premature Menopause. Large doses of pelvic radiation (such as that used to treat cervical cancer) stop the ovaries from functioning and cause the same menopause symptoms as do some chemotherapy drugs. Sometimes this effect is temporary, but often it is permanent. For a more complete discussion, see *Premature Menopause*, pages 336 and 338, and *Premature Menopause: Some Solutions*, page 337.

Vaginal Irritation and Scarring. Since tissues that are irradiated become inflamed, the vagina may feel tender during treatment and for a few weeks afterward. However, as long as she does not experience heavy bleeding or pain, a woman can have intercourse while receiving pelvic radiation therapy.

Scar tissue tends to form as the inflammation heals, causing the vagina to narrow and lose elasticity so that it may not enlarge as much during intercourse as it once did. One way to avoid this is to have sexual intercourse at least three or four times a week or to use a vaginal dilator to stretch the vagina until intercourse becomes comfortable.

By using a vaginal dilator several times a week, you can prevent scar tissue from tightening the vagina. A vaginal dilator is a plastic or rubber tube a bit smaller than an erect penis. Available only by doctor's prescription, dilators stretch out the vagina, keeping it a normal size and making intercourse and gynecologic exams more comfortable.

Pain from Ulceration. A less common complication is a radiation ulcer or sore spot in the vagina that causes pain during sexual activity. Although the ulcer can take months to heal, it will eventually disappear.

Effects of Hormone Therapy and Surgery on Sexuality

Some people with breast, prostate, or uterine cancer receive treatment with sex hormones. Although the hormones help treat the cancer, they generally alter sexual functioning in some way.

For Men

If prostate cancer has spread, it is necessary to block testosterone from nourishing the cancer cells by either removing the testicles, taking hormones, or both. For men, loss of desire is the principal effect of hormone therapy on sexuality. Most men also have trouble getting or keeping an erection or reaching an orgasm, but some have a desire for sex even though they have erection problems. Other men stay sexually active for many years.

For Women

Tamoxifen (Nolvadex) and progestins prevent cancer cells from using estrogen, which can stimulate certain types of breast and endometrial cancer cells. These hormones can cause some menopausal symptoms, including hot flashes. Because tamoxifen actually acts like a weak form of estrogen on vaginal tissues, in menopausal women it can have the positive impact of increasing vaginal lubrication.

The hormones themselves can sometimes decrease sexual desire. Women with breast cancer are sometimes treated with androgens (so-called male hormones) when other hormone treatments no longer work. Androgen treatments can boost a woman's sexual desire but, in large doses, can also deepen her voice, cause acne, and increase facial hair. Although these virilizing effects can be upsetting, they are not usually severe enough to be very noticeable at the doses used for cancer treatment. It is helpful to keep in mind that the androgen is being given to control the cancer.

INFORM

YOURSELF

Lost Sexual Desire: Is Androgen Replacement for You?

Androgens are the hormones believed to control sexual desire in both men and women. Testosterone is a common androgen, and although many people think of it as a male hormone, women's bodies also produce and use it, although in lesser quantities.

For Men

For men experiencing a loss of desire or erection problems, a blood test can determine whether testosterone levels are normal. If they are low, which is rare, replacement therapy can be helpful in restoring sexual desire. An injection or patch is more effective than hormone pills.

Since a replacement testosterone dosage is designed to return the androgen level to normal and no higher, there are no known risks associated with it. Those men who have prostate cancer or a history of prostate cancer, however, must avoid testosterone, since it can accelerate the growth of prostate cancer cells.

For Women

According to some experts, many women who go through menopause prematurely have low testosterone levels and thus lose some desire for sex. If a blood test reveals that this is the problem, testosterone replacement may be a possibility. A small dose, about one-tenth that used to treat men, may boost sexual desire without causing any virilizing effects like lowering your voice or causing facial hair to grow.

Keep in mind that testosterone only restores desire. It does not relieve other symptoms of menopause, such as vaginal dryness or loss of elasticity. There are some minor risks for women taking testosterone. It can have a mildly negative impact on your cholesterol level and produce oily skin. It also is risky for women with some types of breast cancer to take testosterone or any hormones that might make the cancer grow. The benefits and safety of testosterone replacement are still somewhat controversial.

Coping with Specific Cancers and Procedures That Affect Female Sexuality and Fertility

Hysterectomy

A hysterectomy is usually done to treat cancer of the uterus or ovary. Although the uterus, the cervix, and an inch or two of the deep vagina are removed, the woman is still able to feel sexual pleasure. Particularly for women of childbearing age, however, the operation can be emotionally difficult, since they are no longer able to have children as a result. If both ovaries are removed from a premenopausal woman, premature menopause will result. Sometimes in younger women, one ovary will be left in place to prevent this.

Although several popular self-help books have suggested that a large percentage of women have problems becoming aroused or reaching orgasm after having a hysterectomy, no scientific data substantiate this. Women find that the area around the clitoris and the lining of the vagina remain as sensitive as they were before the surgery, even after a radical hysterectomy, which includes removing part of the upper vagina.

Coping Tips. Removal of the uterus, cervix, or ovaries doesn't affect a woman's ability to have an orgasm. But when a radical hysterectomy is done, an inch

Female Sexual Problems Caused by Cancer Treatment

Treatment	Low Sexual Desire	Less Vaginal Moisture	Reduced Vaginal Size	Painful Intercourse	Trouble Reaching Orgasm	Infertility
Chemotherapy	Sometimes	Often	Sometimes	Often	Rarely	Often
Pelvic radiation therapy	Rarely	Often	Often	Often	Rarely	Often
Radical hysterectomy	Rarely	Often*	Often	Rarely	Rarely	Always
Radical cystectomy	Rarely	Often*	Always	Sometimes	Rarely	Always
Abdominoperineal (A-P) resection	Rarely	Often*	Sometimes	Sometimes	Rarely	Sometimes
Total pelvic exenteration with vaginal reconstruction	Sometimes	Always	Sometimes	Sometimes	Sometimes	Always
Radical vulvectomy	Rarely	Never	Sometimes	Often	Sometimes	Never
Conization of the cervix	Never	Never	Never	Rarely	Never	Rarely
Oophorectomy (removal of one tube and ovary)	Rarely	Never*	Never*	Rarely	Never	Rarely
Oophorectomy (removal of both tubes and ovaries)	Rarely	Often*	Sometimes*	Sometimes*	Rarely	Always
Mastectomy or radiation to the breast	Rarely	Never	Never	Never	Rarely	Never
Antiestrogen therapy for the breast or uterine cancer	Sometimes	Rarely	Rarely	Rarely	Rarely	Rarely
Androgen therapy	Never	Never	Never	Never	Never	Uncertain

*Vaginal dryness and size changes should not occur if one ovary is left in or if hormone replacement therapy is given. It is advisable to use birth control to avoid the possibility of pregnancy at this time.

or two of the deep vagina is removed, and complete penetration may not be possible. Extra time spent on foreplay makes the most of the natural deepening of the vagina that occurs with sexual excitement. But if the vagina still feels short, a woman can close her hands around the base of her partner's penis to give him the feeling of more depth during thrusting. Another method is to put lubricating gel on the tops of the woman's thighs and around the outer genitals and to squeeze the thighs together during intercourse.

Radical Cystectomy

A cystectomy is surgery to control bladder cancer. During a cystectomy the bladder, uterus, ovaries, fallopian tubes, cervix, urethra, and the front wall of the vagina are removed. (Urine exits the body through an ostomy, or opening, in the abdomen.) Although the clitoris remains intact, a surgeon must reconstruct the vagina to enable the woman to have intercourse again. One type of vaginal reconstruction makes the vagina narrower, and the other makes it shorter. Although both can result in painful intercourse initially, most women find that it becomes less uncomfortable over time.

It is important to discuss the advantages and disadvantages of both types of reconstruction with the doctor before the surgery. Recently, surgeons have begun to try to spare more of the vaginal tissue when they perform cystectomies.

Coping with Painful Intercourse. Pain during intercourse can be eased by using lubricants or vaginal dilators, taking prescribed replacement hormones, or using estrogen creams, if appropriate. If intercourse is painful, you may also want to try different intercourse positions to find the one that is most comfortable.

Most women do not realize that they are contributing to the pain by tensing the muscles around the vaginal entrance. The fear that penetration will hurt causes a reflex of muscle tension. These muscles are called the pubococcygeal, or PC, muscles. They form a ring around the outer third of the vagina, closest to the entrance. Fortunately, there are exercises you can practice that will help you learn to relax these muscles.

Radical Vulvectomy

A radical vulvectomy removes a woman's entire outer genital area, including the inner and outer lips of the vulva, the clitoris, and often the lymph nodes that drain the vulva. The sexual consequences can be considerable, as the vulva contributes greatly to a woman's sexual pleasure. Even though the outer third of the vagina, which remains intact, has numerous nerve endings, many women find they have trouble reaching an orgasm without the clitoris. Also, the scarring that results from the surgery can narrow the vaginal opening and make penetration difficult.

Some women may lose sexual interest because they fear that the changes in the appearance of the area around their genitals will disturb their partner, especially for those who enjoy oral sex. If the surgery included removal of lymph nodes in the groin, unsightly leg swelling can also be a continuing problem.

Coping Tips. In some cases, a surgeon can reconstruct the contours of the vulva. Vaginal dilators can be used to stretch the vaginal opening, or in severe cases, skin grafting can widen the entrance.

Increasingly, surgeons have been able to spare a woman's sexual functioning by removing only the tumor and adjoining tissue, rather than by performing such radical surgery.

Total Pelvic Exenteration

Removal of the pelvic organs—the uterus, ovaries, bladder, rectum, and vagina—is called total pelvic exenteration. The outer genitals—the vulva and the clitoris—are not removed. This radical pelvic surgery can alter a woman's sexual pleasure and ability to achieve orgasm, even though the sensitive vulva may remain. The vagina must be completely reconstructed to make intercourse possible. The most widely accepted reconstruction procedure uses muscle and skin from the inner thigh to create a closed tube the same size and shape as the vagina. Since the nerves remain attached, the reconstructed vagina is sensitive to touch, but it does not become moist with arousal. Women may have to learn through experience to find intercourse erotic with a reconstructed vagina. Most women also have a colostomy and a urinary ostomy, unless they have internal reconstruction work.

Coping Tips. Even after total pelvic exenteration, it is possible, with determination and motivation, to return to sexual activity. A sex therapist can help. Because the outer genitals, including the clitoris, are usually not removed, some women find they can still feel pleasure and reach an orgasm when the outer genitals are caressed.

Mastectomy

Although a mastectomy (the removal of one or both breasts) does not directly influence a woman's ability to have sex, she may feel inhibited or lack interest in sex if she is embarrassed by her body or afraid of turning off her partner. Women who enjoy stimulation of their breasts may have trouble enjoying caressing of the remaining breast. When both breasts are removed or reconstructed, women may need to shift their focus to other erotic zones to achieve sexual arousal.

A partial mastectomy may reduce nipple sensation, depending on the location and extent of surgery. A reconstructed breast and nipple do not have the same sensitivity to touch as the natural breast does, but women often find that they develop more pleasurable feelings over time.

Coping Tips. If breast caressing becomes less pleasurable, couples can experiment to find other sensitive parts of the body. Spending more time on caressing the body and being creative with various kinds of touch can help.

Some women feel more comfortable wearing a breast prosthesis and lingerie during sex. Others find the prosthesis awkward or feel no need to conceal their scar.

Women who have had a radical mastectomy may have problems when resting their own weight on their chest or arm, or it may be uncomfortable when their partner rests on them. Supporting these areas with pillows during sex may help.

Coping with Specific Cancers and Procedures That Affect Male Sexuality and Fertility

Radical Pelvic Surgery

Radical pelvic surgery varies depending on the type of cancer being treated. Some operations cause more erection problems than others. For example, recovery of full erections after total pelvic exenteration (removal of the prostate, seminal vesicles, bladder, and rectum) is unheard of, but the surgery is so rare that no statistics are available. After removal of the bladder (cystectomy), some men recover erections firm enough for vaginal intercourse. At least 15 percent who have standard prostatectomies regain their ability to have complete erections. Erections are more likely to be recovered after abdominoperineal (AP) resection (removal of the lower colon and rectum).

Since radical surgery can damage the nerves that control blood flow to the penis, it may be difficult for men either to achieve or to maintain an erection. In the past decade, nerve-sparing techniques have been developed for radical prostatectomy and are also sometimes used with radical cystectomy or AP resection. After a nerve-sparing prostatectomy, many men may eventually recover adequate erections. Sometimes these erections are not completely firm, however. Recovery often takes up to a year or even two to be as complete as possible.

Operations that interfere with blood flow to the penis also affect the ability to have a complete erection. In time, new blood vessels develop, which helps restore circulation.

Coping Tips. The recovery of erections varies from person to person and depends on the man's age, how good his erections were before surgery, and the extent of surgery necessary. In general, younger men, especially those under the ages of 50 to 60, and men who had good erections before their cancer surgery are more likely to regain full erections than older men are. If a man had difficulties before the operation because of health problems or old age, he will most likely have problems after surgery.

Radical prostatectomy and radical cystectomy also result in a loss of semen production. Although orgasm occurs, nothing is emitted, a phenomenon known as dry orgasm. Some men consider dry orgasms less satisfying, whereas others say they feel completely normal. Most people can't tell the

INFORM

YOURSELF

Male Sexual Problems Caused by Cancer Treatment

Treatment	Low Sexual Desire	Erection Problems	Lack of Orgasm	Dry Orgasm	Weaker Orgasm	Infertility
Chemotherapy	Sometimes	Rarely	Rarely	Rarely	Rarely	Often
Pelvic radiation therapy	Rarely	Sometimes	Rarely	Rarely	Sometimes	Often
Retroperitoneal lymph node dissection	Rarely	Rarely	Rarely	Often	Sometimes	Often
Abdominoperineal (A-P) resection	Rarely	Often	Rarely	Often	Sometimes	Sometimes*
Radical prostatectomy	Rarely	Often	Rarely	Always	Sometimes	Always***
Radical cystectomy	Rarely	Often	Rarely	Always	Sometimes	Always***
Total pelvic exenteration	Rarely	Often	Rarely	Always	Sometimes	Always
Partial penectomy	Rarely	Rarely	Rarely	Never	Rarely	Never
Total penectomy	Rarely	Always	Sometimes	Never	Sometimes	Usually*
Orchiectomy (removal of one testicle)	Rarely	Rarely	Never	Never	Never	Rarely**
Orchiectomy (removal of both testicles)	Often	Often	Sometimes	Sometimes	Sometimes	Always
Hormone therapy for prostate cancer	Often	Often	Sometimes	Sometimes	Sometimes	Always

*Artificial insemination of a spouse with the man's own semen may be possible.

**Infertile only if remaining testicle is not normal.

*** In vitro fertilization using sperm cells retrieved directly from the testicles may be possible, however.

difference during intercourse and no pleasure is lost. The man will not be able to father children, however, although high-technology in vitro fertilization with sperm cells retrieved directly from the testicles may be possible.

An AP resection for colon cancer also can cause a dry orgasm, but for a different reason. Sometimes retrograde ejaculation occurs. Because of surgery-related nerve damage, the valve between the bladder and urethra, which is normally tightly closed during emission, stays open. As a result, the semen goes backward into the bladder instead of out through the penis. Since the semen mixes with the urine, it is not unusual to have cloudy-looking urine after this type of ejaculation. If the man wants to have children, the sperm can sometimes be recovered from the urine and used to make a woman pregnant. Some medications may also restore normal ejaculation temporarily when attempting pregnancy. Retrograde ejaculation is not painful.

Sometimes the nerve damage is more severe, and there is no emission at all; the prostate and seminal vesicles are "paralyzed." Infertility treatments may still be useful, however, and orgasm remains pleasurable.

Orgasms may be weaker after pelvic surgery and premature ejaculation (reaching a climax too quickly) is not unusual among men who have erection problems. It may help to slow down the excitement phase of sex.

Testicular Surgery

The sexual and reproductive consequences of surgery for testicular cancer depend on whether one or both testicles are removed.

Coping with the Loss of One Testicle. Testicular cancer almost always affects only one testicle, and so only the abnormal one is removed. Since the remaining testicle compensates for the loss of testosterone, this surgery usually does not physically affect a man's sexual desire.

Because one side of the sac looks empty, some men feel embarrassed in front of their partners or in the locker room. A testicular prosthesis, a silicone gel-filled sac that looks and feels like a testicle, can be implanted.

Coping with the Loss of Two Testicles. Both testicles are sometimes removed from those men whose prostate cancer has spread, to stop the production of testosterone that nourishes the cancer. In this case, the cords at the tops of the testicles are left so that the sacs do not look empty. Since the testicles produce most of a man's testosterone, this surgery can greatly reduce his sexual desire and ability to achieve and maintain erections.

Coping with Lymph Node Dissections for Testicular Cancer (Retroperitoneal Lymphadenectomy). Men with testicular cancer often have surgery to remove the lymph nodes to which the cancer can spread. This surgery frequently damages the nerves that control emission, causing a dry orgasm. As with AP resection, the problem may be due to retrograde ejaculation or to total paralysis of the emission phase. Again, orgasm is still pleasurable.

Because men with testicular cancer are usually young and have not completed their families, surgeons may either try to avoid doing a lymph node dissection, or they may remove less tissue, making it more likely that crucial nerves will be spared.

Penectomy

If a man has a partial penectomy, which removes only the end of the penis, he can still have an erection, orgasm, and normal ejaculation. If a total penectomy is required, the entire penis is removed. Since the remaining tissues around the genitals still have nerve endings, a man can still experience erotic sensations when the scrotum, the skin behind the scrotum, or the area surrounding the surgical scars is caressed. He can have an orgasm and ejaculate through the opening created for his urinary tube (called a perineal urethrostomy).

Coping Tips. Despite his loss, a motivated man can learn to reach orgasm through sexual fantasies, erotic pictures and stories, or sensitive touching around the scrotum. He can also please his partner in many ways without a penis, using his fingers, oral sex, or a vibrator.

INFORM

YOURSELF

Can Your Sexual and Reproductive Functioning Be Spared?

When faced with a cancer treatment that can damage your sexual or reproductive functioning, be assertive with your health care team in asking whether an alternative procedure is available. In general, radical procedures remove an entire organ. More localized procedures leave some of the organ or tissue and possibly more of its functioning intact.

You must weigh the importance of maintaining your full sexual and reproductive capability and intact appearance against the ability of the treatment to eliminate or control the cancer. Men can bank their sperm to be frozen and used later to father children. Researchers currently are developing the ability to freeze a woman's unfertilized eggs or ovarian tissue. At present only fertilized embryos, produced by in vitro fertilization, can be successfully frozen and thawed. Those men or women who wish to have children may be willing to postpone treatment to allow for sperm banking or in vitro (test-tube) fertilization, if that's an option, or to risk a less drastic procedure that may have a somewhat lower cure rate until they are able to have a family.

For Men

If you have been told you need radical surgery, ask your doctor whether you are a candidate for a procedure that spares the nerves responsible for erection or emission.

Cancer of the penis is most common in elderly men who may have already stopped having sex because of other health problems. Whether the amputation is partial or total, however, this operation can devastate a man's self-image, so sexual or psychological counseling may be helpful.

For Women

Preserving the breast through lumpectomy or having a mastectomy followed by a breast reconstruction can help women with breast cancer feel more whole and attractive, even though most reconstructive procedures eliminate breast sensation entirely.

If you have vulvar cancer, ask your doctor whether you are a good candidate for a local excision that removes only the tumor and some of the surrounding tissue instead of the whole vulva. This type of surgery is less disfiguring, results in less scarring and less painful intercourse, and removes less sensitive tissue, so that sexual pleasure is preserved. Avoiding a groin node dissection also saves considerable discomfort and disfigurement.

For early-stage cervical cancer, a hysterectomy that leaves the ovaries intact is usually as effective as radiation therapy. Neither treatment can preserve a woman's fertility. Some studies indicate that women who undergo a hysterectomy have fewer sexual difficulties than do women who have radiation therapy.

Other Surgeries' Effects on Sex

Several surgical procedures may alter your body in ways that do not directly affect your ability to perform or respond sexually but that can cause embarrassment or physical awkwardness in intimate situations. For example, operations on the face can cause changes in appearance that are very hard for you and others to deal with (see Chapter 20).

Other types of surgery do necessitate some kinds of personal care before making love, however, for which specific advice follows.

Urostomy or Colostomy

Both a urostomy (removal of the tubes through which urine leaves the body) and a colostomy (removal of the colon) result in the often permanent need to wear an ostomy bag to collect urine and feces. Some people are comfortable making love with the ostomy bag exposed, but others like to cover it up. Either way, the bag should be emptied and sealed before lovemaking, to reduce the chance of leakage. If the bag does leak, jump in the shower together and try again. Some people use a pouch cover to make the bag look less medical. You can get urinary ostomy pouches made in a smaller size for short-term use during sexual activity. If you have had a colostomy, you may be able to irrigate and regulate your bowel movements so that you can wear a small stoma cap instead of a pouch. You can also avoid eating gas-forming foods. Women can wear sexy lingerie to cover the bag, and men can wear a T-shirt.

For some people, touching the ostomy can feel erotic. Too much rubbing or touching, however, can tear or irritate the stoma and should be avoided.

And no objects should be placed in a stoma. Most people are more comfortable during sex if the partner's weight is off the ostomy. Sometimes a small pillow can be used to shift the partner's weight away from the appliance.

Laryngectomy

Since they can no longer breathe through their mouth following a laryngectomy, removal of the voice box, many people worry about how their partners will feel about kissing them. Embarrassment and worry about odors coming from the tube in their neck also can make people lose interest in sex.

Some people find wearing perfume or aftershave and avoiding spicy foods reduce the odors from the stoma. Most people like to wear a stoma cover in their neck during lovemaking. Since talking requires effort and can lessen some of the emotional overtones during lovemaking, communicating any needs and desires before intercourse or through touch while making love can help things go more smoothly.

Limb Amputation

Although the need to become accustomed to the appearance of a limb stump is obvious and may for a while affect one's body image and self-esteem, there are practical considerations that may help facilitate lovemaking. Pillows can be used to support the remaining part of a limb, but some couples find that the prosthesis helps in positioning and makes movement easier. Many people also experience phantom limb sensations or pain. When there is actual discomfort, pain-relieving medication may be helpful.

Maintaining or Restoring Your Sex Life

For everyone—those with and without cancer—keeping a sex life going depends on a lot more than the physical ability to perform sexually. But having cancer adds its own issues, which need to be understood and worked through by you and your partner.

How Do You Feel About Your Body?

The first order of business for many people is to restore their self-esteem and body image (see Chapter 20). Many people find that once they get used to seeing themselves naked in a mirror, they can accept themselves as they are and feel more at ease in a sexual situation.

Sexual difficulties resulting from cancer treatment can, of course, jar your self-image. Fear of pain during intercourse or anxiety about erections can interfere with your sexual image. Learning what can be done to relieve the problems, communicating with your partner, and finding new ways of expressing love and intimacy all can help reassure you that you are still a vital, sexual person.

You may have come to the point that staying sexually active is not so important to you. You may not want to go through the pain or the ordeal involved. This does not mean you are less of a person or less loveable. Talking to your partner and understanding that you still have love and support are important to restoring your sense of wholeness and well being. As long as you both feel comfortable about it, you can find other ways of staying intimate.

Talk!

Good communication is essential. Cancer puts a lot of strain on each partner in a relationship and on the relationship itself, whether it is long standing or relatively new. There is much you will need to talk about—each other's fears, needs, anger, yearnings, anguish, and hopes. For example, many partners of people with cancer are afraid to initiate sexual contact for fear of causing pain. Their reluctance often comes across as cold and standoffish and can hurt the very sensitive feelings of the person with cancer. Open discussion can eliminate an unfounded concern or allow both of you to work out more comfortable ways of being close and giving pleasure.

Understand What You Can and Cannot Do

People with cancer and their partners often think that sex will make the cancer worse or make it recur. Some people avoid sex because they think the cancer is contagious. These myths, though common, are untrue. Talking honestly with a doctor or sex therapist can help couples gain a better understanding of what they can and cannot do before, during, and after treatment. The questions on page 355 can help you ask your doctor about the effects of your treatment on your sexuality and what, if any, activities you should avoid at particular phases of treatment.

Take It Easy

Don't expect to "pick up where you left off" sexually. Schedule private time together, and make it relaxed, romantic, and special. Start the lovemaking slowly by gently touching each other's bodies, but not the genitals or breasts yet. Concentrate on the feelings of pleasure you are having. Many couples prefer to caress each other for a long while, gradually adding genital touching and building up the excitement over days or even weeks before resuming intercourse. And if intercourse is no longer possible or desired, you will have learned much about bringing pleasure to yourself and your partner.

Change Your Routine

Many couples have a favorite position for lovemaking or a routine for their sexual activity. Cancer treatment may cause changes that mean you need to find new ways to be comfortable and to please each other. If your movement is restricted or you are no longer comfortable in your usual lovemaking positions, experiment to find new positions. There is no right or wrong way. Each couple needs to decide what is right for them.

Keep in mind that it is possible to show physical affection and experience sexual pleasure in ways other than conventional intercourse. Intimate touching, for example, remains pleasurable regardless of the type of cancer treatment you've undergone. Women with vaginal dryness and men with erection problems can still reach orgasm through touching.

Sexual intercourse or physical pleasure is not at the top of everyone's agenda, however. Nonsexual touching—hugging, cuddling, or holding hands—is equally important and keeps couples feeling intimate with each other.

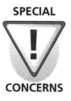

SPECIAL

CONCERNS

When Not to Have Sex

Your doctor will tell you when you can resume sexual activity after surgery. But whenever you are in doubt about whether sex might be harmful or hazardous, ask your doctor. The following are situations in which sexual activity may pose a risk.

- Bleeding in the genital area or urinary tract. If bleeding becomes heavier after sex, it's best to stop having intercourse until the cause has been identified and treated.

- Infection may be a threat when the immune system is suppressed, such as when the white blood cell count is low as a result of chemotherapy or radiation therapy. Ask your doctor if you're concerned about sexual contact.

- If a male partner has any signs of sexually transmitted diseases such as a strange sore on his penis or whitish fluid (other than semen) at the opening at the tip. Also, do not engage in unprotected sex if you or your partner have other sex partners.

Sex and the Single Person

It is not unusual for single people to worry about being rejected by future lovers because of cancer. You may be concerned about the way in which your partner will react to any changes in body appearance. Also important are the anxieties that can keep a single person who has had cancer from committing to a relationship afterward. Fear of not being able to have children because of possible infertility, fear of not living to see future children grow up, or fear of becoming a burden to a future spouse makes single people afraid of drawing someone they love into an uncertain future.

It is important to have honest and open communication with any current or future partner, but finding a good time to discuss mastectomy scars, an ostomy bag, or a sexual problem can be difficult while dating. Bringing up these concerns too soon may scare the person away. But waiting too long may make the other person feel mistrusted or duped. Most people find it is best to wait until a sense of trust has developed and they feel liked and accepted (see also page 436, *Single with Cancer,* in Chapter 26).

QUESTIONS

TO ASK

Questions to Ask Your Doctor
About the Effects of Treatments on Sex

Health care professionals seldom bring up the topic of sex. Sometimes they are too busy; sometimes they are too uncomfortable or embarrassed to bring it up. You should, however, try to fight whatever embarrassment you feel and talk to your doctor or nurse about sex. The more you know about what sexual changes to expect, the better you can cope with what happens. Everyone has the right to know about his or her own sexual health. Here are some questions to ask:

- How will this treatment (surgery, chemotherapy, radiation) affect my desire for sex?

- How will this treatment affect my ability to feel pleasure when my genital areas are touched?

- How will this treatment affect my ability to reach an orgasm?

- Am I likely to have pain during sex as a result of this treatment?

- How will this treatment affect my ability to have an erection and ejaculate semen?

- Will this treatment make me menopausal or interfere with my taking replacement estrogen after menopause?

- How will this treatment affect my ability to have children in the future?

- Will the effects be temporary or permanent?

- What will I look like? Can you show me pictures?

- Are any alternatives or options available to me?

- Is there any reason that I should not have sex while undergoing treatment?

Where to Go for Help

A proper diagnosis will determine whether sexual difficulties are caused by physical or emotional problems or both. If sexual problems continue after treatment has ended, it can be helpful to talk to a professional. Some people get referrals from their oncologist, gynecologist, urologist, family doctor, social worker, or nurse. Here are other options to try:

- A sexual rehabilitation program in a cancer center. This option may be available only for those treated at that center. Ask the social services department in the hospital in which you were treated whether such a program is available there, or for a referral to another one.

- Sexual dysfunction clinics. Some medical schools and private practice groups run comprehensive clinics to diagnose and treat sexual problems. They vary in the range of services and health care specialists they offer.

- Urologists. These specialists have skills in treating erection problems.

- Gynecologists. A gynecologist with special expertise in treating pelvic pain, menopause, or cancer may be available in your community.

- Sex therapists. Although most states have no laws regulating this field, a sex therapist should be a trained, certified mental health professional with additional training in sex therapy. A qualified sex therapist never suggests having sex with you or observing you having sex.

INFORM

YOURSELF

For Further Assistance

The following are some professional societies that give referrals. Ask for a therapist who is familiar with the sexual difficulties caused by cancer and its treatment.

- American Association of Sex Educators, Counselors, and Therapists (AASECT), P.O. Box 5488, Richmond, VA 23220-0488; www.aasect.org.

- Marital therapists or other mental health professionals. Frequently the source of a sexual problem after the onset of cancer is in the relationship. It can help to work on these and other personal issues that may be interfering. Remember, too, that any problems you had before probably will continue or even grow worse under the added pressure of illness. Sex therapists frequently also specialize in marital counseling.

- A support group of others with cancer or of people with your type of cancer. Confide in others who have been through the same experience and seek their practical advice.

Managing Disabilities and Limitations

Cancer treatment causes almost everyone to experience some change in their physical being and ability to care for themselves. The effects may range from trivial to overwhelming, from temporary inconvenience to lifelong disability. Therapy can alter a body function, appearance, or both, possibly affecting the way you speak, walk, eat, eliminate, or perform an activity that you once took for granted.

The way in which these changes affect any individual varies enormously. A young woman with breast cancer, for example, may not face the same problems as a postmenopausal woman with the same disease, and neither of them has the same needs as a man with a colostomy or a child whose leg must be amputated. This is why one of the basic principles of rehabilitation medicine—a specialty concerned with enabling people to attain their full functioning potential—is that you must help plan your therapy. The main purpose of rehabilitation is to enable a person to function from day to day and to regain as much independence as possible and do the things that are important to you. The circumstances of your illness and the ongoing changes in your physical ability are always incorporated into the rehabilitation plan.

What Rehabilitation Can Do for You

The objectives of rehabilitation were summed up by the National Cancer Institute as part of a broad effort to improve the quality of life for people with cancer:

*   *Psychological adjustment:* overcoming anger and fear, developing a positive attitude, learning how to relax, and becoming secure enough to express yourself sexually (see Chapters 21 and 27).

- *Physical functioning:* coping with side effects; recognizing your strengths and limitations; learning new skills in daily functioning; adapting to the loss of limbs, organs, or capabilities; maintaining good nutrition; and getting enough exercise (see Chapters 18 and 19).

- *Vocational counseling:* arranging for productive work and recreation, recovering socially, getting your support system in place, and renewing or establishing contacts with friends (see Chapter 8).

- An effective rehabilitation plan always recognizes challenges to self-esteem and personal relationships (see Chapters 20, 26, and 28).

When Rehabilitation Begins

The time just after your diagnosis is crucial for obtaining psychological support, learning about your illness, developing coping skills, and preparing yourself for what is ahead. Learning about your potential for recovery early on can help relieve some of the fear and anxiety you may feel about your treatment and your future. Knowing what to expect, what you can do to recover as rapidly and fully as possible, and how to make the best of your situation can greatly diminish your fear of the unknown and the tendency to imagine the worst. Information, learning the self-care that might be necessary, and early preparation can be enormously helpful.

Many people find that accepting their diagnosis and becoming comfortable with changes to their bodies is easier when they are shown that living with a disability need not be as terrible as they may fear. For example, getting a clear explanation of what happens when you have an ostomy (a surgically created opening in the abdomen for waste elimination) allows you to feel a sense of control in a situation in which the loss of this body function is a central concern. For this reason, surgeons typically invite an ostomy specialist, called an enterostomal or stoma therapist, to talk with their patients before such surgery.

Who Needs Rehabilitation?

Nearly everyone who has been treated for cancer needs some rehabilitation, even if it only involves getting help in regaining strength after bed rest.

The following are some examples of specific difficulties that extensive, focused rehabilitation can address:

- *Head and neck cancer:* swallowing, eating, drinking, maintaining adequate food and water intake, talking, and appearance.

- *Cancer of the uterus, ovary, vulva, or vagina:* changes in internal or external anatomy, fear of the loss of femininity and of one's partner's reaction, compromised sexual function, and loss of childbearing ability.

- *Cancer of the bowel or bladder:* loss of voluntary control, adequate food and water intake, dietary changes, feelings of social isolation or stigma, sexual difficulties because of anatomic changes, difficulty in traveling and interference with hobbies, work, and recreation.

People with advanced cancer of any type are usually better able to cope with its emotional demands when they can care for themselves as much as possible. Rehabilitation goals can include relieving symptoms that diminish well being, making the environment safe and workable, and ensuring physical and emotional support.

Getting the Help You Need

Although rehabilitation is a widely accepted aspect of cancer treatment, not all doctors recommend it or make sure that those who need it get it. And other obstacles may exist as well. Community hospitals don't always have the necessary resources. Medical care professionals may be able to offer several aspects of care, but a specific person may not be responsible for making a rehabilitation plan.

If your oncologist or hospital social worker cannot help, the local unit of the American Cancer Society (ACS) may be of assistance.

The Team Approach

Rehabilitation calls for the coordinated efforts of a team of specialists, usually led by a physiatrist—a doctor who specializes in rehabilitation techniques. He or she is trained to diagnose and treat neuromuscular and musculoskeletal disorders and can design therapies to restore mobility or compensate for its limitations. A physiatrist also prescribes treatment provided by physical therapists and other members of the team, such as exercise instruction, fitting and training in how to use braces or artificial limbs, breathing assistance, and counseling.

INFORM

YOURSELF

Who Does What

Depending on your situation, your team may include one or several of the following:

- *Physiatrists*, doctors who specialize in rehabilitation medicine.

- *Physical therapists*, who teach exercises and other physical techniques for overcoming disabilities and using artificial limbs or braces, evaluate muscle strength and range of movement in joints, and teach hygienic self-care.

- *Occupational therapists*, who assess the ability to perform daily functions and instruct patients on how to use special techniques and tools to compensate for their disabilities.

- *Respiratory therapists*, who treat breathing disorders under the direction of a doctor and teach techniques to restore lung function.

- *Oncology nurses*, specially trained to care for people with cancer and to teach them about their care before, during, and after treatment; who plan at-home care and rehabilitation; and who help families deal with social and emotional issues.

- *Social workers*, who help patients and their families plan treatments and services, guide them to community resources, work with physiatrists or physical or occupational therapists in finding vocational or other counselors, and provide emotional support, psychological guidance, and sometimes stress management. They may evaluate your living environment and suggest how to change it to meet your particular physical needs. They may also coordinate community resources.

- *Psychologists*, who assess psychological status and problem-solving skills and suggest ways of handling the many challenges of cancer and its treatment, including self-esteem and sexuality issues, family difficulties, and lifestyle changes. They may provide training in stress management techniques and offer behavioral strategies for dealing with certain aspects of treatment. Psychologists also may help evaluate changes in personality and mental capacity, such as testing memory, perceptual function, and personality.

- *Speech pathologists*, who offer preoperative evaluation and counseling, provide treatment for neurologic communication problems, plan vocal re-education, and train people with defects in the mouth or without a larynx to acquire and use esophageal speech (see the *Learning to Talk* section of this chapter).

- *Nutritionists*, who help you maintain good nutrition while dealing with such problems as weight loss, appetite changes, or taste disorders; offer guidance in planning meals; and teach special techniques for supplementary feedings.

- *Vocational rehabilitation counselors*, who evaluate how cancer and its treatment affect life roles and vocational skills and, when necessary, offer counseling regarding career changes. They may serve as a link to placement and training agencies.

- *Maxillofacial prosthodontists*, dental specialists who create devices to restore swallowing and speech after surgery.

- *Enterostomal therapists*, nurse-specialists who help patients with a stoma (artificial opening) to select collection devices and give instructions on how to use them. Therapists may be certified by the International

Association for Enterostomal Therapy. (Many therapists have ostomies themselves.)

- *Prosthetist-orthotists*, who evaluate, design, fabricate, and fit braces and prostheses (artificial body parts).

- *Recreational therapists*, who help people improve their well being through music, dance, and art.

- *Volunteers*, who have been trained to provide educational information and support. Many volunteers also are cancer survivors, willing to pass along what they have learned about coping with impairments or other difficulties of living with this disease.

Family Helpers

Some of the most important participants on the rehabilitation team are not medical specialists but your loved ones—close personal friends, partners, significant others, and the like. Experience has shown that the people who are most successful in their efforts at recovery and rehabilitation are those whose families make the healthiest adjustment to the cancer, encourage and support efforts toward their recovery, and become involved in rehabilitation whenever appropriate. Nevertheless, people with cancer who are accustomed to being independent may find it especially difficult to share responsibility, let others in on decision-making, or sacrifice some of their freedom (see Chapter 28).

Types of Intervention

Rehabilitation may be preventive, restorative, supportive, or palliative. Some people may need only one kind; others, two or three. For example, a woman undergoing a mastectomy for breast cancer may receive these kinds of rehabilitation care:

- *Preventive,* such as discussion and counseling before treatment, to prepare her for possible complications and to give her emotional support regarding her body image and sexual concerns.

- *Restorative,* which may include exercises to achieve pain-free use of the affected arm as soon as possible after surgery, and possibly reconstructive surgery or breast prosthesis to achieve cosmetic restoration.

- *Supportive,* that is, help in accepting the loss of her breast and coping with fears and anxieties.

She may or may not need the fourth type, palliative rehabilitation, which focuses primarily on pain relief and physical and emotional support for the person with advanced cancer.

Preventive Rehabilitation

There are ways to avoid or minimize some of the effects of cancer and its treatment. For example, bed rest may create problems that may be prevented if steps to protect the skin and stimulate circulation are taken early.

Exercises to Do in Bed

The following movements help maintain the full movement of the joints and gently stretch muscles:

Shoulder Rotation

Lie on your back with knees bent, feet flat on mat. Use as many pillows as you need to feel comfortable. As you progress, you will need to use fewer pillows.

a.   Place pillows on left side, next to your head. Slide left arm out to side so that it is as level with shoulder as possible. Bend elbow to 90°. By rotating the shoulder, allow the back of your hand to rest on pillows without pain. Hold five seconds. Relax. Repeat three times.

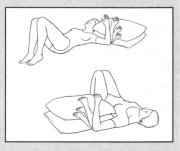

Repeat exercise with right arm.

b.   Position left arm as in exercise (a) above, but place pillows next to ribs on that side. By rotating the shoulder, allow the palm of your hand to rest on pillows without pain. Hold five seconds. Relax. Repeat three times.

Repeat exercise with right arm.

Knee to Chest—Side-Lying

a.   Lie on your right side, with knees slightly bent up toward your chest. Place pillow under your head.

b.   Slide your left knee up to your chest without straining. Lower the knee to the floor.

c.   Gently straighten out the leg so that both the hip and knee are straight. Lower the leg to the floor so that no effort is used to hold it. Return the leg to the starting position.

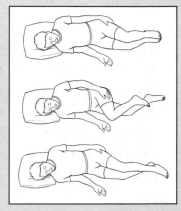

Repeat 3 times.
Turn onto your left side and repeat exercise 3 times.

Shoulder Flexion

Sit in a straight-back chair with your feet flat on floor, or lie on your back with your knees bent and feet flat on the mat.

Cradle your left arm with your right arm. Slowly raise both arms overhead as far as possible. Allow your right arm to do most of the work. Do not go past point of pain. Hold five seconds. Relax. Repeat three times.

Reverse arms and repeat exercise three times.

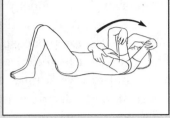

Hip Adductor Stretching—Back-Lying

a. Lie on your back with your knees bent and feet flat on the mat.

b. Hook your right foot behind your left heel. Let your right leg fall gently to the right. Hold for one to five seconds. Return to the starting position and repeat with your left leg.

Repeat three times on each side.

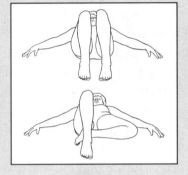

Abdominal Strengthening—Back-Lying

a. Lie on your back with your knees bent and feet flat on mat. Breathe in deeply.

b. Forcefully blow out through pursed lips; pull in your stomach muscles while blowing out. This forced exhalation should take approximately two seconds longer than the inhalation.

Repeat six times.

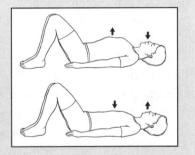

Knee to Chest—Back-Lying

a. Lie on your back with your knees bent and feet flat on mat.

b. Raise your right knee up to your chest as far as possible without straining or using your hands, and then return the foot to the floor with the knee bent.

c. Slide your heel along the mat until the leg is straight. Gently roll the leg from side to side.

Return to starting position. Repeat with other leg.

Repeat six times with each leg.

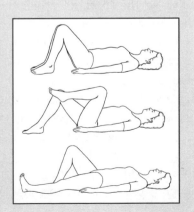

Immobility. Inactivity causes your muscles and other body systems to deteriorate. You may become weak, and your muscles may tighten and lose their elasticity, further impairing mobility and slowing recovery (see Chapter 19).

Maintaining joint mobility through exercises helps prevent joint stiffness and contractures. A physical therapist can provide specific exercises to do in and out of bed (appropriately placed pillows relieve pressure on the hips and tailbone). Using a footboard and back-of-the-leg splints and doing certain exercises in bed several times a day is a preventive strategy. If necessary, a therapist may use electric muscle stimulation, a painless method in which electrodes are placed on the skin over the muscles to stimulate them to contract.

Soft mattresses and even trying to make yourself more comfortable by pillows under your knees or behind your neck may aggravate some of the side effects of prolonged bed rest or create other problems, including backaches. Keeping your knees bent for long periods in bed immobilizes leg muscles in a shortened position, further limiting your mobility.

When your normal activity is limited—particularly if you must stay in bed for long periods of time—a physical therapist can teach you and/or the person caring for you several techniques to maintain joint flexibility.

Pretreatment Counseling. Today cancer specialists can anticipate with some precision what lies ahead. For example, if you must have your larynx removed, you should be advised of the several kinds of artificial or aided speech available and encouraged to talk to a specialist about which one might be most appropriate or easiest for you to use.

If you are having an arm or leg amputated, you'll need to know about phantom limb sensation. Everyone who has a limb amputated can expect to experience this sensation in the space where his or her limb once was. Counseling can help prepare you for this sensation. Phantom limb pain occurs in about one-third of patients. Pretreatment counseling also can help those with head and neck cancer. For example, the teeth are particularly susceptible to damage from radiation therapy. The radiation alters the flow of saliva so that bacteria proliferate and contribute to tooth decay. A dental checkup before radiotherapy, with prophylactic treatment if time permits, can prevent cavities. Any essential tooth extractions should be done and allowed to heal before radiation therapy. A program of preventive oral hygiene can maintain the health of the mouth and teeth and lessen the danger of bone damage. Fluoride treatments may help prevent decay and the sensitivity to hot, cold, and sweet foods that sometimes occurs.

Counseling before surgery is also necessary for those who are having part of a lung removed, since their breathing may be seriously compromised. Of course, quitting smoking is a primary goal. An uncomplicated recovery also depends on the ability to cough and expectorate fluid from the lungs. There

Arm Rehabilitation After Mastectomy

Lymphedema (swelling) of the arm on the side of the surgery is a potential complication after mastectomy that is not only inconvenient, but can become painful and severely disabling. It can also make the arm more susceptible to infections, which can become quite serious. Preventive steps are based on avoiding excessive use of the arm and protecting the skin and circulation. To do this:

- wear canvas gloves when gardening and rubber gloves when washing dishes

- use a thimble for sewing

- keep sleeves loose

- wash even the smallest break in the skin of the affected arm with soap and water and cover it with a bandage

- use an electric razor if you shave your underarms

- keep your arm elevated when sitting down

- apply a moisturizing body cream several times a day, since dryness encourages skin breaks

- call your doctor if your arm appears red or feels hot or swollen

- try to do small tasks requiring manual dexterity, such as typing, sewing, and knitting, as they may hasten physical rehabilitation

Don't do the following with the affected hand or arm:

- hold a cigarette

- wear restrictive clothing, a wristwatch, or other jewelry

- carry your purse or anything heavy

- cut or pick at cuticles or hangnails

- work around thorny plants or garden without gloves

- reach into a hot oven

- permit injections or vaccinations or blood to be drawn or blood pressure taken

- get sunburned

- perform any task involving balance or depth perception, such as attempting to drive, before you have recovered completely

are methods and exercises to help in learning to cough correctly, expand the remaining lung, and ensure complete filling of the lung with air. It's easier for people to learn breathing exercises before surgery, when they are not hindered by pain from the surgical incision. These techniques help keep the airway clear. Preoperative lessons in effective coughing facilitate drainage, allow sputum to be expelled from the lungs, and keep breathing passages open. Pain at the incision site can be eased with hand splinting, a way of holding the chest, and changing position to aid the draining of bronchial secretions.

Restorative Rehabilitation

Restorative rehabilitation is designed to compensate for changes in appearance and function that result from cancer or its treatment. Examples include reconstructive breast surgery, artificial limbs and joints, electronic aids to speech, and exercises to improve muscle strength and joint mobility. Plastic surgery or prostheses may improve or eliminate disfigurement.

Muscle Problems. Cancer or its treatment can directly affect your muscles. For example, in head and neck cancer, surgery sometimes unavoidably affects the nerve that controls the shoulder muscles, which in turn alter alignment and movement. If the nerve is severed, the shoulder will droop, become painful and weak, and be difficult or impossible to raise. Rehabilitation with both passive and active exercise can greatly improve some aspects of shoulder motion even if it cannot restore full function.

Prosthetic Limbs. Amputation of a limb is a major loss that produces a substantial change in mobility, affecting your ability to care for yourself and your independence. It also significantly changes appearance, which may hinder recovery, because of its impact on body image and self-esteem (see Chapter 20). Fortunately, prosthetic design, limb care, and rehabilitation techniques have become quite advanced, and it now is possible to have a well-fitted, smoothly functioning artificial limb.

The rehabilitation team should confer with your medical and surgical team before the operation. The extent of the amputation will determine how much disability you will experience and how complex and lengthy your rehabilitation will be. Almost everyone who loses a limb is fitted for an artificial one as soon as possible after surgery, allowing adequate time for stump healing and shrinkage. In some cases, the prosthesis must be molded before surgery. And if you are about to lose a leg, you may get instructions in walking or using crutches before your operation, when your balance is normal and pain doesn't interfere. This preoperative gait training will result in your being able to get around quite soon after the operation.

Occupational therapy and training in self-care and dexterity begin soon after an arm amputation. Proper conditioning—including exercises to maintain mobility of the joints near the amputation stump—is essential to using an upper-extremity prosthesis.

Our national enthusiasm for sports has led to some important benefits for amputees. Many have become athletes, and thousands now participate in sports activities. Their determination has helped stimulate research and experimentation to produce some important new devices and aids to activity, for example, energy-storing foot replacements that assist in "pushing off" and devices with specialized grasps for rods, reels, guns, skis, rackets, and gymnastic equipment. The many specialized athletic groups for amputees also are an important source of psychological support and motivation.

Reconstruction. Breasts can be replaced by implants that move and feel like the body's own tissue. The implants may be synthetic—a silicone bag filled with a liquid material such as saline—or your own skin and fat may be used to create a new breast. The breast can be reconstructed at the time of the mastectomy or in a later operation. Because these decisions are complicated and many techniques are available, it's important to consult with at least one specialist—such as a plastic surgeon—before your cancer surgery.

For head and neck cancers, remarkable things can be done with surgery, implantable devices, and prostheses. Healthy tissue from the chest or other parts of the body can be used to repair even large facial defects. Bone "harvested" from the skull or hip can be sculpted to replenish surgically removed bone. Permanently implanted devices can be used to rebuild the nose, cheek-bones, and forehead, and artificial material may be combined with grafted bone to make a new jaw.

If you need reconstructive surgery for any reason, a variety of specialists may confer with your surgeon before the operation to make sure the surgery will be done so as to enable the best possible restoration later. A prosthodontist may make impressions and casts so that any devices or repairs made later will fit, look natural, and feel comfortable. It's important to try to be patient during the restoration, though, since some of the procedures must be done in small steps over a period of time.

Supportive Rehabilitation

Regardless of the extent of your disability—even if it is quite severe—you will benefit from rehabilitation by gaining control of the ordinary activities of life, learning to deal with whatever you confront, and regaining some degree of independence. For example, people with cancer of the central nervous system that leaves them paralyzed and essentially dependent on others can learn to propel an electric wheelchair with a mouth wand, chin control, or breathing apparatus. There now are devices that let them talk on the telephone and control a television set, light switches, call buttons, and other equipment.

Indeed, techniques that promote self-care and mobility are almost unlimited. People who have lost the use of one hand or arm, for example, can learn one-handed techniques and use such aids as shoes with one-handed closures, Velcro fasteners instead of buttons, silverware for one-handed eating, bathtub or shower benches, and long-handled sponges and grabbers. Patients with paralysis, leg amputations, or other mobility difficulties can learn how to use various kinds of wheelchairs or to walk with a four-legged cane, even on stairs, ramps, and uneven ground. An important part of this learning is knowing safety limits, how to get out of trouble (for example, getting up after a fall), and when to ask for assistance.

Learning to Talk. One of the most dramatic forms of supportive rehabilitation is alternative forms of speech for those unable to talk because of brain tumors, tumors that compress the spinal cord, or removal of the larynx. If you have cancer of the larynx, for instance, you may be offered speech rehabilitation by esophageal voice, a voice prosthesis inserted through an opening in the throat, or an electrolarynx, a battery-powered tone generator.

Living with an Ostomy. For many people the worst part of dealing with an ostomy is learning that they are going to need one. The best thing you can do for yourself at the very start is to talk to experts. No question should be left unasked or unanswered. A visit from a member of the United Ostomy Association (UOA; see *Resources* for contact information) can be informative and reassuring. For example, you will learn that at least half the people who have colostomies develop a regular pattern of evacuation so that they don't even need a collection device. You can also train yourself to evacuate on schedule by irrigating the intestinal tract through the stoma.

Your stoma therapist and other health care professionals should give you all the information you need about how to take care of yourself at home, how to get help in your community, and how to go back to your job (unless you have serious medical complications or your work requires heavy, prolonged lifting). You can expect few restrictions on travel, recreational activities, or sports—even swimming—as long as the appliance seal is waterproof.

When treatment for intestinal or genitourinary cancer requires an ostomy, you have to confront not only the loss of your previous elimination function but drastically altered feelings about your body and your identity (see Chapter 20). Supportive rehabilitation can address all these issues.

One-on-One Assistance. Some people find it helpful to meet another person who has had the same kind of cancer and has been trained to counsel others on the emotional and practical aspects of their recovery. Several organizations make such services available, such as the ACS through its *Reach to Recovery* program. *Reach to Recovery* volunteers have had breast cancer and are specially trained to share their knowledge and experiences and support. The UOA, which can provide a volunteer hospital visitor who is about your age and sex and has your kind of ostomy, holds meetings for an exchange of information, moral support, and a discussion of mutual problems. It also provides information and names of people to call for assistance (see *Resources* for contact information).

Laryngectomy clubs that function under the auspices of the International Association of Laryngectomies also promote the exchange of information.

Man to Man, an ACS prostate cancer education and support group, has a visitation component in some areas. Trained volunteers will meet with or arrange a telephone visit in order to provide support and information to men and their partners about prostate cancer.

Vocational Rehabilitation

Medical social workers, physical occupational therapists, and vocational counselors can help ease your transition back into the workforce. They can devise ways to adapt your job to the needs of your physical disability or teach you techniques to make you more efficient and productive. Work issues need to be addressed as early as possible in your rehabilitation. Preparing for your return to work also gives you a tangible goal and motivation for your overall rehabilitation effort.

It is very important to try to avoid feeling defeated by job setbacks or rejections. Negative images of yourself as a "has-been" at work, fear of colleagues and employers, or thoughts about cancer's limiting the horizons of your working life aren't constructive. At least three-fourths of all cancer patients go back to work. Talking with other cancer survivors about their work experiences and how they surmounted particular difficulties is helpful (see *Employment Issues*, pages 373–375.)

Palliative Rehabilitation

Many people with advanced cancer or metastatic disease can live and function well for some time even if they cannot be cured. Palliative rehabilitation is designed to provide comfort, emotional support, assistance in day-to-day functioning, and symptom relief. The main purpose is not to cure, but to improve the quality of life of a person with cancer.

Palliative rehabilitation can transform lives in ways ranging from the very simple and ordinary to the dramatic. On the simplest level, you can learn how to move from bed to chair or wheelchair without help, which makes the difference between being confined to bed and being somewhat more independent. Modifying the home or work environment and learning to use tools adapted to specific disabilities can allow you to work and/or participate in leisure activities. All these efforts can cut down on the need for caretakers or the demands on family members.

More far-reaching steps include total joint replacements for people who are susceptible to fractures. The outcome is often additional months of being able to walk or move comfortably. For some people, a destroyed cervical vertebra can be replaced with an artificial one, providing comfort and preventing helplessness.

Pain relief is an important part of palliative rehabilitation, requiring careful choices by the members of your treatment team (see Chapter 23). They need to take into account the source of your pain, its quality, and its duration; what causes it and what makes it worse; and how it affects your life. It may be mild, moderate, or severe, and it may be relieved by nothing more than heat and aspirin or it may require medication. Like all other aspects of rehabilitation, this requires a customized approach.

Hospice care, which may be considered a part of palliative rehabilitation, has become a good option for those whose cancer is so far advanced that little more can be expected from therapy. Not everyone with advanced cancer needs hospice care, though, and some people don't want it. However, it should be available to all who do. An important advantage and a reason that so many seriously ill people prefer hospice care is that it can allow them to remain at home with their families, rather than in the hospital, to the last (see Chapter 31).

Spiritual solace, whether from a religious adviser or other source, is another vital aspect of palliative rehabilitation for many people. Organized religion became directly involved in cancer care almost twenty years ago when the ACS started offering educational programs for clergy and produced its first training film on pastoral care.

If you are a member of a nonreligious group with a significant spiritual component, such as Alcoholics Anonymous and/or other twelve-step programs, it's helpful to stay involved and active, as these groups have proven to be a source of strength during major life crises.

Home Care

Lengthy hospital stays are discouraged these days. Much of a person's care during treatment, recovery, and rehabilitation takes place at home. Typically family, friends, neighbors, and even some volunteer groups can provide assistance. But when professional health care is needed because a person requires it, there are home care organizations that can help, as well as independent providers.

What You Need

Your doctor and social worker can help you and your family determine what type of services you need and the types of providers and agencies that provide skilled home care and supplies. The following are a list of possibilities, but it does not encompass all of the 20,000 home health care agencies available in the United States.

- *Homemaker and home care aide agencies.* People recommended by these agencies will help assist you with basic functions and household maintenance. For instance, they can prepare meals and assist you in bathing and dressing. They may do housekeeping and/or serve as companions. In some states, these agencies are licensed.

- *Pharmaceutical and infusion therapy companies.* People receiving intravenous infusions or nutritional support receive instruction from nurses. These companies provide the supplies and professional services needed to maintain the therapy.

- *Medical equipment and supply dealers.* These companies deliver—and in some cases install—equipment and instruct people how to use it. In general, they do not provide direct care. They can supply equipment ranging from respirators and wheelchairs to wound care supplies.

- *Staffing registries and private-duty agencies.* Nurses, homemakers, home care aids, and company contact information are all available through these employment agencies.

- *Independent providers.* Independent providers are independent nurses, homemakers, home care aides, and companions who are privately employed.

- *Hospice care.* This team of health care professionals and volunteers are trained to care for those who are not expected to recover and support their families. They are available twenty-four hours a day to help keep a person cared for at home comfortable and free of pain. Many hospice programs are licensed by the state and Medicare certified (see Chapter 31).

Interviewing a Home Care Agency

Although most states require licensing of home care agencies, not all do. Furthermore, not all agencies ask to be certified by an accrediting organization such as the Joint Commission on Accreditation of Healthcare Organizations (JCAHO). This is a not-for-profit group that evaluates organizations and programs to assess the quality of their services. Contact your State Office on Aging or your state health insurance counseling program for more information. If you are thinking of working with a home health agency, ask your state insurance office for a recent inspection or "survey" report.

QUESTIONS

TO ASK

Here are some important questions to ask before accepting help from an agency, company, or program:

- Is this program Medicare certified? Programs that are certified have met the federal minimum requirements for patient care and management.

- Is the program licensed by the state (if your state requires licensing)?

- Are written statements provided that outline services, eligibility criteria, costs, payment procedure, employee job descriptions, malpractice, and liability insurance?

- How long has the agency been in business?

- Can you obtain references from health care professionals (your doctor, for instance)? It's wise to check with the Better Business Bureau, the local Consumer Bureau, or the State Attorney General's office to see if there have been complaints filed against the agency or program.

- Is the agency flexible in applying its policies to you?

- Will the agency assess your situation to determine if Medicare will cover the cost?

- Will the agency create an individualized care plan in writing for you? Will the plan be updated as your needs change?

- Will a nurse or social worker come to your home to evaluate the type of services needed?

- Will the nurse or social worker consult with those professionals involved in your care, such as your doctor, social worker, nurses? Will they consult with your family?

- Does the agency or program train, supervise, and monitor its caregivers?

- Is there a contact person at the agency that you can call with questions and complaints?

- How are problems resolved?

- Is it necessary for you to have a primary caregiver among your family or friends? What responsibilities must they assume?

- Is confidentiality about your case and private life assured?

- How is payment and billing handled? Are all financial arrangements made in writing?

- If equipment is being used, will someone be provided by the dealer or company to teach you how to use it and to maintain the equipment in your home?

- Is there a twenty-four hour number to call with questions and complaints?

- Do the staff people have a caring, competent attitude? Do they speak in language you can easily understand and avoid complicated medical terminology?

- How quickly can the agency initiate the service you need?

- If you have to be hospitalized, what are the agency's policies regarding your care?

- Does the agency explain your rights and responsibilities? Federal law requires that you be informed of your rights as a patient.

Employment Issues

In our society, work provides not only financial support but also a sense of identity and self-worth. People with cancer have the same rights as everyone else to employment befitting their skills, training, and experience. You should not have to accept jobs you never would have considered before your illness; and hiring, promotion, and treatment in the workplace should depend entirely on ability and qualifications. In reality, however, cancer survivors face many employment and workplace discrimination issues for which outside assistance is necessary and available. You may want to begin by contacting your local chapter of the ACS (see *Resources* for contact information).

People with cancer often face a less than ideal situation when they return to work or seek employment. They may feel "locked into" jobs they would like to leave but can't because they're afraid they will never be hired if they have to reveal their cancer on a new job application. Others continue to work at jobs that aren't satisfying or are physically too demanding, or they continue to work beyond a previously planned early retirement date because of financial need.

In addition, despite generally improved attitudes toward an understanding of cancer, some prejudices and wariness in the workplace remain, perhaps produced or exaggerated by competitiveness and economic pressures and fears.

Employers and coworkers may react out of a vague fear or uneasiness about cancer in the abstract, as some kind of lurking, unspecified danger. Many people are bothered by it as an unpleasant reminder of their own mortality. And some people just don't know what to say or how to treat you (see Chapters 26 and 28).

Employers' attitudes are hard to assess, but some may be afraid of lower production or financial losses because of your diminished capability or the occasional need to take time off from work for treatment. Despite these concerns, a Metropolitan Life survey shows that the absentee rate for people with cancer doesn't differ from that of other workers.

Current Legal Protection

Some people with job problems related to cancer are protected by federal legislation such as the Americans with Disabilities Act (ADA). According to the ADA, it is unlawful to discriminate in employment against a person with a disability who is qualified for the job. It is also unlawful to discriminate against someone whose family member has a disability, and it prohibits employers from taking any action against a person who is advocating for their rights under the ADA. An employer is also required to make reasonable accommodations for an applicant or employee with a disability, from making the workplace accessible to job restructuring to modifying work schedules. Employers are prohibited from asking job applicants about their disability, including if they have or ever have had cancer.

The U.S. Equal Employment Opportunity Commission (EEOC), along with state and local agencies, enforces the employment part of the ADA. Since 1994, the ADA includes employers with fifteen or more employees. Although the ADA does not specify which medical conditions are considered disabilities, between 1992, when the law was implemented, and 1998, 2.4 percent of the charges resolved under it have related to people with cancer. Information about the ADA is available through a toll-free hotline at 800-514-0301.

Nearly all states have laws pertaining to employing people with various illnesses, including some that are specifically aimed at cancer. Some court decisions have been helpful. For example, a ruling in California requires employers to provide reasonable accommodation for medical appointments, including long-term chemotherapy or radiation therapy. Federal law protects you from having your health insurance policy automatically canceled if you lose or leave your job. The Consolidated Omnibus Reconciliation Act (COBRA) allows employees to buy health insurance back from their employers (who have more than twenty employees) even though they no longer work there or their hours are reduced.

Although the vocational counselor on your rehabilitation team can help with some of your job-related legal questions, you may have to take some initiative in finding out what laws or interpretations of the law may affect you and how you can deal with any grievances.

Vocational Counseling

You may not realize how much your feelings of security and self-worth depend on your being active, productive, and capable of taking care of yourself and others. A loss of self-esteem can be magnified by physical disability or the demands of recovery that make you dependent on family and friends for financial support.

It's vital to find ways of returning to productive work in some capacity. If you cannot return to your job, you may have to learn a new skill, go back to school, or establish a work-at-home career. Vocational counselors and others on the rehabilitation team can help match your skills with available jobs or assist you with job training if necessary.

The Pain Challenge

Pain is one of the most feared aspects of cancer, but about 90 percent of people with cancer pain can get relief. Today, there are many different kinds of methods available that can help relieve cancer pain. Most people with cancer can continue to work, rest, play, and enjoy the company of family and friends, hobbies, and other pleasurable activities relatively pain-free.

For far too long, the importance of managing cancer pain was overlooked. Pain was seen as something to be endured—an inevitable consequence of the disease process. Now research provides growing evidence that pain can be controlled in the great majority of cases, although it is often undertreated.

This chapter explores the causes and effects of cancer pain. It explores how you can communicate with others about your discomfort and how you and your health care team can work together to ease the burden of pain and achieve the highest possible quality of life. It also describes the basic approaches to pain relief: the pharmacologic (medicines), surgical, anesthetic, neurologic, and mind-body methods typically incorporated in a treatment plan.

As you consider the possibilities for pain relief and discuss them with your caregivers, remember that you have a right to accept or reject any treatment that is proposed. Also realize that if you experience pain caused by cancer or its therapies, you have the right to expect relief. If your pain relief therapy is inadequate, you need to say so.

What Is Pain?

Pain is the body's way of telling the brain that something is wrong. Thousands of nerve endings throughout the body send signals along nerves to the brain, which then processes the sensory information as pain. On one level, pain may simply be considered any sensation that hurts.

Pain may be acute or chronic. Acute pain is severe and lasts a relatively short time. It is usually a sign that body tissue is being injured in some way, and the pain generally disappears when the injury heals. Chronic pain may range from mild to severe and is present in some degree for long periods of time.

Cancer causes pain when the disease invades bones, muscles, or blood vessels. Pain also occurs if the cancer presses on nerves, blocks hollow organs such as the bowel, pinches blood vessels, or produces inflammation. The treatments aimed at the cancer may sometimes cause pain as well.

Pain has many dimensions. The longer the physical pain persists, the greater the suffering it causes in virtually all aspects of life. Unrelieved pain makes it hard to carry out many of the basic activities of life, such as dressing, eating, and walking. It can cause you to feel anxious, angry, or depressed. It strips away personal dignity and can result in hopelessness. In a vicious cycle, pain may make it impossible for some people to comply with the treatment for their cancer—the very treatment that holds some promise for relieving their pain.

Fear of Pain

When you first learned you had cancer, you may have assumed that you would have pain. Although pain is indeed a common complication of certain kinds of cancer, it is not inevitable. In fact, most early cancers do not cause pain.

Fear often gives rise to myths, and fear of cancer pain is no exception. Even if pain does develop in the early stages of cancer, it is by no means certain that it will get worse. Often the treatment that removes or shrinks tumors also relieves pain. Nor is pain a sign that the cancer is incurable.

A New Awareness of Pain

According to a 1992 survey of 1,200 cancer doctors, only 50 percent believed that pain control in their hospitals was adequate, and 85 percent believed that patients were undermedicated for pain. Many steps were immediately taken to remedy this situation. The National Cancer Institute began giving grants to support projects whose goal is to raise awareness of the need for better pain management. Programs now exist in most states to educate health care professionals (and also people with cancer) about undertreated pain. These programs alert people to the problem, describe options for pain control, and work to make cancer pain relief a high priority.

The Joint Commission on Accreditation of Healthcare Organizations (JCAHO), an independent nonprofit organization which evaluates and accredits more than 19,500 health care organizations in the United States, has developed new pain management standards for hospitals. The standards require health care facilities to observe patients' rights in appropriate assessment and management of pain, and the JCAHO suggests specific methods of implementing a commitment to pain management.

Many hospitals are revising patient charts to track the severity of pain and the results of pain control strategies. Pain is now considered a vital sign, and monitoring it is considered as significant as checking body temperature and heartbeat.

Medical schools are making pain treatment part of the training program for oncologists. Such training is essential in changing attitudes and bringing new pain control strategies into the mainstream. Schools of nursing have incorporated pain in their curricula to teach all nurses about the importance of pain relief.

Today, depending on the circumstances, the professionals involved in pain assessment and treatment may include oncologists, nurses, anesthesiologists, home health care providers, psychiatrists, psychologists, social workers, and therapists versed in complementary techniques such as hypnosis and biofeedback. (See *The Pain Control Team* on page 381.)

Legislation for Pain Control

A range of legislative efforts are currently underway in Congress and various state houses that may significantly affect the ways in which the public, providers, and health systems understand the issue of cancer pain control and obtain and use appropriate and adequate cancer pain treatment. Among the legislative issues currently being addressed are coverage, adequate reimbursement for pain control, access to pain specialists, and support for health professional education about and adoption of nationwide guidelines by the Agency for Healthcare Research and Quality (AHRQ).

Support for legislation for pain control medication reimbursement by private payers and Medicare/Medicaid will help to ensure access to pain treatment for all Americans. Advocacy for additional research funding for agencies that conduct cancer pain research will ensure that knowledge and understanding of pain control issues will continue to improve.

At the state level, legislation has been passed that has affected the quality of pain management. In 1994, residents of the state of Oregon voted narrowly to approve the Death with Dignity Act. The law currently allows doctors to actively and intentionally assist terminally ill patients with ending their lives, which is very controversial. The American Cancer Society (ACS) has a long-standing policy against doctor-assisted suicide because it violates one of the most basic doctrine of medical practice: do no harm. Therefore, the ACS opposes the Oregon Death with Dignity Act. In fact, a number of the ACS offices have actively and consistently opposed state-based measures that would permit assisted suicide in their respective states.

Research shows that untreated or undertreated pain is often a major factor in a patient's decision to take a life-ending action. Pain need not be a reason to consider ending life because it can be successfully relieved in almost all cases of people with cancer or other serious illnesses. The assurance of adequate pain and symptom management will not only improve the quality of life for people with cancer, but will prevent requests for doctor-assisted suicide. Forty-six percent of patients requesting doctor-assisted suicide in Oregon since November 1997 decided not to end their lives once they had been provided adequate pain relief. This demonstrates the need for actively addressing pain and symptom management.

At the federal level, several members of Congress have introduced legislation addressing a variety of issues related to pain management. In 1999, the Pain Relief Promotion Act (PRPA) was introduced, but no action has been taken on the bill thus far. If passed into law, it would affect not only the lives of people in pain but the way health care professionals treat pain. The goal of the PRPA is to promote pain management without permitting doctors to participate in assisted suicide or euthanasia. It was written to override the Death with Dignity Act; however, the legislation could have unintended, but serious negative consequences for the management of pain and palliative care.

The PRPA would ban the use of federally controlled substances (such as opioids) for doctor-assisted suicide and place the responsibility of determining what is considered legitimate medical practice using controlled substances with the Drug Enforcement Agency (DEA). The bill also includes provisions relating to pain management and health professional education and training in an attempt to clarify the important need for pain and symptom management.

The Experience of Pain

Your perceptions affect the way in which you experience pain. Cultures and individuals have different pain thresholds and different ways of expressing the pain they feel.

It's Personal

Several factors influence each individual's experience with pain, affecting the ways in which patients feel pain and react to the pain experience. For example, some people with cancer may feel they should downplay the extent of their pain. It may be partly the result of cultural conditioning. In some cultures it is common to practice a stiff upper lip philosophy of enduring hardship. But the motto, "No pain, no gain" is not applicable to cancer pain. There is nothing to be gained from suffering through the pain associated with cancer.

Life experience also plays a part in the experience of pain. Your ability to cope with challenge, your level of emotional maturity, your attitudes toward doctors and medications, and the impact of the illness on your life goals all influence your perception of pain. And clearly, social support—love and understanding from family and friends—makes a big difference.

Psychological factors such as fears and worries about cancer and about death can also influence your perception of pain. If you believe that you have good control over your situation and that you're aware of your limits and what steps you can take to feel better, you may experience less pain than a person who doesn't have such confidence. But if you worry a lot, you may be tense, anxious, and unable to sleep. Insomnia and fatigue can worsen the pain.

Being aware of the meaning you attach to pain can translate directly into better pain management. In some cases, counseling can help uncover troublesome beliefs about pain. For example, someone who sees pain as a punishment or a lesson from God may benefit from talking with a member of the clergy or other spiritual counselor. Be open and honest about any such feelings; others may help you cope with your concerns.

Why It Hurts

The pain associated with cancer may result from the tumor itself, the cancer treatments, complications of the disease, or a combination of all three. Over the course of the illness, the quality of the pain—as well as what is causing it—may change. Your pain relief choices will be determined by the cause of discomfort and whether or not the cause is temporary.

Most complaints are a direct reflection of the tumor's growth and spread. When cancer cells invade bones or vital organs or press on nerves or blood vessels, they may cause pain. Pain may also result from the effects of the various hormones and other chemicals the body produces in response to cancer.

Cancer treatments may cause a variety of uncomfortable sensations. Surgery, of course, is a major trauma to the body, and strong medications are temporarily needed to reduce pain. As the body begins to heal, the discomfort usually diminishes, and medications are given less often and in lower doses. However, some types of pain related to surgery persist long after the wounds have healed and may require long-term pain relief.

Side effects can also cause discomfort or pain. For example, certain chemotherapy drugs may cause a burning sensation in the hands or feet and skin irritation and breakdown. Depending on the treatment site, radiation therapy may produce uncomfortable sensory changes that last for several months.

Cancer can suppress the immune system, increasing the chances of infection. Local irritation and soreness may be symptoms of infection in the affected area.

Simply being confined to bed may lead to complications from bedsores to constipation, all of which are uncomfortable. The emotional stress of coping with such confinement can lead to muscle tension, which causes pain. Precautions can be taken to prevent these complications, but if these complications do occur, each symptom should be promptly addressed.

A small percentage of people sometimes have another illness or disorder in addition to cancer that produces pain, such as migraine headaches, osteoporosis, or degenerative disk disease. Although these conditions may complicate the cancer treatment, the health care team must address any patient discomfort.

INFORM

YOURSELF

The Pain Control Team

Decisions about pain relief are always subject to re-evaluation. If one approach does not bring comfort, other options almost always exist. However, to ensure an active role in decision-making, it's important that you or a close family member learn as much about pain relief strategies as possible. Education is also critical to overcoming the myths and misunderstandings surrounding cancer pain and its management.

Whatever the plan, continuity of care is crucial to its success. Oncologists, oncology nurses, and primary care professionals must work with social workers, therapists, and any other caregivers on the team to provide consistent and aggressive pain relief in the hospital and at home. If care is fragmented, confusion will result. For example, it can be confusing if the primary care doctor is unaware of the approaches recommended by the hospital staff or if a home care worker is unaware of treatments or dosages that are known to work best.

Of course, the most important person on the pain control team is you. The more involved you are in your own care, the more you will understand your perceptions, which will make you better able to communicate your feelings and bring your pain under control.

Communicating Your Pain

Pain is subjective—it can't be measured by objective tests—so patients' accounts of their pain are crucial to relieving it.

Not every person with cancer is comfortable discussing pain. Some people put up a brave front to protect loved ones from knowing how much they are suffering. Others may not want to distract their health care team from the task at hand—namely, addressing the cancer itself—by asking for pain relief. And some people may fear that pain treatment will cause further suffering or complications, such as addiction to opioids (drugs derived from opium that have sedative effects; also called narcotics).

The best thing to do is to speak up. Tell others what you're experiencing so they can help you. The person who feels pain is the best source of information about it: how bad it is, where it is located, what relieves it, and what doesn't. All too often, though, there is a wide gap between the way a person experiences pain and the way others perceive that pain. One study found that doctors and nurses consistently rated patients' pain as less intense than did the patients themselves. In fact, nurses and the people in their care agreed on the level of severity only about 7 percent of the time. No one knows where and how you hurt better than you do. If you can communicate clearly, there's a better chance that your care providers can determine what is causing the problem. That, in turn, improves the odds that you'll obtain the relief you need.

Pain can be described in a number of ways. The type of cancer involved, the part of the body affected, the combination of treatments you receive, and even your work life and support network have some bearing on the extent and impact of pain and its management. People may describe similar levels of pain in different ways. For example, one person may refer to a level of pain as "agonizing" and "severe" while another may say the same level of pain is "stinging" and "occasional." Caregivers should note any changes in an individual's descriptions of pain over time and be alert to any worsening pain.

How Long It Lasts

One of the chief characteristics of pain is how long it lasts. Acute pain appears suddenly and recedes fairly quickly. Someone in acute pain may experience not only painful sensations, but also rapid heartbeat and an increase in blood pressure. He or she may wince and rub the affected area. Such pain may come from the cancer itself, usually from the swelling of a tumor. When the tumor is removed or made to shrink, most people experience dramatic pain relief. Analgesic medications, taken as needed, can provide relief.

Acute pain can also be a response to cancer therapy. Many people find it easier to bear acute pain when they learn that it comes and goes in a predictable way and that the benefits of treatment greatly outweigh any drawbacks.

Chronic pain lasts more or less continuously for several months. Like acute pain, it can be caused by the disease itself or may be a consequence of the treatment. The pain may grow more severe as time passes, or it may persist at a constant level. Of course, the longer it lasts, the greater its impact on your quality of life.

Over time, chronic pain can give rise to emotional difficulties. Chronic pain can produce mood changes or depression, irritability, disturbed sleep, reduced appetite, and difficulty concentrating. Such pain can lead to changes in personality, lifestyle, and ability to function. Robbed of the ability to enjoy even simple daily activities, a person may lose hope of recovering. But the resulting fear of death only increases the overall level of pain and suffering.

Fortunately, cancer pain is readily treated. Morphine and other opioids are very effective, even over long periods of time. The risk of becoming addicted to opioids for the treatment of cancer pain is quite low; a fear of addition should not cause people to avoid taking opioids (see pages 390–393, *Opioid Analgesics*).

Where It Is

Pain can originate from a particular place, such as when a tumor affects nerves in a specific area. This is known as focal pain. Pain sensations can also spread out along the length of a nerve, causing what is known as radiating (or radicular) pain. But some parts of the body, including some of the internal organs and tissues, do not have pain receptors. When something goes wrong in these areas, the brain reacts by responding as though the pain is occurring somewhere else along the same nerve network. For example, gallbladder disease often produces pain in the right shoulder area. This is known as referred pain. Knowing that pain sensations may not actually arise at the site of the problem helps in determining the type of treatment needed. For example, anesthesia or surgical approaches may be more appropriate for focal pain, whereas medications may be more effective for referred pain.

What Type It Is

Another way to characterize pain is by the changes it produces in the body. Most cancer-related pain is physical, or organic, in nature. (So-called psycho-somatic pain, originating in the mind, is rare in people with cancer, although psychological distress certainly contributes to the severity of pain.)

There are three types of organic pain. *Somatic pain* affects the pain receptors and typically causes you to feel a constant dull or aching sensation in a specific area. Examples are metastatic bone pain, pain felt along a surgical incision, and musculoskeletal pain.

Sometimes pain arises from the stretching and enlarging of tissues or organ structures in the abdominal cavity. This is known as *visceral pain*. Such pain is usually less focused and tends to be referred to distant locations. People often describe visceral pain as a deep squeezing or pressured feeling. If it comes on suddenly, it may lead to nausea, vomiting, and sweating.

A third type of organic pain, *neuropathic pain*, arises from damage to nerves from either the cancer or its treatment. People often describe neuro-pathic pain as severe burning, stabbing, viselike, or shooting pain.

A Picture of Pain

A complete assessment of pain is much like a diagnostic procedure. It involves a discussion during which you describe your situation and undergo an examination to evaluate your physical condition.

Explain How You Feel

The nurse or doctor asks questions about the history of your pain as well as other important details about your illness. Typical questions include:

- How bad is your pain?

- Where do you feel it?

- When did it begin?

- What does it feel like?

- Is it constant? Does it vary? Is it worse at some times of day than others?

- How long does it last?

- How does it affect your ability to carry out your activities?

- What have you done to relieve the pain?

- What has (and hasn't) worked in the past to relieve pain?

There are a number of ways to assess the intensity of pain. One of the easiest is to describe the level of the pain on a scale of 0 to 10. As a measure of severity, for instance, 0 might represent no pain at all and 10 might indicate the worst pain you can imagine. Such numbers are highly subjective—one person's 7 might be another person's 4. What is important, though, is the consistency of your responses over time.

The pattern of pain is also relevant. It helps to know, for example, if the pain is constant or if it comes and goes; if it changes throughout the day or is usually the same in intensity and location; if certain activities (such as moving your arms, breathing, swallowing, standing up, or lying down) trigger painful feelings. Especially valuable is a verbal description of the pain. Such descriptions provide clues to what is happening inside the body (see box on page 385).

To arrive at a true measure of your pain, your doctor or nurse should also ask about its psychological and social impact. They will want to know about the degree of suffering, about its effect on your mood, the extent of physical disability it causes, how you function with your family or on the job, and what concerns you may have such as finances, work, and so on. Sometimes these questions are best answered by a spouse or other close relative or friend. It helps enormously if someone who knows you well and can talk about the impact of your pain can be present for the assessment. If you are incapacitated or otherwise unable to speak, the presence of such an ally is essential.

The Physical Exam

A doctor or nurse may look for signs of inflammation or tenderness and check vital signs, since heart rate (pulse) and blood pressure may increase during pain. These signs are not useful, however, when attempting to measure the amount of pain, nor will pain show up on an x-ray or under a microscope.

INFORM

YOURSELF

Words for Describing Pain

Flickering	Jumping	Pricking	Sharp
Quivering	Flashing	Boring	Cutting
Pulsing	Shooting	Drilling	Lacerating
Throbbing		Stabbing	
Beating			
Pounding			
Pinching	Tugging	Hot	Tingling
Pressing	Pulling	Burning	Itchy
Gnawing	Wrenching	Scalding	Smarting
Cramping		Searing	Stinging
Crushing			
Dull	Tender	Tiring	Sickening
Sore	Rasping	Exhausting	Suffocating
Hurting	Splitting		
Aching			
Heavy			
Fearful	Punishing	Wretched	Annoying
Frightful	Grueling	Blinding	Troublesome
Terrifying	Cruel		Miserable
	Vicious		Intense
	Killing		Unbearable
Spreading	Tight	Cool	Nagging
Radiating	Numb	Cold	Nauseating
Penetrating	Drawing	Freezing	Agonizing
Piercing	Squeezing		Dreadful
	Tearing		Torturing

Even so, certain imaging procedures can help pinpoint the cause of pain or reveal the extent of tissue injury or damage. Computerized tomography (CT) scans, for example, can reveal changes in bones and certain soft tissues. Magnetic resonance imaging (MRI) helps evaluate damage to the vertebrae, spinal cord compression, or the metastasis of cancer cells to the brain. In many cases, these procedures may not be necessary to obtain the information needed to carry out treatment.

Keep a Pain Log

It can be difficult to remember when you experience pain, the nature of pain at particular times, what you did to relieve pain, and what you were doing when it occurred. Keeping a daily pain log can help you communicate with your caregivers and keep track of which pain relief methods work best. Here is a sample page for one day.

Time	Severity from 1 (very mild) to 10 (never worse)	Description (choose from list on page 385)	What you were doing when it began (such as walking, sleeping)	Name and amount of medication taken	Nondrug techniques you tried (such as meditation, heat)
Midnight					
1 a.m.					
2 a.m.					
3 a.m.					
4 a.m.					
5 a.m.					
6 a.m.					
7 a.m.					
8 a.m.					
9 a.m.					
10 a.m.					
11 a.m.					
Noon					
1 p.m.					
2 p.m.					
3 p.m.					
4 p.m.					
5 p.m.					
6 p.m.					
7 p.m.					
8 p.m.					
9 p.m.					
10 p.m.					
11 p.m.					

To the greatest extent possible, health professionals should provide relief for people in pain at the time of the assessment, before proceeding. Pain is not an excuse for not doing a careful work-up, particularly since the results of the assessment will determine a course of action that might relieve it.

Taking Control of Pain

Pain control (or pain management) means treating pain aggressively to provide the maximum degree of relief possible. This usually means treatment with medications and other methods, such as surgery. But it also includes techniques that improve the quality of life and the ability to work, enjoy recreation, and function as normally as possible. It may involve psychological therapy, training in relaxation techniques, and a number of other strategies that do not require medications.

Current studies are determining what approaches work best for people with different types of cancer. New federal guidelines for relieving cancer pain have been published, and nearly every state has launched a cancer pain relief initiative to promote awareness of pain control strategies. Education is helping overcome myths and misunderstandings that doctors and nurses as well as patients have maintained in regard to pain treatment. In addition, the importance of mind-body approaches to pain (such as certain relaxation techniques, imagery, and hypnosis) is being recognized by health professionals in traditional hospital settings.

In many instances, cancer therapy removes or shrinks the tumor and thus eliminates the source of the pain. The basic cancer treatments can also be palliative—that is, prescribed for pain relief. Radiation eases pain in more than half the cases and is usually the fastest and most effective strategy for specific types of pain, such as pain caused by bone metastases. Surgery, such as tumor removal, drainage of abscesses, or treatment of bowel obstruction, also can ease pain.

Chemotherapy has palliative value, but it is unpredictable; its effects are often delayed; and it carries the risk of side effects. But if the best treatment for the cancer is chemotherapy, then it has a good chance of relieving the pain if the cancer is responding to the medication.

Medication Options

Seventy to ninety percent of people with cancer who have pain find relief through the use of analgesics, agents that relieve pain without causing a loss of consciousness. The other strategies, used alone or in combination with analgesics, can help most of the remaining people in pain.

A few years ago, the World Health Organization (WHO) became concerned that not enough was being done to treat pain in people with cancer. After

TIPS AND

ADVICE

Pain Control Strategies

- Anticipate pain if possible, and respond to it quickly. If you can prevent pain from developing or becoming severe, pain relief will be more effective and your doses of medication may be lower.

- Don't try to tough it out or wait until the pain becomes unbearable before seeking relief. Generally, the worse the pain is, the longer it takes to get relief.

- Don't be afraid to admit you have pain. Only you know how you feel. Communicating to family members and caregivers about your pain is essential. Don't worry about being seen as a complainer or a difficult patient. Pain relief is vital to managing cancer, and unless others know about your situation, they can't help you as much as you may need.

- Resist comparing your situation with someone else's. Your pain, like your cancer, is unique, and so is the treatment you require.

- Try to follow your doctor's orders. You may need to take a medication at certain intervals, even if you're not in much pain at the time, to get the most benefit.

- Let people know if you're not getting the relief you expected. The effects of cancer on your body can change from day to day, and a medication that worked in the past may not continue to be effective. Don't wait for your next appointment before letting your doctor know if the pain therapy isn't working.

- Take note of and immediately report any side effects of the pain treatment.

studying the problem, the WHO devised a "ladder" approach to pain management. As shown in the box on page 389, the ladder image conveys the basic plan for using pain relieving medicines: start with the simplest and gradually proceed to the most powerful opioids until a satisfactory level of relief is reached.

Nonopioid Analgesics

In many cases of mild to moderate pain, nonopioid drugs such as acetaminophen, aspirin, and ibuprofen provide good relief. This is especially true if you are able to "stay on top of the pain," meaning you are able to anticipate the need for medication and take it as directed before the pain becomes severe.

Like other pain relievers, nonopioid analgesics work by affecting the nervous system. However, unlike opioids, which dull the central nervous

Pain Ladder

The first step on the ladder is the use of nonopioid analgesics, such as aspirin or acetaminophen, and non-steroidal anti-inflammatory drugs (NSAIDs), such as ibuprofen and naproxen. These are used alone or with adjuvant medications— that is, additional drugs that are usually pre-scribed for a specific complaint other than pain, but in combination with the analgesic can enhance the pain relief

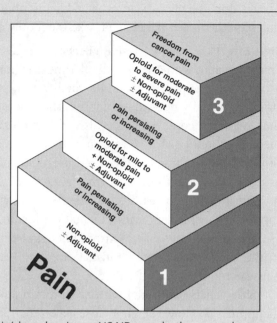

effect. If none of the nonopioid analgesics or NSAIDs work, the second step is to try a weak opioid in addition as needed. (An opioid is a natural or synthetic drug that has a morphine-like action.) If high doses of this regimen are not adequate, the third step is to use a potent opioid, usually morphine, with or without NSAIDs or other adjuvants.

Reprinted with permission of the World Health Organization. From Cancer Pain Relief and Palliative Care. Report of a WHO Expert Committee. Geneva Switzerland: World Health Organization, ©1990.

system, these pain relievers as a rule do not cause drowsiness. They have few serious side effects (although they can have some; see page 390). They provide temporary relief, usually for about three or four hours, although some may be longer lasting. The choice of nonopioid analgesics includes acetaminophen (Tylenol is a well-known brand) and the nonsteroidal anti-inflammatory drugs (NSAIDs) such as ibuprofen (Motrin, Advil, Rufen, Nuprin) and naproxen (Naprosyn, Anaprox, Aleve). Some people cannot tolerate the NSAIDs because of gastrointestinal side effects. Numerous kinds of NSAIDs are available, some over-the-counter, some by prescription only. One NSAID may effectively relieve pain for one person, whereas another type may not, so switching medications can be helpful.

Treatment with nonopioid analgesics generally begins with low doses, which may be increased over two or three weeks. These medications have what is known as a ceiling dose, beyond which increased doses do not do any good. In this way, they differ from opioids, which do provide more relief at higher doses. Always drink plenty of water when taking nonopioid analgesics, and even if you purchase them over the counter, take them only as your doctor suggests.

Side Effects. The risk of side effects increases with the dose of nonopioid analgesic and with the length of time the medication is taken. Although aspirin is generally a very safe medication, it can cause bleeding in the stomach, usually noticed as blood in the stools or unexplained bruising. For that reason, people who are also using anticancer drugs that may cause bleeding should not take aspirin. Others who should avoid aspirin include those taking steroids, such as prednisone; those taking blood thinners, such as Coumadin; and those who are allergic to aspirin or have a history of ulcers or gout. In children, aspirin may cause Reye's syndrome, a serious illness that can lead to respiratory arrest, mental confusion, coma, and death. Therefore, children should not take aspirin. Other side effects of aspirin include ringing in the ears, hearing loss, unusual sweating, rapid breathing and heartbeat, nausea, vomiting, and diarrhea.

Side effects associated with acetaminophen are rare, which accounts for its popularity. However, large doses taken daily for a long period of time may result in liver or kidney damage.

NSAIDs are generally safe but can cause nausea, vomiting, indigestion, and constipation. They also interfere with blood clotting, so people with low platelet counts should not take them. Other potential side effects of NSAIDs are dizziness, headache, ringing in the ears, fluid retention, dry mouth, and increased heart rate.

TIPS AND

ADVICE

Comparison of Some Nonopioid Analgesics

	Reduce pain, fever	Reduce inflammation, pain of swollen joints	Can irritate stomach	Can affect blood clotting	Can cause Reye's syndrome	Can worsen kidney problems
Aspirin	Yes	Yes	Yes	Yes	Yes	No
Acetaminophen	Yes	No	No	No	No	No
Ibuprofen	Yes	Yes	Yes	Yes	No	Yes
Naproxen	Yes	Yes	Yes	Yes	No	Yes

Opioid Analgesics

If treatment with nonopioid analgesics does not bring sufficient pain relief, the next step on the ladder is the use of opioids. Unfortunately, opioids have become associated with drug addicts and traffic in illegal "street" drugs. Furthermore, myths and misunderstandings about opioids have led to the underuse of these drugs, which are exceedingly valuable in relieving cancer pain. Recently, though—in large part because of the experience gained from the hospice movement in England—health professionals have come to recognize the benefits of long-term use of opioid analgesics.

Opioids (the word comes from the Greek term for numbness) range in strength from mild to strong. Some, such as codeine, can be either mild or strong, depending on their dosages and how they are used. As a rule, the low strength products work only about as well and for as long as aspirin does.

Opioids can be given alone, but some are used in combination with nonopioid analgesics. These medications are usually given by mouth, but some are given as intravenous (IV) injections or as rectal suppositories if you have difficulty swallowing. A long-lasting (twelve-hour) form of morphine also is available.

There is no best choice of medications, nor is there any such thing as a standard dose of opioids. Each person in treatment has different needs, a different level of pain, and a different threshold for tolerating medication and its adverse effects.

Morphine is considered the gold standard of opioid pain relief. Morphine (MS Contin, Oramorph) or a related medication called hydromorphone (Dilaudid) is frequently the first choice for treating moderate to severe pain, especially among the elderly with severe cancer-related pain. Other opioids frequently used are levorphanol (Levo-Dromoran), methadone (Dolophine), or oxycodone (an ingredient in Percodan and Percocet).

Opioid Analgesics

Mild	Strong	
Codeine	Fentanyl	Morphine
Hydrocodone	Hydromorphone	Methadone
Oxycodone	Levorphanol	Oxymorphone
Propoxyphene		

TIPS AND

ADVICE

Generally, doctors begin by prescribing low doses of opioids and increase the dose until pain is relieved or unpleasant side effects begin. If at that point the pain has not been relieved, the doctor may prescribe another kind of opioid or add a nonopioid analgesic plus some other adjuvant medication.

Research has shown that usually the best treatment plan is giving a fixed dose of opioid every four hours around the clock, plus additional "rescue doses" of a short-acting opioid if the person has what is called "breakthrough" pain. This strategy has several advantages. Most important, of course, is that it effectively controls pain. It also provides additional relief should something happen that suddenly increases the level of pain. Furthermore, it means that you can get relief without having to request it. This eases the feelings of guilt, awkwardness, hesitation, and responsibility that can accompany constant requests for more relief.

Side Effects and Other Concerns. One problem in using opioids is that different medications produce pain relief at different dosages. For instance, 10 milligrams of one medication might have the same effect as 100 milligrams of another. The method of delivery can also make a difference: injections, tablets, and patches allow morphine to enter the bloodstream at different rates and may provide relief for varying periods of time. Morphine taken orally, for example, must pass through the stomach before it can enter the bloodstream and find its way to the pain receptors. Controlled-release (CR) morphine releases morphine over a period of twelve hours.

Changing the route of administration or the type of opioid may cause the health care professional to undermedicate for pain. Today, however, cancer care professionals are becoming more aware of the need to provide equianalgesia—in other words, to continue to achieve pain relief by compensating for changes in types of medications or routes of administration.

Gastrointestinal Side Effects. Although side effects are a less serious problem than the underuse of analgesics, they are fairly common, especially at higher doses. Constipation is a common side effect of opioids. These medications reduce the intestines' motility, or movement, which makes it harder to move the bowels and results in dry, hard stools. Other problems associated with cancer and its treatment, such as reduced activity, poor appetite, and weakness, can contribute to the constipation. The likelihood of constipation can be decreased by eating high-fiber foods (fruits, vegetables, oatmeal, stewed prunes, prune juice, bran cereal, or added bran) and by drinking eight to ten glasses of water a day. Exercise helps too. Health care professionals may suggest the use of a stool softener combined with a laxative, such as magnesium hydroxide (Phillips Milk of Magnesia). Before starting your opioid, talk with your doctor or nurse about what you can do to prevent the constipation.

Low-grade nausea is an infrequent side effect, but it can be problematic for the patient who is receiving treatment (such as chemotherapy) that causes nausea and vomiting. Some steps that may help with the nausea include staying in bed for about an hour after receiving pain medication; taking small sips of water and avoiding food until the nausea passes; and avoiding the smell of foods. If a person's symptoms warrant it, antinausea medication may be prescribed.

Sedation. Opioids can produce drowsiness and sometimes sedation, depending on the medication and the dose. Sometimes, though, sleepiness is a direct result of pain relief; freed from discomfort, you are at last able to catch up on much-needed rest. In these cases, the drowsiness disappears after a few days. If not, it may help to switch to another kind of opioid drug.

Respiratory Depression. Respiratory depression is the slowing down of breathing, and it can be the most disconcerting of all the side effects. Family members become very concerned when respirations decrease. Respiratory depression is not a common side effect, and the risk usually diminishes over time.

Other Problems. Other side effects include dry mouth and itching. Urinary retention can develop, especially in people with prostate or pelvic cancers. Changing the medication or discontinuing any adjuvant medications that can contribute to such problems, such as antidepressants, can minimize these side effects. Opioids such as methadone and levorphanol have a long half-life (the time it takes for the dose to break down in the body). The doctor will take this into account when changing from these medications to other opioids.

Fear of Addiction

Perhaps the most important point to be made in this chapter is that people who take opioids to relieve pain caused by a medical disease are not addicts, nor are they at serious risk of becoming addicts, no matter how much of the medication they take or how often they take it.

An irrational fear of addiction causes many health professionals to resist administering opioids, many people with cancer pain to fear taking them, and many well-meaning friends and family members to pressure their loved ones not to comply with the treatment when opioids are prescribed. One survey found that nearly half of people with cancer-related pain were reluctant to report their suffering, apparently out of concern that they would be given opioids. Half were also afraid to take pain medications as prescribed. This fear of addiction, which is almost totally unfounded, prevents many people with cancer from achieving the degree of pain relief to which they are entitled.

A big part of the problem is confusion over the meaning of the terms *tolerance, dependency,* and *addiction*.

Tolerance. Opioid drugs commonly produce tolerance, which means that you may need to take higher doses to achieve the same effects you once experienced. Many people remain comfortable on stable doses of opioids for long periods of time, but others notice that their usual doses of pain relief don't last as long as they used to. This is one sign that they are developing a tolerance to the pain medication, which might happen because the disease is progressing or because they are under increased psychological distress. In any case, the medically correct pain control strategy for people who have become tolerant of opioid pain relief is to increase the dose or the frequency with which the medication is given. Unlike nonopioid analgesics, opioids have no ceiling dose, and large amounts of the medication are sometimes needed to achieve adequate pain relief. Another approach to pain control in someone who has developed a tolerance is switching to a different type of opioid.

Although opioid users become tolerant of a medication's effects and increase their use, it's important to remember that tolerance alone does not mean they are becoming addicted.

Many doctors and nurses still do not understand that tolerance differs from addiction (although increased education is improving the situation). Therefore, if health care professionals see that a patient is becoming tolerant of an opioid, they may reduce its use. These care-givers may have the mistaken notion that if "too much" of the medication is used now, the medication will not work later when the person "really needs it." The flaw in this argument is the assumption that people with cancer "really need" an opioid only when their pain is not relieved by other strategies.

Dependence. Dependence on pain relief, on the other hand, is a different issue. There are two types of dependence: physical and psychological.

Physical dependence is a normal, predictable, and not very serious result of using opioids. People who take high enough doses of a medication for a long enough time will likely become physically dependent on it. The most notable sign of dependency is that when a person suddenly stops taking the medication, he or she experiences withdrawal symptoms: agitation, fear, chills, sweating, shaking, sleeplessness, and worsening of pain. As bad as it sounds, the withdrawal syndrome can be easily avoided and managed well by slowly reducing the use of opioids over time. Note that even though opioid addicts may become physically dependent on a medication, *physical dependence is not addiction.*

Psychological dependence is what most experts today mean when they speak of addiction. Addicts take drugs to satisfy physical, emotional, and psychological needs, not to solve a medical problem. Their lives become centered on obtaining and taking drugs. And they keep taking drugs despite serious financial, legal, or health consequences.

The use of an opioid is only one factor in developing a psychological dependence; a person's social, economic, and psychiatric backgrounds also play critical roles. Unless someone has a history of drug abuse, there is little risk that a patient being treated for a painful medical illness like cancer is at risk of developing a psychological addiction to an opioid drug. Indeed, the incidence of psychological dependence among cancer patients is rare. According to a report in the *New England Journal of Medicine*, for which

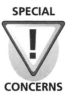

SPECIAL

CONCERNS

The Myths About Opioids

- "Opioids pose a strong risk of addiction." False. The risk of addiction is less than one in 3,000. Unfortunately, the misplaced fear of addiction often means that these drugs are not employed as frequently as they should be or in adequate doses to provide pain relief.

- "Opioids produce euphoria, which inevitably leads to being hooked." Not true. People taking opioids for pain relief seldom report feeling euphoric. Even if they do, it is unlikely that they will continue to seek drugs for their euphoric effects after the pain has gone away.

- "People are given morphine only when they're at death's door." Not true. In good cancer management, opioids are administered as soon as pain becomes moderately severe. As the ladder strategy suggests, opioids are an appropriate treatment when nonopioids alone fail to provide the amount and duration of relief the person needs.

- "Morphine doesn't work when taken by mouth." False. This belief originated from some faulty studies done some years ago. In fact, oral morphine is very effective. (Injected opioids may work faster at lower doses, however.)

- "Heroin is a better opioid than morphine." Untrue. Anyway, the body converts heroin to morphine.

- "People always need high doses of opioids." Wrong. Every person is different. Effective doses of morphine can range from 5 to 180 mg every four hours. Most people require only moderate doses; in fact, many people with advanced cancer and chronic severe pain need no more than 20 mg every four hours, no matter how long the therapy lasts.

- "I'll die of an overdose." Not likely. Many people fear opioids because of news reports about drug users who die of overdoses. Even though the doses required for adequate pain relief are sometimes high, they are rarely, if ever, large enough to cause death. Death among substance abusers usually occurs when they take outrageously high doses or consume dangerous combinations of substances, such as heroin and cocaine. And addicts often take illegal opioids manufactured by amateur scientists—compounds that contain impurities or are "cut" with adulterating substances such as talcum powder.

- "There's a limit to the effective dose of an opioid." Not so. The stronger the pain is, the more of an opioid is required for relief. Again, NSAIDs do have a ceiling dose, but opioids can be used in increasing amounts until they bring the pain under control. Furthermore, increasing the dose (often a necessary step in managing the pain of progressive cancer) does not increase the already minimal risk of addiction.

- "People taking opioids always need to take antinausea drugs." Some do, especially in the beginning. Women are more prone to experience nausea than men. But in most cases, the antinausea therapy can be stopped after a few days.

- "People should take morphine only when they feel the need." No. The best strategy is to take regular doses around the clock, rather than on an as needed, or prn, basis.

researchers reviewed the records of nearly 12,000 hospital patients with pain who had no history of drug addiction and who were treated with opioids, the scientists found that only four out of these many thousands developed a psychological dependence—a risk of about three hundredths of 1 percent.

Adjuvant Medications

In many instances, medications that treat a variety of complaints other than pain can enhance the effectiveness of analgesic therapy. Scientists are not sure why this is true, and they lack solid evidence as to which adjuvant medications work best for people with various kinds of cancer. Still, adjuvant medications often have a greater effect than nonopioid or opioid analgesics alone.

Tricyclic Antidepressants. Tricyclic antidepressants enhance the activity of various neurotransmitters in the brain and can be very useful medications for managing pain. Tricyclics such as amitryptyline (Elavil, Endep), doxepin (Adapin, Sinequan), and imipramine (Tofranil) are especially effective for relieving the dull, burning pain that results from nerve infiltration by cancer cells. The doses needed for pain relief are lower than those used in treating depression.

Anticonvulsants. Carbamazepine (Tegretol) and other anticonvulsants relieve the sharp stabbing or burning pains of tumors pressing on nerves, especially those in the head and neck. Such pain is notoriously resistant to opioids. These medications also are used to manage pain following surgical injury and for people with stump pain or pain in the lower extremities.

Corticosteroids. For many people, dexamethasone (Decadron), used in treating back pain due to compression of the spinal cord, produces significant relief and lowers the need for analgesic medications. Prednisone (Deltasone) relieves pain in people with advanced cancer.

Other steroids may help people with bony metastases or nerve infiltration. Steroids can also have positive effects on appetite and mood, and there is some evidence that they may work directly against certain kinds of tumors. Accordingly, people with advanced cancer who receive steroids often need lower doses of opioids to control pain.

Adjuvant Medications for Cancer Pain

Type of Medication	Example(s)	Uses
Tricyclic antidepressants	Amitriptyline, doxepin, imipramine	Dull, burning pain due to nerve infiltration
Anticonvulsants	Carbamazepine, phenytoin, clonazepam	Stabbing pain due to nerve infiltration or compression, surgical injury, stump pain
Corticosteroids	Prednisone	Advanced cancer
	Dexamethasone	Back pain due to spinal cord compression, diffuse bony metastases, nerve infiltration
Antianxiety medications	Haloperidol, diazepam, Lorazepam, alprazolam	Reduce opioid doses, psychosis, or delirium

INFORM

YOURSELF

How Medications Are Given

Over the course of their illness, many people need to take pain medications via a number of different routes—most need two routes. The way that the medications are administered can make a big difference in the way they work against pain. For example, medications given orally or rectally may take longer to take effect. Many people become anxious and distressed while waiting for the medication to work. This is a concern when an individual is making decisions about medications, particularly when he or she is transferred home from the hospital or to a hospice. Caregivers and family members should therefore be aware that the way in which medications are given can change the degree of pain relief.

As a rule, chronic pain is best treated orally. This route is easier, cheaper, and safer, and it generally provides longer relief than other routes. People who do not have to be attached to tubes and poles in order to receive pain relief remain more mobile and can participate more fully in life than they otherwise could. Medications taken orally are generally given in higher doses than those given by other means, because the medication must pass through the stomach's acidic environment before it can be absorbed into the bloodstream. Morphine is available in an elixir form, which can be swallowed or absorbed through the mucous membrane of the mouth. The latter method may be the route of choice for people who have difficulty swallowing.

Other routes can be used if medications cannot be taken by mouth—for example, an intestinal obstruction or nausea and vomiting following chemotherapy will temporarily rule out oral medications. Intranasal medications, which are absorbed through the nasal membranes, or transdermal medications, which are absorbed through the skin, are sometimes an option for people who have difficulty receiving injections.

Injection directly into the spinal canal (epidural or intrathecal administration) puts the medication closer to its target, the nervous system. As a result, less of the medication circulates to the brain, which reduces the risk of side effects.

Morphine and other opioids are available as suppositories so that they can be administered through the rectum.

INFORM

YOURSELF

Routes of Administration

- Oral (swallowed)

- Sublingual (under the tongue)

- Continuous infusion

- Subcutaneous (under the skin)

- Intravenous (through a vein)

- Epidural (injected into a space along the spinal cord)

- Intrathecal (injected into the spinal canal)

- Rectal (suppositories)

- Intranasal (into the nose)

- Transdermal (skin patch)

Self-Administered Pain Therapy

One of the most commonly used approaches to cancer pain management allows you to administer medications to yourself at the rate and dosage you choose. Patient-controlled analgesia (PCA) is common in many cancer care facilities. PCA (sometimes called demand or self-administered analgesia) uses an electronic pump attached to a drug reservoir and a timing device. A tube is connected to a small needle inserted under the skin or into a vein. When you feel pain, you press a button on the pump and receive a preset dose of medication. The timer is adjustable so that no more than a certain amount of medication can be taken over a given time. For example, it may be set to release no more than four doses of a medication in an hour, no matter how many times you press the button. PCA is often used after surgery or for anyone with severe pain.

Although some experts question whether this approach will prove cost effective in the long run, studies have found that people who self-medicate tend to be discharged earlier and may suffer fewer chronic pain problems later. People who can control their pain themselves may use lower total doses of medications than would have been prescribed by their caregivers. And most people prefer this arrangement to being stuck with a needle every few hours. If nothing else, PCA provides a psychological edge, because pain is easier to bear if you know it can be addressed instantly and whenever you want.

Thanks to advances in technology, many people today can use miniature pumps that fit into a fanny pack, backpack, or purse and deliver a continuous infusion of analgesic medication. One device even straps to the wrist like a watch. You can thus enjoy the benefits of pain relief while continuing your daily activities.

Nerve Surgery

For many people, medicine and nondrug treatments help relieve pain. If these approaches aren't effective, other treatments are available, including nerve blocks whereby pain medicine is injected into or around a nerve or into the spine to block the pain, and neurosurgery, where pain nerves are cut to relieve the pain.

Neurosurgery (nerve surgery) is performed when pain relief from a cancer treatment or from the use of analgesics is inadequate. The goal of nerve surgery is to interrupt the pathway along which pain signals travel to the brain. The process (sometimes called neuroablation) cuts or destroys part of the pain nerve fibers. Such procedures are expensive because they are usually performed by highly skilled experts at special treatment centers. Only those with clearly localized pain are likely to benefit from this procedure; moreover, serious risks are involved, including the temporary or permanent loss of feeling or motor control in some parts of the body.

Anesthetics

Anesthetic techniques may help people with well-defined local pain caused by a tumor that is infiltrating surrounding tissue. Some anesthetic methods work for short periods of time; others, such as cryoanalgesia, or freezing, can cause permanent nerve blockage. Some people whose pain does not respond to other approaches may benefit from these techniques.

A drawback of this strategy is that many nerves may need to be blocked to achieve adequate relief. Up to 13 percent of people may suffer permanent side effects such as urinary or rectal incontinence, motor weakness, or abnormal tingling or burning sensations (paresthesias).

Most anesthesia techniques block nerves. For example, pain in the chest wall and abdominal wall can be relieved by interrupting the nerves that exit from the spinal cord to supply these sites. Pain in the legs, groin, and low back can be helped by infusing medications into the epidural or intrathecal spaces to numb the nerves that receive pain signals from these sites. Patients with upper abdominal pain from pancreatic cancer can get good relief from interruption of the nerves near the pancreas.

Continuous epidural infusion is used when the pain is difficult to treat, as in cases of advanced metastatic disease involving the pelvis and lower body. Either an infusion pump delivers the medication to the spinal column through a catheter, or a small reservoir is surgically implanted in the body to dispense the medication in small doses over time. The advantage of this method is that it provides effective relief without disrupting the function of the muscles and nerves.

Stimulating Nerves

Blocking the nerves is one way to reduce pain. Another is to stimulate the nerves with signals that are not painful, such as gentle vibrations. This technique is believed to crowd out the painful feelings and keep them from traveling along the spinal cord to the brain. In a way, it's like flooding a switchboard with telephone calls to prevent other calls from getting through. Nerve stimulation is very safe, but it seems to work best only in the short term; long-lasting pain relief is rare.

Common techniques include stimulating the skin with pressure, friction, temperature change, or chemicals. The simplest and most widely used method is counterirritation, such as brisk rubbing of the painful area, often following the use of a cooling spray.

Acupuncture

According to a National Institutes of Health (NIH) expert panel consisting of scientists, researchers, and health care professionals, acupuncture is an effective treatment for nausea caused by chemotherapy drugs and for postoperative pain. Some evidence suggests that acupuncture may lessen the need for conventional pain relieving medicines.

Acupuncture is a technique in which very thin needles of varying lengths are inserted through the skin to stimulate specific nerves. In traditional acupuncture, specially trained practitioners insert needles at specific locations, called acupoints, which are believed to control specific areas of pain sensation. Needles usually remain in place for less than thirty minutes. Skilled acupuncturists cause virtually no pain. Once inserted, the acupuncturist may twirl the needles and apply heat or a weak electrical current to enhance the effects of therapy. In acupressure, a popular variation of acupuncture, therapists press on acupoints with their fingers instead of using needles. This technique is used by itself or as part of a larger system of manual healing such as shiatsu massage.

Although it originated 2,000 to 3,000 years ago, acupuncture remains an important component of current traditional Chinese medicine. In China, acupuncture is used as an anesthetic during surgery and is believed to have the power to cure diseases and relieve symptoms of illness. Some practitioners claim that acupuncture relieves pain by stimulating the production of endorphins—natural substances in the body responsible for relieving pain. In the United States and Europe, it is used primarily to control pain and relieve disease symptoms such as nausea.

Many other conditions have been treated by acupuncture. The WHO, for example, has listed more than forty diseases that lend themselves to acupuncture treatment. They noted that the list is based on clinical experience rather than research findings. The NIH states that acupuncture may be useful as an adjunct treatment (used in addition to the main treatment) for conditions such as addiction, stroke rehabilitation, headache, menstrual cramps, tennis elbow, fibromyalgia, myofacial pain, osteoarthritis, low back pain, carpal tunnel syndrome, and asthma. However, further research is needed to determine the effectiveness for its use with these and other conditions.

Acupuncture is considered an effective treatment when used to treat conditions for which it has been proven to be effective (e.g., chemotherapy nausea and vomiting, and postoperative pain). However, the NIH has not specifically recommended using acupuncture for cancer pain.

Most doctors believe acupuncture is safe as long as the needles used are sterile and the therapy is conducted by a trained professional. The American Academy of Medical Acupuncture maintains a current referral list of doctors who practice acupuncture. Medicare does not cover acupuncture, but it is covered by some private health insurance plans and health maintenance organizations.

Transcutaneous Electrical Nerve Stimulation

Transcutaneous electrical nerve stimulation (TENS) is a method of pain relief in which a special device transmits electrical impulses through electrodes to an area of the body that is in pain. The resulting relief can be substantial, but the effect usually lasts only as long as the machine is turned on. Supporters claim that TENS is an effective method for relieving acute pain caused by surgery, migraines, injuries, arthritis, tendonitis, bursitis, chronic wounds, cancer, and other sources. Some people with cancer, particularly those with mild neuropathic pain (pain related to nerve tissue damage), may benefit from TENS for brief periods of time. TENS may also be more effective when used with analgesics (pain medicines). Although there is some evidence that TENS may offer short-term pain relief for some people, the long-term benefits have not been proven. After a few months, or even days, many people no longer get relief. A variation on TENS is the surgical implantation of a small electrode to produce stimulation.

TENS is used widely by physical therapists and other medical practitioners, but can also be performed at home by patients using a portable TENS system. There are more than one hundred types of TENS units approved for use by the U.S. Food and Drug Administration. A prescription is needed to obtain a system, so if you are interested in obtaining a home TENS unit, you will need to talk to your doctor or physical therapist.

TENS is generally considered safe. However, electrical current that is too intense can burn the skin. The electrodes should not be placed over the eyes, heart, brain, or front of the throat. People with heart problems should not use TENS. The effects of long-term use of TENS on fetuses is unknown, therefore pregnant women should not undergo the therapy.

Physical Therapy

The value of physical therapy techniques is often overlooked in the treatment of cancer pain. For example, a surgical corset can relieve back pain in people with progressive vertebral disease. Arm or shoulder splints ease pain due to nerve infiltration in those regions. Physical therapy can prevent or delay muscle contractions or frozen joints in people who are partly immobilized. Massage, muscle stretching, or the use of hot or cold compresses can prevent muscle pain. Apart from their physical benefits, these techniques offer some degree of self-control over pain, which can lead to psychological benefits and greater independence.

Pain and the Mind, Body, and Spirit

Complementary methods such as massage therapy, yoga, and meditation are also referred to as nondrug or noninvasive treatments. These techniques rely heavily on the ability of the mind to influence responses to pain.

Relaxation exercises, for example, may help reduce pain. Music or television may distract you from pain. Talk to your doctors and nurses about these treatments. They will be able to give you more information and discuss how the techniques may help relieve your pain.

Mind-body strategies increase your sense of personal control over pain. They help reduce feelings of hopelessness and helplessness and offer a calming diversion of attention. As yet, few studies have explored the role of such techniques in managing cancer-related pain, although recent research has found that hypnosis can be very effective. Experience suggests that for many people these methods can be an important adjunct to an overall program of pain therapy. Most likely to benefit are those with:

- *intermittent,* predictable pain such as that associated with treatment procedures

- *incidental* pain associated with metastatic bone disease that flares up during movement

- *chronic* pain accompanied by anxiety

Your health care professional may recommend that you try some of these treatments along with your medicine to give you even more pain relief. Your loved ones may want to help you to use these treatments. Keep in mind that these treatments will help to make your medicines work better and relieve other symptoms, but they should not be used instead of your medicine.

The following techniques include methods that focus on the connections between the mind, body, and spirit, and their power for healing, as well as methods that involve touching, manipulating, or moving the body. When used along with conventional treatment, many of these methods can help relieve pain or improve your quality of life. You may use these treatments along with your regular medicine:

- biofeedback

- distraction

- hypnosis

- imagery and visualization

- meditation

- music therapy

- prayer and other spiritual practices

- relaxation exercises

- yoga

Because many of these techniques are helpful in managing a number of cancer symptoms in addition to pain, they are discussed in greater detail in Chapter 27.

Cognitive and Behavioral Techniques. Cognitive and behavioral strategies help you learn to divert your attention from your pain, improve your ability to tolerate it, and increase your feelings of control over your situation. Cognitive techniques include learning about the disease, discovering distraction techniques, and focusing your mind through controlled mental imagery. In cognitive therapy you learn healthier ways to think about your illness and interpret its meaning in your life.

A word about imagery: this cognitive method can help you fill your mind with beautiful or soothing pictures, allowing you to disconnect temporarily from pain. Such a strategy may have tremendous value. Despite the message of certain popular books and articles, however, imagery is not a treatment for the cancer itself. It has not proved effective in shrinking tumors or eliminating metastatic cells.

Behavioral methods help eliminate behaviors such as the tensing of muscles that may contribute to the severity of pain. Some behavioral strategies teach skills to help you cope with pain and modify your reactions to it. These techniques are especially effective in managing acute pain arising from cancer procedures and as adjuncts to an overall program of chronic pain therapy.

Perhaps the most important and basic cognitive-behavioral techniques are relaxation and distraction. As mentioned, muscular tension—which can arise directly from the pain or from the fear of anticipating future pain—makes the experience of pain worse. The ability to relax, then, is an essential survival skill. When you relax, you break the vicious cycle of pain-anxiety-tension-pain. You waste less energy, are able to sleep better, feel less anxious, and can benefit more from other methods of pain relief. Approaches to relaxation include breathing exercises, biofeedback, music therapy, medication, massage, and imagery (see Chapter 27).

Psychiatric Therapy

Chronic pain can make anyone vulnerable to severe depression. Short-term supportive psychotherapy provides education and emotional support and helps everyone, family members included, adapt to the difficult situation. Therapy can help you identify your strong points, determine what methods of coping work best, and learn new skills. In addition, a therapist may recommend medications to reduce anxiety or feelings of depression. As noted earlier, some antidepressant medications also relieve pain when used as adjuvants to analgesics.

Insisting on Pain Relief

Not everyone with cancer has pain. Of those who do, most can find relief through treatment with medications alone or with a combination of medications, surgical procedures, and psychological strategies. Opioids, including morphine, are extremely valuable weapons, but because of fear and misunderstandings, they are too often underused in the fight against cancer pain. Fortunately, that picture is changing.

People with cancer, including those near the end of life, have the right to insist on the highest possible quality of life when dealing with their disease. They are entitled to request and receive aggressive pain management. Cancer care is not complete until pain is under control.

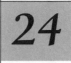
Fatigue

Fatigue is a symptom of cancer, a side effect of treatment, and a reaction to the physical and emotional stresses of survival. According to some estimates, as many as nine out of ten people with cancer must cope with fatigue at some point during treatment. For most people, recovery brings relief from this invisible side effect, but for a few, tiring easily and adjusting to compensate for a lack of energy becomes the "new normal." Treatment-related fatigue—the feeling that you just can't do the things you normally do or want to do—is the most common side effect of cancer treatment, but until recently one of the most overlooked. In fact, doctors sometimes fail to prepare patients for this side effect at all. Some experts say that current awareness of the problem is at the same stage of knowledge that cancer-related pain control was five to eight years ago. Through the efforts of those who have experienced this demoralizing side effect and health care professionals concerned about the lack of recognition given to the problems of fatigue, the topic is now the subject of research, professional publications, continuing education for health professionals, and patient education. Some cancer centers even provide self-assessment questionnaires to help patients assess fatigue and monitor it along with other side effects during the course of treatment.

Fatigue can affect a person's quality of life during and after treatment as seriously as the other more obvious side effects of nausea and vomiting and pain. It, too, may interfere with the most basic functions of life. Recently, two large studies found that fatigue far outranks pain, nausea and vomiting, and depression in terms of being the most bothersome and long-lasting side effect.

The Invisible Side Effect

People vary enormously in their experience of fatigue, but in general, cancer-related fatigue feels different than the tiredness and even exhaustion that everyone feels from time to time. Some people undergoing cancer treatment complain of a lethargic feeling that causes them to curtail their activities for a short time. Some people experience mild tiredness that is annoying but manageable and is resolved within a few weeks after treatment. But for others, fatigue is overwhelming—it comes on suddenly and lasts for several months after treatment. These people describe their feeling as "beyond tired," "unrelenting tiredness," or "feeling like a dishrag all the time." Some say simply, "I get tired for no reason." Regardless of its severity or duration, cancer fatigue is different from everyday tiredness in that it may not be relieved by rest.

Because people have a tendency to try and keep up their normal activities even though they're undergoing physically challenging treatments, they may ignore the signs of fatigue. This is a warning that you need to slow down, rest, curtail your responsibilities, or ask for help. Being aware of what is happening can help you cope and adjust to it. And, according to experts in treating cancer-related fatigue, being informed may diminish stress and anxiety, both of which can make fatigue worse.

INFORM

YOURSELF

Signs of Fatigue:

- feeling like you have no energy
- sleeping more than usual
- not wanting to do normal activities
- loss of interest in people or things
- decreased attention to personal appearance
- feeling tired even after sleeping
- lack of sexual desire
- difficulty concentrating
- difficulty learning new information
- clumsiness
- poor memory
- feeling irritable or impatient
- lack of interest in daily activities

Why Am I So Tired?

How and why fatigue occurs is not clearly understood. Some experts believe it is related to an increase in metabolic wastes due to rapid cell destruction. In fact, some experts say that the most common cause of cancer-related fatigue is the tumor itself. It may cause fatigue by directly affecting metabolism.

There are many different possible causes of cancer-related fatigue, such as the cancer itself, sleep disturbances, and excessive inactivity. The following are possible causes of fatigue during treatment.

Combination Cancer Treatment

Fatigue is common with chemotherapy, radiation therapy, and biological therapy. Chemotherapy and radiation therapy can cause fatigue because of destruction of rapidly dividing cells, especially the cells in the bone marrow affecting the red blood cells that can result in anemia. Rapid cell growth and death also produce an accumulation of cell by-products, which can increase the energy needed to repair when the body tries to repair damaged tissue. The mental fatigue occurring with biological therapy is not clearly understood. Many of the causes of fatigue discussed in this section are directly related to cancer treatment.

Dehydration

Diarrhea or vomiting after any cancer treatment can lead to an imbalance in electrolytes—such as sodium, magnesium, and calcium—circulating in the bloodstream. Weakness is a warning sign of electrolyte imbalance, which can be corrected with special drinks (see Chapter 18) or with intravenous fluids containing electrolytes. Even after the immediate problem of dehydration is corrected, it's important to maintain good nutrition and drink a sufficient amount of water to compensate for fluid losses.

Anemia

There are several causes of anemia, a condition in which a person's red blood cell count is lower than normal. Fatigue is the hallmark symptom of anemia. Blood loss is an obvious potential cause of anemia. But the condition can also be caused by malnutrition, severe organ dysfunction, certain drugs that lead to iron deficiency, chemotherapy, and other treatments.

Treatment for anemia depends on the cause of the problem. Of course, correcting the cause of any internal bleeding is essential. Improving the nutrient value of the diet can help replenish iron stores. (Iron is needed to make hemoglobin, the oxygen-carrying component of red blood cells.) Replacement of deficiencies such as iron or folic acid may improve the anemia. Transfusion may be needed for an acute blood loss or a new medicine called epoetin alpha can help increase the hemoglobin level, thus resolving some cancer-related anemia.

Infection

Infection is a common cause of fatigue and can make a person who is already feeling weak and tired even worse. When the immune system is stimulated to resist infection, fatigue-causing cytokines flood the system. Obviously, combating the infection is the first step toward diminishing fatigue.

Medications

Some drugs have energy-depleting side effects, for example, pain medications, antinausea drugs, and certain antidepressants. The problem may be avoided by reducing the drug dose or changing to another drug that is less likely to cause you to feel sleepy. Although the degree of sedation varies, taking multiple medicines with numerous side effects may compound fatigue symptoms. Ask your doctor if the medicines you are taking could add to your fatigue.

Pain

Physical discomfort is an important cause of fatigue. The tension and strain of dealing with pain is exhausting. Pain interferes with restful sleep. And pain gets in the way of participating in other activities that might be relaxing, distracting, or energizing. In fact, studies are underway to determine to what extent cancer-related fatigue is affected by inactivity (whether the result of pain or something else) and the resulting muscle wasting.

Treating the cause of the pain is essential. It's also important to administer pain relieving medicines before the pain becomes severe and in sufficient amounts to allow a person uninterrupted sleep (see Chapter 23).

Stress, Anxiety, and Depression

Stress and anxiety can perpetuate or worsen fatigue—if worries keep you from sleeping, you become more tired. Wendy S. Harpham, M.D., a doctor who is a long-term cancer survivor, has studied fatigue, and she describes a cycle of anxiety, depression, and fatigue. The fatigue triggers a cascade of problems—some practical, some social and financial, and some emotional. Concern about these problems interferes with day-to-day functioning, sleeping, and resting, which makes the fatigue worse. And the worsening fatigue makes you feel more anxious and depressed.

Dr. Harpham writes that breaking the cycle requires knowledge, hope, and action. Of course, the cause of the fatigue must be treated, but it's also important to learn how to cope with it, perhaps adjusting to the limitations of cancer treatments and their aftermath, and seeking support (see Chapters 26 and 27).

Nutrition

Specific factors such as changes in metabolism, the tumor's competition for nutrients, poor appetite, nausea/vomiting, and diarrhea or bowel obstruction can result in fatigue. Changes in the ability to process nutrients, increased energy requirements, and decreased intake of food and fluids can also affect cancer-related fatigue.

Overexertion

It's difficult for some people who have cancer to acknowledge that they cannot keep up with their usual activities and so they attempt to keep up with their usual work, social, and family schedules. You may even take on more responsibilities than you had before your diagnosis in order to keep busy and distract yourself from the situation. Keeping busy can be a helpful coping tool, to a certain extent. But when exertion saps your physical energy, you can become exhausted.

Fatigue expert Dr. Harpham advises people with cancer to lie down and rest *before* getting to the point of feeling unwell. If you think of needing rest not as a loss, she says, but as a way to regain control, it may ease the frustration you feel at having to take a break or a nap.

TIPS AND

ADVICE

When to Call the Doctor:

- if you are too tired to get out of bed for more than a twenty-four hour period

- if you become confused

- if your fatigue becomes progressively worse

Treating Fatigue

Undergoing a medical evaluation to determine the cause of fatigue is the first step in treating fatigue. Determining the underlying cause will allow your doctor to treat it, if possible, and will offer you an understanding of what is going on and, to a degree, what can be expected. Some people say that understanding the cause of their fatigue helps them cope with it. Changes in one's day-to-day life can help control fatigue and may prevent it from becoming debilitating. When fatigue can't be significantly diminished, it may be necessary to make some lifestyle changes.

Correct Any Medical Problems

If the underlying cause of fatigue is identified, it should be treated if possible. For example, if you are anemic, it's important to correct the anemia. Medication side effects should be controlled or prevented, and dehydration and electrolyte imbalances should all be corrected.

Rest

You may be able to avoid fatigue by taking the steps previously described, but another important approach to managing fatigue is resting *before* you become overly tired. A good night's sleep is important, but so are frequent short naps and breaks during the day. This may mean making a change in your work schedule or the family's routine. But don't overdo the rest because too much rest can decrease your energy level. If you have trouble sleeping, talk with your doctor.

Conserve your energy for the activities that are most important to you, and ask for help with those that leave you feeling drained. For example, if preparing a meal leaves you too tired to enjoy it with your family, ask a friend or family member to help. Ask a neighbor to pick up groceries for you during his or her own grocery shopping. Schedule activities throughout the day rather than all at once. Recruit friends, family, and neighbors to help, and delegate as much as you can. Stay as active as you can but just remember the short breaks and spread your activities out during the day.

Eat Well

It can be difficult to stay well nourished and hydrated, particularly when undergoing treatments such as chemotherapy (see Chapter 18). Still, it's important to try to eat healthy foods even though you may not be able to eat very much so that what you do consume delivers essential nutrients. Remember to drink plenty of fluids as well. If you are having difficulty eating, discuss this with your doctor or nurse. They may ask you to see a dietitian who can help with your diet and meal planning.

Exercise

Stretching, yoga, walking, and swimming are physical activities that combat fatigue by stimulating the muscles and circulatory system without putting stress on the joints. In one study of women with breast cancer, women who exercised experienced less fatigue than nonexercising patients did, and those who didn't exercise experienced increased fatigue. Physical exercise also has emotional benefits, improving mood, self-confidence, and well being (see Chapter 19).

One note of caution when exercising to counteract fatigue: be sure to rest between periods of physical exertion. Muscles require at least a day to recover from strenuous exercise. Keep in mind that the normal routine of physical activity that you may have kept up before cancer and its treatment may feel strenuous for some time afterward. Don't be tempted to push too hard to prove you are still strong.

Keep in mind that if you are having trouble relaxing and are feeling stressed about being tired, your muscles will be tense and unable to recover adequately from exercise.

25

Cancer Emergencies

When a primary cancer or metastasis involves a vital organ, puts pressure on it, or otherwise alters its function, serious—sometimes life-threatening—problems can occur. How aggressively the emergency is treated depends on several factors. For example, when control of the cancer is likely, treating the underlying condition causing the complication may not only relieve the distressing symptom, it may improve the person's quality of life and perhaps prolong his or her survival. Even if the disease is advanced and treatment of the cancer has failed, procedures that relieve the emergency can prolong life as well as make the person with cancer more comfortable. In situations where there is no possibility of prolonging life, emergency measures may still be taken to ease the discomfort.

As in any medical crisis, an awareness of the warning signs of distress and quick action can help resolve a problem before it becomes life-threatening. Most complications related to cancer can be treated, and if hospitalization is necessary, the person with cancer is usually able to return home once the crisis is resolved.

Symptoms often begin in subtle, barely noticeable ways and progress through stages of severity and urgency. A person who knows what to look for is in a good position to seek treatment before a complication becomes a full-blown emergency. Obviously people with advanced cancer and their families need to talk with the doctor in order to become aware of warning signs and symptoms. But anyone undergoing cancer treatment should feel comfortable calling the doctor or nurse if they are concerned about any physical sensation or mental state that seems out of the ordinary. Certain cancers or sites of metastases, as you will learn, increase the risk of particular problems. Being familiar with your own risks may mean the difference between paying prompt attention to a troubling complication and resolving a true emergency.

The following are some cancer emergencies that may complicate treatment. You should contact your doctor if you experience the warning signs of any conditions listed below. This discussion is not meant to alarm or paint a picture of the worst-case scenario, but to inform you of symptoms that should not be ignored and their possible causes. These situations can usually be managed, and the earlier they are addressed the better.

Excess Fluid Near the Heart

When fluid accumulates between the pericardium—the fibrous sac that contains the heart and the great vessels that lead into and from it—and the heart itself, pressure is placed on the heart, compromising its function. This situation, known as pericardial effusion, prevents the heart from pumping out a normal amount of blood, so that the circulatory system—including the heart—is in crisis. The amount of fluid within the sac can soar from the normal ounce or so to as much as a liter. When an excessive amount of fluid accumulates so rapidly that the body is unable to cope with it, the condition is called cardiac tamponade. This emergency requires immediate action.

The most common cause of cardiac tamponade is cancer. Approximately 75 percent of pericardial effusion cases are complications from lymphoma, leukemia, and cancers of the lung and breast. Sometimes a tumor pressing directly on the pericardium causes the condition.

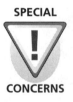

SPECIAL

CONCERNS

WARNING SIGNS

Symptoms of cardiac tamponade vary according to how the body adjusts to and compensates for the pressure on the heart. The following are some common signs and symptoms:

- chest pain

- increased pulse rate (pulse may also be difficult to feel)

- fingernails may turn blue

- anxiety, restlessness, and confusion

- fatigue and shortness of breath

- veins of the neck may become enlarged

- stomach may swell

- decreased urination

- coughing or difficulty swallowing

A few of the diagnostic tests that may be done to precisely diagnose the cause and extent of the problem are CT scan, chest x-ray, MRI, electrocardiography, and echocardiography. Withdrawing fluid through a needle placed into the pericardium is both a diagnostic test and a treatment, since removing just an ounce and a half of fluid can provide relief.

The emergency measures taken for pleural effusion and cardiac tamponade are similar. In both situations the goal is to remove the excess fluid, prevent more fluid from accumulating, and keep other complications of impaired heart function to a minimum. Oxygen is given to relieve symptoms. Bedrest and sitting up in bed help take strain off the heart. Drugs are administered to maintain blood pressure and increase urine flow.

Removing the fluid from the sac is called pericardiocentesis. It is done at the person's bedside using a local anesthetic. A tiny catheter may be left in place for a day or so to continue draining fluid as it accumulates. A cardiac monitor and other equipment continually monitor the heart during the procedure and afterward. Nurses will also be watching for any signs of further complications. Needless to say, this is a tense and stressful situation, so the person undergoing the procedure is given sedatives and may stay in an intensive care unit.

To prevent fluid from accumulating again—and it does so in about half of those who have pericardiocentesis—drugs are injected into the catheter over the course of a day or two. These drugs cause a slight inflammation within the pericardium, which closes the hole in the pericardium.

Eventually the cause of the fluid accumulation—usually the underlying cancer—must be treated. Chemotherapy and radiation therapy to the pericardium may be prescribed.

Blood-Related Complications

The most common emergency involving the blood is a combination of abnormal clotting followed by bleeding called disseminated intravascular coagulation (DIC). When DIC occurs, blood clots initially form too easily, and many small clots occur in the tiny blood vessels that supply the organs. The body's attempts to maintain healthy clot formation are overwhelmed and the opposite situation—hemorrhaging, or bleeding—follows.

Experts are not certain how common DIC is because it may not be detected unless bleeding is severe. However, it's estimated that DIC affects about 10 percent of people with cancer.

DIC can be acute, which usually requires immediate treatment, or chronic. The acute type of DIC often affects those with acute leukemia, when DIC can occur before or during chemotherapy or as a result of a person's receiving infusions of blood products. Those with solid tumors of the breast and prostate are most likely to experience DIC, but cancers of the lung, stomach, and pancreas are also commonly associated with the complication.

DIC is most often triggered by an infection, but the cancer itself is sometimes responsible. Liver cancer or liver metastasis, for example, increases the risk of DIC, since the liver is involved in replacing blood-clotting factors.

The tiny clots that form as part of DIC rarely cause noticeable symptoms, and even the bleeding that follows may not be detected until it becomes severe. By that time, DIC can be fatal. Noticing its early warning signs, therefore, is critical.

SPECIAL

CONCERNS

WARNING SIGNS

The symptoms of DIC vary depending on whether the condition is acute or chronic. The following are some common signs and symptoms:

- bleeding from the nose, gums, or a skin injury (people with acute DIC may bleed from several different places simultaneously)

- failure of blood to clot after blood is drawn

- blood in the urine or in the stool

- painful joints (can be a symptom of bleeding into the joints)

- unusually heavy or prolonged menstrual periods

- confusion, lethargy, dizziness, and even coma or seizures (indications that there is bleeding into the brain)

You or your caregivers need to be alert to signs of bleeding into the tissues. Any unusual bruise, tiny red spots or raised rash on the skin, or blue color in the extremities should be reported to your doctor or nurse immediately.

There is no single test for DIC, but an alert doctor can detect the problem and successfully treat it by considering the symptoms and measuring various substances in the blood, such as clotting factors.

It is essential to treat the underlying cause, if it can be determined. Immediate symptom relief includes oxygen therapy, replacing fluid and blood lost, and providing blood components. Treating the clotting aspect of DIC is also important. Because of the emergency nature of acute DIC and the continuous monitoring the treatment requires, a person with this complication is usually cared for in the intensive care unit until clotting factors are normal and bleeding has stopped.

Septic Shock

When infectious agents invade the body, a fever almost always develops, which can cause a rapid heartbeat and increased breathing rates. The infection can progress, involving the entire body and if not treated appropriately, it can become severe, causing an emergency condition called septic shock. Septic shock indicates that there is severe sepsis, or infection involving the entire body—blood pressure plummets and vital organs begin to fail.

Septic shock is the number one cause of death in intensive care units in the United States. While any type of infection can cause septic shock, bacterial infection is most often at fault. People with cancer are at especially high risk because their immune functions are already compromised and chemotherapy, radiation therapy, or the cancer itself hampers their normal defenses.

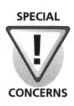

SPECIAL

CONCERNS

WARNING SIGNS

Classic signs of septic shock include:

- chills and fever

- low blood pressure

- rapid heart and breathing rates

- confusion or disorientation

- decreased urination

- nausea and vomiting

Tests of various body functions provide essential information about the person's condition. Doctors use blood tests to identify the organism causing the underlying infection. Blood tests reveal other signs: an increase in the number of white blood cells and an absence of white blood cells if the patient is receiving cancer treatment that affects the cells of the blood. Platelets can also be affected with septic shock, and anemia is common. Blood sugar levels increase, but may drop below normal if septic shock persists.

Preventing septic shock requires careful observation anytime there is an infection or the possibility of one, and you should report any of the symptoms described above to the doctor immediately. If you develop septic shock, the goal of treatment is maintaining vital functions until the infection is brought under control with antibiotics. Fluids must be replaced, which will also increase blood pressure and help the heart work more efficiently. Oxygen is needed to sustain function of the organs. Sometimes steroids are used to diminish the inflammatory response, but their use is controversial. Hospitalization is necessary for providing oxygen, replacing fluid, and closely monitoring someone with septic shock.

Spinal Cord Compression

Pressure on the spinal cord from a primary tumor within the spinal cord or, more commonly, from the extension of vertebral metastases, affects only about 5 percent of people with cancer. Although this complication is rare, it's important to be aware of it because of the risk of paralysis. Certainly anyone who has bone metastases or is at risk of cancer spreading to the bone needs to recognize the early warning signs.

The spinal cord extends from the base of the brain to the top of the lumbar vertebrae that form the middle portion of the spinal column. The spinal cord is surrounded by the bony vertebral column, and the nerves within the spinal cord carry sensory impulses to the brain that convey messages from the brain to the muscles that control movement.

The bones of the skeleton are the third most frequent site of cancer metastasis, and the spine is the most common location of skeletal metastasis. (Breast, lung, and prostate cancers are most often associated with bone metastasis.) When spinal compression occurs, it is usually in the area of the thoracic vertebrae of the upper portion of the spine, but it can occur anywhere.

SPECIAL

!

CONCERNS

WARNING SIGNS

The symptoms of spinal cord compression usually reflect where the tumor or metastatic lesion is located. Initial back pain may be followed or accompanied by weakness and a diminished sensation. Below are further symptom details:

- Back pain is the most noticeable warning of spinal cord compression, and it often begins days to weeks before the condition becomes severe. The pain may move from one area to another as nerves along the spinal column are irritated. It may feel like a constrictive band around the upper back. Or the pain may radiate down the arms or legs. This pain is distinctive from the pain of a slipped disc or other benign cause in that lying down provides no relief. A person with spinal cord compression may actually find it difficult to sleep lying in bed, preferring instead to sleep in a recliner or chair.

- Numbness or a "pins-and-needles" feeling below the waist is another symptom of spinal cord compression. Someone who experiences weakness from this complication (a stiffness or heaviness when climbing stairs or getting out of a chair, for example) typically has a spinal cord that is more than 75 percent compressed. If the compression progresses, a person may lose the ability to sense temperature, pressure, and/or vibration. Eventually bladder and bowel control will be affected as well.

Destruction or collapse of the vertebrae by metastases can be detected on an x-ray, but MRI is the preferred way to diagnose spinal cord compression. It's safer, because unlike tests such as myelography, no dye injection is needed. Also, if an MRI of the entire spine is done, multiple lesions can be detected; about 10 to 30 percent of people with spinal cord compression have more than one site of metastasis.

Spinal cord compression is considered an emergency because immediate treatment is needed to preserve the function of the nerves in the spinal cord, prevent paralysis, and, if the vertebrae of the neck are involved, to avoid respiratory arrest.

Steroids are used to reduce edema in the spinal cord as well as relieve pain and improve nerve function. Radiation therapy is given to shrink the metastases. In recent years, advances in surgical techniques have made it possible to surgically remove a tumor, but surgery does involve some risks, particularly postoperative complications such as infection, bleeding, and leaking of spinal fluid.

Tumors that are sensitive to anticancer drugs, such as Hodgkin's and non-Hodgkin's lymphoma, may benefit from chemotherapy. Also, bisphosphonates, which prevent bone resorption, may reduce the risk of spinal cord compression, particularly in those with metastatic breast cancer and myeloma.

Medication, warm baths, hydrotherapy, and massage can help relieve pain from spinal cord compression (see Chapter 23).

Hormone-Related Syndromes

A malignancy or cancer metasasis sometimes has wide-ranging effects that may lead to a chronic condition and/or an emergency situation. For example, some tumors cause the abnormal secretion of hormones that affect systems quite a distance from the original cancer site. The diseases that result are called paraneoplastic syndromes. Although their occurrence is rare, when paraneoplastic syndromes do occur as a result of cancer, one of the most common is *syndrome of inappropriate antidiuretic hormone* (SIADH).

In the healthy person, antidiuretic hormone (ADH) is secreted by the pituitary gland at the base of the brain when there is a shift in the amount of water needed in the bloodstream. The hormone helps to regulate the kidneys, which will reabsorb water if it is needed by the body. The amount of ADH secreted is sometimes increased, for example, when an otherwise healthy person is in pain, is bleeding, or has undergone some kind of trauma.

SIADH may occur when a malignancy secretes ADH and/or another form of ADH called arginine vasopressin. (Sometimes the term *syndrome of inappropriate diuresis* [SIAD] is used since ADH may not be the only abnormal hormone secreted. The results of SIADH and SIAD are the same.) The hormone signals the kidneys to conserve fluid, even though it's not really necessary, and the urine becomes very concentrated. The retained water accumulates within the body's cells, which ultimately may be especially dangerous to organs such as the brain. Swelling in the brain can cause death if not treated.

SIADH is rare and affects only about 1 to 2 percent of people with cancer. It usually occurs in those with small cell lung cancer but may affect those with cancers of the pancreas, duodenum, esophagus, colon, brain, head and neck (especially cancer in the mouth and throat), ovaries and prostate; acute and chronic leukemia; mesothelioma; sarcoma; Hodgkin's disease; and lymphosarcoma. The cancers appear to have the ability to make, store, and release ADH. SIADH is also a risk when the person with cancer develops an infection, such as pneumonia or tuberculosis, is in pain and receiving morphine, is suffering from emotional stress, or is receiving chemotherapy drugs such as vincristine, vinblastine, and cyclophosphamide. General anesthesia and nausea also cause secretion of ADH. Some people's heart tissue may secrete a hormone that has a similar effect to that of ADH.

Because SIADH may be life-threatening, people with lung cancer—particularly small cell lung cancer—their family members, and their caregivers need to be alert to the early warning signs, vague though these signs often are. As the condition progresses, the signs become more obvious.

SPECIAL

CONCERNS

WARNING SIGNS

The following are indications of abnormally low levels of sodium in the blood that result when too much sodium is lost in the urine:

- nausea

- weakness

- muscle cramps

- headaches

- anorexia

- confusion

- lethargy

Treatment varies according to the amount of sodium lost. In mild cases, restricting fluid, treating the underlying cancer, and discontinuing a medication that may be at fault will resolve the situation. Severely affected people are treated in the intensive care unit, where they can be frequently monitored. They may be given intravenous sodium and furosimide (Lasix), a potent diuretic.

Metabolic Problems

A side effect of treatment such as chemotherapy is that cellular debris from dead cancer cells enters the bloodstream within a short time. In some people a series of metabolic problems result that can lead to heart, kidney, and/or lung complications. A combination of these complications is known as tumor lysis syndrome (TLS).

The more cells that are killed, the greater the danger of TLS. Those with many cancer cells, such as those with high-grade lymphoma or acute leukemia, may be hospitalized for their treatment so they can be monitored closely for signs of TLS. Studies have shown that those with cancer in many lymph nodes, an enlarged spleen, kidney problems, or many metastases are also at increased risk of this complication. High blood levels of an enzyme called lactic dehydrogenase (LDH) or uric acid and a high white blood cell count are risk factors, too.

As the body attempts to get rid of the cellular debris, some of the waste—such as the genetic material from the cells—is converted by the liver into chemicals normally found in the body in smaller amounts, such as uric acid. There is also an increase in minerals such as potassium and phosphorus, which seriously upsets the body's chemistry and causes the kidneys to malfunction and the electrical system of the heart to slow. The gastrointestinal system, the nervous system, and the muscular system are also affected.

WARNING SIGNS

SPECIAL

CONCERNS

The symptoms of TLS vary depending on the stage of the syndrome. The symptoms of the early stages of TLS include:

- tiredness

- loss of appetite

- nausea

- muscle weakness

- cramps

- pain over the kidneys

- vomiting and diarrhea

Symptoms become more severe if the situation progresses. They may include:

- mild numbness sometimes leading to muscle irritability and finally convulsions

- memory loss

- hallucinations

- drop in heart rate and blood pressure (after initially increasing)

Oncologists are well aware that people who receive chemotherapy for rapidly developing cancers are at risk for TLS, which is one reason why they measure the amount of uric acid, calcium, phosphorous, and other minerals before treatment begins. TLS is best prevented and treated by keeping the person well hydrated so they urinate frequently and by identifying mineral imbalances early and correcting them. Allopurinol, a medication that prevents uric acid from being formed, is given both to prevent the syndrome and treat it. Attempting to keep the urine alkaline with drugs or intravenous sodium bicarbonate is a controversial remedy. In severe situations dialysis to compensate for the failing kidneys may be necessary.

Blockage of the Superior Vena Cava

The superior vena cava is one of three vessels through which blood flows from the body into the upper right chamber or atrium of the heart. All the blood from the upper part of the body returns to the heart through this one large vein, so any change in pressure in the veins of the head, neck, upper arms, or chest can inhibit blood flow through the superior vena cava. A blockage from a tumor or blood clot anywhere along this vital route can also slow blood flow, with serious consequences. The most common blockage is caused by compression from a primary or metastatic tumor in the mediastinum (breastbone).

The syndrome that results—superior vena cava syndrome (SVCS)—is not usually fatal and so may not be considered a true emergency unless there is swelling of the brain or difficulty breathing. SVCS occurs mostly in people with cancer, particularly those with lung cancer, lymphoma involving the mediastinum, metastatic breast cancer, and advanced lung cancer. The incidence is relatively rare, however, affecting only about 3 to 4 percent of patients.

When the superior vena cava is blocked, blood pools in the vessel and eventually may be forced to flow through other veins into the right atrium. However, since the vessels here are so much smaller than the vena cava, less blood can enter the heart and a series of serious problems may result. Since the heart is receiving less blood, it puts out less blood, which affects the delivery of oxygen to all parts of the body. Furthermore, the increased pressure in the blood vessels causes fluid to collect in the sac that contains the heart as well as in the lungs. The face, neck, upper chest, and upper arms may swell. Eventually the walls of the blood vessels are damaged, and the blood itself may be altered.

A chest x-ray can confirm SVCS in most cases. A CT scan can provide even more detailed information about the area around the mediastinum and the condition of the blood vessels.

Treatment depends on the cause of the obstruction and the person's prognosis. For instance, if a blood clot has formed next to a catheter that is delivering chemotherapy, a drug to dissolve the clot can be injected. If the cause is a tumor, radiation therapy or chemotherapy may be used to shrink it. Surgery can be done to insert a stint, or tube, to keep the vein open and relieve the obstruction. Sometimes the obstruction can be bypassed with an operation in which a section of vein from the leg is used to create a new passageway from another major vein of the neck or shoulder directly to the atrium of the heart.

Immediate treatment usually involves relieving the symptoms with oxygen, bed rest, and drugs such as steroids and diuretics to relieve swelling.

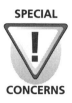

SPECIAL

CONCERNS

WARNING SIGNS

The initial symptoms of SVCS are usually vague and generalized (as they are with most cancer emergencies). The following are some of the most common symptoms:

- shortness of breath

- dry cough

- dizziness

- feeling of fullness in the upper body (that is relieved when lying down or bending over)

- neck vein may appear enlarged

- veins of the chest and arms sometimes appear more prominent than usual

- noticeable swelling of the face and around the eyes

- face may look flushed or tinged with blue

Symptoms become more severe and obvious if the condition progresses. The following are signs of airway obstruction and swelling of the brain:

- vision problems

- difficulty breathing

- hoarseness

- confusion

- diminished consciousness

Future Complications

As more people continue to live longer with cancer, it's expected that the incidence of complications and emergencies will increase. Although cancer emergencies are stressful, uncomfortable, and often frightening, many can be treated successfully, particularly if the problem is detected before acute illness occurs.

26

Coping with Your Cancer

Not so many years ago, coping with cancer meant preparing for the end. Today, most men, women, and children who have cancer also have a future. Cure rates continue to improve, and people with cancer are living longer. For them as well as for their families, coping means learning to maintain the highest quality of life while living with a chronic illness. And that means preserving self-esteem and being able to find significance and pleasure in life, being comfortable, and enjoying important relationships in the face of the emotional and practical challenges of living with cancer, which can be enormous—and sometimes overwhelming—from the start.

No two people or families deal with the cancer experience in the same way. All come with their own history of handling crisis, threat, and challenge. Yet as more attention is paid to helping individuals and families cope with cancer, researchers report that most people do cope remarkably well, whether the cancer is advanced, successfully cured, or becomes chronic. A number of people with cancer and those close to them even report that the experience helped them improve the quality of their lives. These people say that through this experience, which they would never have wished upon themselves or their families, they were able to find new meaning in life, solidify relationships, and discover what is important to them and what is not.

Through the study of how individual people and their networks of family and friends confront the problems that cancer creates, much has been learned about styles of coping and how they help or hinder. The chapters that focus on coping in this book provide help for people with cancer and those who are important to them, including children, to comprehend and bolster their own ways of dealing with the crisis and challenge of cancer (see also Chapters 27 and 28).

Factors in Coping

Coping refers to how a person or a family comes to terms with an illness, makes decisions and solves problems as they occur, and adapts to life changes while still feeling good about themselves. A person who copes well with cancer and a person who doesn't will have very different experiences, even if they have the same type of cancer progressing in a similar way.

The following are a number of coping factors from which you can determine your style of dealing with cancer and its effects on your life. There is no "right" approach. However, you may be able to look at these factors and decide if some of the ways in which you are trying to manage may be causing other problems or may simply not be working.

Emotions

It is normal and appropriate to experience a range of difficult and mixed feelings throughout your illness and recovery, such as anxiety, anger, depression, guilt, sadness, worry, fear, hopelessness, and grief. Working through your feelings is essential to successful coping, which allows you to proceed with treatment and recovery. Anyone who experiences continual, overwhelming distress after learning their cancer diagnosis, for example, will be unable to focus on gathering information about their cancer and treatment or make critical decisions. Someone who feels unremitting rage (at the unfairness of it all, at God, at the terrible disruption of present opportunities and future plans) may blame doctors and treatment providers and refuse to follow medical advice or alienate those trying to help. During treatment, a woman or man who is distressed at losing hair because of chemotherapy may avoid the company of others, who could serve as an important distraction and source of support during the difficult weeks of treatment.

Such people, and indeed anyone with cancer, can benefit from learning emotional regulation or distress-tolerance skills, as well as techniques to manage anxiety (see Chapter 27). Cancer is a new kind of stress or series of stresses that most people aren't prepared for, and you may need to learn new ways of handling your emotions, thought processes, and behaviors. If your distress is overwhelming, counseling can be helpful (see Chapter 8).

Coping with emotions does not mean pretending that you're not upset when you actually are. Never feel that you must bottle up your feelings, be ashamed of them, or feel "positive" all the time. Talking with another person about your feelings, writing in a journal, and finding some quiet time for yourself may all be important. Some people find that quiet, introspective activities such as yoga or meditation improve their sense of well being.

Flexibility

In general, those who cope well are flexible, so they can adapt more easily to uncertainty and change. No one wants to have an ostomy. However, someone who can grieve for the loss of the natural elimination function following surgery but accept the change as a way of getting on with living will achieve a much higher quality of life than someone who can't accept his or her altered body. Someone whose self-image is based on being the family breadwinner and who can't stand having a spouse or child assume this role during his or her illness will suffer far more distress than will someone who perceives that adapting to the changing circumstances is for the good of all.

Control

Having a sense of control over what happens to you and those you love makes a difficult experience easier to bear. Gathering information about the illness, choosing doctors and hospitals, participating in treatment decisions, and knowing what to expect can counteract feelings that you are at the mercy of others and of fate and that nothing can be done to improve the situation. Learning that you can control pain, symptoms, and side effects can be extremely empowering. However, it is important to be realistic about your efforts. You don't have to relentlessly gather information, ask question after question, and make all the decisions. Rather, you can gain control by making sure you have a treatment team that you can trust to recommend and provide the best care for your situation.

It's possible to gather too much information, however, and feel inundated with too many details. Also, coping by seeking information may work well during the diagnostic and treatment phases of illness but may be less effective for dealing with uncertainty after the treatment ends.

Similarly, staying in control of what is happening by being extremely vigilant about symptoms and side effects can become problematic during periods of remission or recovery for those who have become highly sensitive to every bodily sensation.

It is important to be able to distinguish what you can control from what you cannot. Try to focus on what you can change and you will have a greater sense of control.

People who cannot tolerate the changes taking place in their bodies will suffer stress and anxiety just when they need to devote their energy to taking care of themselves.

Hopefulness and a Positive Outlook

Hope has been called "probably the single most important factor needed for living with cancer." Hoping for the best possible outcome often motivates people to take good care of themselves and to follow medical advice. Men and women who are hopeful usually look on the bright side to see the glass as half full rather than half empty. They therefore can find meaning in situations in which others would find less to live for. Because they believe that things will work out, they attempt to solve the problems that occur. And because they try, they accomplish more than those who don't make an effort.

People who can find something good or meaningful in even the most difficult experiences and who can concentrate on what they still have rather than on what they've lost often feel spiritually enriched, more involved in their daily lives, and more connected to others. They also report that living with cancer has made them better people, showed them who and what really matters, and helped them appreciate life more.

The ability to see something positive in most experiences can be learned. To kindle hope, look around your life and find the smallest things that are worth living for. Set short-term goals that you can achieve, such as attending a child's or grandchild's recital, being around people you care for, or doing something you enjoy during a comfortable hour.

Try to take one day at a time and "live in the now." Focus on what is meaningful and enjoyable in the present rather than on what you risk losing in the future. When you have a bad day, don't read more meaning into it than when you have a good day.

Some people initiate positive changes in their lifestyle during this time. If you've been sedentary, you might start a walking program (see Chapter 19) or pay more attention to eating a nutritious diet (see Chapter 18).

But beware of any coercion you may feel, from yourself or others, that you must feel positive and cheerful about what is happening to you or to force a coping style on yourself that just isn't you. Don't fake it. Keeping your true feelings inside and feeling guilty about them will make it much harder to cope with what's going on, to deal with other people honestly and intimately, and to get the help you need. Much of the pressure to be positive comes from the unfounded belief that emotions are what made you sick and what will prevent you from getting better.

Trying to keep a hopeful, positive attitude and making each day count often lessens the impact of cancer on you and those close to you and may make it easier to solve problems. But it will not make a difference between illness and recovery. Similarly, less than perfect coping skills will not trigger a recurrence.

Feeling hopeless, powerless, and convinced that you have nothing to live for can be a sign of depression. Depression can be treated and hope restored even in gravely ill people (see Chapter 27). Although a fatalistic, resigned attitude cannot foster a fighting spirit or a high quality of life in the early stages of illness, such a coping style is the way some tolerate the approaching end of life.

Having a positive attitude is not the same as wishful thinking, which is simply pretending that something good is going to happen rather than doing something about it (see page 427, *Denial*).

Fighting Spirit

People with a fighting spirit take on cancer as a battle to be won. At times they may be angry and hostile, just as warriors are, but they direct that energy into finding out everything they can about their illness and demanding to have the best possible care and, of course, to be involved in decisions. They rush headlong toward every hurdle in their path. They believe that they have power over what happens to them and use all "weapons" at hand. With their sense of entitlement, they are not necessarily "good" patients or easy to get along with. They don't passively agree to everything that happens to them, and they forcefully insist on what they want even if it's inconvenient. But they do tend to get the best out of their health care system because they insist on it.

Even if you are not by nature a fighter, with your permission a friend or family member who is can accomplish as much on your behalf.

TIPS AND

ADVICE

I Can Cope

The American Cancer Society (ACS) has designed three types of courses to help people with cancer and their families understand the emotional challenges of cancer. By helping people understand various aspects of their cancer experience and develop the necessary skills for coping with the different tasks before them, the ACS believes they will make informed decisions about their care with their doctors and become partners with the members of their health care team.

The courses are available in communities throughout the United States and in some other countries. Health care professionals who have completed the ACS training program conduct the courses, with the exception of the option modules, which may be facilitated by people knowledgeable in the topics.

Classic Course

For eight weeks, participants meet weekly for two hours. Topics covered include cancer information and questions about human anatomy, cancer diagnosis, treatment, side effects, new research, communication, emotions, sexuality, self-esteem, and community resources. The program provides facts, encouragement, practical hints through presentation and class discussions. There is no charge for attending the classes.

Compact Course

The sixteen-hour classic course has been condensed to eight hours for those who cannot make the commitment the longer course requires. Because it's shorter, there is less group interaction and more self-motivated learning is required.

Option Modules

These single-topic, two-hour sessions focus on a specific aspect of cancer, such as pain relief or financial concerns. Sessions are developed as needs are identified. The modules may be offered to those who have attended the Classic or Compact Course, or they may be freestanding, one-shot seminars.

Problem Solving

There are many ways to approach the problems that cancer presents. At one extreme is the style of "taking the bull by the horns" and seeking information and opinions, evaluating the options, setting priorities, considering advantages and disadvantages, and ultimately making choices. If one way doesn't work, the people who employ this problem-solving style try another. Although not everyone can meet this ideal—particularly when feeling ill, anxious, isolated, or sapped of strength—attempting to confront both large and everyday problems as they occur keeps them from getting out of hand (see pages 428–429, *How to Make an Informed Decision*).

Good problem solvers attempt to reduce problems to a manageable size and solve the larger challenges one step at a time.

The other extreme—doing nothing and passively letting things happen— is rarely satisfying and usually creates more problems, which become harder to resolve.

It often is easier to take a team approach (see Chapter 6). Even if someone else is the information-gatherer or decision-maker, be sure to make clear your personal opinions and preferences or risk getting stuck with solutions that aren't suitable for you.

Of course, not all problems can be resolved. "Nevertheless, more problems are solved by awareness and acceptance than by disavowal, avoidance, and denial," observed a psychiatrist who has studied coping in people with cancer.

Denial

Denial—the ability to proceed as if you or a family member doesn't have cancer—can be either a helpful or a harmful coping style, depending on the behavior it produces. Denial is destructive when, for instance, a person with a lump or troubling symptoms delays going to a doctor because "there's nothing wrong with me." People who exhibit this kind of maladaptive denial may not show up for treatment, seek or retain information that they need to know, ask questions, make necessary plans for themselves or others for whom they are responsible, and sometimes may not experience the emotions that are appropriate to their situation.

Family members or friends who are in denial don't visit or pretend everything is just fine when they do, don't listen, don't provide needed help, and thus strain the relationship. They are in denial because the reality is too terrifying for them to confront.

But the ability to keep the frightening truth at some distance can also be beneficial, as long as you do what needs to be done. Minimizing the seriousness of your diagnosis can provide time for the reality to sink in while you seek second opinions and settle on a treatment plan. Making plans for the future, even if others think they're unrealistic, can be motivating and interesting, as long as you don't set yourself up to fail (see page 433, *Coping with Disappointment and Frustration*). Going about your life at home or at work as if you or someone close to you doesn't have cancer or as if it's not serious can minimize your fear and anxiety and contribute to a high quality of life. But make sure you do what needs to be done to solve the real-life problems that, denial or no denial, won't go away.

TIPS AND

ADVICE

How to Make an Informed Decision

When there's a lot on your mind, it's hard to focus on one problem at a time. It often helps to write things down. Use the following chart to organize your thoughts and to help you take the necessary steps to reach a decision. Write your responses on a separate piece of paper.

1. What are the problems I need to resolve now? (List all that come to mind, in any order.)

2. How important are these problems? (To set priorities, number each item on your list, from most important to least important right now.)

3. Beginning with my highest-priority problem, what are all the alternative solutions I can think of? (List all that come to mind, in any order.)

4. Do I need more information about any of them or about other possible solutions?

    If you answered yes to this question, what can you do or who can you ask to find out more?

5. What are the advantages and disadvantages of each alternative I have thought of? (List all that apply.)

	Advantages	Disadvantages
Solution 1		

	Advantages	**Disadvantages**
Solution 2		
Solution 3		

6. Considering all the advantages and disadvantages, which option seems to make most sense?

7. Whose help or contribution do I need in order to implement this choice?

8. What do I need to do now to get it going?

9. When will I take the first step? (Set a realistic schedule.)

10. I still can't seem to make up my mind or take action. What's bothering me? (Write down everything that comes to mind. Then relax and try again when you're ready.)

Repeat steps 3 through 10 for every problem on your list, in order of importance.

People with cancer as well as their family members need to be aware, however, that the desire to play down the seriousness of the illness may prevent others from providing emotional or practical support. In the past, family members and sometimes medical staff would not tell the patient the truth. In this situation, patients were not given the opportunity to make an informed decision about what would happen to them nor were they able to take care of unfinished business. Now the pendulum has swung in the other direction. Each person should be allowed to deal with "the truth" in his or her own way.

Support

Seeking the support, assistance, and companionship of other people is critical in coping with cancer. Can you open up to others, ask for help, share your concerns? Many people with cancer have no one close to them. Others would rather keep the diagnosis to themselves or be alone rather than endure uncaring or frightened reactions of others toward their illness (see page 434, *Stigma and Unfortunate Reactions from Other People*). Even those who find that others rally around them when they or a family member is ill can benefit from self-help, group support, and professional assistance available for people with cancer. One of the principal advantages of support groups is help with coping (see Chapter 8).

Faith and spirituality can be an enormous source of strength to people in crisis. For those who already participate in an organized religion, meeting the challenges of cancer sometimes deepens their faith. For those who have not contemplated their beliefs before, this may be a time to seek support and solace in some spiritual practice. Most spiritual organizations have ministers or counselors with special training in helping people cope with cancer.

TIPS AND

ADVICE

Forget Your Troubles?

Yes, when you can. Sure, there's plenty to worry about with cancer. But try not to dwell on what can't be changed. And by all means, permit yourself full enjoyment at those times when you're feeling okay. Have fun. Relish a good laugh. Reward yourself after each step you complete in your treatment. Activities that take your mind off your illness may help. Continue your enjoyable activities. And if you cannot, find new activities. Take walks with your friends or listen to your favorite music. Taking on a new interest or challenge can also give you a sense of accomplishment that helps relieve stress.

Compliment yourself and others for everyone's endurance, determination, strength, and caring. Celebrate birthdays, holidays, and anniversaries just as before.

Besides providing some relief from the concerns of cancer treatment and recovery, these moments of enjoyment and reward can energize you to get through difficult times.

Coping Challenges

Although the cancer experience is rarely the same for any two people, there are predictable critical periods that challenge everyone's emotional resources. If at any time during your illness your efforts at coping seem to fail, help is always available. Ask for it. Social workers, nurses, your doctor, a pastor, or a chaplain are good people to start with.

Diagnosis

Diagnosis is, of course, a time of enormous shock for most people, except perhaps some who are elderly or have already been in compromised health for a long time. Despite their great emotional distress, all people need to absorb complicated information and make weighty decisions quickly, a task for which most of us, even in the best of health, would not feel equipped. The need for others' support is great at a time when many people are hesitant to share the news or wish to retreat into themselves. Joining a support group or talking with people who have been through this experience can be very helpful.

Treatment

When their treatment commences, many people are faced with having to reorganize their family lives and work responsibilities and to deal with insurance and finances, all while preparing to deal with effects of surgery, radiation, chemotherapy, and or other treatments. Those who have a difficult time enduring the treatments, emotionally or physically, may be tempted not to continue and, instead, to "let nature take its course." Body image, self-esteem, and intimate relationships may be sorely challenged, and many people feel at this stage that they will never be themselves again. But these are not insurmountable problems.

Coping with the side effects of even the most aggressive treatments is much easier for those who have explored in advance all the new developments in pain and symptom control that have become available in recent years. Some of these methods and technologies may even help prevent unnecessary discomfort and disability. But because they are relatively new, they may not be routinely offered to people who do not know about them and seek them out.

Resuming Normal Routines When Treatment Ends

The end of treatment is a cause for celebration, and some people plan a special event to mark this turning point in their lives. Although the emphasis is on the "end" of a physically and emotionally demanding experience, this is also a new beginning. And it's also a period of transition with challenges of its own.

For instance, although the active treatment is behind you, there may still be an uncertainty about the future and long-term or permanent physical disabilities that you and your family must manage. Now that the immediate crisis is over, those close to you may start letting feelings surface that they thought were too upsetting to express before. Tensions may arise as you attempt to take back some of the responsibilities that you had been forced to relinquish. Working through these challenges together as a family can bring you to a new and gratifying level of intimacy with your loved ones, but it may not come easily. Still, cancer survivors say that they often discover the strength and unity of their families.

Children may find it especially difficult to deal with the change that your cancer has brought into their lives. Since they may not be able to identify or articulate their concerns, fears, and anger, they may express them in unhealthy ways. Reassure them (in a way that is appropriate for their age) that you understand that they are upset and that such feelings are a normal reaction to all that they have been through. If there are permanent changes in their lives as a result of your cancer, be as straightforward as you can about what they can expect. Children need to see the world as stable and predictable, and you can help by giving their lives structure and safety in every area possible.

On a personal level, you may find yourself confronting some surprising emotions. Though you may be thrilled to be regaining your independence, be prepared, too, for feeling a little let down as the attention shifts away from you and onto other issues and people. You may even feel abandoned and as though you're facing the future alone. Those with lasting disabilities may find adjusting to their limitations especially difficult, as medical and personal support is no longer so constant. And there is a natural grieving period for the loss of what once was taken for granted.

This period of powerful emotions will pass, so be patient with yourself and try not to inflict self-blame for not "getting over this" more quickly. It's possible that with the pain and suffering of your treatment behind you, negative feelings that you couldn't acknowledge before may now come forth. The same coping skills that helped you deal with the diagnosis can be helpful now as well—doing relaxation exercises, keeping a journal, and taking part in support groups are not just emergency measures. And, as before, if you experience any of the warning signs of depression (see Chapter 27), seek help.

Recurrence and Relapse

The return of your cancer produces the same shock and distress of the initial diagnosis, but now your faith that you can win this battle may falter—even though this is not necessarily the medical reality. Some people blame themselves, as if they could have prevented it with a different sort of behavior or attitude. Even for those who coped well with the initial round of treatment, having to go through it all again, perhaps even more aggressively, can be discouraging. And whatever success you may have had at establishing new directions or taking up where you left off may now come to a halt.

In addition, all the practical problems of being in treatment return, and your supporters may not be as available to help out this time around. They may be exhausted by their initial efforts or so frightened that they can't face you. (For more information about recurrence, see Chapter 30).

Those who enter clinical trials face still other coping challenges, not least of which is dealing with the uncertainty of a treatment that might not be as effective as other treatments. They must also deal with a treatment that has not yet proved to be successful.

Coping with Disappointment and Frustration

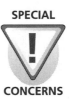

SPECIAL

CONCERNS

Most disappointment and frustration evolve from unmet expectations. What you hope for is up to you. But if you spend all your time worrying about the worst possible outcomes of tests or treatments, you will sap your energy, deplete your strength for dealing with whatever the results may be, and waste precious time that you could use for fun or productivity. And worry won't change the outcome.

You must believe in yourself so that even if things don't go well, you can survive those times with your spirit alive, ready for the next challenge.

WARNING SIGNS

- You are constantly looking into the future, to the total exclusion of the present, (or conversely, you completely block out anything to do with the future because you might be disappointed).

- You keep pretending that everything will be all right, when inside you feel just the opposite.

- You avoid positive feelings because you fear being let down.

- You are setting unrealistic goals and then sinking emotionally because you are unable to meet them.

- You feel that only a physical change will make you feel better emotionally.

Advancing Illness

Maintaining hope while undergoing treatments and their side effects is a major challenge, especially for those who lack information about the purpose and consequences of continuing treatment. For example, many people are confused between interventions that could cure their cancer and those that relieve symptoms.

Accepting that your life span is limited yet still has meaning is a fundamental coping task. You and your family may be afraid to talk about it and to make appropriate decisions; as a result you may feel distant from one another, frightened, and unprepared.

Pain and other unpleasant symptoms and physical limitations can leave you and your family feeling helpless and overwhelmed. Those people whose coping style is not assertive may not insist on receiving adequate relief, for which many approaches are available.

Information about options and financing for continuing care at this stage of illness is of prime importance. Support groups, social workers, oncology nurses, and the other sources of formal support can be very important (see Chapter 8). Emotionally and spiritually, groups can help improve your quality of life, alleviate your anxiety and depression, and help maintain your feelings of self-worth and well being, to which everyone is entitled at all stages of life.

Stigma and Unfortunate Reactions from Other People

Of all the coping challenges to prepare for when living the best you can with cancer, there's one that catches nearly everybody by surprise: the distancing, insensitive, hurtful, and sometimes rude reactions of other people. It seems inexplicable that at a time when you would expect your relatives, friends, neighbors, coworkers, and acquaintances to turn out in force, some never call or visit. Others won't get too close to you; still others seem to blame you for your illness; and some who do visit are nervous and uncomfortable and won't mention your illness. Some just don't know what to say.

The best way to cope with such behavior and to protect your feelings is to understand that many people are afraid of cancer and of their own vulnerability. Hard as it may seem to comprehend, their reaction has little to do with you personally.

Cancer still carries a stigma in some people's minds, and so they may feel embarrassed or uncomfortable around you or they may pick up on your own worries that you are no longer "socially acceptable." But beyond the stigma is the fear that many people have of their own mortality, which may be triggered by your illness or that of a family member. Or they may be so afraid of their own pain in seeing you suffer or of losing you that they pretend you don't exist, deny that you're ill, or withdraw emotionally from you.

When, What, and Whom to Tell

Telling anyone, from new acquaintances to potential employers, that you have or have had cancer is fraught with risks, from ostracism to outright discrimination. Before telling anyone, however, examine your own feelings about the illness. If you feel down deep that you are "tainted" or unworthy because of your sickness, you will probably communicate these feelings to others and may influence their response.

Dealing with Other People's Reactions

"Get cancer and you'll find out who your friends really are," many people say who have been through it. Indeed, besides continually reminding yourself that others' unfortunate reactions are not a reflection on you, a good coping strategy is to let go of the people who disappoint you and turn toward those who come through for you. You may find that some of the most understanding and helpful people are those who have had a serious illness themselves and have no fear of reaching out to you. Support and self-help groups may be good ways of finding people—potential new friends, if you're open to it—who have had such an experience.

Joining such groups may indirectly improve your relationships with those close to you. At times, your family and friends may react insensitively simply because they are so stressed by the disruptions to their own daily lives that they may have limited tolerance for more difficult talk about cancer. Your counterparts in the support group, however, share your intense need to analyze facts and feelings.

Other coping strategies include the following:

- Educate others about cancer. Let them know it's not catching, for example, or a certain death sentence. Accurate information is always a good way to counteract fear and ignorance that fuel inappropriate responses.

- If the person is important to you, try to talk about your feelings of disappointment or letdown. Tell the person how he or she can help.

- Encourage others to be there in whatever small ways they can. Ask for something that this person is good at, like choosing interesting books or videos, helping you figure out a bank statement or insurance bill, fixing a leaky faucet, or just talking on the telephone.

- Talk about what it's like to have cancer. Some people may be avoiding you because they don't know what to ask or to say or are afraid to bring anything up that may be painful to you. Encourage them to ask questions.

- Understand and forgive. Rather than expending precious energy in anger or hurt feelings, compassion for the person's fear or discomfort may make you feel better.

In Your Personal Life

It probably makes little sense not to tell your friends and family members that you have or have had cancer. Concealing it can be very stressful at a time when you need their emotional and practical support. How they react to you will be a test of your relationship, of course.

Sharing the information with casual or new acquaintances can be quite difficult. Consider how the other person might interpret or respond to the information. Is his or her response likely to be hurtful or helpful?

TIPS AND

ADVICE

Single with Cancer

It can be especially difficult for single people who want to go on about their lives as if they have been untouched by the disease to know what and when to tell people, especially new romantic partners. Here's what Susan Nessim, cancer survivor and founder of the Cancervive support group, and co-author Judith Ellis suggest in their book *Cancervive: The Challenge of Life After Cancer:*

There is certainly nothing wrong with being forthright; it allows you to set the stage for an honest and sincere relationship. If this approach results in high attrition in your romantic life, however, you might rethink your tactics. It could be that you are using this "first strike" approach as a way of protecting yourself or perhaps you are using your history of cancer as a way of testing the other person. "I've had cancer; take me or leave me" is the message implicit in this approach. Try to determine what is motivating your need to tell potential partners of your illness.

On the other side of this issue are the survivors who have found that honesty is not the best policy—at least not on the first or second date. Experience has shown them that most people are threatened when confronted with the topic of cancer early on in a relationship. It could be that you are hitting your friend with too much too soon—before both of you have had a chance to establish bonds of affection and trust.

There is another advantage to waiting. If somewhere down the road, the two of you part ways, you will have a better idea as to whether it was cancer or simply "bad chemistry" that caused the romance to sputter out. For many survivors, it is important to make this distinction. But that's hard to do if you have made a point of revealing your cancer early in the game.

The issue of disclosure is a personal one, only you can know if and when to share this part of who you are. Most survivors say it all comes down to sizing up the other person and then gauging whether the relationship has potential for longevity.

At Work

Although it may not be wise to volunteer a cancer history at a job interview because employers may fear that you will not be productive or that you will increase their health insurance costs, always tell the truth if you are asked about your medical history. Provide a brief explanation of the illness and your recovery. Express confidence in your skills, outlook, and energy. Don't over-explain or the interviewer may think that you're trying to conceal something. Be aware that there are laws protecting people with cancer against illegal discrimination, and if you need assistance in understanding the laws in your state, your local chapter of the American Cancer Society can help (see also Chapter 22).

Even if you have no problem getting or keeping a job, be prepared for ignorant and fearful attitudes of coworkers. Educating them about the illness and demonstrating how well you have come through it may help. If you have a new job, you may want to size up your coworkers before confiding in them, in the same way you would before revealing any personal information. If your company has a Human Resources office and your cancer history is already known, ask for their help in distributing information about cancer should you run into unpleasant reactions.

For your own sake, remember that most people at work know somebody with cancer, probably in their own families. In other words, you're not the only one on the planet with this disease. If you can talk about your history comfortably, you may well encourage their respect, and they may turn to you when they need information.

27

Coping with Stress, Fear, Anxiety, and Depression

Dealing with the emotions triggered by having cancer is as important to a person's comfort and recovery as managing the physical symptoms. Stress, fear, anxiety, sadness, confusion, and feelings of helplessness or depression are common at all stages of the illness, beginning with the first feeling that something might be wrong. At the very least, these reactions can lower pain tolerance and make the treatments harder to endure, diminishing quality of life, the strength or desire to fight the illness, and the ability to make the best decisions.

Claims that negative attitudes cause cancer have not been proven. Indeed, studies of stress and cancer have lead to conflicting results. Chronic, unremitting stress does suppress the immune system, but there is no definitive evidence that any stress-reduction technique such as imagery, hypnosis, or relaxation affects survival.

On the other hand, research does suggest that participation in support groups and educational interventions helps reduce tension, anxiety, and fatigue, increases compliance with treatment, and improves the quality of life for people with cancer.

Normal or Not

It is normal for someone with cancer to experience emotional upheavals for short periods of time, especially around crisis points, such as the time of diagnosis, the beginning or end of treatment, the anniversary of the treatment, or learning that the cancer has advanced. There are techniques that can make this emotional discomfort easier to tolerate when you are distressed.

Unremitting or severe mental anguish, despair, or the desire to die are not normal feelings. And having cancer does not mean you should resign yourself to feeling at the end of your rope. Anyone who tells you, "Of course you're depressed—you have cancer" is misinformed. Even among those with advanced illness, extreme mental anguish and the wish to die are symptoms of clinical depression, a condition that can be treated. Painful, continuing psychological states that last for several weeks can be relieved and treatment should always be investigated. Regaining a sense of mastery is critical to maintaining a good quality of life that can be yours at every stage of illness.

Anxiety

Anxiety is an emotional response to fear. When you are anxious, your body responds as if it is under physical attack. Your heart beats faster, your blood pressure increases, muscles tense, and stress hormones such as adrenaline are released into the system. Ordinarily, when the perceived danger passes, these systems return to normal. But in chronic stress, the body remains in a state of arousal, and over time, this can affect the immune system. Among anxiety's many mind and body symptoms are muscle tension, sweaty palms, pounding heart, difficulty breathing, racing pulse, headaches, jitteriness, irritability, upset stomach, excessive worrying, difficulty concentrating, indecision, and panic.

Anxiety can occur at many critical junctures throughout the cancer experience. Diagnosis and recurrence are potentially the most anxious times for people with cancer. Many fear being disabled, disfigured, or dependent; losing income or significant relationships; losing control or experiencing pain; or dying. Sometimes the anxiety associated with these fears is mixed with depressed feelings, and it can be hard to sort them all out. If you are having difficulty, it may be advisable to consult a mental health professional who is knowledgeable about cancer care (see page 440, *Getting Help*).

Anxiety that you may have suffered before your cancer diagnosis may increase or recur under the strain of being sick. Anyone with a history of phobias or panic disorders is advised to consult a mental health professional before treatment begins to plan strategies for managing the situations that trigger these reactions. Stress inoculation, as such a preventive approach is called, has been shown to reduce distress and maximize coping.

Anticipatory Anxiety

Fear of treatment, doctor visits, and tests may also produce anxiety. Anticipatory anxiety refers to the distress and associated physical symptoms that occur before surgery and such procedures as needle biopsies, endoscopies, sigmoidoscopies, radiation treatment, chemotherapy, and scans. Magnetic resonance imaging (MRI) requires that you lie immobilized in a narrow cylinder for a prolonged period, and people with even mild claustrophobia may become apprehensive in such circumstances. Before chemotherapy, many people experience anticipatory anxiety in the form of nausea and vomiting.

Physical Causes

Hormone-secreting tumors found in cancers of the pancreas, lungs, thyroid, and adrenal glands often produce anxiety and sometimes even panic. Anxiety also is associated with liver cancer and with certain cancer-fighting drugs, including the corticosteroids. In such instances, doctors may prescribe antianxiety medication (a tranquilizer) that is compatible with other aspects of the treatment.

Inadequately controlled pain produces overwhelming anxiety that the suffering will be prolonged. Often simply adjusting the pain medication can help relieve this distress, as can the numerous techniques of behavioral medicine, described later in this chapter, that help you deal with pain (see Chapter 23).

Getting Help

Ups and downs in mood are expected for anyone who is coping with a life-threatening disease. Action to reduce anxiety is always recommended to control unpleasant emotions, reduce tension, and provide a sense of direction, control, and hope. Some mind-body techniques ease mild anxiety, but if the bad feelings and physical symptoms last longer than two weeks, are getting worse, become overwhelming, or are preventing you from taking an active role in your care, professional help is needed.

Behavioral techniques, counseling, and/or medication may be prescribed to help you feel more comfortable, relaxed, and able to cope. Mild antianxiety medications, such as diazepam (Valium), and a number of mind-body techniques, including progressive relaxation, systematic desensitization, distraction, guided imagery, and hypnosis, have also been used successfully to manage these symptoms.

Depression

As with intermittent anxiety, occasional depressed feelings are not unusual in people living with cancer. Depression that does not go away, however, can and should be treated. Symptoms include unremitting sadness, feelings of loss, hopelessness, irritability, irregular sleep patterns (insomnia or sleeping too much), difficulty concentrating, a desire to be alone, and diminished interest in sex.

Appetite and weight changes and a lack of vim and vigor are key symptoms of depression as well, but they are also common symptoms of cancer and its treatment. Many people with cancer and sometimes even their caregivers assume that these changes mean the cancer is worsening, but that is not always the case. In fact, depression can be the sole culprit, and with appropriate treatment the depression will lift, taking these alarming symptoms with it and giving you much more hope and satisfaction in your day-to-day life.

Depression and Loss

Learning that you have cancer almost always produces feelings of loss, anger, and fear. These emotions may deepen when the treatment ends or if the cancer becomes advanced. Sometimes a depressed mood is triggered by a form of cancer or cancer treatment that strikes at a basic source of your identity or self-esteem. For example, a woman who has a mastectomy or a hysterectomy may experience a blow to her sense of herself as a woman. Or, having a prostate gland removed or irradiated might undermine a man's self-concept; or bone cancer could challenge a professional athlete's meaning in life. Many people become sad or even despondent in response to disfiguring treatments or to hair loss from chemotherapy (see Chapter 20).

Physical Factors

A depressed mood may also have a physical origin. For example, depression is a common symptom of pancreatic cancer and certain brain cancers and, like anxiety, is a side effect of inadequately controlled pain. Pain can have a depressing effect, and in turn, a depressed mood makes pain harder to tolerate.

Systemic imbalances, such as thyroid problems or nutritional deficiencies, may cause mood changes. Some anticancer medications have a depressive effect. So do some of the medications prescribed to control nausea. Steroid drugs may cause emotional upsets ranging from minor mood swings to severe depression and suicidal feelings.

Getting Help

It is not always easy to tell whether a depressed mood is associated with the cancer itself or its treatment, or whether it is a temporary emotional reaction that is adaptive under the circumstances, or a sign of a more serious clinical depression that may have nothing to do with the cancer. A thorough diagnosis by a mental health professional who is knowledgeable about cancer is essential if symptoms last longer than two weeks; if feelings of guilt or hopelessness arise, or self-esteem plummets; or if you have a prior history of depression. If you are unable to eat or sleep for several days, call your doctor. Thoughts of suicide demand immediate attention. Any prolonged depression destroys the quality of life that you are entitled to at any stage of illness, even at the end of life. It also robs you of the ability to make reasoned, sensible decisions.

SPECIAL

!

CONCERNS

Recognizing Depression

Being depressed is different from just being sad. Depression permeates your whole existence and causes an emotional paralysis that can devastate you if you're not prepared. The symptoms of clinical depression are listed below. Family and friends should be alert for these symptoms in someone with cancer and help him or her seek an evaluation for depression when indicated.

Symptoms of clinical depression include the following:

- persistent sadness or "empty" feelings
- loss of interest or pleasure in usual activities
- loss of energy, feeling "slowed down"
- insomnia, restless sleep, or much more sleep than usual
- eating disturbances (loss of appetite or overeating)
- inability to make decisions or concentrate
- feelings of worthlessness or hopelessness
- irritability
- excessive crying
- chronic aches and pains for no apparent reason
- thoughts of death or suicide, suicide attempts

Call the doctor if:

- you have thoughts of death or suicide
- you cannot eat or sleep and continually feel uninterested in activities of daily living
- you feel like you are unable to breathe, are sweating, and feel restless
- you are unable to experience pleasure in anything

Sometimes one or more of the many types of antidepressant medications can relieve the symptoms. Likewise, counseling or psychotherapy alone can be an effective approach for some people. More often, however, persistent, severe depression is best managed through a combination of medication, counseling, mind-body interventions, and/or group support.

Although any medical doctor can prescribe antidepressants, a psychiatrist generally has more experience in administering such medications and monitoring their potential interaction with cancer and cancer treatments. Your oncologist, social worker, or psychologist can provide a referral.

Dealing with Depression

When you're depressed, you become thoroughly convinced that your glass is half empty and draining fast: you are sure there is no hope that you will ever feel better. Attempting to change that attitude helps restore the ability to take pleasure in life and in the people who care for you.

Here are some suggestions for developing a positive attitude. Try them as an exercise even if you're convinced they won't help. Remember, when you're depressed, you believe that nothing will be of benefit. That's the depression talking. As mentioned before, if you have thoughts of suicide or death, if you cannot sleep or eat, or if you feel apathy about everything, call your doctor right away.

- Resist thinking about what you've lost. Concentrate on what you still have left and what you have gained by your experiences. You may find you have a great deal to offer others.

- Keep your mind active. Push yourself to go to movies. Read. Listen to music. Enjoy the company of interesting, stimulating people. Try to spend less time dwelling on your own situation. Distract yourself.

- Exercise to the extent that you can. Physical activity is among the best antidotes to depression. Even if your depressed mood returns later, at least you'll know there's something you can do to make yourself feel better for a while.

- Listen to audiotapes that concentrate on positive images. Even if you're not sure they will help—or that you can get well—listen anyway. At least you'll be spending your time in a positive environment.

- Practice relaxation techniques.

- Don't expect too much of yourself. Reward yourself for positive thoughts and activities. But don't be too hard on yourself if you give in to depression now and then. Just gently and persistently draw yourself away from it when you can.

- Know that you're not alone. People who are depressed tend to withdraw from others, which makes them feel even more isolated. Even if you think that you don't have the energy for company or that nobody would want to be with you, stay involved with other people. If there's no one you feel close to or if the people in your life seem unresponsive, join a support group for people with cancer, who will understand how you feel.

- Talk about feelings and fears you and your family members may be having.

- Use prayer or other types of spiritual support.

- Ask for counseling and guidance from a psychiatrist, social worker, pastoral counselor, or psychologist who is knowledgeable about cancer. Your doctor or the social work department at the hospital at which you are being treated can be a good source for information, assistance, or referrals.

- Talk with your doctor about antianxiety or antidepressant medication.

Help for Depressed People with Advanced Cancer. People with advanced cancer are particularly vulnerable to depression. Supportive psychotherapy combined with spiritual counseling can be beneficial, along with antidepressant or stimulant medications and behavioral techniques such as music therapy. Taking small but significant actions, such as talking with family and friends, taping recollections, or writing a living will can help shake some fears and feelings of futility and restore a sense of living fully in the time remaining.

Mind-Body Medicine

The burgeoning field of mind-body medicine, which focuses on the interplay of thoughts, emotions, and health, offers an array of noninvasive behavioral techniques to help deal with the physical effects, side effects, and mental stresses of having cancer. These methods are almost always used in conjunction with medication, counseling, and group support.

Relaxation therapy, meditation, and hypnosis are just a few approaches that are now often included in mainstream cancer care (see Chapter 17). Wherever you are in the disease process, mind-body techniques can help improve your mood and therefore the quality of your life. If you are relaxed and free of distress, you will be better able to focus your attention on important decisions you may have to make concerning your care. There is evidence that people who feel they are actively managing their treatment have less pain.

It also is important to encourage family members and others on your support team to learn these techniques. Not only will they be able to help you in your efforts, but they, too, will benefit.

The exercises or therapies in this chapter involve some form of physical or mental relaxation, and you may find they can help you better deal with the emotional stresses resulting from the effects of treatment or pressures of responsibilities at home. You have the power to change how you respond to stress by practicing many of these techniques. In general, all of these therapies promote healing, improve mood, and enhance the quality of your life.

Books, videos, and web sites offer information on many of these different techniques. You can usually find a class on some of these methods at fitness and community centers in your area. Some hospitals and health centers offer training in these techniques. If these are not enough to help you cope, consider taking advantage of psychosocial support services available in your area (see *Resources*).

Setting Goals

Mind-body techniques are safe and, in many cases, are easy to learn to do on your own. But like any interventions, they are most effective as part of a well-supervised comprehensive treatment plan. A social worker, psychiatrist, psychologist, psychiatric nurse, or other mental health care professional with expertise in cancer care and behavioral medicine can suggest a program of techniques for relieving stress, emotional symptoms, pain, and unpleasant treatment side effects and can act as a coach in helping you learn to use them. Be sure your oncologist is aware of any techniques you try, particularly self-help methods. If he or she is not supportive, have your counselor call and discuss with the doctor the importance of these techniques.

The method that will be most beneficial depends on your medical condition, your personality, how active or sedentary you are, and your treatment goals. For example, are you trying to relieve short-term pain? To learn to distract yourself during an uncomfortable test or procedure? To overcome a fear of needles? Or do you have a larger goal—perhaps to use the experience of having cancer as an opportunity to learn positive coping skills and more adaptive mental habits?

Some of the methods outlined here, such as hypnosis and systematic desensitization, require a professional to serve as your guide, at least initially. In most cases, you will be given audiotapes and other tools so you can continue practicing on your own. Other methods, such as distraction (diverting your mind from tension and discomfort) are easy to learn without professional help.

Expressive Therapies

These techniques involve harnessing the healing power of the arts (visual, performing, and literary) and creative expression. Expressive therapies are used as a way of identifying and expressing feelings. They tap into experiences on many levels through the senses including verbal, visual, hearing, and touch. A variety of methods are used, such as painting, drawing, music, dance, and writing. Music and dance therapy provide outlets for feelings and improve mood and well being. Other therapies based in the arts have similar benefits. Several expressive therapies are highlighted below.

Art Therapy. Art therapy involves the use of creative activities to express emotions through the many media of the visual arts. Using clay, paints, and collages, you can create a painting, drawing, mask, sculpture, or other art pieces that express your feelings about cancer. Using art provides a way for people to come to terms with emotional conflicts, increase self-awareness, and express unspoken and often unconscious concerns about their cancer. This therapy views the creative act as healing, which helps to reduce stress, fear, and anxiety. Art therapy may also be used to distract people whose illnesses or treatments cause pain.

Many medical centers and hospitals include art therapy as part of their inpatient care. Art therapists work with people individually or in groups. The job of the art therapist is to help people express themselves through their creations. Although uncomfortable feelings may be stirred up at times, this is considered part of the healing process.

Dance Therapy. Dance therapy is the therapeutic use of movement to improve the mental and physical well being of a person. It focuses on the connection between the mind and body to promote health and healing. Dance therapy is based on the belief that the mind and body work together. Through dance, it is thought people can identify and express their innermost emotions, bringing those feelings to the surface. Some people claim that this can create a sense of renewal, unity, and completeness.

Dance therapists help people develop a nonverbal language that offers information about what is going on in their bodies. The therapist observes a person's movements to make an assessment and then designs a program to help the specific condition. The frequency and level of difficulty of the therapy is usually tailored to meet the needs of the participants.

Dance therapy is used in a variety of settings with people who have social, emotional, cognitive, or physical concerns. It is often used as a part of the recovery process for people with chronic illness. Dance therapists work with individuals and groups, as well as entire families.

Journaling. Consider keeping a journal. Writing down your experiences and your emotions can help you come to terms with your situation. You might use your journal to reflect on the impact of cancer on your life. It's also a way to express any feelings of anger, confusion, joy, or guilt in a healthy way. It may even help you keep up with symptoms and treatment.

A journal should not be a burden or something you feel you have to do. When writing in a journal, do not worry about grammar or complete sentences. You may even find that you doodle or draw notes in your journal. Use a computer to journal if it is easier for you.

Remind your family that a journal is private. If you want to, share certain parts of your journal with others to help express yourself. You might even want a trusted friend or counselor to comment on certain passages. Gaining insight into your thoughts and feelings will help you cope.

Feelings Journal

Acknowledging your feelings and working through them is a healing process. Being honest with yourself and others and giving yourself permission to feel and express negative feelings is usually the most helpful thing to do. You can complete the sentences below to help you explore your reactions to many of the situations you are likely to face.

- When I first found out I had cancer, I felt _____
  _____.

- I wish that I _____
  _____.

- I can make this come true by doing _____
  _____.

- One of the things that I worry about most is _____
  _____.

- What would make me feel better is _____
  _____.

- When I tell others about my condition _____
  _____.

- I feel closest to people when _____
  _____.

- Other people see me as _____
  _____.

- I would like other people to see me as _____
  _____.

- When I get angry _____
  _____.

- When things get to be too much, I _____
  _____.

- I would like to handle things by _____
  _____.

- I couldn't get along without _____
  _____.

- The best times are _____
  _____.

- What I like most about myself is _____
  _____.

Music Therapy. Music therapy is a method that consists of the active or passive use of music in order to promote healing and enhance one's quality of life. There is some evidence that when used along with standard treatment, music therapy can help to reduce pain and anxiety and relieve chemotherapy-induced nausea and vomiting. It may also relieve stress and provide an overall sense of well being. Some studies have found that music therapy can lower heart rate, blood pressure, and breathing rate. Some medical experts believe it can aid healing, improve physical movement, and enrich a person's quality of life. There is some evidence that music therapy reduces high blood pressure, rapid heartbeat, depression, and sleeplessness.

Music therapists design music sessions for individuals and groups based on individual needs and tastes. Some aspects of music therapy include music improvisation, receptive music listening, songwriting, lyric discussion, imagery, music performance, and learning through music. Individuals can also perform their own music therapy at home by listening to music or sounds that help relieve their symptoms. Music therapy can be conducted in a variety of places, including hospitals, cancer centers, hospices, at home, or anywhere people can benefit from its calming or stimulating effects. Many rehabilitation departments employ music, art, and dance therapists to help people recover from physical problems caused by cancer therapy.

Mind, Body, and Spirit Techniques

The following exercises or therapies involve some form of physical or mental relaxation, and you may find that they can help you better deal with the emotional stresses resulting from the effects of treatment or pressures of responsibilities at home. You have the power to change how you respond to stress by practicing many of these techniques. In general, all of these therapies promote healing, improve mood, and enhance the quality of your life.

Aromatherapy. Aromatherapy is the use of essential oils—fragrant substances distilled from plants—to alter mood or improve health. Aromatherapy is promoted as a natural way to help people cope with chronic pain, depression, and stress, and to produce a feeling of well being. Some evidence suggests that these effects may be real.

There are approximately forty essential oils commonly used in aromatherapy. These highly concentrated aromatic substances are either inhaled or applied as oils during massage. Essential oils should never be taken internally. Also, people should avoid exposure for a long period of time. You can apply the oils yourself, or a practitioner can apply them. Many aromatherapists in the United States are trained as massage therapists, psychologists, social workers, or chiropractors who use the oils as part of their practice.

Biofeedback. Biofeedback is a treatment method that uses monitoring devices to help people consciously regulate physiological processes that are usually controlled automatically, such as heart rate, blood pressure, temperature, perspiration, and muscle tension. It has been approved by an independent panel convened by the National Institutes of Health (NIH) as a useful complementary therapy for treating chronic pain and insomnia. It can also regulate or alter other physical functions that may be causing discomfort.

With the guidance of a biofeedback therapist, patients use various monitoring devices to measure information that controls their bodily processes. Patients can adjust their thinking and other mental processes in order to control bodily functions, such as heart rate, temperature, perspiration, blood flow, brain activity, or muscle tension. The process is repeated as often as necessary until patients can reliably use conscious thought to change physical functions.

Hypnosis. Hypnosis is an effective tool for reducing blood pressure, pain, anxiety, nausea, vomiting, phobias, and aversions to certain cancer treatments. It is a method of putting people in a state of restful alertness that helps them focus on a certain problem or symptom. People who are hypnotized have selective attention and are able to achieve a state of heightened concentration while blocking out distractions. This allows people to be open to images, suggestions, and ideas for resolving issues and improving their quality of life. Hypnosis is one of several relaxation methods that have been approved by an independent panel convened by the NIH as a useful complementary therapy for treating chronic pain.

There are many different types of hypnotic techniques. However, most hypnosis begins with an induction. While a person is sitting or lying quietly, the hypnotherapist talks in gentle, soothing tones, describes images, and repeats a series of verbal suggestions that allows people to become relaxed, yet deeply absorbed and focused on their awareness. People under hypnosis may appear to be asleep, but they are actually in an altered state of concentration and can focus on a specific goal.

Contrary to what many believe, people under hypnosis are not under the control of the hypnotherapist, nor can they be made to do something they wouldn't ordinarily do. Hypnosis is not brainwashing, and ideas are not "planted" in people's minds to make people do things against their will. Quite the opposite is true. Hypnosis is used to help people gain more control over their actions, emotions, and bodies.

People who practice hypnosis are licensed. It is important to be hypnotized by a trained professional. People can also be taught how to hypnotize themselves. Ask your doctor or social worker for a referral, or contact the American Society of Clinical Hypnosis (630-980-4740 or www.asch.net).

Commercial relaxation tapes are widely available in bookstores or by mail order, but many people find a familiar voice more soothing. An individualized tape is particularly effective; a therapist or counselor can make one using images and instructions that are especially meaningful to you.

TIPS AND

ADVICE

Body Scan

Body scan is a basic relaxation exercise for everyone. Focusing on each part of your body in turn and relaxing your muscles one by one helps you develop more awareness of how your body feels when it is tense and when it is relaxed so that you can quickly sense and release tension. Until you have learned the exercise, you might have someone read the instructions aloud as you perform them. Or you can tape the instructions in advance. Plan to spend about fifteen to twenty minutes on the exercise, but avoid it immediately after meals.

Find a comfortable position. This usually means lying on your back with your legs slightly apart, letting your feet fall outward, and your arms resting at your sides with your palms up or down. You can also sit in a chair or stool if that's more comfortable, with your feet flat on the floor and your hands resting lightly on your thighs or arms of the chair or between your legs. Loosen any tight clothing, particularly your waistband or anything that constricts your breathing.

Close your eyes. Begin to take slow, deep breaths with your mouth closed. When your breathing is relaxed, mentally begin to scan your whole body for tension, as follows: each time you inhale, focus on a body part (your foot, for example). Think about whether that part of your body is tense or relaxed. What does that feel like? Then as you exhale, release any tension that you locate in that area. What does it feel like now?

Begin with your left foot. Focus on the sole of your foot, then the toes, then move slowly to the instep, the top of your foot, your ankle. Slowly scan upward to your calf, your knee, your thigh. Then repeat the process on your right leg.

When you reach the top of your right thigh, turn your attention to your torso. Be aware of any tension in your buttocks, the small of your back, your hips, your abdomen, your stomach. Then move upward, scanning your chest, heart area, lungs, and the top of your chest.

Now focus on your left hand, starting at the fingertips and working upward through your fingers, hand, wrist, forearm, elbow, upper arm, shoulder. Slowly shift your attention to your right hand and repeat the process. When you have finished scanning your right shoulder, turn to your neck, your throat, then your face, scanning your mouth, nose, ears, eyes. Slowly move up your forehead to your scalp, and then imagine any remaining tension being released through the top of your head.

Now, keeping your eyes closed, spend a few minutes lying or sitting quietly, letting your body sink deeper and deeper into a relaxed state. Notice what it feels like to have your body and mind deeply relaxed. Then, when you are ready, take a few deep breaths and slowly open your eyes. Repeat this exercise once or twice a day and at bedtime.

Imagery/Visualization. Visual imagery is a relaxation technique that involves mental exercises designed to enable the mind to influence the health, performance, and well being of the body. One common technique, guided imagery, involves visualizing a specific image or goal to be achieved and then imagining achieving that goal. Athletes often use visual imagery to help improve their performance.

Some people with cancer have found that imagery can reduce nausea and vomiting associated with chemotherapy, relieve stress, enhance the immune system, facilitate weight gain, combat depression, and lessen pain. Imagery and visualization are also useful to help decrease anxiety about tests and procedures that you may undergo. For example, using imagery to relax will keep your veins from constricting when you are having an IV.

There are many different imagery techniques. They can be self-taught with the help of books or learning tapes, or they can be practiced under the guidance of a trained therapist. Imagery sessions with a health professional may last twenty to thirty minutes. The more you practice these exercises, the more you will be able to reduce your stress.

Alternative therapies that recommend using active imagery to attack the cancer itself have received a lot of attention. But so far, there is no evidence that imagery alone can alter the course of the disease.

Passive imagery. In passive imagery, once you are in a relaxed state, you look at the visual images or other sense impressions that spontaneously appear in your mind. When carried out under the guidance of a therapist, this exercise can be helpful in uncovering fears or resistances that might be interfering with your treatment, including concerns from money worries to fear of dying.

Active imagery. A more widely used approach is active imagery, in which you consciously choose the images, conjuring up sensory impressions to quell anxiety, lift depression, induce sleep or deep relaxation, manage physical symptoms, prepare yourself for surgery or treatment, or achieve other goals. Studies show that the body responds physiologically to mental images as if they were real events. Therefore, envisioning yourself lying in a grassy meadow on a warm summer day can have the same beneficial relaxing effect as actually being there.

Guided imagery. In guided imagery, a therapist leads you through the process, or you can listen to taped instructions. The therapist may make a special tape with instructions and images that are particularly evocative for you, or may recommend ones for you to buy. Generally, in the first part of the exercise you settle into a deeply relaxed state. To do this, you might be asked to envision yourself in a place with peaceful associations: a beach, the woods, a mountaintop, a flower garden, a lake, or perhaps a special spot remembered from childhood. Alternatively, you might simply visualize a color, such as sky blue,

Focused Breathing

Deep, rhythmic breathing can relax the body and focus the mind, helping to relieve anxiety, depressed feelings, pain, and fatigue. The following is a simple exercise based on a yoga technique (see pages 457–458, *Yoga*). Plan to spend about five to ten minutes on it, once or twice a day and whenever you are feeling stressed.

Sit up straight in a chair with your legs uncrossed and your feet flat on the floor, or, if you prefer, sit cross-legged on a cushion, or lie flat if that is more comfortable for you.

Inhale slowly and deeply, breathing through your nose and keeping your mouth closed.

Imagine your breath filling up your lower abdomen, then your stomach, then your chest. Then slowly release all the air, pausing briefly before beginning the next inhalation.

As you continue breathing, be aware of the breath coming in and out your nose, of your abdomen expanding and contracting, of your diaphragm rising and falling. You do not need to control your breathing. Just observe it as it becomes steadier and deeper and more relaxed.

or a pleasing aroma—your favorite perfume, perhaps. Then other images will be introduced, related to what you want to achieve.

When the goal is to manage pain, many people find it useful to transform the pain into a more tolerable sensation, such as heat or cold or tingling. One person might imagine trailing his hands in a cool mountain stream or running them under a sprinkler; another might see herself warming her hands in front of a crackling campfire or burying them in her cat's fur.

Some people prefer to experience their pain as an integral part of their imagined scenario—pretending, for example, that the pain is the sweet agony of running a marathon or of crashing into another player in a hockey game. Others might opt to rise above the pain with an image of floating on a mattress of fluffy white clouds.

Just as athletes use imagery to rehearse successful outcomes—seeing themselves performing all the movements necessary to clearing the high hurdles, for example—you can use it to envision clearing a treatment hurdle, such as enduring a diagnostic test, chemotherapy, or surgery, with a minimum of discomfort and a prompt recovery. To control the nausea associated with chemotherapy, for example, you might envision yourself driving to the hospital, walking confidently down the corridor, being hooked up to the IV, and then having the chemo flow into your arm like beautiful liquid gold.

Guided imagery can also help you rehearse a positive outcome to a difficult emotional scene. Perhaps you want to tell your family that you are frightened about having cancer and need them to be more supportive, or you want to tell your boss that you have cancer and will need time off for treatment. Visualize yourself taking every step necessary to tell them what you need.

TIPS AND ADVICE

Visual Imagery Exercise

These exercises may be done sitting up or lying down. Choose a quiet place with minimal distractions. Try to get as comfortable as possible, but do not cross your arms and legs because that may cut off circulation and cause numbness or tingling. You can close your eyes at any time. If you choose to keep your eyes open, fix your gaze on one spot in the room and continue to stare at it throughout the exercise. Feel free to shift your body at any time during the exercise to become more comfortable. You can ask someone to read the instructions to you or you can record the instructions for yourself.

Now allow your attention to shift to your breathing. Breathe in through your nose and out through your mouth. Breathe slowly and deeply from your diaphragm. Feel your abdomen moving out when you inhale and moving in when you exhale. Continue to take deep, comfortable breaths. Do not force your breath, just observe your slow, steady, rhythmic breathing. With each breath, allow yourself to breathe more slowly and deeply. Each time you exhale, relax your muscles and imagine that you are blowing away all your tension, anxiety, fear, or confusion. Each time you inhale, imagine you are taking in healing breaths of relaxation. You can choose a word, idea, or image to help you deepen that feeling of relaxation as you continue to breathe deeply. If any distracting thoughts come to mind, just let them drift away and focus your attention on your breathing.

Now let yourself go to a very relaxing place. Choose a place where you feel most calm and most at peace. It could be a place you've been to before or a place you'd like to visit. Imagine going down six steps and at the bottom of the steps you move into this very relaxing and peaceful place. Notice everything around you in this place. Notice all the sights, smells, and feelings that are there. Let yourself be absorbed and comforted in this special place. This is where you feel safe, whole, and protected. Experience this feeling deep in your muscles, your skin, your bones, and throughout your body. You may sense your body becoming still, like the surface of calm water that reflects the sky. You may experience a sense of warmth like being embraced in a soft blanket. Allow yourself to take in all the comforting feelings as you enjoy your special place.

After you take a few moments to enjoy your relaxing, healing place, gradually let yourself walk back up the six steps. You can always go back to your special image or place; it will always be there for you. But, for now, it's time to come back to this place where you will carry your comforting feelings within you. Begin by counting backwards from six and working your way back to the top. Six, five—you're becoming more aware of the sounds around you in the room. Four, three—feeling more alert, awake, and refreshed. Two, one—you are now back in the room feeling deeply relaxed, but alert and ready to face the rest of the day. Slowly open your eyes if you haven't already.

Massage. Massage involves the manipulation, rubbing, and kneading of the body's muscle and soft tissue. It has been shown to decrease stress, anxiety, depression, insomnia, pain, and relax muscles. Many people find that massage brings a temporary feeling of well being and relaxation.

There are many different massage techniques. Massage strokes can vary from light and shallow to firm and deep. Gentle massage therapy can relieve joint stiffness, as well as stimulate circulation and help maintain muscle tone. This is particularly useful if your cancer is limiting your ability to exercise and stay active.

Some people worry that massage might make their cancer spread. Although there is some evidence that deep massage could break off bits of a tumor, gentle stroking that avoids the tumor area is not likely to be harmful. In any case, always check with your oncologist before receiving any kind of bodywork or massage.

The type of massage you choose will depend on the needs of the individual and the style of the massage therapist. If a person has a particular complaint, the therapist may focus on the area of pain or discomfort. Typical massage therapy sessions last from thirty minutes to one hour. Seek out a trained and licensed professional massage therapist.

Prayer and Other Spiritual Practices. Spirituality is generally described as an awareness of something greater than the individual self and is usually expressed through religion and/or prayer. Studies have found that spirituality and religion are very important to the quality of life for some people with cancer. Intercessory prayer (praying for others) may be an effective addition to standard medical care. The benefits of prayer may include reduction of stress and anxiety, promotion of a more positive outlook, and the strengthening of the will to live.

Proponents of spirituality claim that prayer can decrease the negative effects of disease, speed recovery, and increase the effectiveness of medical treatments. Religious attendance has been associated with improvement of various health conditions such as heart disease, hypertension, stroke, colitis, uterine and other cancers, as well as overall health status.

Many medical institutions and practitioners include spirituality and prayer as important components of healing. In addition, hospitals have chapels, and they contract with ministers, rabbis, and voluntary organizations to serve the spiritual needs of people with cancer.

Relaxation Exercises. Relaxation exercises are used to manage anxiety, reduce muscle tension and fatigue, relieve pain, increase energy, and enhance other pain relief methods. Relaxation exercises can be learned through tapes and books that are widely available, which provide step-by-step instructions for a variety of relaxation techniques.

Being able to relax both body and mind is one of the most useful skills for managing the discomfort associated with cancer and stress. There are many different types of relaxation techniques (including visual imagery). Studies show that when you are rested and relaxed, you may need less pain medication. Relaxation also helps the body counter the effects of stress by reducing muscle tension and lowering blood pressure and heart rate.

You can use progressive muscle relaxation—relaxing the body part by part (see page 450, *Body Scan*)—to dispel anxiety while awaiting treatment or surgery, to aid sleep, to relieve pain, or to enter a deeply relaxed state for imagery work or hypnosis. Progressive muscle relaxation increases the awareness of how to identify tension in the body and the ability to relax specific muscle groups throughout the body.

Deep abdominal breathing involves learning how to breathe from the lower part of the abdomen. Many people breathe from the chest rather than the abdomen, which is less effective in creating a state of relaxation. Slow rhythmic breathing begins by staring at an object, or closing the eyes and concentrating on breathing or on a peaceful scene. Taking long, slow, deep, relaxed breaths is an easy way to calm down during a procedure or stressful time.

Autogenic training is a technique used to teach the mind and body to respond to positive messages that are repeated to oneself. Autogenic phrases help people to monitor themselves by focusing their awareness on the connection between verbal commands and physical relaxation.

The relaxation response, by Herbert Benson, M.D., is a form of meditation that involves sitting comfortably in a quiet place and repeating a mantra silently.

Relaxation Exercise

Many people with cancer have found relaxation techniques helpful. These techniques can be used anytime—even for short periods of time. Practice relaxation once a day, but not within an hour after a meal since digestion may interfere with the ability to relax certain muscles.

TIPS AND

ADVICE

1. Sit quietly in a comfortable position (such as in an easy chair or sofa) and practice this exercise when you are not feeling rushed.

2. Close your eyes if you feel comfortable doing so.

3. Deeply relax your muscles, beginning with the face and going throughout the entire body (shoulders, chest, arms, hands, stomach, legs) and ending with the feet. Allow the tension to "flow out through your feet."

    Now concentrate your attention on your head, and relax your head even further by thinking, "I'm going to let all the tension flow out of my head. I'm letting go of the tension, and I'm letting warm feelings of relaxation smooth out the muscles in my head and face. I'm becoming more relaxed."

    Repeat these same steps for different parts of your body: your shoulders, arms, hands, chest, abdomen, legs, and feet. Do this slowly—spend enough time to feel more relaxed before going on to the next part of the body.

4. When your body feels very relaxed, concentrate on your breathing. Become aware of how rhythmic and deep your breathing has become. Breathe slowly and deeply. Breathe through your nose. As you breathe out, say the word "calm" silently to yourself. Slowly take a breath in. Now slowly let it out and silently say "calm" to yourself. Repeat this with every breath. It helps you to relax more if you concentrate on just this one word "calm." Continue breathing deeply, becoming more and more relaxed.

5. Continue this exercise for ten to fifteen minutes. Remain relaxed and breathing slowly. At the end of the exercise, open your eyes slowly to become adjusted to the light in the room, and sit quietly for a few minutes.

    When it is over, ask yourself how relaxed you became and if there were any problems. One problem can be drifting and distracting thoughts. If this happens at the next session, think to yourself, "Let relaxation happen at its own pace." If a distracting thought occurs, let it pass. Let it fly away like a bird. Don't fight it. Concentrate more on the word "calm." Let the thought drift by and repeat "calm" over and over again as your breathing gets slower and deeper—as you relax more and more.

6. Do these exercises regularly—once a day is best. In the beginning, it may help to have someone else give you the instructions. You can record these instructions on an inexpensive tape recorder and play them when you are relaxing. If you prefer, you can record yourself giving the instructions and use that.

Choose a relaxation position that is comfortable for you.

7. When practicing, choose a time when you will not be disturbed. Tell the other people in your household what you are doing and ask them to be quiet during the exercise.

8. After you become skilled at this exercise, you will find that it is easy to apply when you are getting tense. For example, if you are feeling tense while waiting to see the doctor or for a treatment, you can easily close your eyes for a few minutes and use this exercise to relax and feel calm.

9. It's a good idea to learn this relaxation technique early—before anxiety becomes severe. It can then help to keep severe anxiety from happening.

Tai Chi. Tai chi is an ancient Chinese activity that was introduced to reverse the tenseness that came from practicing the martial arts. It was developed to help the warrior relax and not be on the offensive all the time. The purpose was to mediate the effect of the martial arts on the inner self, especially the effects of anger. It is a mind-body, self-healing system that uses movement, meditation, and breathing to improve health and well being. Tai chi is based on the philosophy of Taoism, a Chinese belief system first developed in the sixth century B.C. Its slow, graceful movements, accompanied by rhythmic breathing, relax the body as well as the mind. Tai chi relies entirely on technique rather than strength or power. It requires learning a number of different forms or movement groups.

Research has shown that tai chi is useful as a form of exercise that may improve posture, balance, muscle mass and tone, flexibility, stamina, and strength in older adults. Tai chi is also recognized as a method to reduce stress and lower heart rate and blood pressure.

People who practice the deep breathing and physical movements of tai chi claim that it makes them feel more relaxed, agile, and younger. This general sense of well being is said to reduce stress and lower blood pressure. Practitioners claim it is particularly suited for older adults or for others who are not physically strong or healthy.

Tai chi is taught in many health clubs, schools, and recreational facilities. Practitioners believe that daily practice is necessary in order to get the most benefit from tai chi. Once an individual has mastered a form, it can be practiced at home.

Yoga. Yoga is a form of nonaerobic exercise that involves a program of precise posture and breathing activities. It can be a useful method to enhance a person's quality of life and help relieve some symptoms associated with chronic diseases such as cancer, arthritis, and heart disease, and can lead to increased relaxation and physical fitness.

People who practice yoga claim that it leads to a state of physical health, relaxation, happiness, peace, and tranquility. There is some evidence showing that yoga can lower stress, increase strength, and provide a good form of exercise. Proponents also claim that yoga can be used to eliminate insomnia and increase stamina.

There are different variations and aspects of yoga. The most common form of yoga involves the use of movement, breathing exercises, and meditation to achieve a connection with the mind, body, and spirit. The goal of yoga is perfect concentration to attain the ancient Hindu ideal of samadhi—separation of pure consciousness from the outside world through the development of intuitive insight.

Practitioners say yoga should be done either at the beginning or the end of the day. A typical session can last from twenty minutes to one hour. A session may include guided relaxation, meditation, and sometimes visualization. It often ends with the chanting of a mantra (a meaningful word or phrase) to achieve a deeper state of relaxation. Yoga requires several sessions a week in order to become proficient. Yoga can be practiced at home without an instructor, or in adult education classes or classes usually offered at health clubs and community centers. There are also numerous books and videotapes available on yoga.

Cognitive Therapies

Cognitive techniques focus on helping people gain a sense of control over the way they think about things. Such strategies seek to change patterns of negative thinking, replace irrational ideas, ease worries, and reduce mental stress.

Cognitive Restructuring. This is a method that helps people change faulty thought patterns. Cognitive restructuring techniques involve identifying negative thoughts, feelings, or fears and replacing them with constructive or realistic ones. These strategies are based on the theory that what leads to emotional consequences is not what happens to you in life, but how you interpret it. The techniques help you review your habitual ways of responding to stress and modify your coping style by thinking through the problem differently.

There are many different kinds of cognitive restructuring techniques. Identifying critical thoughts and irrational beliefs is the key to understanding how to change these patterns. You can teach yourself to develop an internal dialogue and change any automatic negative thinking into rational responses. One way to do this is to record your negative thoughts, list how they make you feel, and write a rational response to the situation.

Distraction. One of the easiest and most useful coping methods for handling short-term discomfort is the use of distraction. If you have ever daydreamed

Cognitive Restructuring Techniques

Situation	Feelings	Thoughts	Evidence	Alternate Response
Explain what happened that was upsetting.	Describe how you felt after it happened and the intensity of the feeling (1 = weak, 10 = strong).	Write down any negative things you told yourself or thoughts you had.	Is there any validity to the irrational beliefs? Provide examples.	Write down other things you can tell yourself to counter-balance the negative thoughts.
• *I was late and missed my appoint- ment.*	• *Stupid (8)* • *Frustrated (6)*	• *I never do anything right.*	• *That's not true, there are a lot of things I do right.*	• *I am usually on time.* • *Next time I will be on schedule.*

in a meeting, counted sheep, worn headphones to avoid the boredom of exercise or a bus ride, or kept busy to avoid thinking about something unpleasant, you are an old hand at distraction. Distraction involves a wide range of techniques, from imagery and thought stopping to watching or listening to music, movies, and tapes. The goal is to direct your awareness away from the physical or emotional distress you are feeling. This technique does not require much energy, so it may be very useful when you are tired. It can be used to manage anxiety before surgery or treatments, control nausea or vomiting, handle acute (short-term) pain, manage treatment-related phobias (e.g., fear of needles or MRIs), or stop repetitive, negative thoughts.

Any activity that occupies your attention can be used for distraction. If you enjoy working with your hands, crafts such as needlework, model building, or painting may be useful. Losing yourself in a good book might divert your mind from the pain. Going to a movie or watching television are also good distraction methods. If your concentration is diminished, try math games, like subtracting 47 from 1,000, or counting back from a certain number. Slow, rhythmic breathing can be used for distraction as well as relaxation. You may find it helpful to listen to relatively fast music through a headset or earphones. To help keep your attention on the music, tap out the rhythm or adjust the volume. If the mere smell of the hospital's chemotherapy wing makes you ill, you can distract yourself by taking along a small bottle of perfume or a scented oil to smell when you feel nauseated.

Graded Task Assignments. This method is used to identify a goal and then to list small steps to achieve it. For example, the demands of treatment can make it difficult to keep in touch with friends. When your treatment is over, you'll want to resume these friendships but may feel overwhelmed by the task of trying to rebuild your life.

First, identify your goal: to reconnect with your support system. Then give yourself graded task assignments—specific, manageable steps toward that goal. You might make a list of people with whom you've lost touch and then call one friend a day. The next tasks might be to make one lunch date a week, to go on that date, and to talk with a friend about how things are going. Step by step, you can reach your goal without exhausting yourself physically or emotionally.

Thought Stopping. Cancer raises many fears and it is hard not to worry about everything from your physical health to medical expenses, work, and family pressures. But constant worrying can hinder your quality of life and healing efforts. The technique of thought stopping is a tool used for many years by behavior therapists and psychologists. It is a simple self-help tool that is used for interrupting repetitive or unpleasant thoughts.

First, identify the thought you want to stop (for example, "I'm not a good parent," or "How will I ever get through this?"). Then, every time you have this thought, visualize a big red stop sign (or another image that means "halt" to you) and say "Stop!" loudly and firmly to yourself. Some people wear a rubber band around their wrists and snap it every time the intrusive thought arises. Practice this exercise until it becomes automatic. Then whenever the thought pops up, so will the image, and your inner voice will silently command the thought to stop.

Issues for Families and Friends

Cancer affects everyone close to the person who becomes ill—the spouse, children, parents, friends, partner, and lover who constitute the modern-day family. The disease changes the individual and alters the family. Be prepared: the cumulative stresses will challenge even the best-functioning families or circle of friends. But, depending on how everyone responds, cancer can also bring them closer and provide a deepened appreciation of life and of one another.

What to Expect

Coping crises for the family tend to mirror those for the individual (see Chapter 26), beginning with the shock of the diagnosis, the need to make life-altering decisions rapidly, the extraordinary disruption to life of entering active treatment, and the readjustment to life after treatment.

Not everyone reacts in the same way to the distress, of course, or adjusts on the same timetable. For example, the person with cancer may already have made peace with some loss of physical functioning, while a spouse or child is still wishing that things were the same as they were before. And each person has his or her own concerns. The adult children of a cancer patient may struggle with their sometimes-conflicting responsibilities toward their parents and their own children, for instance. Friends may be troubled by concerns about their own health or mortality. Spouses may feel overwhelmed by practical matters, not the least of them financial.

Although there is no one way of coping with cancer in the family that works for everyone, generally the adjustment is easier when all are involved from the start. Everyone, including children (as will be explained later in the chapter), should receive accurate information about the illness and its treatment. Being included in the information and education process and feeling that everyone has a role helps family members comprehend the physical and emotional challenges of the cancer experience, feel more in control, provide support where it counts, and make informed decisions on behalf of all.

Coping Styles

An important element in coping is understanding what to expect from the illness, the treatment, yourself, and everyone else. Everybody has his or her own coping style, and so thinking about how you usually function in a crisis, separately and together, can help forestall surprises.

Some family members, for example, deal with difficulty in their personal lives by throwing themselves into their jobs or hobbies, becoming less available to their families. Although this style may help them escape their distress, it can be misunderstood by others in the family as uncaring, and it may indeed prove inconvenient for those who have to fill in at home or at the hospital. Others, in order to manage their own anxiety, attempt to take control of all information gathering and decision-making, thereby leaving the person with cancer with little voice.

In some families, crisis causes fighting and blaming. Some draw closer to one another, perhaps feeling more of a sense of purpose than when life returns to normal. Some reach out to others for support, whereas others draw in and away from the outside world.

Threats to a family often make everyone behave immaturely. Even among grown siblings, old rivalries may surface and threaten the cooperation so necessary at this time. Groups in which everyone is very involved with and dependent on one another may feel more at a loss than do those whose members are more autonomous.

Common Dilemmas

Understanding how each family member copes with crisis may help you plan for cancer's effects on family life. Confusion, anger, frustration, anxiety, guilt, or depression can result from any or all of the following.

Role Changes. Almost invariably after a diagnosis of cancer, one or more people in the group must take over the duties of the person who is ill. Over time, the new responsibilities, on top of what may already be a full load, can be a great burden for adults and children alike.

The families that seem to adapt best have always been flexible about who does what. When both spouses have worked and shared household chores, by design or necessity, they have probably had to learn how to fill in for one another. But in those families in which each member has had a specific, fixed role and the boundaries have rarely overlapped—such as those with the tradition that the man works and the woman keeps house—the adjustment is likely to be more difficult.

Burnout Alert

TIPS AND ADVICE

Caring for someone who is sick, taking over his or her responsibilities, having to change habits and routines, and worrying about what will happen results in fatigue at the very least. At the most, the combined pressures lead to resentment, guilt, exhaustion, depression, even physical illness, and an inability to continue to care for your loved one or friend. This condition is sometimes called burnout.

Recognize the Signs

- You're exhausted all the time.

- You can't fall asleep, sleep through the night, or get up in the morning.

- You've pulled away from your friends and lost interest in the activities that used to bring pleasure.

- You feel guilty that you're not doing enough or that you don't want to do even more.

- You worry that you don't really care anymore for the person you're caring for.

- You are easily irritated by people who tell you that you should take care of yourself.

- You think the only relief you can get right now is from alcohol, drugs, food, or cigarettes.

- You don't feel well.

- You're sure that nothing good is ever going to happen again; you feel numb; and you don't care.

What to Do

Above all, you must recognize the importance of your own respite and resist feeling guilty for thinking of yourself.

You may need to learn to delegate some of the responsibilities that you think you "should" be doing yourself. Insist, if need be, that out-of-town family members provide their fair share of assistance.

Divide up responsibilities according to each person's strengths, interests, and personalities; some people are better at dealing with paperwork than providing a soothing presence at the bedside, for example. Some may be good at dealing with medical personnel and taking notes, and others can run errands or cook meals. Those who may be unable or unwilling to contribute time might help out financially.

Ask friends, neighbors, people in your church or synagogue, or others in your informal support network for whatever help they can provide. People are often glad to be asked.

Recognize your limits and forgive yourself for not being perfect and for not being able to do more for your loved one than is humanly possible.

Practice stress reduction techniques, anything from taking a hot bath to getting some exercise to practicing the relaxation and meditation techniques (see Chapter 27).

Distract yourself. There's no reason to focus all your thoughts on your friend's or loved one's illness—in fact, there's every reason not to. Go out to dinner or the movies. Have a good laugh. Goof off. Play games. Go on a vacation, if only for a day. Remember that if you lighten up, you'll take better care of the person with cancer and make him or her feel less guilty. Sick people are often highly sensitive to the body language and unexpressed feelings of those taking care of them.

Recognize and deal with your depression. Problems with sleeping and eating, irritability, negativity, hopelessness, and loss of energy all are symptomatic of depression. Although these feelings and symptoms tend to occur at times of intense distress, if they become your constant companions after the crisis is over, you need to address them for your own health and ability to function.

Shifting the balance of power can be trying too. Frequently, one person in the family is the decision-maker or the one on whom everybody relies in a crisis. So when illness strikes this dominant individual, life can be chaotic while everybody tries to sort out who's "in charge." But it can ultimately bring a family closer when those who have been kept in the background are allowed to demonstrate their competence.

For most people, self-esteem is defined at least in part by the roles they fulfill in life. For the sick family member, giving up these roles, even for a short time, can be an enormous loss. It may be possible to exchange some responsibilities—trading the bill paying for the lawn mowing, for example— to enable the person with cancer to feel useful while taking some of the load off those who have been picking up the slack.

It helps to be able to call on others in the extended family or in the community to take over the additional responsibilities. Families that have always prided themselves on their complete self-sufficiency may find coping difficult unless they reach out. When asking for assistance, be specific about what you want and when you want it.

Disruption of Routines. Most people follow fixed routines in their daily lives, patterns that provide structure and predictability. But when cancer is diagnosed, these usual ways of doing things are thrown up in the air. Everyone has to accommodate the demands of the illness and the treatment schedule, yet at the same time, each person has daily responsibilities that may conflict with the needs of the person with cancer. Such disruptions are especially difficult for children, who often react to even minor changes in meal and bedtimes and types of food and to who helps with homework and who takes them to school.

Never underestimate the amount of stress that results from the conflicts between daily needs of each family member and those of the person with cancer, and don't be surprised if at times someone is feeling angry, resentful, or guilty. A grown son may feel that he's being petty about wanting to golf rather than going to the hospital. Likewise, a wife may feel guilty for wishing to go to lunch with friends rather than stay home taking care of her husband. But the desire to relax and enjoy yourself is understandable. Indeed, finding some way to schedule "time off" from a loved one's illness may be essential to avoid burnout.

Future Plans. Every family has dreams and hopes at every stage of life. Perhaps one of the most difficult coping challenges, therefore, is accepting a future that has suddenly become unpredictable, in which all that you've worked for or dreamed about may not come true, at least not in the way you had hoped or within the time frame you had set. Rather than concentrate on what hopes may be lost, try to manage for the time being by setting new short-term goals and making plans for now that you know you can complete. You can continue to add steps to the plan as the course of the illness and the potential for recovery become clearer.

An illness that threatens your ability to pursue important personal goals—such as new career responsibilities, a young adult's planned move away from home, retirement plans—tests the strength of marriage and family bonds. To resolve this potential crisis, try to avoid all-or-nothing solutions, such as forfeiting plans forever. There may be a way to negotiate a temporary compromise among all those whose needs conflict. For example, a child who was about to go away to college and who is now needed at home, or whose family needs the tuition money for expenses, may be able to postpone admission and enroll for one year in a local, less expensive community college.

These conflicts can produce difficult, mixed feelings of guilt and anger. Here you're supposed to be fully supportive of the person who's ill, and all you can do is think of yourself. But you've got important needs of your own, right? At times like these, outside perspectives, from a support group or religious or psychological counselor, can be a great relief.

Relationship Conflicts. Couples, family members, and friends who have forgotten how much they mean to one another may well be brought closer by the experience of cancer. But it can also be the straw that breaks the camel's back: relationships that were deeply troubled to begin with may not survive. Conflicts and problems that existed before the illness could get worse.

Much depends on your individual and collective style of functioning. Stress can bring out the best or worst in people, usually both. Similarly, it reveals the strengths and vulnerabilities in any relationship.

Loss of Physical Intimacy. For everyone in the network of family and friends, maintaining physical intimacy is important to your sense of closeness. But some people may be afraid of touching or hugging the sick person, perhaps out of a deep-seated fear that the illness is "catching" or simply because the changes to the loved one's body are upsetting. Intimate partners may be concerned that sex will injure the person who is ill or recovering. Or sometimes people with cancer are so upset with their own appearance that they reject physical closeness. If such is the case, intimate partners should be aware that their willingness to look at the changes in their loved ones' bodies and to touch them will contribute greatly to their renewed self-acceptance (see Chapter 20).

Although cancer and its treatment can profoundly affect sexuality, a return to some form of physical intimacy is virtually always possible. But couples must confront the issues (see Chapter 21).

The Importance of Communication

The ability to talk and listen to one another is essential to finding solutions to the challenges cancer presents to a couple, family, or group. But even if all have communicated reasonably well before, cancer produces complex and intense feelings that can be difficult to talk about. Family members often use silence as a shield to protect themselves or the person with cancer from their fears. Often they don't want to trouble each other with upsetting thoughts or feelings. Unfortunately, withholding or denying genuine feelings engenders stress and tension and creates an unfortunate distance.

Of course, people have different communication needs at various times. The person with cancer may want to talk about the progress of the illness, but a friend or spouse may not be ready to acknowledge what is happening. Or the significant others may be trying to manage their own fears at a time when the sick person is feeling more positive and hopeful. Parents may want to have a long talk about the illness and its consequences with children living at

Couples and Cancer: How Are We Doing?

It may help to ask yourself questions such as these:

- Does one of you deal with difficult feelings by distancing yourself emotionally or physically from the person who needs you?

- Does one of you tend to minimize a threat, act overly cheerful all the time, or refuse to acknowledge there's a problem?

- Are you resentful that your needs are being pushed under the rug because of the illness?

- Do you tend to blame one another when something terrible happens?

- Does one of you seem unrealistically optimistic or pessimistic in ways that cause conflict and distance?

- Do you feel that your or your partner's level of anxiety or emotionality is hurting your relationship?

- Was your relationship or family life so troubled or chaotic before the diagnosis that you thought it couldn't get any worse—but it did?

- Is the illness so much on your minds that there's just nothing else you can talk about anymore?

- Do you have difficulty talking to and listening to one another?

- Do you feel that cancer has trapped you in a relationship that you wish to escape?

  Answering yes to any of these might mean you could use some help, together or separately, to deal with the stresses and strains of cancer.

home; children, however, can generally tolerate intense emotions only briefly but may need to revisit them repeatedly over time.

Family members frequently differ in their communication styles. Many men have been raised not to share their feelings; women may be less inclined toward silence. These are broad generalizations, but if family members' ways of sharing feelings and information conflict, each member will experience greater stress in times of crisis if he or she cannot find a way to talk about it.

What to Do

It is better not to try to protect one another but, rather, to have the courage to discuss any concerns and to listen to each other. As research among women who have had mastectomies has shown, the type of support they most valued was their husbands' willingness to listen to them and to talk about the disease.

Cancer in the Morton Family

Henry Morton had just retired from his oil-supply business, which he had founded nearly fifty years before; then he was diagnosed with melanoma. Henry had always been proud of "never being sick a day in my life." His wife of forty-eight years, Janelle, and their four adult children had also relied on Henry's strength and hardiness and had never pressured him to get regular medical checkups, since he was always in such good health.

Henry had definitely been the head of the family and its chief decision-maker, although Beth, his eldest child who now ran the family business, had come to be the unofficial second in command. Janelle—who had always depended on Henry and, later, her children—was shattered and lost. She felt incompetent to express an opinion about what course of action to take, as did all the children except Beth. Beth insisted on gathering information and getting more opinions, but Henry wouldn't hear of it. He followed the advice of the surgeon to whom their family doctor referred him and had surgery within days.

The family gathered at his bedside. "It was like a wake," Beth remembers. Everyone felt bereft contemplating the potential loss of the family linchpin. Beth was the only one of the siblings who lived in the same city, and she began to feel that she was the only responsible one of the lot—an old resentment. For their part, her sisters and brother felt pushed around by her constant attempts to organize who was going to be at home or at the hospital helping. Yet her siblings, under the pressure of their first family crisis, among themselves blamed Beth for not having forced their father to take better care of his health, so that his cancer would have been discovered at an earlier stage.

None of the Mortons—not even Beth or Henry himself—asked the doctors about the prognosis. The medical team took the lead from the family and did not force information on them that they did not want to know about the odds against a cure when the cancer was discovered so late. They did encourage Henry to seek regular checkups, which he did.

Henry recovered well from the surgery, and the family followed him, acting as if nothing serious had happened—just a bad scare. At the next Christmas gathering, about six months after the surgery, the siblings were able to talk about how childish they had acted with one another and vowed to forgive and forget.

They were careful not to refer to their father's illness in front of their mother, for fear that she would worry about a recurrence and become depressed. Janelle, however, was extremely anxious about her husband's health but felt that there was no one she could talk to about it. Whenever she tried to raise her concerns with Beth, her daughter would rush to reassure her that everything would be all right. In her isolation and fear, Janelle grew depressed, waiting for "the other shoe to drop."

The first metastasis was discovered nearly a year later, which stripped away the family facade that everything was just fine and that Henry would live forever. This time Henry was willing to let Beth do more research on his behalf and include the whole family in decisions that had to be made. For the first time since he had become ill, they all began to share their concerns, which freed them to express their love for one another more openly. The hospital oncology team encouraged Janelle to join a spouse support group, which she did readily and gratefully.

Beth, who had just had her third child and continued to head the family business, tried again to organize how her siblings would help their parents. This time her brother and sisters were more sensitive to her need to feel in control and recognized that they were used to letting her do all the work. They worked out their responsibilities among themselves and scheduled visits so that one of them would be in town at all times to give support to their parents and to Beth. They even gave Beth a birthday present of a weekend at a spa for her and her husband. Her sisters came to take care of the children.

Everyone in the family wanted to visit so frequently, with their spouses and children, that they began to recognize that the pressure was too great on Henry to entertain them, which was his style. Although the cancer had now spread to Henry's brain, he continued to believe that it was in remission. His sons became convinced that Henry should "face the truth," but the rest of the family, with the help of hospital social workers, were able to convince them that as long as his affairs were in good order, Henry was entitled to his optimism.

It was Beth's idea to have a fiftieth wedding anniversary party for her parents. They hired a caterer and invited relatives and longtime friends. Beth and her brother and sisters told each invited guest that there was only one rule for the evening: talk about happy times. Despite how ill Henry looked, there was to be no grief.

"I think it was the happiest night of my life," Beth says. "I wouldn't have believed that even though Daddy was so weak, so much joy could exist in one room. I learned things about my dad and mom that I had never known, how inspiring they had been as a young couple to their friends and family, how my dad had started his brother in business, so many things!"

"As the evening went on, Dad no longer looked ill or changed to any of us in the room, I'm sure of that. We all were ageless, immortal, happy in our love for one another. What greater meaning could come out of any life?" Henry remains at home, receiving hospice care. He enjoys the company of his family, and they have found renewal in one another.

Everyone in the circle of family or friends needs to try to take in what the other person is saying without judging or minimizing his or her feelings, or providing false reassurances. When you don't know how to respond, say so, and continue listening. If you lack a solution to a difficult problem, you often don't need to say anything other than to acknowledge that you hear what the other person is saying and are willing to think about it. If the other person seems lost for words, simply ask a question.

Schedule frequent family meetings in which you air all your concerns, large and small, and solve problems before they grow unwieldy. If family members are separated by distance, try to get together frequently. Or send videotapes or audiotapes in which you address one another directly.

Support groups for families of people with cancer provide an important forum. You can unload troubling feelings and concerns in a safe environment and at the same time get feedback about how to approach difficult subjects and solve problems.

Turning to helping professionals—social workers, nurses, psychiatrists, clergy, psychologists—to facilitate communication can also provide needed relief and enable growth through crisis. In families that have had numerous difficulties before the onset of illness, as well as those that have become over- whelmed dealing with the cancer, outside help may be the lifeline they need.

Helping Children Adjust to Cancer in the Family

When cancer strikes families with dependent children, parents often want to protect them as long as possible from the harsh "adult" realities. Or they are so wrapped up in dealing with the illness and treatment that they don't have time to spend with the children. In any case, even very small children will know that something is terribly wrong. They perceive their parents' moods and anxieties, unusual absences, secrecy, and even the slightest alterations in the daily routines that regulate their lives. Children are good lie detectors, often better than adults. But if they aren't given an honest explanation, they will arrive at their own conclusions, which spring from their imaginations and immature intellects. Very often children feel rejected and conclude that Mommy or Daddy is away, secretive, or staying in bed because he or she doesn't love them anymore or as punishment for their "bad" behavior.

The way parents cope with these emotional and practical disruptions sets the stage for how their children deal with them. Cancer may be the first family crisis the children have faced. How youngsters adapt is important to their social and emotional development and can influence how they will deal with difficulty in the future. If they've already experienced loss or serious illness in the family constel- lation, their previous fears and anxieties will probably affect their coping now.

On the parents' side, the fact that they have to help their children adjust can be a powerful incentive to manage themselves as constructively as

Don't Avoid It—Talk About It

The great strain of dealing with cancer can disrupt the communication even within families that are used to being open with one another. Conversation can become stiff and awkward, particularly when family members become overprotective of one another. All too commonly, they are reluctant to talk about the disease and its effects with the person who has it and with others closely involved. Those who feel uncomfortable with the subject may avoid it at all costs, even switching off the television if the word cancer is mentioned. Many people fear that if they talk about death, they will sound like they have given up, which would upset or depress the person with cancer.

- Drop the charade! It won't work, and it's a handicap.

- Be kind to yourself, understand that the stress of your situation has led to your overprotective attitudes and actions.

- Realize that you are not really protecting the person with cancer. People have an innate sense of physical self and usually are aware of their own states of health—sometimes even before the diagnoses are made. Keeping secrets or avoiding the subject is just silencing any form of communication you may be able to have.

- Understand that being honest does not mean being blunt or tactless or unkind. It means discussing real events and projected events and sharing emotional reactions to those events.

- Start slowly. Discussions about truly important issues—no matter what they may be—are always difficult. So don't rush. And don't let silences scare you away from the issues. It's often hard to find the right words to describe feelings.

- Listen. Don't interpret another's response and then change it into something it wasn't meant to be. If you're uncertain about the meaning of what's said to you, ask for clarification.

- Be honest. Don't pretend that you're not concerned or afraid or angry if you are. Try to explain what you are really feeling to the person with cancer or another family member. Allow that person to help you.

- Talking about death can be hard for everyone. The point is to talk about your feelings. "I am afraid of losing you" is a way to express your concern that your loved one may die. The important thing is to let each other know how much you care.

- If it seems useful, seek help from a nonfamily member to guide conversations that are difficult for you.

possible. If they are not overwhelmed by the current crisis, they may welcome being able to shift their focus to their youngsters, with whom they may feel a greater sense of effectiveness and control.

Tell Them

As with adults, information demystifies cancer and helps children feel less helpless. Thus, the first and most important step is to give the children accurate information about the illness immediately. Tell them the name of the disease, where it is located, and how it will be treated. Keep them posted throughout the illness about what is going on in the present and what is likely to happen in the near future.

A parent or relative who is very close to the children should convey the news, in familiar surroundings.

Explain the effects of the illness and the side effects of the treatment such as fatigue, hair loss, weight loss, surgical alterations, and moods, so that the children are not left to fantasize why these things are happening.

How you tell them will depend on their age, of course. Use simple, age-appropriate language based on what is really happening. Begin by asking a child what he or she understands or thinks about the illness. Using dolls or drawing pictures can help, but don't use fairy tales to help little ones understand, because stories can stimulate children's imaginations to follow unforeseen directions. To be certain that the child understands what you've said, ask at a later time what he or she knows about your situation. You can then clarify any misunderstandings and fill in significant knowledge gaps. Encourage children to tell you what they believe cancer is and how it will affect you and their lives.

When you discuss your treatment, let the child know what side effects are likely to happen, how cancer might affect his or her day-to-day life, and when life is likely to return to normal. Children need to know if you will be able to help with homework, participate in the car pool, or coach the Little League team. If you can't fulfill a responsibility, discuss with them what's being done to make alternative arrangements and what people might be filling in for you until you're better.

Remember that children are familiar with being sick, going to doctors, and taking medicines. But be careful about saying things such as, "It's like when you had a sore throat and had to go to the doctor," because they might conclude that their sore throat caused the parent's illness or that the next time their throat hurts, it means that they have cancer.

Although a child may not respond right away, be prepared to answer whatever questions come up and allow him or her to react emotionally. Keep in mind that a child may react more to how you are behaving than to what you are saying.

Parents often avoid useful discussions with their children because they're afraid of such pointed and difficult questions as "Will you die?" The answers to all questions should be honest but as optimistic and focused on hope as the situation allows. For example, a parent might say, "Some people with cancer get all better and some don't. I'm trying my best to get better." Or, "That's really not something you need to worry about right now. I'll tell you if I think that's a possibility." Responses like these are balanced.

When death is a possibility, parents need to acknowledge how difficult it is to live with uncertainty and to emphasize their determination to confront whatever happens together as a family. Be sure to let children know when death is near, and if possible, allow a final leave-taking.

Children need continuous reassurance that they'll be safe, secure, and loved. Because cancer and its treatment necessitate frequent absences from home, and leaving youngsters in the care of others for periods of time, reassure them that you have made plans for their care and that they are not being abandoned. Let them know that as a parent, you are going to make sure that they are all right, no matter what happens.

Regardless of age, anger is one of the most common reactions to the turmoil created by cancer. It's also one of the most difficult to express because it's considered such an unacceptable emotion. When children are unable to express their anger it will come out in other ways. Allow a child to be angry and acknowledge the cause of the feeling. A child who is angry because of a disappointment might be told, "I know you're upset that I missed your school play last month," or "I know you're upset that you haven't been able to get to your piano lesson because I couldn't drive you." While you want a child to express anger, you also need to maintain normal discipline with regard to their behavior. Children need to know their limits, especially at times of upheaval. If you sense anger is behind some misbehavior, and your child is unwilling to talk about it, at least encourage him or her to vent feelings in other ways. Any activity that expends energy—kicking a soccer ball around the back yard, punching a pillow, or drawing a picture of what is making them mad and then tearing it to pieces—may help.

It is important to let children know that the parent's illness is not their fault. Children dwell at the center of their small universes and often think that bad things happen because they were naughty.

Keep in mind that communicating with young people about cancer is not a one-time event; it is an ongoing process. Should the illness go into an extended remission, continue as a chronic problem, or recur, children will require updates tailored to their own changing understanding and emotional needs.

You may want to ask a social worker, school counselor, or other parents in your position how they have explained cancer to children that are your youngsters' ages. In any case, tell your child's teachers about the illness so that they can be alert to problems that crop up in school as a result.

What They Can Do

Children often must take on additional chores and responsibilities when a parent is ill. Providing tasks for them can help them feel involved and necessary in the parent's recovery, at a time when children often feel left out. Small children can bring the mail to the parent or paint pictures to send to the hospital, for example.

Older children will probably have to help out more than usual around the house or even take jobs to contribute to the family finances. Especially if there is no other adult living at home, they may even have to assume parental roles that they are not prepared for, such as cooking or caring for younger siblings. This can be a great burden at a time when they are learning to be independent. Even more than adult helpers, teenagers need time off and frequent expressions of appreciation.

Life as Normal

Life is anything but normal when a parent has cancer. Seeing to children's emotional and physical needs can be extraordinarily difficult in the face of illness-related absences or disability. This is especially true in a single-parent household or if the other parent has to work extra hours to compensate for lost earnings or increased costs. It may be necessary to call on friends and relatives to provide childcare. Childcare can be a parent's greatest problem even in the best of times, and if adequate supervision for children cannot be found now, investigate community resources (see Chapter 8).

When you return home, plan activities that don't demand a lot of energy but allow you to have time with your child. Reading a book together or playing a board game let children know that you are still in charge and that they are not alone. Don't forget to take time to simply cuddle. Children may feel sad that you can no longer do the activities together that you once did. Hugging and soothing words can help them adjust to that loss.

Because of the many disruptions, maintaining children's normal routines and allowing them their usual activities in and out of school are important. This gives a sense of security that is needed to stay on track developmentally. Adolescents, in particular, need to spend time with their peers and have their privacy.

Signs of Problems

Any distressing family situation or threat to their security is likely to be revealed in children's behavior at home, in school, and with friends. Kids who were having problems before will probably have a worse time now, so counseling may be needed to help them manage their increased distress without prolonged consequences for their schoolwork and peer relationships.

Children of all ages may have trouble sleeping or have nightmares, lose their appetites, develop physical complaints, become unusually quiet or fearful, and/or begin to fail at tasks at which they are usually successful.

Becky's Mom Has Cancer

When Maureen Tyler was diagnosed with breast cancer, her daughter, Becky, had just turned 5 and was about to enter kindergarten. Becky was too young to understand any threat to her mother's life, although she heard the fear in her parents' voices as they discussed the diagnosis.

Maureen sat down with Becky and told her about the lump in her breast. Becky knew that she had been breast-fed as a baby, and it was hard for her to understand that this nurturing part of her mother had something wrong with it. Her mother let her feel the lump and explained that Grandma would come to take care of Becky while she was in the hospital to have the breast with the lump taken away. She also explained that she would be tired for a while after she came back from the hospital but that she would still be the same loving mommy except for the change in one part of her body.

That night, when Becky's father put her to bed, she asked him to tell her the whole story again, and they acted it out with teddy bears. When her mother left for the hospital, Becky clung to her for a minute and then patted her mother's breast and said goodbye to it.

Because she was so young, Becky was not allowed to visit her mother in the hospital, but she and her grandmother drove by it and looked up, trying to imagine which window was Mommy's. Her mother called her every evening on the telephone, and Becky drew lots of pictures expressing her childlike understanding of what had happened.

When her mother came home, she tired easily, and Becky had to learn to bring her mother a glass of water or the morning mail. She also had to learn to play alone more. She wanted to see where the surgery had been, and she touched the scar gently. She continued to reenact the surgery from time to time with her teddy bears, but gradually she lost interest as Mommy seemed more like her old self.

Preschool and School-Age Children. When a parent has been diagnosed with cancer, small children often regress, resume bedwetting, become clingy, talk baby talk, refuse to go to day care, and so on. School-age children may resist going to school, have problems with schoolwork, or develop difficulties in relationships with siblings and peers. Because they now rely so much on the well parent, they may also react strongly, perhaps angrily, when the well parent cries or otherwise seems fragile. They may not seem as sympathetic or supportive as parents might hope them to be. Indeed, they may be furious at the sick parent and critical of his or her changed appearance and failure to attend to their needs.

Teenagers. Adolescents, as befits their complex developmental period, can have a range of complicated reactions. In the process of testing their parents' limits and breaking away, they may feel very ambivalent about their sick parent, wanting to help and yet feeling angry and guilty about wanting to flee. Their reaction can be especially difficult for them, and everybody around them, if they were not getting along with the parent before the illness.

More aware than younger children of cancer news in the media and developmentally able to think of the future, teens may be extremely frightened of death and loss. They may feel utterly alone and abandoned. More capable of empathy, older adolescents may feel overwhelmed by the parents' pain and their own helplessness in dealing with it. So as a result, some may become aloof, while others become anxiously overinvolved in the parent's care.

Some more mature teens cope as adults do, seeking and evaluating information and turning to friends and counselors for help. Some, however, may act out aggressively and destructively, whereas others may begin to fail in school, even if they've been trying to keep up. They may start developing headaches, rashes, and other psychosomatic problems. Some may abandon their social outlets and retreat into their rooms.

What to Do

Always inform teachers that there's cancer in the family so that they can keep track of how the children are performing and report any problems. Any significant changes in their behavior that persist for more than a couple of weeks are warning signs that children are having difficulty. And if children start talking about wanting to die or suddenly begin giving away favorite possessions, seek help from a mental health professional immediately.

Additional attention from their parents may be all that young children need to get them back on track. Talk to them, try to get them to verbalize their feelings, and always express your love. Remember that kids need to know that the surviving parent will be there to take care of them.

When problems persist or are destructive, a parent or other responsible adult must intervene. Always try to determine the children's understanding of the illness. Despite your best attempts, they may have imagined something that is deeply disturbing to them. This may be true even for older children. If your child's distress is not relieved by talking with you and other family members, if his or her behavior seems extreme, or if the expected regression and misbehavior is persistent, a consultation with a professional may help.

Even with less severe problems, talking to the school guidance counselor or seeking help through the social work department at your hospital or through other resources can relieve the pressure on you when your own capacity to cope with your children's reactions is limited. Ask about support groups just for children of parents with cancer.

There's Something to Celebrate

Celebrating holidays and family occasions and milestones—religious rituals, birthdays, graduations, athletic or academic accomplishments, steps in the parent's recovery—and pursuing shared activities as a group take on increased significance when there's cancer in the family. Allowing yourselves to mark important events and to channel your energies away from fear and sadness offers a welcome distraction from the serious concerns that have probably been dominating your family life.

Most of all, celebrations are a way to recall how much you mean to one another, to bolster hope and restore energy, and to confirm that each person in the family is special. You'll see that even if one of you is ill, you have a future as a family. And memories last forever.

29

The Financial Costs

You may be concerned about the toll your cancer will take on your finances. Unfortunately, the need to attend to money matters comes at a time when you are already on an emotional high-wire because of your cancer. If you are physically unable to manage or concentrate on financial issues, you may become frustrated and fearful that you won't be able to keep up with important details. After all, you want your top priority to be recovery, not money and insurance.

Money and insurance issues can be stressful to deal with even when a person is healthy. There are many different types of insurance, managed care plans, government-sponsored programs, and health maintenance organization networks to consider, each with different restrictions. Health care is constantly changing and medical care costs are continually rising, adding to the challenge. It's stressful to deal with managing a budget and facing unexpected, out-of-pocket costs that are not covered by insurance, such as childcare, housekeeping services, or travel for treatment.

Remember: at each stage in your diagnosis, treatment, and recovery, others can help you cope with finances and insurance. Perhaps a friend or family member can temporarily take over the chore of paying regular bills and helping to manage your personal finances. (Experts do caution, however, that the people with cancer not turn over *all* financial responsibility to anyone during this time unless absolutely necessary.) Hospitals, clinics, and doctor's offices usually have someone who can complete claims forms for insurance coverage or reimbursement. A case manager or financial assistance planner at the hospital or clinic can help you gain access to financial resources. If finances are strained, ask a hospital financial counselor, social worker, or case manager for assistance. Often arrangements can be made if the hospital is aware of your situation.

Those without insurance are especially vulnerable when faced with a diagnosis of cancer. If you are without insurance, you may need to ask for help from trusted friends and family or a group you belong to, such as a church or a professional organization (see *What to Do If You Don't Have Insurance*, pages 488–490).

What a Social Worker Can Do for You

Because of changes in the health care system, such as early discharge, and the financial strains that illness creates for many Americans, social workers have become even more important resources. Throughout this chapter, you will notice that you are referred to the social worker for help in locating programs that may help you financially or community resources that can provide services. Social workers may also advise you about working with insurance companies to get the services you need.

INFORM

YOURSELF

Assessing Your Situation

It's important to keep meticulous records noting every dollar spent for health care, from the first visit to the doctor when cancer is detected, throughout treatment, recovery, and rehabilitation. This includes not just doctor and hospital bills, but payment for services that you can no longer do yourself, travel expenses, over-the-counter medications as well as prescription drug costs, health care supplies, and so on. Keeping documents and receipts will enable you to be reimbursed for some expenses and perhaps allow you to receive a tax deduction. It can also help if questions arise regarding hospital or doctor billings.

Preparing a financial plan for your cancer and treatment is not so different from making a regular budget. Part of evaluating your finances is assessing your savings and investments as well as planning your estate. However, now you will need to consider how cancer and its treatment are related to your income, benefits, and needs.

When you evaluate your financial situation, consider the many issues addressed in this chapter and the avenues of help that are available. If you are a working person, first evaluate your income in light of your job situation, considering the time you will need to undergo treatment, the expected recovery period, and whether you will be able to return to your full working capacity. If you are disabled, you need to determine how much money you will receive from your disability plan and how long the benefits will last (see Chapter 22).

The Federal Consumer Information Center offers information about managing debt and many other topics. You can call them toll free at 800-688-9889 or 800-326-2996 (TDD), or visit their web site at www.pueblo.gsa.gov. You can also contact the American Cancer Society (ACS) at 800-ACS-2345 (www.cancer.org) or contact your local unit for information on services and resources in your community.

When debt cannot be managed and medical expenses have overwhelmed financial resources, some people consider declaring bankruptcy. If you ever find yourself in this position, talk to a lawyer or seek advice from a legal aid clinic or other nonprofit agency, such as Consumer Credit Counseling.

Professional Advice

A financial planner isn't a health care provider, but by guiding you and your family through this challenging time, her or she may be a helpful—if not necessary—part of your health care team. Relieving your concerns may relieve the stress and anxiety caused by this potential financial health crisis.

A financial planner reviews all of your finances, including your income, investments, expenses (medical as well as living costs), benefits, and taxes, and helps you plan for the present and the future. The planner also helps you formulate your goals and design a realistic plan to achieve them. Of course, a financial planner is also of tremendous help to those who are not ill. For example, a recent survey found that households with an annual income of less than $100,000 that had financial plans saved twice as much as families with a similar income who didn't have a plan. For people facing a costly, potentially chronic illness such as cancer, a financial planner is especially useful. It's important, however, to select a planner who is skilled in handling the issues and needs you are facing.

Finding a Financial Planner. You can begin by asking your doctor, social worker, and others involved in your care if they can recommend a financial planner. Your lawyer or accountant may make recommendations, too. If you participate in a support group, ask the other members for referrals. Sometimes other people with cancer who have worked with financial planners can give you a recommendation. The National Endowment for Financial Education has collaborated with the ACS in developing a program about finance management for people with cancer. Call ACS (800-ACS-2345) for more information about the program and materials (called *Taking Charge of Money Matters*).

Gather a few recommendations and research several planners so you can choose the right one for you. If finding a financial planner is beyond your abilities at this time, ask for help. A trusted friend or family member can assist you in your search, perhaps making calls, gathering references, and doing preliminary interviews. See the *Resources* section at the end of this book for contact information for organizations that can provide information about financial assistance.

Narrowing Down the List. Before meeting with planners, you will want to obtain information about the person's background in writing. They should be able to provide a resume and/or biography with references, so that you or the person assisting you can do a preliminary background check. If there are some planners you call who cannot provide you with all of the information you need to feel confident in their abilities, cross them off your list.

The information you need to know about the financial planner is the person's level of education; professional credentials, such as the Certified Financial Planner (CFP®) designation; membership in professional groups; licenses, such as for selling stocks, insurance, or real estate; and type of clientele. Remember that it's always best to work with a planner who has helped clients with backgrounds or circumstances similar to your own, so consider whether or not the planner has worked with people with cancer. And, most important, make sure you know how the planner expects to be paid.

You should plan to interview the planner in more detail during the initial meeting (for which you should not be charged). Asking specific questions will help you learn if the financial planner is knowledgeable and experienced, and if he or she clearly understands your situation. You will also be able to judge if the planner is more interested in selling financial products than in helping you. This is the time to determine if the planner's approach fits your needs and if you feel comfortable with the person. One of the most important questions you need to be able to answer at the interview is, do you feel confident in this person's judgments? Depending on your situation and your health, you may want to have a trusted friend or family member with you when you interview your potential financial planner. Those who will be affected by your finances need to have a clear understanding of what is involved.

Groups exist to oversee financial professionals. They can tell you if the planner you're considering was ever subject to a disciplinary action. See the *Resources* section for contact information.

Making a Financial Plan

Whether you work with a financial planner on your own or with a trusted advisor, you will need to methodically review and evaluate your income, your financial resources, potential sources of assistance, insurance and benefits, and expenses. Financial planning also includes planning your estate— something everyone should do regardless of state of health. Your spouse and possibly children need to be involved in designing your financial plan because they will be affected by it. A spouse who has never handled money before may need encouragement to learn about financial matters. And it's

Questions to Ask a Financial Planner

As you ask some of the following questions, jot down the answers to consider later. You might ask to record the interview so you can review it later.

- Can you describe your typical client?

- Have you ever worked with a client who has cancer? Or have you helped with the finances of a family member or friend who has cancer?

- How would your planning advice to me differ from a typical financial planning client?

- Do you feel comfortable dealing with this issue?

- What would be the issues you see as most important in my particular situation? Describe the financial planning process you would take me through.

- Are you familiar with all aspects of medical coverage, disability benefits, life insurance, accelerated benefits, and viatical settlements?

- Are you familiar with the employee rights of cancer patients?

- Do you prepare written plans? How detailed are they?

- How often will you review my finances?

- How often should I talk with you?

- What do you expect from me?

- Do you recommend specific products? How do you decide how my money should be divided?

- Describe your investment style or philosophy. Do you specialize in certain types of investments? Do you exclude any types?

- What type of investment strategy would you recommend for someone in my situation?

- How are you paid? How are your fees determined (fee, commission from the sale of financial products, fee plus commission)?

- Have you ever been disciplined by a regulatory group?

- If our relationship doesn't work out, how would we end it?

important to have someone with whom you can discuss troublesome questions such as, "Which bill should I pay first?"

Involving children is a delicate matter because it involves other issues. For instance, it might seem to you that having them see how you handle money gives up some of your authority as a parent and, of course, privacy. On the other hand, the benefit is that they will know you trust them and feel that they are helping in your recovery. Also, it's an educational experience for them. If at some point in the future they need to be involved with your financial matters, they will not experience any surprises.

Estimating Expenses

Make a list of expected expenses. Think big: base your numbers on the highest possible expenses. That way you'll be prepared for any costs that come along.

A good plan allows for the unexpected—the worst-case scenario. In cancer treatment that includes planning for the highest out-of-pocket expenses, travel costs, the longest possible hospital stay, the increasingly high costs of prescription drugs, experimental treatments that won't be covered by your insurance, home health care costs, and not being able to work.

Consider every possible need. You aren't likely to overlook the cost of prescription drugs and lost income, but don't forget that your living expenses are likely to increase as well. They may include the cost of special diets, cosmetics, wigs or hairpieces, cleaning services, physical changes in your home, and professional services—not just home health care providers, but the cost of an attorney, financial advisor, and therapist or counselor as well.

If you have not been in counseling before, you may not realize that you may experience a need for this kind of help when you have cancer. Counseling may help you deal with the issues and feelings that arise because of your cancer diagnosis and treatment. It may not be covered by your insurance plan, but it's worth making this cost part of your budget.

These costs may be difficult to estimate, so speak with your doctor and social worker about those that you can't evaluate on your own.

Income. The most important source of income for many people is their salary. It's also possibly the greatest expense in terms of loss. You will need to carefully review your employee benefits (unless you are self-employed) and your rights. (See Chapter 22 for more information on work-related issues.)

Although it's important to have cash on hand or easily accessible to cover medical bills, remember that the profit from selling stocks and some bonds will be included in your taxable income.

Savings and Investments. A person with cancer may want to put six months to a year's worth of regular and medical expenses into investments that can easily be converted into cash, if possible, such as a money market account at a bank or a money market mutual fund. In terms of making investments, this is not the time to consider making high-risk investments or to think about long-term growth. Short-term and limited-term investments that can provide income are wise choices now.

Estate Planning. Estate planning is a good idea for everyone, not just people with cancer. Your house, car, jewelry, life insurance policies, retirement funds, and savings are all part of your estate. Setting up specific plans for your estate will give you peace of mind. You'll know that your intentions will be carried out when you die and that you will be in control of your health care at all stages of your life. Estate planning documents include a will and an advance directive. An advance directive is a legal document that specifies a power of attorney for health care (also called a durable power of attorney for health care or health care proxy) and may include a living will. (See Chapter 31 for information about advance directives.)

An estate attorney can discuss your needs and draw up the appropriate documents. Trusts, which protect your assets from taxes and probate costs, may be necessary. If your finances are simple, wills and advance directives can be drafted at a legal clinic or nonprofit groups that can help.

Resources

Thinking through your potential financial needs and assessing your resources may be the last thing on your mind as you cope with cancer. But if you approach the challenge in a systematic way, it's likely to be less intimidating and stressful. There are a variety of sources of insurance, income, and options for assistance that may be open to you. You should be aware of all your options.

Medical Insurance

Insurance is your most important asset, since over time it may reimburse as much as $1 million of your health care costs. Knowing what your plan covers will ease your mind and may help you more accurately estimate out-of-pocket expenses. Read your insurance plan carefully now. Call your insurance company and ask the customer service or claims department any questions you have. (If you belong to an HMO, the information or patient services center can answer inquiries.) If you don't understand your medical coverage, call and ask for an explanation in writing. If an employer provides your insurance coverage, you can also talk with the human resources department. Confirm what you're told with the insurance company. Some hospitals also have a financial aid counselor, oncology social worker, or patient advocate who can help you understand your policy.

As you read over your policy, you'll be reminded of your deductible—another out-of-pocket cost. Also know what portion of the costs—the coinsurance—you will be responsible for paying. For example, the plan may cover 80 percent of the approved cost of a treatment. You pay the other 20 percent of the approved cost. Some doctors, however, charge more than the approved cost of treatment and you are expected to pay this additional cost also.

Some managed care plans, such as HMOs, have you pay a small dollar amount each time you go to the doctor. The amount you are charged is called the copayment, or copay. With this type of plan, you also might pay a small amount for prescription drugs. Copays can add up over time if you are seeing several doctors a week or needing many prescriptions. Again, it's wise to estimate how much you will spend weekly on copays, then budget for these amounts. Your policy will also explain if you have a "pre-existing condition exclusion period." That means that if you had a health problem (such as cancer) before you joined the plan, you will have to wait a certain period of time (usually no more than a year) before the insurer will cover the cost of that problem. According to new rules about exclusion periods, they don't apply to you if you have had medical coverage for eighteen months, you have already met a pre-existing condition exclusion period, and you have not been without health coverage for more than sixty-two days.

You will also want to look carefully to determine if your medical plan covers prescription drugs, counseling, home care, and investigative treatments. Knowing in advance the costs that you must pay out-of-pocket will get you thinking about low-cost solutions for certain expenses. For example, prescription drugs, which can become quite expensive, may be available in a generic equivalent. Or an alternative and less costly drug may be available. There may be a patient assistance program from the pharmaceutical company that will provide free drugs. This information is available at the Pharmaceutical Research and Manufactures of America (PhRMA; www.phrma.org), or your doctor or nurse may be able to help you research companies that provide drugs free of charge. Some hospitals have a patient assistant fund that can help with the cost of drugs. Some doctors are able to dispense free samples of drugs.

Some insurance plans provide additional coverage under a "catastrophic illness" clause. Check to see if your policy has this clause.

Some plans have a "stop-loss," "breakpoint," or "out-of-pocket" limit. This is the most you will have to spend per person each year. For example, an insurance company may have a stop-loss of $5,000. After you have paid the $5,000 in deductibles and similar costs, the insurance company will pay 100 percent of the covered expenses for the rest of the year. Some insurance plans are discontinued if you're unable to work. Read your benefits book to see if your employer continues to pay the cost of your medical insurance if you are disabled (see Chapter 22).

Insurance plans vary with regard to experimental treatments. If your doctor recommends a treatment that is under study, you have a few options. Ask if the treatment is part of a clinical trial. If it is, or could be, some of the care may be free of charge. To learn more about clinical trials, contact the National Cancer Institute at 800-4-CANCER (www.cancer.gov).

Some medical plans decide whether to pay for experimental therapies individually. Ask for your doctor's help when submitting paperwork about the treatment to your insurance company. It may help if your doctor includes studies supporting the therapy, its benefits, and its acceptance by the medical community. If your claim is turned down, try again. If turned down again, ask if your medical plan has an appeals process. If you still have to pay for some or all of the treatment, try to negotiate for a lower cost.

Read your medical plan to see if or how home care is provided. Also, find out how many visits a year are covered by your plan and how many hours make up a visit. Most plans cover only skilled care, which must be medically necessary and prescribed by a doctor. The kind of home care that often is needed is custodial care—someone to help with the activities of daily living. Custodial care is often not considered medically necessary and may not be covered.

When Your Insurance Company Won't Pay. If you feel that a claim has been unfairly denied, first discuss it with the doctor's office or the hospital claims

QUESTIONS

TO ASK

What Does My Insurance Cover?

You may want to ask your insurance agent the following questions as you evaluate your options:

- Is there a toll-free number I can call to get information? Is it important to speak to the same person each time I call?

- Does my policy have a monetary limit on benefits?

- Will my hospital stay be covered?

- How do I find out if a procedure is covered? Who do I call?

- If I want to see a doctor who is out of network, will that be covered?

- Are the costs of participating in a clinical trial covered?

- Does my policy cover all my expenses through several rounds of chemotherapy or radiation?

- Does my policy cover recurrence and subsequent treatment?

- Are counseling services covered by my policy?

- How many home care visits a year are covered?

- Is custodial care covered?

- Does my policy cover reconstructive surgery?

- Which treatments are covered under this policy?

- Does my policy cover treatments for medical problems that may result from reconstructive surgery?

office. The problem may relate to the language in the policy or an interpretation of it.

A customer service representative or case manager at the insurance company may also be helpful. Sometimes the problem can be easily resolved, such as if the "coding" on the claim was wrong. But if an appeal is necessary, the case manager can explain the appeal process to you. In fact, a case manager can be helpful to you in many ways, so it's worthwhile developing a good working relationship with him or her.

If there is no coding or language problem, your first step is to resubmit the claim along with a copy of the letter denying your coverage. If the claim is still denied, here is what you may need to do:

- Do not pay until the matter is resolved.

- Submit the claim a third time and request another review.

- Speak with a supervisor, who may be able to change the decision.

- Appeal the denial in writing and explain why the claim should be paid. (Ask members of your health care team for help with this official appeal if you need it.)

- Ask for a written response to your appeal.

- Keep the original copies of correspondence. Make and keep copies of medical records.

- Keep a log of dated calls, names of those you speak to, and specifics of conversations about the denial.

- Consult the consumer services division of your state insurance department or commission. (Complaint forms are available on many state insurance departments' web sites. The National Association of Insurance Commissioners web site at www.naic.org may supply you with more information.)

- Continue attempts to resolve the matter.

- Think about taking legal action.

To file a complaint about an HMO, contact the U.S. Health Care Financing Administration (each region of the country has a different contact number; www.hcfa.gov).

The U.S. Department of Labor, Pension and Welfare Benefits Administration can help you file a claim related to a private employer, union self-insurance, or self-financed plan (800-998-7542; www.dol.gov/dol/pwba).

Medicaid complaints may be directed to your state department of social services or medical assistance services.

Medicare complaints may be filed with the U.S. Social Security Administration (800-772-1213; www.ssa.gov). The U.S. Department of Veterans Affairs (877-222-VETS; www.va.gov) handles complaints about veterans' benefits.

Taking Your Insurance with You. Under the Consolidated Omnibus Budget Reconciliation Act (COBRA), you can keep your insurance for eighteen months after you leave a company or become a part-time worker, provided your company has twenty or more employees. Your employer must notify you in writing about the COBRA option and if you want it, you must activate its coverage within sixty days. However, you must then pay for the full cost (at the employer's group rate) of coverage plus up to 2 percent to cover administrative costs. If you leave your job because you are disabled, you can stay on COBRA for an additional eleven months. If you leave your job for other reasons and become disabled within sixty days, you can remain on COBRA for the entire twenty-nine months (eighteen months basic COBRA plus the additional eleven months). This is the waiting period for Medicare, so if you apply for Social Security as soon as you become disabled, you can have access to Medicare when COBRA runs out.

COBRA also helps you qualify for a private health care policy. For example, if you stay on COBRA until it runs out, you cannot be turned down from buying a private health care policy. Also, the insurance company cannot make you prove insurability or face a preexisting condition exclusion period. You'll need to buy the private policy within sixty-two days from the date COBRA runs out. (If you wait too long, you may be able to get a state-sponsored plan, which is available for hard-to-insure people.)

Some medical plans offer "disability extension of benefits," which covers the cost of continuing treatment for a disabling illness for some time (usually one year, if you lose your medical coverage). For instance, if your insurance lapses while you are on disability, the cost of your continued treatment is covered and you don't pay a premium during this time.

What to Do If You Don't Have Insurance. Getting a job with a large company that offers good benefits is one solution, but be careful to read their medical plan's policy regarding preexisting conditions. You may also qualify for one of the programs listed below. Hospital financial counselors and social workers are acquainted with government programs and will be able to help you determine what, if any, programs may offer you assistance.

Medicaid. This government program is available to those with income and assets below a certain level, which varies from state to state. Since not all health care providers accept Medicaid, choices and possibly quality of care may be limited. Examples of those eligible for Medicaid are: low-income families with children, Supplemental Security Income (SSI) recipients, infants born to Medicaid-eligible pregnant women or children under age 6, and pregnant women whose income is below the family poverty level. People receiving Medicare may receive help for their out-of-pocket expenses from their state Medicaid program.

Medicare. This government program is available to those who meet a very strict definition of disability and therefore qualify for Social Security benefits. You qualify for Medicare after twenty-nine months of disability or reaching the age of 65.

Medicare provides basic health coverage, but it doesn't apply to all of your medical expenses. It is divided into two parts: Part A, which is free, pays for hospital care, home health care, hospice care, and care in Medicare-certified nursing facilities. Part B covers diagnostic studies, doctor's services, durable medical equipment used at home, and ambulance transportation.

Most health care providers do accept Medicare. Medicare options now include the following:

- **Health Maintenance Organization (HMO).** In a Medicare HMO, you go only to the doctors and hospitals it includes. Your primary doctor must approve the majority of services before you receive them.

- **Preferred Provider Organization (PPO).** In a PPO, you choose doctors and hospitals from within a network. The medical providers who agree to become part of the network charge lower fees to plan members than non–plan members.

- **Point of Service (POS).** A POS plan combines the features of an HMO and PPO, but is less restrictive. You can choose doctors and hospitals outside the network, but your costs will be lower if you stay within the network.

Before choosing one of the managed care forms of Medicare, read through the plan to be sure you'll be happy with your choice of doctors and hospitals. To learn about the various Medicare options, check with your state's insurance commission or review various consumer-oriented publications.

Medigap. There are ten Medigap plans, identified by letters A through J, and they are offered in all fifty states. Plan A is the core plan. The others contain the features of Plan A, plus other benefits. However, not all insurance carriers offer all ten plans. Check with several companies to see which plan offers the benefits you need at a price that is affordable for you. These are add-on policies that become available within six months of going on Medicare.

Veterans' benefits. Veterans qualify for benefits from the government. These benefits are changing and the number of veterans' medical facilities is declining, so contact the Department of Veterans Affairs for details. Veterans and their dependents and survivors also may participate in the Civilian Health and Medical Program of the Uniformed Services (CHAMPUS) or as it is now called, TRICARE Standard. This program shares the cost of professional home care services, social work and counseling services, medications, and many other costs.

The Hill-Burton program. The federal government provides funds to hospitals and other medical facilities so that free or low-cost services are available to those who cannot pay their medical costs. However, services covered by other government programs—such as Medicare and Medicaid—or by some insurance policies, aren't covered by Hill-Burton. Eligibility is based on family size and income. Income is based on your earnings for the previous year or your income from the last three months multiplied by four, whichever is less.

The Older Americans Act (OAA). This act, which is currently being reauthorized by Congress, is designed to enable frail and disabled people 60 years old and older to remain independent. The OAA covers some home care services, such as aides, meal delivery, and escort and shopping services. The funds are granted based on social and financial need. For more information, visit the Administration on Aging web page (www.aoa.dhhs.gov).

Community organizations. Civic and religious organizations may offer financial assistance for people with cancer. The Salvation Army, United Way, Lutheran Social Services, and Catholic Social Services are organizations to investigate (they may be found in the phone book yellow pages under "Social Service Organizations"). Churches and synagogues may also offer other services such as transportation, childcare, and home care services that can help relieve the financial burden of out-of-pocket expenses. The ACS also can tell you about numerous organizations that support the person with cancer.

Borrowing from friends and family. A close friend or family member may be willing to loan you money, especially if you outline a repayment period and an interest rate that at least meets the minimum federal rate. (To find out what it is, go to the IRS web site at www.irs.ustreas.gov.) If you follow this route, put the agreement in writing to avoid misunderstandings about the terms. The interest on family loans may be taxable, so you and the person making the loan should discuss this with an accountant. If you don't think you will be able to repay the loan, ask for a gift instead. Any individual, including a relative, can give you a tax-free gift of up to $10,000 a year, and a couple can give up to $20,000. One way to avoid reaching this limit is for others to directly pay your medical facility bill. (The gift does not provide a tax deduction for the person offering the gift.)

Guaranteed Access Programs. A number of states sell comprehensive health insurance to those of their residents who have difficulty getting coverage. These state programs, sometimes called risk pools, help people who have been denied coverage. They are not for the indigent, and in fact, the insurance typically costs more than regular insurance. The HIPAA (Health Insurance Portability and Accountability Act of 1996) provides nationwide standards and a guarantee of access to health insurance coverage.

Programs vary from one state to another, but in general they are nonprofit associations with a board of directors. The board contracts with an established insurance company to collect premiums and pay claims and administrate the program on a day-to-day basis. Insurance benefits vary, but risk pools typically offer benefits that are comparable to basic private market plans—80/20 major medical and outpatient coverage and a choice of deductible and copayments. Maximum lifetime benefits vary by state from as low as $250,000 to $1 million (and may even have no cap).

Group plan issuers may deny, exclude, or limit an enrollee's benefits arising from a preexisting condition for no more than twelve months following the effective date of coverage. This waiting period may be waived for people who have had continual coverage previously.

Although this insurance is costly, there is a cap on the premium that varies from state to state. Some state risk pools do have a subsidy for lower income, medically uninsurable people. Contact ACS (800-ACS-2345) for a current list of states and the companies that run their Guaranteed Access programs or call your state department of insurance.

Long-Term Disability Insurance

Private disability insurance plans may pay 60 to 70 percent of your monthly income if you are unable to work. It's important to review your policy carefully to determine how it defines disability, what the preexisting condition exclusion period is, and whether or not your premiums are waived during your illness. You also need to know the monthly benefit amount, the benefit period, the waiting period, and its taxability status. The hospital financial counselor or social worker can help you determine whether your policy affects your access to government-provided disability income.

Your life insurance policy may include something called a "waiver of premium." This generally means that the insurance company pays the policy's premium if you become disabled.

Insurance to cover credit card bills if you become disabled is also available (see page 494, under *Credit Insurance*).

Social Security Disability Income (SSDI). If you have been working for many years, you have contributed to Social Security and qualify for disability benefits if you meet their narrow definition of disability. (If you're rejected, try again, since many cases are approved after appeal.) Benefits do not begin until the sixth full month of disability. Your income has nothing to do with whether you qualify for SSDI. To find out how to apply, call the Social Security Administration.

Supplemental Security Income (SSI). If you have not worked much or if your income was very low before you became unable to work, you may be eligible for SSI, provided your assets are below a certain level. You must be disabled, over age 65, and/or blind. The monthly income provided by SSI varies from state to state, but it can be as much as $500.

Retirement Plans

If you qualify for a so-called hardship provision, your retirement plan may provide cash before retirement without a penalty. A financial advisor or your employer's human resources office can let you know if this is available to you.

Life Insurance

Life insurance has traditionally been of benefit to the surviving family of a deceased person. Today it can be used to provide cash to the owner of the policy. This may be a good option particularly for those whose children are grown and no longer rely on the person who holds the policy for support. There are several methods for obtaining cash in this way, but be certain to get expert advice before you do so.

Cash Value Life Insurance Policy Loans. If you have this type of policy, you may be able to get a loan on the cash value of your policy or even withdraw some of the cash value. It's wise to seek expert tax and insurance advice, since tax issues could arise. Also, realize that the type of insurance that most employers provide to their workers is "term insurance." Although a loan might be raised on a term policy, this type of policy does not have cash value.

Loans. You may be able to use your life insurance as the basis for getting a loan. The loan is paid off at your death. If you are trying to qualify for a program such as SSI (where your income is used to judge your eligibility), a loan is a good idea. The money from the loan isn't counted as part of your total income.

Accelerated Death Benefits. Some policies offer a predeath payment for those with a life expectancy that is less than one year. Check with your insurer to see if it offers this type of program. Keep in mind that receiving accelerated death benefits may keep you from qualifying for some government programs.

Viatical Loans or Settlements. You also may be able to borrow against your life insurance policy through a company that makes viatical loans. The interest charged is likely to be high. However, loan proceeds can be set up so that you could still qualify for government programs like SSI. It's important to use the loan proceeds to pay for medical costs. If the money is used to bolster a bank or savings account, you may not qualify for some government programs. However, the viatical funds are income tax free if the legislative rules about terminal illness are met.

This way of taking a loan against one's life insurance policy or selling it for cash is also called a "living benefit." This option is usually made available only if a doctor certifies that the person with cancer has a terminal condition and is expected to live less than several years. Usually the person who considers the option is unable to work and has limited income.

A viatical loan or settlement will ease the stress of your financial concerns, but be aware of these disadvantages:

• Your heirs will receive no insurance money from your policy.

• You may not make the best trade available.

• Once a policy is sold, the sale is usually not reversible.

A viatical payment is usually between 60 and 80 percent of the face value of the policy. The original insurance company may offer more money, sometimes as much as 95 percent of the face value of the policy. It is usually tax free, and the holder of the policy can use the money in any way he or she wants.

Those with a term policy may be able to take a loan on the policy. Sometimes a loan may be raised from a third party using the life insurance policy as collateral. For more information, contact the National Viatical Association or the Viatical Association of America (see the *Resources* section).

Credit and Loans

Credit or loans may provide temporary solutions. If you already have credit card balances that you cannot pay, you can try to consolidate your balance to a card that charges a low interest rate. If you find you are unable to make even the minimum payments, call the credit card company and explain your situation. It may be useful to contact a Consumer Credit Counseling office (see *Resources*).

If you don't already have credit (e.g., credit cards, home equity lines of credit, a home equity loan), establish it as soon as you can. Try to get overdraft protection on your checking account. Although it's recommended that you not use these sources of credit except in emergencies, you'll want to know how much credit you can access before the need for it arises. For example, if your doctor recommends an experimental treatment not covered by your insurance, having credit will allow you to pursue this option. Also, you may find the lag time between submitting a claim and receiving the check from your insurer quite long. Having credit will allow you to pay the bills promptly. In some cases, you may want to pay your doctor bills with a credit card.

Your first step in getting credit is to check your credit profile. Contact one of the three major reporting agencies (Equifax, Experian, Transunion) in order to get a copy of your credit profile.

Some lending companies will loan money to terminally ill people, using the person's insurance policy as collateral. The loan is repaid from the proceeds of the policy after the person's death and the remaining value of the policy is paid to the beneficiary.

Credit Insurance. When using credit, consider applying for types of insurance called credit life and credit disability. If you already have credit, you may be able to get this insurance simply by calling the credit card company or lender. If you die without this protection, the money from your estate will first go toward paying off these debts. Any remaining estate funds will then go to your heirs.

The amount that you would pay for these types of insurance is based on how much you owe. If you owe a large amount, the insurance could be costly. Most financial advisors do not recommend that the average consumer have these insurance coverages, but they are options to consider if you're being treated for cancer.

Credit life insurance pays off the balance on a credit card or loan if you die. It is very simple to get credit life insurance on a credit card. Few credit card companies ever ask you medical questions. However, larger loans, such as mortgages and car loans, can be difficult to insure.

Credit disability insurance pays your minimum monthly payment for a period of time, usually a year. Generally, you don't have to prove your ability to be insured. However, there is often a preexisting condition exclusion period that is typically six months long. To receive the benefit, you must have the coverage for six months before becoming disabled from a preexisting condition. If you became disabled during the first six months, credit disability would not pay.

Home Equity Conversion

Home equity conversion allows homeowners over age 62 to convert part of their homes' equity into cash. The most common type is a "reverse mortgage," which is a loan against your home that doesn't have to be repaid as long as you live there. The cash can pay medical bills and other expenses. The loan can be repaid in the future if the borrower sells the home, dies, or moves. However, a reverse mortgage may disqualify you from some government programs, so discuss this option with a financial advisor to determine if this is worthwhile for you. The AARP and other nonprofit consumer groups may also be able to provide information about home equity conversion.

Staying on Top of the Bills and Claims

It's very important to submit claims for all your medical expenses, even when you are uncertain about your coverage. You or the person handling your finances needs to establish a system of tracking expenses and claims. Keeping accurate and complete records of claims submitted, pending, and paid will help you know when you've reached your deductible (if you have one) and your reimbursement limit. Keep copies of everything—letters of medical necessity, bills, receipts, requests for sick leave, and correspondence with insurance companies. If you discuss the specifics of your employee benefits package with human resources, ask that person to put the answers in writing and sign it.

Submit your bills as you receive them. If you can't pay your bills, ask the hospital financial counselor, caseworker, or social worker for help. They can often make payment arrangements with you.

If you have problems getting a claim covered by an insurance company, ask for help from the doctor's office or the hospital claims office. Problems may relate to the language in the policy or an interpretation of it, so be aware of the exact language that supports the coverage denial. Also, an insurance company representative can explain the appeal process for a disputed claim.

Breast Cancer and the Medically Underserved

In 2000, the Breast and Cervical Cancer Treatment Act was signed into law. This act enhances the National Breast and Cervical Cancer Early Detection Program (NBCCEDP) by providing funds to pay for treatment associated with breast and cervical cancer in medically underserved populations. Implementation of this new option will help women focus their energies on fighting their disease instead of worrying about how to pay for treatment. As in the Early Detection Program, individual states must adopt the Breast and Cervical Cancer Treatment Act in order to receive matching federal funds. For more information on this program, please contact the CDC (888-842-6355; www.cdc.gov/cancer).

INFORM

YOURSELF

Advancing Illness

30

Metastasis and Recurrence

The initial course of therapy is successful for about half the people diagnosed with a malignancy. These people never have to fight another battle with the disease.

But in some situations, cancer has spread, or metastasized, from the primary site to another part of the body by the time cancer is diagnosed. For example, if a man has lung cancer that has spread to the brain at the time of diagnosis, his treatment will be very different from a man whose lung cancer has not spread to the brain. But if metastasis is found after initial treatment, the cancer care team explores treatment possibilities in order to attempt to control the cancer as long as possible and preserve a good quality of life for the person.

In other cases someone may enjoy a period of remission when he or she is cancer free for some time after the initial treatment. If the cancer recurs after this time, it does not mean, however, that controlling it is impossible.

Whether the disease metastasized before treatment began or has recurred, much can be done to continue the battle and maintain a satisfactory quality of life with surgery, chemotherapy, radiation therapy, and/or biological therapy. Optimism, hope, and effective coping strategies are great allies as well. This chapter will discuss a "second stage" of treatment and all of the feelings and emotions that accompany realization of a metastasis or recurrence.

Understanding the Language

The terms used to describe the various transitions in cancer development have different connotations that can sometimes be confusing. The meaning can be clouded, too, by the person—a doctor or a layperson—who uses them.

CANCER BASICS

Words You May Hear

- The name of a tumor or cancer typically refers to its site of origin, that is, the place or organ where it initially developed. For example, a malignancy in the lung is called lung cancer, and even if those cells spread to the liver, the cancer is still called lung cancer or sometimes lung cancer metastatic to the liver or metastatic lung cancer to the liver. Cancer terms also convey information about a tumor's location in other ways: a *primary tumor* is an original tumor. The primary site is the location of the original tumor.

- A *secondary tumor* is the result of the spread of cancer either by extension or via the blood or lymphatic system. A secondary site is the location of cancer cells or a tumor at a site other than the primary one.

- A *localized cancer* is a tumor still in one organ, and a localized recurrence is one or more tumors that recur in the original site but with no involvement of nearby lymph nodes or tissue.

- A *regional cancer* refers to the spread of the original cancer to the nearest lymph nodes.

- A *direct extension* is a cancer that has grown, or extended, directly from the original tumor to the surrounding area.

- *Metastatic cancer* indicates that cancer cells from the original tumor are elsewhere in the body, having spread through the blood or lymphatic vessels from the original or primary site.

- A *recurrence* is any reemergence of a tumor after a treatment that initially removed or destroyed all the recognized tumor cells. A recurrence may occur: in the original site (local recurrence) and not involve metastases, in the nearby lymph nodes or adjacent soft tissues (regional recurrence), or in organs or tissues far removed from the initial tumor site (distant recurrence).

- *Remission* is a disease-free interval. The cancer can be in remission for months or years. (Of course, if the cancer never grows back, a person is said to be cured.) If cancer recurs at all, the most likely period is within the first two years following treatment.

- *Advanced cancer* is sometimes medically defined as cancer that has affected at least one organ to the point that it is not functioning well. It may or may not involve metastases or recurrence. The term is more commonly used to describe a cancer that for all practical purposes is incurable and usually indicates that life expectancy is limited, but people with advanced cancer may sometimes live much longer.

It's important for you and your oncologist to speak the same language, so don't hesitate to ask exactly what he or she means by terms like advanced, spread, and recurrence.

How Cancer Spreads

Although malignant tumors grow at different rates and spread in different ways, cancer either spreads directly from the primary tumor to surrounding areas or when cancer cells enter the blood and/or lymph vessels and metastasize to other organs. The latter metastatic process typically progresses in a series of somewhat predictable steps. This sequence of events is called the metastatic cascade. It's important to understand the phenomenon because doctors may refer to one or more of these steps and the factors that influence it when discussing treatment options.

Dormant State

Cancer cells vary in their aggressiveness and tendency to spread, depending on their type and location. Your oncologist makes a treatment recommendation based on his or her knowledge of the likelihood that a particular cancer will spread. The information considered includes the type of cancer, its stage when it was diagnosed, specific characteristics of the cells identified by the pathologist (see Chapter 5), and your general condition. A malignancy may develop slowly and remain inactive for years. Prostate cancer, for example, is usually a slow-growing cancer, so some men who have it die of old age or from other causes before their cancer causes any symptoms or is detected. In general—but not always—as the cancer cells multiply and the tumor grows larger, the likelihood of metastasis increases.

Growth Phase

As a tumor grows, a blood supply develops to nourish the increasing mass. These new blood vessels also give the cells access to the body's general circulation. The process of forming new capillaries to connect the tumor to nearby blood vessels is called neovascularization. Currently, researchers are investigating various ways of assessing a tumor's blood supply or evaluating angiogenesis, the creation of new blood vessels, as a measure of a tumor's potential to metastasize. Researchers are also trying to determine whether angiogenesis can be used as a guide to predict outcomes and create new treatments.

Invasion

Cancer cells spread to areas of the body beyond the original tumor in two ways. Most commonly, single cells break away from the initial tumor and enter the surrounding blood vessels. Clumps of cancer cells accumulate and lodge in the tiny capillaries close to the primary site; some cells manage to enter the general circulation; and others enter the nearby lymphatic system as lymph flows in and out of the bloodstream.

Those cancer cells that enter the circulatory and lymphatic systems follow the paths of those vessels and often travel, or metastasize, to predictable sites in the body. For example, cancer cells eventually make their way to the lungs and the liver because these are the main organs through which blood flows, carrying with it the cancer cells. Wherever the cancer cells settle, they continue growing and form what are called colony tumors.

Although this metastatic process seems very orderly, some patterns cannot be explained by mapping the route of the circulatory or lymphatic vessels. Some cancers find and invade specific sites in what is called a homing pattern. One theory is that cancer cells have certain substances that interact with the cells of certain organs and not others. Or it may be that some organs release chemicals that stimulate the growth of cancer cells that lodge in them. Learning more about the metastatic process will eventually yield important treatment strategies.

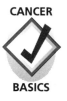

CANCER

BASICS

Invasion of Prostate Cancer into Surrounding Tissue

Cancer cells do not have to enter the blood or lymphatic vessels for spread to occur. Sometimes cancer spreads directly to the tissue adjacent to the primary site. This local spreading is similar to the way ivy grows on a wall. A tumor in the prostate, for example, may grow large enough to extend outside the prostate gland into the surrounding tissue.

Metastasis: A Second Tumor

Once the invading cells reach receptive tissue, some of them develop into secondary tumors (metastases). To ensure the cells' survival, secondary tumors, like the primary tumor, develop a new blood supply.

With the exception of nonmelanoma skin cancers, about one-third of people have metastases detected at the time their cancer is first diagnosed. Another third have metastases that are too small to be detected at the time of diagnoses. These so-called micrometastases will eventually grow large enough to be detected by the usual diagnostic tests or cause symptoms. This is why after surgery to remove a primary tumor, additional treatment called adjuvant therapy—radiation or chemotherapy—is sometimes recommended, even when there is no evidence of metastasis (see Chapters 9 and 15). Furthermore, studies have shown that chemotherapy and/or radiation therapy may be much more effective against micrometastases than either treatment is when the secondary tumors are large enough to be detected.

Map of the Lymph System

The lymph system consists of capillaries and larger vessels, glands known as lymph nodes, and several organs: the spleen, tonsils, and thymus. A clear fluid, called lymph, flows through the capillaries and vessels, which branch throughout the entire body. When cancer cells enter this fluid, they usually become trapped in the nodes and are prevented from spreading further, but sometimes they make their way to distant organs. The illustration shows the network of lymph capillaries and the location of the major lymph nodes and organs.

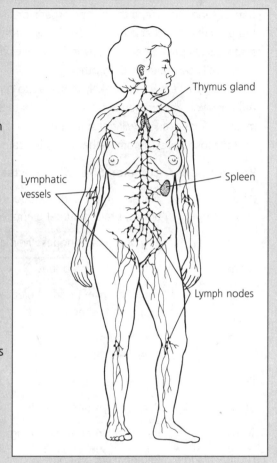

CANCER BASICS

Thymus gland

Lymphatic vessels

Spleen

Lymph nodes

Spotting—and Stopping—Wandering Cells

Staging—determining the amount and location of disease—is done at the time of diagnosis of the primary tumor. A series of tests called a metastatic workup will be done to determine the extent of disease beyond the region of the primary tumor. Some metastatic workup tests are done at the time of diagnosis, and some are performed for the first time at subsequent checkups. They may be repeated if symptoms of spread or recurrence appear (see Chapter 5).

At the time of diagnosis, your oncologist may order tests such as various x-rays and scans to detect metastatic tumors. Occasionally other tests, such as examination of certain body fluids or even a biopsy may be done to identify cancer cells. Which tests are necessary and the extent of the evaluation to detect possible metastases depend on the site and stage of the cancer. Doctors do not always agree on the choice, timeliness, or usefulness of the tests. Nevertheless, managed care providers may require a certain sequence of tests.

CANCER

BASICS

Where Cancer Goes

Cancer tends to spread to specific organs or tissues, usually depending on the path the blood and lymph vessels take from the original site. Also, some tissues provide a more favorable environment in which certain tumor cells can flourish than others.

Some cancers are more likely to spread to certain organs than others. Although you will be monitored for spread to these organs, this does not mean that your cancer will not spread to other sites. Be alert and tell your doctor about any symptoms—they could indicate that your cancer has spread.

Primary Tumor	Common Sites of Metastasis*
Breast	Axillary lymph nodes, opposite breast, lungs, liver, bones, brain, adrenal glands, and ovaries
Colon	Regional lymph nodes, liver, and lungs
Kidney	Lungs, liver, and bones
Lung	Regional lymph nodes, pleura, diaphragm, liver, bones, brain, and adrenal glands
Ovary	Peritoneum, regional lymph nodes, uterus, omentum, intestines, lungs, and liver
Prostate	Bones of spine and pelvis, regional lymph nodes
Stomach	Regional lymph nodes, liver, and lungs
Testis	Regional lymph nodes, lungs, and liver
Urinary bladder	Regional lymph nodes, bones, lungs, peritoneum, pleura, liver, and brain
Uterus	Regional lymph nodes, lungs, and liver

*This does not include organs that may be affected by direct extension of the cancer from its original site.

Preventing New Cancers

Unfortunately, although you have already been diagnosed with a cancer, you may develop other cancers. It is important that you undergo those tests that are known to detect early cancer of the breast, prostate, colon and rectum, and cervix (see Chapter 4). And, of course, it's helpful to follow the recommendations usually given to avoid cancer in the first place, which usually requires making lifestyle changes (see Chapter 2).

Some of these changes are well known. Smokers who break the habit reduce their risk of not only lung cancer but also cancers of the mouth, throat, esophagus, larynx, pancreas, kidney, and bladder. Eating a diet rich in fiber, as found in fruits and grains, helps reduce the risk of colon cancer. Physical activity and a diet rich in fruits and vegetables help control weight and may reduce the risk of endometrial, breast, and colon cancers. Protecting yourself from exposure to the sun lowers the chances of developing skin cancer.

Recurrence: When Cancer Comes Back

A remission may last for decades, but some people experience a recurrence of disease within a few years of the treatment of the original cancer. Of course, no matter how well prepared you may be, hearing your doctor say that the cancer has returned is extremely distressing, and you are immediately forced to confront and cope again with powerful emotions.

You should expect to shed tears of grief over losing your health. If you had a difficult time with the treatment when your cancer was first diagnosed, you may be distraught at having to repeat the process. Some people express feelings of betrayal, by a body that appeared to be healthy, by a medical system that seemed to have failed, by treatments that now seem to have been ineffective. Doubts arise about what treatment can accomplish, and feelings of guilt or self-blame are common. You may question whether you did something to cause the recurrence or didn't do something to improve your resistance to the disease. It's important to dispel these feelings of guilt or irresponsibility by understanding that you have done nothing to cause the cancer metastases or recurrence.

Those who have been through this time of profound disappointment and emotional turmoil and the professionals who have cared for them say that realizing that these myriad feelings are normal is the first step in coping with them.

Keeping Up the Fight

Survivors of cancer suggest that for many people, thinking of the disease as a long-term, chronic condition can help in coping with the fear of recurrence. That is, instead of thinking that you had a cancer that might return at any moment, you should regard yourself as having a cancer that can be managed by taking care of yourself and following your doctor's advice.

You can learn to live with and adjust to having cancer, just as a person learns to live with other serious conditions such as diabetes or high blood pressure. If your disease is in remission, it's essential to follow your doctor's recommended schedule of follow-up visits to detect any signs of metastasis or recurrence. You may be given certain physical exams and blood tests, x-rays, and CT or MRI scans. In addition, your oncologist may request that you have other procedures, not because he or she is worried about anything new, but because these are the steps to follow in managing a chronic condition.

It often is easier to make lifestyle changes, such as altering your diet or stopping smoking, if you think of them as a way to keep yourself in the best possible condition given the challenges of your health history. And if your cancer should return, you will know about it early and take the next appropriate steps for your care. Cancer survivors often say that keeping fully abreast of their conditions throughout their illness is crucial to gaining control of their fear and anxiety and allowing them to make important decisions about their future treatment.

Dealing with the Bad News

Hearing that cancer has reached an advanced stage obviously is a shock. You no longer can deny the existence of the disease, as so often happens after the initial diagnosis. Gradually, though, your expectations will shift. You may find yourself becoming more cautious about your prognosis. Rather than believing the disease will not affect your life span, you may begin to see the future as finite because of your cancer.

Most people who face cancer learn that the battle is as much a mental one as a physical one. For many, greater knowledge about their disease, treatment choices, and prognosis can boost their capacities to handle any setbacks. Those who seem to cope best are the best informed, and recent studies suggest a link between improved survival and effective coping skills (see Chapter 27).

Sharing the Stress

Enlisting support from family and friends may never be quite so important. Old issues may resurface, accompanied by new concerns and fears. Being reassured and supported by close friends and loved ones is the best foundation for handling a recurrence and the even more difficult challenges of advanced disease (see Chapter 8).

People who have been in remission for a long time sometimes have problems asking for help again. No matter how caring the support was the first time around, relying on others once more can generate feelings of failure and fear of being a burden. It's a difficult time for family members and friends as well. They may be hesitant to approach you and worry that they will do or say something wrong. They may also have a hard time coming to terms with their own feelings about your illness (see Chapter 28).

This is why the best way to get support is to ask directly, and in an open and trusting way, for whatever you need. You must be very clear about what you want, and those offering support should be equally clear about what they can give. Everyone should realize that needs—and someone's ability to fulfill them—may change as the situation changes.

Care at the End of Life

Supportive care is concerned with the physical, psychosocial, and spiritual issues of the patient with cancer and the family during cancer treatment. It addresses those interventions used to support patients during the effects caused by treatment, such as nausea and vomiting, pain, mucositis, infection, fatigue, and bleeding. This supportive care is also called symptom management, or managing symptoms caused by the treatment.

Supportive care extends into the cancer experience when it is no longer possible to significantly alter the course of a person's cancer. At no time should anyone ever be told that "there is nothing more we can do." Indeed, something can always be done to relieve symptoms, ease distress, provide comfort, and in other ways improve the quality of life of someone with advanced cancer. This, too, is a type of supportive care called palliative care or end-of-life care. Treatment initiated at this time is designed to help you maintain the best possible level of physical, emotional, mental, spiritual, and social life—regardless of how far your disease has progressed.

Palliative care is concerned with providing maximum quality of life at the time when the cancer can no longer be cured. It can include such interventions as radiation therapy for bone pain, pain control with medications, control of nausea and vomiting, and so on. It is made up of those interventions aimed at comfort and support. When the cancer is no longer responsive to curative treatment, this care is also called end-of-life care or supportive care.

Hospice care is used to mean a specific approach to end-of-life care during the final stages of life, when it is clear that the time remaining is limited.

One of the most important things that you or those close to you can do is to discover what kind of care and assistance is available and to make sure you get it. You can discuss your feelings and needs with your primary caregivers and come to an understanding about how you want to be treated. Many experts think that these discussions should start at the time of diagnosis and continue throughout the course of the disease. Keep in mind, too, that supportive care—that is, care aimed at controlling symptoms and improving the quality of life—is important at any stage of the disease.

The Crucial Turning Point

Deciding to shift the focus of treatment from cure to comfort can be extremely difficult. People with cancer, their families, and even their doctors often have trouble accepting that the therapy directed against the disease is not going to halt it. The reasons for coming to this conclusion include the following:

- The treatment's side effects are debilitating.

- The disease is not responding to treatment.

- The treatment has a detrimental effect on life quality.

When the conclusion is reached that treatment cannot stop the disease, the usual response is to discontinue ineffective treatments and to give greater attention to managing symptoms such as pain, nausea, and anxiety. Sometimes these measures may involve surgery, chemotherapy, or radiation therapy, but with the purpose of palliation, or control, and not cure. It is important to learn both what a treatment can accomplish at this time and what cannot be accomplished.

You may have to make a number of decisions concerning this shift from treatment focused on curing the disease to palliative therapy directed toward controlling symptoms and maintaining a good quality of life. Some choices are difficult, partly because others may see the issue from different points of view and react according to their own needs, concerns, or fears. For example, some doctors are trained to take an aggressive stance against disease and so are uncomfortable about doing anything that seems like "giving up." Family members may have similar beliefs. The final decisions must rest with you, but your family and your primary care doctor and oncologist should also discuss the issues honestly and help reach a consensus.

Quality of Life

The terms quality of life and meaningful life have a variety of meanings. No specific standard or set of guidelines regarding quality of life is widely accepted by the lay public or medical or psychiatric communities. The common notion of a "good" quality of life often includes such things as independence, full functioning of body and senses, and freedom from anxiety. But quality of life is really a very personal issue. For a person with advanced cancer, though, a reasonable quality of life requires at the very least: relief from pain and other uncomfortable symptoms; relief from anxiety and depression, including the fear of pain; and a sense of security that assistance will be readily available whenever needed. All are possible.

For you, acceptable life quality may also require being treated with the respect and consideration that would be expected if you were not sick. It may mean maintaining your personal integrity and self-worth and a sense of meaning and purpose, such as continuing to be consulted on family and perhaps business issues. It may hinge on having some sense of control over events. You may want only a little authority, preferring to feel that others are taking charge and thus freeing you from having to make difficult decisions. Or you may prefer to stay in charge. A good supportive care program should provide just the degree of control that each person needs, which may mean helping overcontrollers to relax their grip a little and accept needed help.

QUESTIONS

TO ASK

Questions to Ask About Treatment

When deciding whether it is appropriate to continue treatment targeted against the disease or to focus the treatment on symptom control and maintaining the quality of life, you and your family can discuss the following questions with your doctor, caregivers, and family:

- Is it possible for this treatment to cure the disease?

- Will the treatment slow the progress of the disease?

- Will the treatment improve the quality of my life?

Care and Communication

Most supportive care is provided in your home, sometimes with intermittent visits to the hospital or a specialty unit if fine-tuning of treatment to control symptoms is required. Your private doctor and/or the doctors of your community hospital may supervise this care. In addition, some hospitals and cancer centers now have hospice and/or supportive care teams. In most cases, your day-to-day palliative care needs will be managed by a nurse working closely with your doctor and other members of the team. Since your relationship with your nurse is critical, he or she must be skilled in pain management, symptom control, and end-of-life issues. This person is often your link to the others involved in your care and—most important—can help you communicate what is happening so that you can get what you need.

One of the most important aspects of hospice care is its emphasis on communication. It isn't always easy to talk to professionals about your day-to-day or even moment-to-moment difficulties and needs. For one thing, you may be anxious and frightened. Many people with advanced cancer constantly monitor their bodies for any sign of something wrong. They worry about what's going to happen later. Although these fears are not unusual, many feel uncomfortable mentioning such things to others. Your caregiver can deal with each worry specifically and concretely, keeping you informed of the treatments and choices available to you. Getting a more realistic idea of your future can provide some relief from worry and make a big difference in both your physical and emotional conditions.

You may not know how to talk about your symptoms. You've never had this experience before, so you have no practice in communicating in these circumstances. Your caregivers can teach you how.

Sometimes other people have to learn new ways of communicating too. In some families, especially among married couples, it is common for one person to be the "communicator." If your husband (or wife, son, daughter, or friend) has usually spoken for you, it may be especially hard for you to speak for yourself now. The other person can continue to be your spokesperson as long as you are able to discuss things clearly with that person and he or she learns how to describe your experience to your caregivers.

Relieving Symptoms

Palliative care specialists have focused considerable attention on what kind of support can best improve the well being of people with advanced cancer. Their concerns are controlling symptoms and maintaining a reasonable quality of life for you and your family.

Pain

One of the first things people with advanced cancer worry about is pain. But cancer does not always cause pain. Although 60 percent of people with advanced cancer have some pain, it can be controlled (see Chapter 23).

Gastrointestinal Problems

Nausea and vomiting may be associated with the disease or with the medicines used to control symptoms. Your health care team will evaluate the symptom and arrive at an appropriate treatment.

Constipation can occur with pain medicines, so a program of treatment to prevent or relieve it is started at the same time as the pain medicine. Constipation is a common cause of distress in people receiving opioids (narcotics) for pain, and it should be treated as aggressively as the pain itself.

Dry Mouth

A dry mouth is a common side effect of certain drugs. It can be relieved in several ways. Cleaning your mouth and rinsing it with water every two hours; using a room humidifier; sucking on ice cubes, lemon candy, pineapple pieces, or frozen tonic water; and chewing sugarless gum are some solutions. It is important that a nurse or doctor examine your mouth periodically for signs of infection, which may also cause your mouth to feel dry.

**TIPS AND
ADVICE**

Talking About Your Needs

People can't help you if they don't know what you need or want. Be specific. For example, it's not enough just to say, "I'm nauseated." Instead, you are encouraged to supply specific details. You might say, "I don't feel nauseated when I lie still, but as soon as I move my head I get sick and vomit." Or, "I vomit once, twice, five times a day. The color is green. I'm always nauseated when I feel upset." This tells your caregiver what may be contributing to your nausea and helps him or her determine what medicine or other measures, such as relaxation techniques, are most likely to relieve the discomfort. "The pain is worse" could mean anything from a little more discomfort all the way to severe. Caregivers can respond more effectively if you say instead, "The pain is mild when I keep still but becomes severe when I try to walk. The pain is in my hip and back." Or, "The pain is worse when I wake up in the morning and improves during the day after I take my pain medication and walk around." Some caregivers encourage you to rate the intensity of your pain on a scale of 0 to 10, or they may give you a list of words to help you describe your problem more precisely (see Chapter 23).

Respiratory Problems

If you cough or have some shortness of breath, your doctor and nurse will evaluate the symptom and start appropriate treatment to make you more comfortable. Sometimes you will be given medicine to help your cough; at other times you will be given medicine to dry the secretions. Sometimes oxygen is helpful; sometimes morphine in combination with other medication is used. The important thing is to let those who care for you know you have some breathing problems so that the symptom can be relieved.

Loss of Appetite

One of the most distressing accompaniments of advanced cancer may be loss of appetite. Some people develop an aversion to certain foods and/or eat less.

Others begin to hate meat, fish, chicken, and eggs. Still others stop liking foods that have always been their favorites. A nurse or nutritionist can tell you how to make meals more attractive and suggest appropriate substitutes. For example, those who no longer enjoy eating meat may get their protein from yogurt or cheese. Frequent, small meals may be more appetizing than large, three-course ones. Cold foods are often more acceptable than hot. Foods with strong aromas can be avoided. People who don't feel like eating in the morning may be more interested by the afternoon. Poor oral hygiene, often a factor in eating problems, can be overcome with proper instruction in mouth care. Sometimes dentures that no longer fit properly can impede a person's ability to eat.

Remember that eating less is normal at the end of life and should not become a focus of stress for the family (see Chapter 18).

Sleeplessness

Sleep-wake patterns may change when people are sick or nearing the end of their life. You may sleep more during the day, when others are around and you feel more secure than in the silence of the night. Again, it is important to find out the cause of the sleeplessness. Is it because of pain, anxiety, other symptoms, or depression? Once the cause is known, appropriate steps can be taken, such as providing better pain control, taking a sedative, airing fears, listening to relaxation tapes at night, and/or keeping a night light on.

Weakness and Fatigue

As the illness progresses, a generalized weakness can make you and your care-givers feel discouraged. Weakness and fatigue can be caused by many things, including the progression of the disease, certain treatments, or depression. Once again, understanding the cause of these symptoms is essential to obtaining appropriate treatment, which is the function of the palliative care team. Some things are reversible; others are not. Pacing yourself and setting goals that can be achieved can be helpful (see Chapter 24).

Forms of Treatment

It is important to understand that the same treatments given when cure was the goal—surgery, chemotherapy, and radiation therapy—may be used in advanced cancer solely to relieve symptoms or to prevent complications (see Chapter 9). This is the time for you and your family to discuss with your oncologist the goals, risks, and benefits of palliative treatment. What are the side effects, and how long will they last; what are the benefits, and how long will they last? When you have the answers, you can decide. Remember that although the decision is yours, many people can help you make it. Many of these treatments are not burdensome and can make a big difference in your quality of life. For example, radiation therapy to reduce the size of a tumor pressing on a nerve and causing pain can be helpful. Chemotherapy can also be used in some instances to reduce the size of a tumor and relieve pain.

Always ask your doctor whether this treatment will improve your quality of life or whether its side effects will diminish it and, therefore, outweigh the benefit.

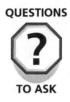

QUESTIONS

TO ASK

Choosing a Treatment

When a doctor recommends medication, surgery, chemotherapy, radiation therapy, or another treatment to relieve symptoms, you may want to ask such questions as the following:

- Will this treatment prolong my life?

- Will this treatment improve the quality of my life?

- Will it do both?

- Will it do neither?

Home Care and Hospital Care Compared

In a major national survey, 86 percent of the people questioned said that if they had advanced disease with no likelihood of cure, they would rather be cared for at home or in the home of a family member than at a hospital. The same percentage said they would be interested in a comprehensive program of care at home by doctors, nurses, counselors, or other health care professionals. When choosing between supportive care in a hospital (or other inpatient facility) or at home, you need to understand the advantages and disadvantages of each. It is a very personal decision that depends on a great many variables. Furthermore, there is no right or wrong choice, only what feels best for you.

A hospital or nursing home has nurse support twenty-four hours a day. At home, a nurse may visit you once or twice a day. In the hospital, you are more separated from your family and familiar surroundings. At home, you are more likely to be at the center of the household. In the hospital, family members can visit and help in modest ways, whereas they must carry the major burden of home care. In each setting, however, you have a team available to you and your family. Your doctor continues to play as important a role in your care as he or she did when the objective of treatment was cure.

Sometimes arrangements can be made to take advantage of both settings at different stages. You and your family should discuss the issues thoroughly with your doctor, nurse, and social worker before you make any decisions. It's important to understand what home care involves. Some families underestimate its difficulties, but others discover that it is well within their capabilities. Including your nurse or social worker in these discussions is important, because your doctor may be unaware of the options available for home care or of the insurance and financial issues.

Hospice Programs

In the Middle Ages, a hospice was a way station for travelers. The term is used today to reflect the philosophy that the final stage of disease is still a part of life's journey. Accepting death is central to the hospice philosophy, yet the emphasis on care reflects the positive aspects of living. Hospice programs continue to provide palliative care, focusing on the last days, weeks, or months of life.

The growth of hospice care is part of a grassroots movement toward social reform that began in the late 1960s. People began to wonder whether life-prolonging technology was valuable or even useful in every instance. They questioned the notion, "If it can be done, it should be done." There was a general movement toward more humane approaches to health care, and values and ethics in medical practice gained new importance. The growing concern with human and social values included a new examination of how to care for people in the final phase of illness.

Professionals and the public alike have come to recognize that too often in the past, people with very advanced disease were allowed to suffer and were isolated when they could have lived relatively well until the end. Some began to express anger and frustration over the widely accepted belief that pain was inevitable. Inspired by St. Christopher's Hospice in England and the pioneering efforts of its founder Cicely Saunders and her colleagues, a variety of special programs have been developed in the United States and Canada for both the inpatient and outpatient care of people with terminal diseases, most often very advanced cancer, and their families.

Hospice care focuses on working with your family to provide home care and on your physical, emotional, and spiritual needs. Although the emphasis is on helping your family take care of you, hospice care is also provided in some nursing homes, hospitals that have hospice units, and independently owned or freestanding hospices. If most of your hospice care will be at home, you may be admitted to a local hospital or hospice unit for a few days to bring a symptom under control or to provide respite for your family. Whatever the setting, hospice care is widely available and is covered by Medicare, Medicaid in over thirty states, the Veterans Administration, and most private insurance plans, HMOs, and other managed care organizations (see Chapter 29).

Many people may be nervous about discontinuing the therapy for their disease because they're afraid their doctor may no longer keep them as a patient. This is the time to make sure that your social worker and nurse are aware of your feelings. They can ensure that you will continue to receive excellent medical care.

Comfort and Communication

One of the greatest differences between hospice and the usual hospital care is that so few things are done "routinely" in a hospice setting. For example, diagnostic tests and procedures are ordered only if the information they provide will lead to measures that will increase your comfort.

People who have used hospice services say that it gave them hope that they would be looked after, without fear of uncontrollable pain or other symptoms. Other advantages that people have mentioned are as follows:

- It's an approach to care that includes the family. Families are encouraged to ask questions and to participate actively in caregiving and decision making.

- Personnel are attuned to details and recognize that you and your family are part of the team. Everyone works together, even though members of the team may have different priorities. For instance, your doctor may be concerned with correctly measuring your response to therapy, but you are more involved in decisions about a distressing family situation. Your family may be worried about the costs of the treatment or managing your care at home. A social worker on the team can be helpful in this case.

- Rules and regulations are relaxed. Instead of making you and your family fit the system, it is adjusted to your needs. If you are in a freestanding hospice or a hospice unit in a hospital, the visiting hours will be flexible.

- Pets are sometimes allowed, as is any activity that doesn't embarrass or disturb other patients.

- The care is highly skilled and compassionate, and it is linked to medical resources. It adds security and keeps people from feeling pushed away or abandoned when cure-related treatments are no longer appropriate or helpful.

- Testing is kept to a minimum. The hospital may be especially fatiguing to people with cancer because typically it is where they are constantly being examined and tested. Caregivers monitor you carefully by talking with you, keeping in touch, and making sure you are comfortable.

- Treatment is focused on relieving distressing symptoms.

- Twenty-four-hour telephone availability is present.

- Care is provided by an interdisciplinary team. All the people involved with your care meet frequently to make sure they are working toward the same goals.

- Nurses participate fully, collaborating with your doctor and social worker in addressing your needs. Specially trained volunteers working with their social work colleagues are available also to help you and your family.

- Finally, spiritual resources are available.

Admission

You may seek to enter a hospice program on your own initiative or be referred by a family member, doctor, social worker, visiting nurse, friend, or clergy member. Typically, there is an initial assessment visit, when a member of the hospice team takes your medical history, evaluates your emotional state and needs, and discusses nursing concerns with you and your family. The admission criteria may vary, but hospices usually accept only those people with a limited life expectancy (usually six months or less). Home hospice programs may require that you live within a defined area; have access to a caregiver among your immediate family, relatives, friends, and neighbors; and want to remain at home during the last stages of your illness. Hospices that are reimbursed by Medicare or Medicaid have similar but slightly more restrictive admission standards.

The Hospice Team

Typically hospice care involves an interdisciplinary team of doctors, nurses, social workers, hospice-certified nursing assistants, clergy, therapists, and volunteers. Not only do members of this team provide care aimed at relieving discomfort and social, emotional, and spiritual services, they also coordinate with each other and communicate with other agencies, health care providers, and even funeral directors.

What makes the hospice team unique is its heightened spiritual component and focus on controlling pain. Another essential part of the hospice approach is recognition of the central role of the family in taking care of their family member.

Body, Mind, and Spirit

People with advanced illness inevitably undergo a psychological crisis, and no person or intervention can eliminate all the distress. But people can be greatly relieved of their loneliness, feelings of vulnerability, practical worries, and spiritual fears and can be helped to cope with their concerns.

In advanced disease, people often turn to their doctors for cure or palliation but seek understanding and consolation elsewhere. Sometimes it helps just to have someone around who makes you physically comfortable and creates a supportive, personally satisfying environment. Of course, your existing support networks—family, friends, clergy, and the like—are vital. But different and special benefits come from talking to those who are not emotionally entangled: your doctor, nurse, social worker, or volunteer trained to serve as a "friendly listener."

People with advanced cancer need to talk. The hospice team can give you opportunities to openly discuss your feelings, especially those that you may not want to reveal to family members for fear of increasing their burden. The team can also help you understand and deal with your family members' discomfort in engaging in these conversations. Respecting your need to talk can be good for them as well as you, because it prevents later feelings of guilt or unfinished business and starts the necessary process of grieving.

Your Family and You

Anticipatory grieving by loved ones can be extremely difficult and painful, but it is a healthy response to advanced illness. Unexpressed or unresolved grief is a frequent source of psychological trouble for family members. Supportive care experts have specific criteria for recognizing the difference between normal and dysfunctional grief.

Under the stress of grief, strains among family members may appear, or old ones may reappear, thus depriving people of mutual support when it is most needed and causing further pain to everyone. Talking openly about such practical matters as obtaining equipment and services in the home, providing for minor children, settling financial affairs, and paying medical bills can eliminate most conflicts. Some people want to talk about their funeral, prayers they'd like said, where they want their ashes scattered, or what they would like to be buried in. This is normal. Various hospice or palliative care team members can help you with each of these concerns.

Occasionally, family members may exhibit unhealthy coping patterns or reactions, such as extreme denial, pathological anxiety, depression, excessive or abnormal grieving, sexual disorders, or other signs of poor adjustment. They can get specialized psychological help from a mental health professional trained to work with the very ill and bereaved (see Chapter 28).

Those who are carrying the largest responsibility for home care may need extra emotional support. Even when everyone in the family may agree that you should be at home, many people are understandably frightened and daunted by the prospect, thinking that they can't possibly learn how to take care of you or have the strength to do it. The supportive caregiver, hospice, or palliative care team can give your family the necessary information and help them deal with these concerns. They also can provide an emotional safety net by listening to your family's fears and frustrations.

To Die in Loving Arms, by Lois B. Morris

My mother, Faye Nathan Borkan, died August 22, 1979, at the age of 67 from cancer that began in her lung and traveled to her liver. This is the story of two weeks of her life, her last two, and how the intervention of some of the kindest people I have ever met made her death worth living.

My mother's illness entered its final stages in early August. She and my father were living in Tucson, Arizona, where they had recently retired. My brother, sister, and I lived in separate locations from coast to coast, and throughout the year we had taken turns being with Mother. I was there when she was hospitalized yet again and it became clear that there was no hope left for recovery. Yet there she lay in the hospital bed while the doctors continued to perform painful tests and useless procedures.

What to do? My family and I, as my mother's condition deteriorated, felt increasingly out of control. At last, a young doctor at the hospital told us, "Call Hillhaven Hospice. They'll help you."

I had heard a little about hospices. A concept imported from England. Places for the terminally ill. A humane way to die.

"They'll help you take care of her at home," the doctor said, "and if you find you can't cope there, you can move her into their facility." He said he would have the hospital social service department contact the hospice on our behalf.

I thanked him gratefully—for the first time in months and months I felt we could do something for Mother.

I went back into her room. "Mother," I said, "how would you like to go home?"

Her eyes opened wide. "Yes!" she said with surprising vigor.

Armed with oxygen and pain medication, my father and I took my mother home, where we were met by her sister Belle. Immediately, Mother's spirits improved. And I felt somewhat more comfortable about returning to my job back East.

My sister, Susan, arrived the day after I left. Shortly, my family's first contact with the hospice was established. A nurse named Joan drove out to assess the situation and to begin so marvelously—almost miraculously—to serve our needs.

Joan's initial advice—after explaining the hospice's home-care, in-patient, and bereavement follow-up services—was that we needed skilled help at home—someone who could handle mother's symptoms and to help prepare meals, to relieve some of the burden so that we could be free to attend to emotional and spiritual needs.

Very matter-of-factly she explained exactly what to expect. She talked about everything from dry lips, to pain, to Mother's rage at becoming increasingly helpless, to incontinence, to coma, to death. Somehow, after a year in which our family faced the inevitable with increasing horror, Joan made it sound acceptable, natural, right.

Joan, as did all hospice personnel, spoke to my mother with honesty, compassion, and love, and she spent a lot of time talking—just talking— to my father and sister.

On her second visit, Joan told Susan and Dad that it was time to say our final goodbyes. "Say the things you never got around to saying, all the things you know she wants to hear. Express your love."

"Mother loved it!" Susan remembers. "She was much more lucid than she'd been for some time. There were a lot of tears—and a lot of smiles."

My brother Gene and I said our goodbyes by phone. Mother responded with sounds of comprehension and by frequently repeating our names.

Now Mother was dying fast. My sister and Joan agreed it was time to move Mother to the hospice. Dad resisted at first, equating the hospice with a nursing home, in his mind the cold place in which his mother had died long before.

Joan suggested that Susan and Dad visit the hospice. "See how it feels," she said.

Immediately upon entering, Susan explains, "There was such a pleasant feeling! Even though each of the fifteen or so patients was dying of cancer, there were signs of life there! A bunch of kids come running out of one of the rooms playing tag. People were smiling. All the doors were open. You had the feeling there was nothing to hide from."

Yes, my father said after Joan had given them a full tour, this was the right place. They went home to talk to Mother, who, after initially refusing to go—she kept saying "hospital!" with repugnance—was convinced by Dad, Susan, and Aunt Belle that she would be much more comfortable there.

Once at the hospice, the family was showered with attention and care. Mother was placed in a room with a view of a peaceful courtyard. The staff doctors and nurses tended immediately to her, paying overwhelming attention, as they did throughout those lost five days, to her comfort. That meant, first of all, treating her pain so that she could be totally free of it yet not so doped up that she had no wits at all about her. The staff observed her constantly, ready at the first sign of any discomfort to drop everything and run to her side.

Very soon after she got there, Mother became frightened. She asked, "What is this place?" Joan answered simply, "This is a hospice, where everybody is very ill like you. We take care of people."

Later, during a moment of consciousness, Mother wet the bed. "Why am I doing this?" she cried out. There was a nurse in the room. "Because *you're ill,"* she answered with a naturalness and simple directness that, Susan reports, relaxed Mother visibly.

Again she became more clearheaded, delighting in recognizing the close friends and family who were gathering to be with her, and each other, during her final hours. The staff attended to the family's needs thoroughly. They encouraged everyone to speak openly, to air their concerns, fears, and worries, to attend to burial and funeral plans, to seek the comfort of our religion, to think of the future. They were exquisitely sensitive.

Susan, who needed to cope with the situation by being "in charge," says, "They didn't deprive me of my role. They understood me." And when Susan mentioned that Mother preferred health foods, they cheerfully made up one of her favorite concoctions according to Susan's precise instructions—though by that time, Mother was beyond eating anything.

The first day, the doctor told the family that death would likely occur within 24 to 48 hours. Gene arrived with his family the next day, at the hospice suggestion allowing his children the run of the place. By the time I arrived two nights later, the kids, eight and three and a half, were very matter of fact about "Grammy." "She doesn't have any teeth anymore," the younger one told me in the car coming from the airport." "She's sleeping." "No, she's not," said the eight-year-old. "She's in a coma."

I asked how she knew that, and she replied, "The nurse told me. That's why her eyes are open. I get to help take care of her."

When I arrived at my mother's bedside, a nurse came up and put her arms around me, that's all, just put her arms around me, and I knew, feeling those arms, that though my mother was dying, it was okay.

Awhile later I turned to leave the room. The nurse urged me to stay. "She's alive," she said "Talk to her. Touch her. Comfort her."

"Can she hear me?" I asked. Though she was moving in the bed, she didn't seem responsive.

"Possibly," the nurse said. "Many people who have come out of comas much deeper than this report having heard everything that was said. Put your lips up close to her ears. Say whatever you want." Then she leaned down, took my mother's hand, and said kindly, "Faye, Lois is here. Now they're all here." My mother made a sound that I still believe was one of recognition and welcome.

I slept at the hospice that night, as my brother had been doing. The next morning, a nurse asked me if there was anything else that I wanted to say to my mother.

"Yes," I said. "I want to tell her to stop fighting, to let go, to be peaceful. But I feel guilty—should I say a thing like that?"

"By all means," said the nurse. "Maybe you'll help her."

So I sat there, urging my mother to be peaceful. I kissed her, stroked her, loved her. I had never felt so close to her since I was a small child. It is a feeling so close, so warm that I know will be with me always.

That afternoon, with only my father and his sister present in the room, my mother very quietly died. The family gathered around her. We sighed and cried. But there was no wailing, no breast beating, no sense of tragedy. Her life had been completed. She had died in loving arms, the same arms that enfolded us all.

After the death, the hospice presence became very discreet. They had seen in all their watchfulness that now we needed each other. Quietly they took care of the final details. When we left a few hours later, I thought our experience with Hillhaven Hospice had ended. But at the funeral two days later, I spotted a hospice nurse and social worker among those who come to pay their respects. "With us all the way," I remember thinking.

And that wasn't the end of it. About six weeks later, when all the attention paid my father was beginning to fade away, a hospice worker phoned my father and asked whether he might like to join a discussion group of widows and widowers weekly at the hospice. Dad gratefully accepted. It's free, and he can attend as long as he wants to.

Recently when I told my father that I was going to write this story, I asked if he could characterize the hospice experience for me.

"Oh," he answered immediately, "it's out of this world!" How right he is.

Hillhaven Hospice, which was operating in Tucson as a freestanding facility at the time this story was written, in 1980, has since closed. Hospice care remains widely available throughout Tucson, however, as elsewhere in the United States.

Certainly home care can be a hardship, especially if the caregiver has a job, children, or other major responsibilities. But many family members discover what's best about themselves in the process, and most find it an enormous comfort to know that they are doing everything they can, that they are deeply involved in making their loved one as comfortable as possible, and that they are really "there" for you.

One of the most difficult situations is that of a person with advanced cancer who has young children. Few parents have experience in knowing how to tell young children what is happening in ways that are appropriate to each child's age. The hospice social worker can help you talk to your children and guide you and your family in the best way to help the youngsters through this period. It's also important to involve school counselors and other key personnel. Parents may benefit from professional advice regarding when and under what circumstances children should visit a parent in the hospital (see also *Helping Children Adjust to Cancer in the Family* in Chapter 28).

QUESTIONS

TO ASK

Making a Decision About Hospice Care

When deciding on a hospice program, ask the hospital, health care agency, nursing home, or independent hospice these questions:

- Are you accredited by a recognized, independent accrediting body, such as the Joint Commission on Accreditation of Health Care Organizations?

- Is the hospice program Medicare certified?

- If a license is required by your state, is the hospice program licensed?

- Does the hospice have a written statement outlining the services it provides? A statement about eligibility criteria? Cost and payment procedures? Employee job descriptions? Malpractice and liability insurance?

- How long has the hospice been serving your community? Can they provide references from professionals who have provided services for them? Ask for specific names and numbers.

- Ask the Better Business Bureau, local Consumer Bureau, or State Attorney General's office, if there have been any complaints about the hospice.

- Does the hospice make an assessment to determine if you or your loved one qualifies for hospice care?

- What are the conditions for admission to the hospice or acceptance by the hospice agency? Are they willing to negotiate over aspects of care that you don't feel comfortable with?

- How quickly does the hospice initiate service? Are there any geographic boundaries?

- How do they plan your care? Is a new plan created for each patient? Are you and your family involved in determining the plan? Is the plan given to you in writing? Can you see a sample care plan?

- Does the hospice offer specialized services, such as nutritional guidance by a dietician? Do they have professional therapists to provide respiratory therapy and physical therapy? Is there a family counselor that can assist your family?

- When hospice care is given at home, is a family primary caregiver required? What responsibilities is that person expected to assume? What do they do for the person who lives alone?

- Does someone from the agency evaluate what services are needed in the home, and does a nurse, social worker, or therapist come to the home to see for him- or herself? Do they consult with the doctor, other health care personnel, and family members?

- Does the agency train, supervise, and monitor its caregivers and are there references on file (two or more should be required)? Are the caregivers licensed and bonded? How often does a supervisor visit?

- How are concerns, complaints, and problems resolved?

- How does the hospice handle payment and billing? (Get all financial arrangements in writing.)

- Is there a written plan for handling, such as power failure, and can you see it? In a situation, such as a natural disaster, can they still deliver home services?

- Does the agency have a twenty-four-hour telephone number to call with questions?

- Does the hospice have a copy of patient's rights and responsibilities information?

In a hospital, nursing home, or freestanding hospice, there are more specific questions to ask, such as:

- Where is the care provided and what are the admission requirements?

- How long can a person stay? What if inpatient care is not needed, but the person cannot return home?

- Can you tour the facility?

- What hospitals provide inpatient care? How does the hospice follow up with those who require such care?

Nearing the End

Experience has shown that many people are better able to deal with the end of life if they are able to acknowledge what is happening. This awareness allows them to resolve old issues and say the things they've always wanted to say to those they love. Finally, it lets people plan and take charge of practical matters, such as providing for their children's education or making certain that their possessions will go to those they wish to have them.

Each person reacts to advanced disease in his or her own way, but often a pattern of emotions follow one another: shock and disbelief that this could be happening, anger that it is happening at this time, a period of mental "bargaining" with God or fate, and finally an acceptance of the reality.

A range of worries often emerges as you begin to imagine the ending of life and what will happen to those you love. You may be concerned about how your family will manage. As your body changes and you become more dependent on others for help, you may worry about becoming a burden or not contributing to the family in the usual way. Sometimes you may feel very alone, that no one could possibly understand what you are going through. This can also be a time for inner growth, leading to a sense of profound peace. As you look back over your life, you may gain insights into yourself and an understanding of some of the events and relationships you experienced.

This is a critical time for clear communication among you, your caregiving staff, and your family. For example, you should let others know whether openly expressing their grief gives you comfort and reassurance of their love or whether it makes you more anxious and distressed. It also is important for family and friends to understand that you may behave differently during these periods of changing emotions. Some people enter a stage of detachment, during which they may seem cool to their family and friends. It will help both you and your family to understand that this is not a real rejection but an attempt to ease away from emotional attachments that are difficult to handle.

Not everyone experiences all these feelings, but when they do arise, it is important to know that ignoring them does not make them go away. Disturbing thoughts often become easier to deal with if you can find a way to express them to someone who is experienced and caring. Various professionals, such as nurses, social workers, chaplains, or psychologists, can listen, help you put your feelings in perspective, and organize any additional help you might wish.

Family and friends also experience a range of emotions. They share the shock and disbelief, the feelings of unfairness and anger, and the overwhelming sense of helplessness to change the outcome. Some may feel guilty for having trouble with these feelings and for wanting the inevitable to be over with. They may be afraid about having to manage alone and begin to realize that the world will never be the same again. If families can reveal their feelings and share what their lives together have meant, it can strengthen relationships and give everyone courage.

The fundamental principle for family and friends during a loved one's late stage of cancer is to be guided by that person's needs and wishes. Some people want to talk about certain topics; others don't. Some want to know that their loved ones are already grieving for them; others are frightened and upset by this. Some of the greatest comfort can come from nonverbal expressions of love, such as a back rub or offering to bring special foods or other treats.

Some of the most significant decisions to be made at this stage are closely related: first, whether to refuse heroic measures for prolonging life, and second, if you are in a hospital, whether to go home for your last days. When considering these options, it is important to remember that there will be various points at which you can change your mind about almost any decision.

Life-Prolonging Measures

In the past, people with advanced disease had few choices. Today, because technology allows extraordinary things to be done to prolong life, people are forced to make extraordinary decisions. Certainly one of the most difficult is deciding whether or not to use life-prolonging measures, including cardiac resuscitation and mechanical breathing assistance in the final stages of life.

Certain measures are carried out routinely unless you have made clear in advance that you don't want them. For example, cardiopulmonary resuscitation (CPR) will be administered in the event of cardiac arrest, unless the doctor in charge—under the patient's agent, health proxy, or surrogate's direction—has issued a "Do Not Resuscitate" order.

In order to encourage people to make decisions about the type and extent of medical care they want—including refusing treatment—the Patient Self-Determination Act (PSDA) was passed in 1990. The PSDA requires that health care agencies ask patients whether they have an advance directive and provide them with educational materials about their rights.

Advance Directive

Many people are concerned about the possibility that they will be unable to make decisions about their care. These people may have their wishes and future health care choices put in writing in what is called an advance directive. This legal document can include a living will and a power of attorney for health care (also called a durable power of attorney for health care). It can be as simple or complex as you need it to be, and can include any specific directions that you want followed. For instance, it can include a statement about whether or not you want to donate your organs for transplantation.

Although the directives may be general, for example, "Do not resuscitate" or "No heroic measures," most experts advise that the documents be quite specific. For example, a directive described by the Harvard Health Letter outlines six different medical situations in which decisions have to be made for people who can no longer speak for themselves. A personal preference regarding each of these can be made specific and clear in a detailed advance directive.

A living will specifies what kind of life-sustaining procedures or artificial life support you do or don't want in a situation in which you may be unable to state your wishes. A life-sustaining procedure or treatment is any mechanical or artificial means that sustains or substitutes for a bodily function and prolongs the dying process when it is clear that recovery is not possible.

These measures may include CPR, use of a breathing device such as a ventilator, medication to alter heart function, and surgical insertion of a feeding tube. It does not include medications or procedures that provide comfort or ease pain.

A power of attorney for health care is a legal document that directs a person chosen by the patient to speak for him or her. This person—also known as a health care proxy, surrogate decision-maker, or agent—can meet with the doctor and other caregivers on the patient's behalf and decide what treatments or procedures to do or not do. Some people name an alternate agent in case the primary agent is unable or unwilling to act when the time comes. The weight of this power is enormous, so it's wise to discuss all your feelings about your care with the agent. If the agent doesn't know your specific wishes in a particular situation, decisions will have to be made based on what he or she thinks you would want.

Only about 15 percent of Americans have advance directives, but every adult should consider making one. It is not reserved for those with a terminal condition. It's important that your doctor, caregivers, and family and/or close friends know that you have an advanced directive. Keep a copy of this document in a safe place and be certain that those close to you know where to find it. Your attorney can also keep a copy.

If for any reason your doctor or the health care agency responsible for your care objects to your advance directive, they must notify you or your family, because they are not required to honor it. To ensure that emergency and hospital personnel know that you do not want a particular life-support procedure, such as CPR, some people cared for at home wear a medical alert bracelet stating that instruction.

Going Home

What used to be the normal course of events—for people to end their days at home in their own beds—has become more rare in this technological era. But like the movement toward palliative and hospice care, it is becoming an increasingly preferred option.

There are definite advantages. Most people are psychologically more comfortable in familiar surroundings, with caring friends and family nearby. Staying home lets you continue to enjoy hobbies or personal projects as long as you are physically able. It gives you greater control over the details of your life, such as sleeping and eating when you are tired or hungry, not when the

A Living Will

SPECIAL

CONCERNS

Living wills differ in every state. The following is an example of a living will for the state of Florida.*

A Declaration made this _____ day of _____ 20_____

I, _____willfully and voluntarily make known my desire that my dying not be artificially prolonged under the circumstances set forth below, and I do hereby declare:

If at any time I have a terminal condition and if my attending or treating doctor and another consulting doctor have determined that there is no medical probability of my recovery from such condition, I direct that life prolonging procedures be withheld or withdrawn when the application of such procedures would serve only to prolong artificially the process of dying, and that I be permitted to die naturally with only the administration of medication or the performance of any medical procedure deemed necessary to provide me with comfort care or to alleviate pain.

It is my intention that this declaration be honored by my family and doctor as the final expression of my legal right to refuse medical or surgical treatment and to accept the consequences for such refusal.

In the event that I have been determined to be unable to provide express and informed consent regarding the withholding, withdrawal, or continuation of life-prolonging procedures, I wish to designate, as my surrogate to carry out the provisions of this declaration:

Name: _____

Address:_____

Zip Code:_____

Phone: _____

I wish to designate the following person as my alternate surrogate, to carry out the provisions of this declaration should my surrogate be unwilling or unable to act on my behalf:

Name: _____

Address:_____

Zip Code:_____

Phone: _____

* Reprinted by permission of Partnership for Caring, Inc.

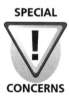

SPECIAL

CONCERNS

Additional Instructions (optional):

I understand the full importance of this declaration, and I am emotionally and mentally competent to make this declaration.

Signed:_____

Witness 1:

Signed:_____

Address:_____

Witness 2:

Signed:_____

Address:_____

SPECIAL

CONCERNS

Designation of Health Care Surrogate

The following is a sample of a form used to designate a health care proxy in the state of Florida.*

Name: _____
           Last   First   Middle Initial

In the event that I have been determined to be incapacitated to provide informed consent for medical treatment and surgical and diagnostic procedures, I wish to designate as my surrogate for health care decisions:

Name: _____

Address:_____

Zip Code:_____

Phone: _____

If my surrogate is unwilling or unable to perform his duties, I wish to designate as my alternate surrogate:

Name: _____

Address:_____

Zip Code:_____

Phone: _____

* Reprinted by permission of Partnership for Caring, Inc.

I fully understand that this designation will permit my designee to make health care decisions and to provide, withhold, or withdraw consent on my behalf; to apply for public benefits to defray the cost of my health care; and to authorize my admission to or transfer from a health care facility.

Additional instructions (optional):

I further affirm that this designation is not being made as a condition of treatment or admission to a health care facility. I will notify and send copy of this document to the following persons other than my surrogate, so they may know who my surrogate is:

Name: _____

Address: _____

Name: _____

Address: _____

Signed: _____

Date: _____

Witness 1:

Signed: _____

Address: _____

Witness 2:

Signed: _____

Address: _____

hospital schedule requires. It makes it easier to refuse or avoid invasive procedures. These things—along with the greater peace and quiet of home—can go a long way toward providing emotional well being. Some people, however, feel safer in the hospital, and that should be respected.

There also are disadvantages. The family may not be available. The needs of the ill person may be too great for family resources. The family may be unable to handle the emotional or physical stress of home care. For some people, being without immediate medical supervision or backup can be frightening. If they have been in the hospital, the doctor who had been caring for them there may not be able to continue as their primary caregiver, and so they may be referred to a new doctor at a crucial time.

QUESTIONS

?

TO ASK

Artificial Nutrition and Hydration

The most important issue, of course, is what you want. But you may not be sure; you may not even know on what basis to make your decision. Some points that may be helpful to discuss when deciding whether to use artificial nutrition and hydration are as follows:

- What is the goal or purpose of artificial feeding? Will it cure or arrest the cancer? Will it prolong life? Will it maintain an acceptable quality of life? Will it make you more comfortable?

- Will it have any benefits?

- What burdens will it create?

- Do your cultural, religious, or personal values affect your choice?

However, hospice care at home is an option that may eliminate or reduce these disadvantages. Another important aid to families is to have a "care plan" provided by the hospital, which outlines a specific schedule of medication and indicates under what circumstances and whom to call for professional assistance. It should also include information on whom to call in an emergency, with backup numbers, and what constitutes an emergency in that person's situation.

Focusing on Comfort

Advanced cancer is emotionally painful for everyone, and some problems associated with it may test the ingenuity, patience, and strength of everyone involved. In general, however, simple remedies, common sense, good nursing care, the liberal use of carefully selected pain relief—anything designed to comfort, not cure—can help reduce your suffering and that of your loved ones. Specialists in palliative care realize that they can't "make everything perfect," but they do have a great many options and alternatives that allow them to make most things much better. The central and most important message of home health care or hospice care providers should be, "We will always do our absolute best for you. If one thing doesn't work well for you, we will try another. You will never be abandoned."

PART VI

Overview of Specific Cancers

How to Use This Overview

Cancer is a disease with at least 100 different forms, depending on where it begins and the tissues and cells it involves. The previous chapters of the book provide information applicable to all types of cancer. This *Overview of Specific Cancers*, which appeared in the first edition of *Informed Decisions* as the *Encyclopedia of Common and Uncommon Cancers*, has been revised to better meet readers' needs for concise overviews of information about specific cancers. It should be a helpful starting point as you learn the basics about cancer types.

Most of the cancers are arranged by site (that is, where they initially occur in the body, such as the skin, breast, kidney, and so on). The sites are organized by physiologic system, and the physiologic systems are organized alphabetically. In general, the cancers that occur within a particular organ system are grouped together. (Thus, for example, all the cancers that affect parts of the digestive system—esophagus, stomach, colon and rectum, liver, and gallbladder—are discussed one after the other.) To locate the entry for a particular cancer, consult the index at the back of the book.

Each *Overview* section begins with information about current incidence and five-year survival rates for cancers of that kind or in that particular site (these figures are based on the year of this publication). Five-year survival rates refer to the percentage of people with cancer who are alive five years after diagnosis. (People who died of another cause are not included in calculating this percentage.) Medical professionals use survival rates in evaluating groups of people with similar diagnoses. Keep in mind that although these estimates may give you an idea of the aggressiveness of the disease, they do not predict how long any individual will live.

In many cases an illustration with explanatory text is also provided to help you understand the basic anatomy involved in a cancer type. Additional categories of information in each entry include the following:

Risk Factors describes factors that increase the risk for developing that type of cancer. You should know, however, that having a risk factor, or even several of them, does not necessarily mean that you will get the disease.

Types of (Specific Cancer) outlines the different types of cancer that originate at that site.

Signs and Symptoms explains ways in which the cancer may give warning.

Diagnostic Tests explains the tests that determine definitively whether cancer is present, where it is present, and its level of development. *Because many of these tests are used to diagnose and stage different cancers, additional details are provided in Chapter 5.*

Treatment explains individual and combination therapies effective in treating the cancer. The choice of treatment depends on many things, such as the type of cancer, location, and stage of disease, as well as age, health status, and personal preferences. Consult your doctor about your unique medical condition.

The *Overview* provides lists and short paragraphs of information. It is not meant to be a comprehensive look at types of cancers; for additional details, instructions, or for more specific information, contact the American Cancer Society (800-ACS-2345; www.cancer.org).

AIDS-Related Cancers

Key Statistics

Acquired immunodeficiency syndrome (AIDS) is caused by the human immunodeficiency virus (HIV). It is estimated that the number of HIV-infected individuals currently ranges from 1 to 2.5 million in the United States and 33 million throughout the world. Over 20 million of these cases are in sub-Saharan Africa. More than 1 million children have been infected with HIV.

In the United States and developed countries, the average time from initial HIV infection to advanced AIDS in an untreated individual is ten years. About 20 percent of people with HIV develop AIDS within five years or less. In 5 to 7 percent of individuals the CD4 cell counts remain normal for ten to fifteen years.

People with advanced stages of AIDS are at risk of developing AIDS-related cancers. AIDS attacks and destroys the body's immune system. Without a fully functional immune system, the individual is at risk for developing a variety of infections and certain types of cancer, including Kaposi's sarcoma, lymphomas, and cervical cancer. About four people out of ten who have AIDS will develop a cancer at some time during their illness. The survival rate from AIDS varies with the stage of the disease. It is approximately 80 percent, but this figure is increasing yearly because of improved treatment and new drugs.

Risk Factors

HIV is acquired through contact with body fluids (such as blood, vaginal secretions, semen, and other body fluids and tissues) from another person with HIV. The virus transfers easily by injection into the bloodstream, by

Certain diseases occur so often in people with AIDS that they are considered "AIDS-defining conditions," which means their presence in a person infected with HIV is a clear sign that full-blown AIDS has developed.

The Centers for Disease Control and Prevention (CDC) has identified certain cancers as AIDS-defining diseases: Kaposi's sarcoma, lymphoma—especially non-Hodgkin's lymphoma and primary central nervous system lymphoma—and invasive cervical cancer, which is cancer of the cervix that has spread to neighboring tissue. Other forms of cancer that may be more likely to develop in people with HIV infection are Hodgkin's disease, anal cancer, oral cancer, and cancer of the testicles. HIV-related cancers tend to be aggressive and often do not respond well to treatment.

rectal intercourse, organ or tissue transplant, and sexual intimacy—the most common method of transfer. HIV infection has occurred in nine groups:

- Individuals who received blood from HIV-positive donors (before 1985);
- Hemophiliacs who received Factor VIII (a blood product) before 1985;
- Men who have intercourse with men who have HIV;
- Women who have intercourse with men who have HIV;
- Men who have intercourse with women who have HIV;
- Intravenous drug users who share needles with individuals who have HIV;
- Children born to mothers who have HIV;
- Children breastfed from mothers with HIV;
- Health care workers who were exposed to blood from patients with HIV at work.

Signs and Symptoms
- Fatigue;
- Headache;
- Muscle and joint pain;
- Intermittent fever;
- Diarrhea;
- Loss of appetite;
- Weight loss;

- Skin problems;

- Neurological symptoms—thirty to fifty percent of individuals have symptoms from infections, cancers, or HIV itself, such as headache and peripheral neuropathy (nerve pain).

Opportunistic Infections

These infections are caused by organisms that rarely cause disease in healthy people, but they can occur commonly in people with AIDS. In the early stages of AIDS, these infections may include oral candidiasis, herpes simplex, shingles, bronchitis, sinusitis, and pneumonia.

In advanced HIV disease, when the immune function is greatly decreased, the person develops serious opportunistic infections and possibly cancer. According to the CDC, any individual with a CD4 lymphocyte count below 200 cells/mm^3 is considered to have AIDS.

Diagnostic Tests

HIV Tests

- HIV enzyme-linked immunosorbent assay (ELISA)—a screening test that shows the antibodies to the virus in the blood;

- Indirect immunofluorescence assay (IFA)—uses a fluorescent dye to detect HIV antibodies in the blood;

- Viral culture methods—involve growing live HIV from infected cells (viral cultures). This was the first method ever used to detect the HIV infection;

- Polymerase chain reaction (PCR)—a highly sensitive test by which the genetic material of a cell is amplified many times to detect HIV viral DNA or RNA (or the genetic material of HIV). This test measures "viral load" (the amount of free virus in the blood) and is used to tell how an infected person is responding to treatment. The "viral load" is expected to go down with treatment.

Laboratory Tests

Laboratory tests that measure the immune function of the individual or serve as markers of the progression of the disease are also important.

- Complete blood cell count (CBC) with white blood cell differentiation;

- Number and percentage of CD4+ T lymphocytes;

- Total immunoglobulins;

- Tests of lymphocyte and monocyte function.

Treatment

Current treatment for HIV/AIDS has three objectives: 1) support the immune system, 2) prevent, control, or eliminate opportunistic infections, and 3) clear the body of HIV. Current research is focusing on finding better antiretroviral drugs, preventive therapies, and treatments of opportunistic infections as ways to restore the damaged immune system.

Antiretroviral Therapy

There are many antiretroviral drugs used today. Many others are in clinical trials to determine their safety and effectiveness. Because of the rapid development of new drugs, the drugs used in HIV treatment are constantly changing.

Zidovudine (ZDV or AZT). This drug stops the formation of DNA. AZT can actually cause some recovery in immune function by increasing the number of helper T cells and decreasing the number of infections. It does not, however, provide a cure.

Reverse Transcriptase Inhibitors. These drugs stop the action of one of the viral enzymes (reverse transcriptase or RT) essential for HIV reproduction. These include abacavir (Ziagen or 159U289), didanosine (Videx or ddI), lamivudine (Epivir or 3TC), stavudine (Zerit or D4T), and zalcitabine (ddC).

Protease Inhibitors. HIV produces an enzyme called protease in the late stages of its reproduction which allows the virus to reproduce. Protease inhibitors block the action of protease. These drugs include Amprenavir (Agenerase), Indinavir (Crixivan—IDV), Nelfinavir (Viracept—AG 1343), Ritonavir (Norvir—ABT 538), Saquinavir (Invirase or RO 318959), and Fortavase.

Combination Therapy

The HIV virus can change its structure and become resistant to drugs, so antiretroviral drugs are often given in combination. An example of one combination is AZT, plus 3TC, plus Indinavir. These are sometimes called "triple combination therapies" or "AIDS drug cocktails."

Treatment of Opportunistic Infections

Infections caused by bacteria, viruses, fungi, or protozoan parasites must be treated and prevented.

Types of AIDS-Related Cancers

The relationship between HIV and these cancers is still not completely understood; however, it is known that the cancers are able to grow rapidly because the individuals who have them have suppressed immune systems.

Unfortunately, cancer in individuals with HIV/AIDS is more difficult to treat than other cancers. This is due to decreased immune function caused by HIV and the decrease in the white blood cell count that results from HIV infection. Individuals with HIV tend to have cancers that are diagnosed at an advanced stage and do not respond as well to treatment.

Each of these cancers is discussed in greater detail in other sections. Here is information about the cancer with regard to AIDS.

Kaposi's Sarcoma

In the past twenty years, the majority of Kaposi's sarcoma (KS) cases have been associated with HIV infection and AIDS in homosexual men. These cases are referred to as AIDS-related KS. It is now known that Kaposi's sarcoma in people with HIV is related to a second viral infection. This virus has been called HHV-8. Its transmission in the United States is usually through male homosexual contact.

In most cases, epidemic KS causes widespread lesions that erupt soon after AIDS develops. Lesions of epidemic KS may arise on the skin and the mouth, and may affect the lymph nodes and other organs—usually the gastrointestinal tract, lung, liver, and spleen. At the time of diagnosis, some people with epidemic KS experience no other symptoms. However, many— even those with no skin lesions—will have swollen lymph nodes, unexplained fever, or weight loss. Eventually, in almost all cases, epidemic KS spreads throughout the body. Extensive lung involvement by KS can be fatal. More often, however, patients die of other AIDS-related complications such as infections. (See *Kaposi's Sarcoma*, pages 565–568, for more information.)

Lymphomas

Non-Hodgkin's lymphoma (NHL) is a cancer that starts in lymphoid tissue and may spread to other organs (see *Non-Hodgkin's Lymphoma*, pages 553–557, for more information). It occurs in 4 to 10 percent of individuals with AIDS and is the second most common cancer associated with HIV disease, after KS.

The non-Hodgkin's lymphomas that typically occur in people with AIDS may be primary central nervous system (CNS) lymphomas—that is, they begin in the brain and spinal cord—or specific types of intermediate and high-grade lymphomas, including Burkitt's lymphoma. Symptoms of CNS lymphoma include seizures, facial paralysis, confusion, memory loss, and lethargy.

The prognosis, or outcome, for patients with HIV-associated NHL depends on lymphocyte (infection-fighting white blood cell) count, the presence of lymphoma in the bone marrow, stage IV NHL, the person's quality of life, and a history of AIDS before diagnosis of NHL.

The best treatment for AIDS-NHL has not been determined. Because AIDS is not a curable disease, treatment is focused on prolonging survival and improving the patient's quality of life.

Studies have shown that AIDS-related lymphomas respond to chemotherapy, with a large percentage of patients responding to a combination of chemotherapy drugs. Treatment with low doses of chemotherapy may be as effective as standard dose treatment.

The use of hematopoietic (blood cell–forming) growth factors and anti-retroviral drugs (drugs that attack the virus) added to chemotherapy treatments shows some promise, but further research is needed.

For patients with primary CNS lymphoma, studies have shown that whole-brain radiation can improve neurologic function, improve the person's quality of life, and improve survival.

Precancerous Changes and Invasive Cervical Cancer

HIV-infected women are at high risk for developing cervical intraepithelial neoplasia (CIN), a cervical precancerous condition, but their risk of developing invasive cervical cancer is even higher. Human papillomavirus (HPV) plays a role in the development of squamous cell carcinoma (SCC) of the cervix in women who are HIV positive. SCC is a cancer that develops in the epithelial tissue that covers and lines the cervix. It begins as an abnormal growth of the cervical cells (CIN). As the disease progresses, the tumor cells become malignant and break through the thin membrane, allowing the cells to invade the uterus and become invasive cervical cancer. (See *Cervical Cancer*, pages 657–660, for more information.)

Women with AIDS and invasive cervical cancer have a greater likelihood of experiencing recurrence of the cancer and a greater likelihood of dying of this disease than HIV-negative women. The lymphocyte count of the woman seems to influence outcome, with a higher count associated with a more favorable outcome.

Standard treatment for CIN is not as effective in HIV-infected women. The likelihood of the disease recurring is high and is associated with the woman's immune function. Women with low lymphocyte counts are at high risk for recurrent disease.

In general, HIV-positive women with good immune function tolerate surgery well. Patients with more advanced disease respond poorly to radiation therapy alone. Chemotherapy has been used in women with advanced or recurrent disease. Close monitoring is essential for toxicities, and antiretroviral drugs are used in women with CD4 counts less than 500.

Anal Cancer

Anal carcinoma is also associated with HPV infection. It is sexually transmitted and occurs most often in homosexual, HIV-infected men. Screening anal pap smears are suggested for HIV-positive homosexual men. The cancer is treated with a combination of chemotherapy (5-FU and mitomycin) and radiation therapy.

Acute Leukemia

Key Statistics

Approximately 12,000 new cases of acute leukemia are diagnosed in adults in the United States each year. About 10,000 of these are acute myelogenous leukemia (AML) and another 1,500 are acute lymphocytic leukemia (ALL). About 21,500 adults and children in the United States die of leukemia each year. Younger adults are more likely to be cured than older ones, and about 20 to 30 percent of adults with AML or ALL can be cured. (See *Childhood Cancers*, pages 584–589, for information about childhood leukemia.)

The five-year survival rate for adults with ALL over the age of 45 is 25 percent for those aged 45 to 54, 20 percent for those aged 55 to 64, and 11 percent for adults aged 65 to 74. For AML, the five-year survival rate is 24 percent for adults aged 45 to 54, 11 percent for those aged 55 to 64, and 5 percent for those aged 65 to 74. The survival rate is much lower for those older than 65.

Risk Factors

- *Smoking.* Smokers have a higher risk of developing AML;

- *Age.* AML is a disease of older people: the average age at diagnosis is 65. ALL is more common among children than adults; the highest incidence is in children under 10, but there is a second peak in adults over 70;

- *Gender.* AML is more common among men than among women;

- *Race.* African Americans are half as likely as Caucasians to develop ALL and have a slightly lower risk for AML as well;

> Bone marrow is the soft inner part of bones and contains the body's blood-forming cells. The cells begin as early "stem" cells that divide and mature into a variety of blood cells: red blood cells, white blood cells, or platelets.
>
> Red blood cells contain hemoglobin, which allows them to carry oxygen from the lungs to all other tissues in the body. Platelets are actually fragments from a type of bone marrow cell called the megakaryocyte. Platelets are important in plugging damaged areas of blood vessels caused by cuts or bruises. White blood cells are important in defending the body against infections. Although there are several types of white cells, the major ones are the granulocytes (also called neutrophils or "polys") and the lymphocytes. The most common adult leukemia, AML, forms in the myeloid cells that are responsible for making granulocytes. ALL develops in cells responsible for making lymphocytes. Lymphocytes are found in many parts of the body because they are the major cells in lymph nodes; but ALL always starts in the bone marrow.

- *Chemical exposures, radiation therapy, and chemotherapy.* People exposed to certain chemicals such as benzene, excessive amounts of radiation (but not from diagnostic x-rays), and certain chemotherapy drugs have an increased risk of leukemia;

- *Genetics.* People with certain genetic disorders, such as Bloom's syndrome, ataxia-telangectasia, and Fanconi's anemia, are at increased risk.

Types of Acute Leukemia

Leukemia is a type of cancer that starts in the blood-forming cells of the bone marrow and quickly moves into the blood. It can then spread to other parts of the body, most commonly the lymph nodes, liver, spleen, brain, spinal cord, and even the skin. Acute means that the leukemia develops quickly and, if not treated, is generally fatal within a few months.

Acute Myelogenous Leukemia

AML arises from the cells responsible for producing blood granulocytes. The leukemia cell is basically a stem cell that fails to mature, so there is an accumulation of these immature cells called "blasts." Several variations of this kind of leukemia exist—the variation depends upon the amount of development of the cells. These range from very undifferentiated leukemias where the cells have not matured at all, to leukemias where the leukemia cells begin to resemble the more mature cells normally found in the bone marrow. A special kind of acute myelogenous leukemia, called acute promyelocytic leukemia, has a very distinctive appearance and treatment.

Acute Lymphoblastic Leukemia

ALL derives from the cells responsible for making lymphocytes, cells responsible for our immune system. They are mostly classified by whether they come from the B line of lymphocytes, the cells responsible for making antibodies, or the T line that is responsible for directly attacking invading organisms.

Signs and Symptoms

Most signs and symptoms of acute leukemia result from a shortage of normal blood cells due to crowding out of normal blood cell–producing bone marrow by the leukemia cells. As a result, people do not have enough properly functioning red blood cells, white blood cells, and blood platelets. Signs and symptoms include:

- Shortness of breath, excessive tiredness, and a "pale" skin color, all due to anemia, a shortage of red blood cells;

- Frequent infections because of a low number of infection-fighting granulocytes;

- Excessive bruising, bleeding, frequent or severe nosebleeds, and bleeding from the gums due to a low blood platelet count (thrombocytopenia);

- Headache, weakness, seizures, vomiting, difficulty in maintaining balance, and blurred vision because of leukemic cells invading the brain;

- Bone or joint pain;

- Enlargement of the liver and spleen because of leukemic infiltration;

- Swollen and painful gums;

- Tiny purplish spots that can look like a common rash;

- Small skin tumors.

Diagnostic Tests

- Blood cell counts and blood cell examination;

- Bone marrow aspiration and biopsy—a needle is used to remove a sample of bone marrow that can be examined for cancer cells; special stains help diagnose the leukemia;

- Lumbar puncture (spinal tap)—a needle is placed in the lower back to obtain a small sample of cerebrospinal fluid, which can be examined for cancer cells;

- Flow cytometry of blood cells—to determine the type of leukemia using special antibodies to detect specific substances on the cell surface or inside the cell;

- Cytogenetics—involves looking at the chromosomes of the leukemia cells, which helps in diagnosis and prognosis;

- X-rays or special scans—may be done to evaluate specific symptoms.

Treatment

Radiation Therapy

Radiation treatment is used to treat leukemia cells in the brain and spinal fluid and in some patients, particularly with ALL, to prevent the leukemia from coming back in these places after chemotherapy. It also plays a role in stem cell transplants.

Chemotherapy

The main treatment for acute leukemia is chemotherapy. Phases of chemotherapy include induction, where treatment is directed to killing most of the leukemia cells; consolidation, where a different kind of chemotherapy is given to kill any remaining leukemia cells; and maintenance, where low doses of chemotherapy are given to ALL patients to prevent the leukemia from coming back.

Remission induction. In AML, this usually involves treatment with two chemotherapy drugs, cytarabine (Ara-C) and an anthracycline drug such as daunorubicin (Cerubidine) or idarubicin (Idamycin). This intensive therapy usually takes place in the hospital. While the treatment typically lasts one week, more hospital time for support will be needed because most of the normal bone marrow cells as well as the leukemic cells will be destroyed. More recently, the U.S. Food and Drug Administration approved treatment of AML with a drug called Mylotarg, which is an antibody against AML cells that has been combined with a chemotherapy agent.

For ALL, the treatment will be an anthracycline combined with vincristine (Oncovin) and prednisone. This causes less bone marrow damage and generally results in shorter hospital stays. Another drug called Gleevec has been found to be helpful in a particular kind of ALL that contains a special chromosome called the Philadelphia chromosome.

Consolidation therapy. This treatment is given after induction of remission to destroy remaining leukemia cells and prevent a relapse. The most common treatment, particularly for adults with AML over age 50, is several courses of high-dose cytarabine chemotherapy. For ALL, several different regimens of multiple drugs are used.

Maintenance therapy. This is used only for patients with ALL and consists of oral methotrexate and mercaptopurine (Purinethol), sometimes with other drugs added.

Central nervous system prophylaxis. Because ALL can come back in the brain or spinal fluid, after remission, these patients are treated with methotrexate delivered by spinal tap into the spinal fluid and sometimes with radiation to the brain.

Stem Cell Transplantation

Stem cell transplantation is sometimes used in younger patients after remission induction, particularly if they have poor prognostic markers (usually determined by the cytogenetics). It is also standard treatment for patients under age 50 who have had a relapse of their leukemia and have gone into a second remission with chemotherapy. (See Chapter 14 for more information on stem cell transplants.)

Treatment of Promyelocytic (M3) Leukemia. Treatment of this subtype of AML differs from usual AML treatment because a nonchemotherapy drug, all-trans retinoic acid (ATRA), a drug related to vitamin A, is also used. Although remission induction is usually possible with ATRA alone, combining the ATRA with chemotherapy produces the best results. Another drug, arsenic trioxide, has also been found to be effective.

Chronic Leukemia

Key Statistics

Approximately 12,800 new cases of the two types of chronic leukemia are diagnosed in the United States each year: 8,100 new cases of chronic lymphocytic leukemia (CLL) and 4,700 new cases of chronic myelogenous leukemia (CML). Hairy cell leukemia is estimated to account for about 2 percent of leukemias each year.

Most chronic leukemias affect adults. The average age of patients with chronic lymphocytic leukemia (CLL) is about 70 years. The average age of patients with chronic myelogenous leukemia (CML) is 50 to 60 years. Patients with hairy cell leukemia (HCL) are most often 50 to 60 years old. About 2 percent of chronic leukemia patients are children (see *Childhood Leukemia,* pages 584–589).

The five-year survival rate for people with CLL is around 75 percent. It is a little higher for younger adults (under age 65) than older adults. For people with CML, the five-year survival is much lower: 44 percent for those aged 45 to 54, 33 percent for patients 55 to 64, and 26 percent for those 65 to 74. The survival rate is even lower for the very elderly.

(See *Acute Leukemia,* pages 541–545, for an explanation of bone marrow, blood cells, and other important aspects of the blood.)

Risk Factors

- *Radiation.* People with high-dose radiation exposure (such as being a survivor of an atomic bomb blast or nuclear reactor accident) have an increased risk of developing CML, but not CLL;

- *Family history.* People with first-degree relatives (parents, siblings, or children) with CLL have a two- to fourfold increased risk for this cancer.

Types of Chronic Leukemia

CLL

CLL is a disease of the lymphocyte, a cell found in the bone marrow as well as lymph nodes and, rarely, other tissues. These cells are generally small, round, and often appear normal. But the major finding in CLL is that their number in the blood is very high. The normal lymphocyte count is up to 5,000 per cubic millimeter of blood while in CLL it often goes to 100,000 or above. The second difference is that these cells are monoclonal. Lymphocytes produce antibodies. Normally they produce a diversity of antibodies, but in CLL the cells all produce the same one. Special tests find that all the cells are completely alike as though they were twins, multiplied many times.

CML

CML is a malignancy of the white blood cell–producing cells of the bone marrow. Instead of maturing completely, the cells form a partly mature form called the myelocyte. This is the characteristic cell of this leukemia. In addition all the other cells of the myeloid cell line are produced so that the blood contains a variety of cells. The count often goes as high as 100,000 to 200,000 and sometimes higher. A second characteristic of CML is that the cells contain an abnormal chromosome called the Philadelphia chromosome.

This abnormal chromosome comes about because of breaks in chromosomes 9 and 22 with the transfer of material between these chromosomes. Chromosome 22 comes out much smaller in this exchange, which is why it was recognized as an abnormal chromosome by doctors in Philadelphia.

Other Types and Subtypes

Hairy Cell Leukemia (HCL). Like chronic lymphocytic leukemia, HCL is a slowly progressing cancer of lymphocytes. HCL cells have fine projections from their surface that make them appear "hairy."

Signs and Symptoms

At least one-fifth of people with chronic leukemia have no symptoms at the time their cancer is diagnosed. Many of the signs and symptoms of chronic leukemia occur because the leukemic cells replace the bone marrow's normal blood-producing cells.

- Fatigue—may be due to anemia or just from a high white blood cell count;
- Anemia (a shortage of red blood cells) causes excessive tiredness, a "pale" color to the skin, and in more serious cases, shortness of breath;
- Infection—pneumonia can be seen in people with CLL;
- A low platelet count—can in rare instances lead to bleeding;
- Enlargement of the spleen;
- Enlargement of lymph nodes.

Diagnostic Tests

- Blood cell counts and blood cell examination;
- Bone marrow aspiration and biopsy with special stains to help diagnose the leukemia—a needle is used to remove a sample of bone marrow that can be examined for cancer cells;
- Flow cytometry of blood cells—to determine the type of leukemia using special antibodies to detect specific substances on the cell surface or inside the cell;
- Cytogenetics—looking at the chromosomes of the leukemia cells, which helps in diagnosis and prognosis;
- X-rays or special scans—may be done to evaluate specific symptoms.

Treatment

Chemotherapy

CML is often treated with a drug called hydroxyurea (Hydrea), a pill that lowers the blood counts and has few side effects, but probably does not prolong life. In the last few years, many doctors have been using alpha interferon, an injection that may prolong life in some patients, but has fairly severe side effects. More recently, the U.S. Food and Drug Administration approved Gleevec, a drug that seems to control the leukemia without many side effects and may prolong life.

CLL is treated with chlorambucil (Leukeran), a drug with few side effects that lowers the white blood cell count but doesn't prolong life. Another drug, fludarabine (Fludar), is more effective in lowering blood counts but has more side effects.

Immunotherapy

A drug called Campath was approved more recently for use in CLL. Campath is a monoclonal antibody directed against the CLL cell.

Radiation Therapy

Radiation is used on rare occasions to shrink swollen organs, particularly the spleen.

Stem Cell Transplantation

For CLL, this is an experimental procedure, but for young patients with CML (under 45), allogeneic stem cell transplant is the treatment of choice. (See Chapter 14 for more information on stem cell transplants.)

Hodgkin's Disease

Key Statistics

Approximately 7,400 new cases of Hodgkin's disease (3,900 men and 3,500 women) are diagnosed in the United States each year and an estimated 1,300 people (700 men and 600 women) die of this disease. Death rates have fallen over 60 percent since the early 1970s because of better treatment.

Hodgkin's disease can occur in both children and adults. It is more common, though, in two age groups: early adulthood (age 15 to 40, usually 25–30) and late adulthood (after age 55). Hodgkin's disease is rare before 5 years of age. From 10 to 15 percent of cases are diagnosed in children 16 years of age and younger.

The five-year survival rate depends on a patient's age, the type of Hodgkin's disease, and its extent, but in general it is around 90 percent.

> The lymph nodes are small, bean-shaped organs found in the neck, underarm, groin, and elsewhere in the body. They are also found inside the chest, abdomen, and pelvis. Lymph nodes make and store infection-fighting white blood cells, called lymphocytes. They are connected throughout the body by lymph vessels (narrow tubes similar to blood vessels). These lymph vessels carry a colorless, watery fluid (lymphatic fluid) that contains lymphocytes. Eventually the lymphatic fluid is emptied into the blood vessels in the left upper chest.
>
> Other components of the lymphatic system include the spleen, the bone marrow, and the thymus. The spleen is an organ in the left side of the upper abdomen. It removes old cells and, if present, other debris from the blood. The bone marrow is the spongy tissue inside the bones that creates new red and white blood cells, including lymphocytes. The thymus is a small organ in the chest that is important during early childhood in development of a special lymphocyte called a T cell.

Risk Factors

- *Infection.* There is a slightly increased rate of Hodgkin's disease in people who have had infectious mononucleosis (sometimes called "mono"), an infection caused by the Epstein-Barr virus. However, there is no evidence of a previous Epstein-Barr virus infection in half of the patients with Hodgkin's disease, so its role is unclear;

- *Immune deficiency.* Slightly higher rates of the disease occur among people with reduced immunity, such as those with the acquired immunodeficiency syndrome (AIDS), organ transplant patients who must take immune system–suppressing drugs, and people with congenital immunodeficiency syndromes;

- *Family history.* Certain families have many family members who develop Hodgkin's disease.

Types of Hodgkin's Disease

Hodgkin's disease, sometimes called Hodgkin's lymphoma, is a cancer that starts in lymphatic tissue, the lymph nodes and related organs that are part of the body's immune and blood-forming systems. Because lymphatic tissue is present in many parts of the body, Hodgkin's disease can start almost anywhere. The cancer cells generally spread through the lymphatic vessels to other lymphatic structures. If it gets into the bloodstream, it can also spread to almost any other part of the body.

Lymphomas are divided into two general types: Hodgkin's disease (named after Dr. Thomas Hodgkin, who first recognized it in 1832) and non-Hodgkin's lymphomas. The cancer cells in Hodgkin's disease are named Reed-Sternberg cells, after the two doctors who first described them in detail. Many scientists believe that these cells are a type of malignant B lymphocyte. (Normal B lymphocytes are the cells that make antibodies that help fight infections.) The different types of Hodgkin's disease are lymphocyte predominance, nodular sclerosis, mixed cellularity, and lymphocyte depletion.

Signs and Symptoms

- Enlarged lymph nodes that may grow very slowly; the most common sites are in the neck, under the arms, and in the chest;

- Fever that may come and go over periods of several days or weeks;

- Drenching night sweats;

- Itching;

- Fatigue;

- Loss of appetite;

- Weight loss.

Diagnostic Tests

- Excisional or incisional biopsy of lymph node—in an excisional biopsy, the entire lesion is removed. An incisional biopsy, which removes only a portion of the affected tissue, is performed on a large or ulcerated lesion or one that appears to grow deeply into the tissue;

- Fine needle aspiration (FNA)—a thin needle is used to withdraw fluid or small samples of tissue from the tumor mass so that cells can be viewed with a microscope;

- CT scan—a rotating x-ray beam creates a series of pictures of the body taken from many angles. It can identify abnormally large lymph nodes and abnormalities of the spleen or other organs that might be due to Hodgkin's disease;

- MRI scan—uses magnetic fields and radio waves instead of x-rays to create images of selected areas of the body;

- Gallium scan—when a special radioactive substance called gallium is injected into a vein, it is taken up by the Hodgkin's disease cells, and is detected by a special type of camera that shows the size and location of the tumors;

- Lymphangiogram—this involves injecting a dye into a lymphatic vessel in the foot to help locate Hodgkin's disease in the abdomen and pelvis;

- Bone marrow biopsy—a needle is used to remove a sample of bone marrow that can be examined for cancer cells;

- Laparotomy—a surgeon cuts into the abdomen, and checks to see if organs contain cancer. The surgeon then biopsies small pieces of tissue and usually removes the spleen.

Treatment

About 90 percent of newly diagnosed patients are cured with chemotherapy and/or radiation therapy. Bone marrow transplantation is being used for certain patients. In most cases except for biopsy and staging, surgery plays little role in the treatment of Hodgkin's disease.

Chemotherapy

Chemotherapy for Hodgkin's disease always involves the use of multiple drugs. Two common examples of combination treatments (see Chapter 15) are MOPP and ABVD. MOPP refers to **m**echlorethamine (Mustargen, or nitrogen mustard), vincristine (**O**ncovin), **p**rocarbazine (Matulane), and **p**rednisone. ABVD refers to doxorubicin (**A**driamycin), **b**leomycin (Blenoxane), **v**inblastine (Velban), and **d**acarbazine (DTIC-Dome). MOPP is no longer commonly used. Most doctors prefer to use ABVD. Chemotherapy is used when the lymphoma is too widespread for radiation alone.

Radiation Therapy

External beam radiation is most useful when the disease is localized to one part of the body or is so bulky that even if chemotherapy is used, it won't get rid of all the disease in the area. Most doctors treat only the known area of disease with radiation. This is called involved field radiation.

After three to six courses of multidrug chemotherapy, involved field radiation may be given to areas of particularly bulky tumors. Radiation therapy may also be given without chemotherapy to the mantle field—the neck, chest, and lymph nodes under the arms. When inverted Y field radiation therapy (to the lymph nodes in the upper abdomen, the spleen, and the lymph nodes in the pelvis) is given together with mantle field radiation, the combination is called total nodal irradiation. ·

Stem Cell Transplantation

Stem cell transplantation with the patient's own cells (called an autologous stem cell transplant) is often used if a patient has relapsed after chemotherapy. (See Chapter 14 for more information on stem cell transplants.)

Hodgkin's Disease in Children

If a child is sexually mature and has reached or almost reached full development of muscles and bone mass, the treatment is usually the same as given to adults. If, however, the child's body growth is still below what will be achieved in adulthood, then chemotherapy will be favored over radiation therapy because radiation will affect bone and muscle growth. In general, the treatment of Hodgkin's disease is similar to that in adults. When radiation treatment is given to children for their Hodgkin's disease, the amount of treatment is kept low. This means that in order to cure children, pediatric oncologists often combine radiation in low doses with chemotherapy. The success of this approach has been excellent with cure rates of 85 to 100 percent of children with more advanced disease.

Non-Hodgkin's Lymphoma

Key Statistics

Approximately 56,200 new cases of non-Hodgkin's lymphoma (31,100 men and 25,100 women), including children, are diagnosed in the United States each year and about 26,300 people (13,800 men and 12,500 women) die of this disease. It is the fifth most common cancer in this country, excluding skin cancers. Since the early 1970s, incidence rates for non-Hodgkin's lymphoma have nearly doubled; during the 1990s, the rate of increase appeared to slow and may be beginning to decline. The increase was a result of both better methods of detection and an actual increase in the number of new cases.

The five-year survival rate for all types of lymphomas combined is around 50 to 60 percent, but because there are so many different types with different prognoses, it is best to consult the REAL classification (see pages 554–555).

Risk Factors

- *Age.* Over 95 percent of non-Hodgkin's lymphoma cases occur in adults. The risk of developing non-Hodgkin's lymphoma increases throughout life, and the elderly have the highest risk;

- *Gender.* Men are affected more often than women;

- *Race.* Caucasians are more affected than other racial groups;

- *Immune deficiency.* The risk of lymphoma is increased by immune deficiency, whether genetically based or acquired (such as AIDS) or caused by taking drugs that suppress the immune system (for example, in people who have had organ transplants);

- *Exposure to radiation*, either because of cancer treatment or inadvertent exposure;

- *Previous treatment* with some chemotherapy drugs;

- *Certain viral infections* and even a bacterial infection of the stomach called *Helicobacter pylori.*

Types of Non-Hodgkin's Lymphoma

Non-Hodgkin's lymphoma is cancer that starts in lymphoid tissue (also called lymphatic tissue). Lymphoid tissue is formed by several types of immune system cells that work together to resist infections (see the callout in *Hodgkin's Disease*, page 549, for information about lymphoid tissue).

There are two main types of lymphomas. Hodgkin's lymphoma or Hodgkin's disease is named after Dr. Thomas Hodgkin, who first described it as a new disease in 1832. All other types of lymphoma are called non-Hodgkin's lymphomas (NHL). These two types of lymphoma can usually be distinguished from each other by examining the cancerous tissue under a microscope. In some cases, additional tests to identify specific chemical components of the lymphoma cells or tests of the cells' DNA may be needed.

The classification of non-Hodgkin's lymphoma seems quite confusing because there are so many types of non-Hodgkin's lymphoma and because several different systems of lymphoma classification have been developed.

The two most widely accepted classifications in the United States are the Working Formulation and the REAL classification. The Working Formulation uses the size and shape of the cancer cells and their pattern of growth within the lymph node to classify lymphomas. Size is described as large or small and shape is described as cleaved (showing folds or indentations) or noncleaved (basically smooth and round). Growth pattern may be follicular (arranged in clusters of cells) or diffuse (a scattered cell distribution). Not every lymphoma is described using all three features (size, shape, and pattern). For example, lymphomas might be described as follicular small-cleaved cell type, diffuse mixed (small and large) cell type, or small noncleaved cell type.

The Working Formulation divides non-Hodgkin's lymphoma into the following categories:

- **Low grade:** small lymphocytic and follicular small cleaved cell; follicular mixed (small cleaved and large cell);

- **Intermediate grade:** follicular, large cell; diffuse small cleaved cell; diffuse mixed (small and large cell); diffuse large cell;

- **High grade:** immunoblastic; lymphoblastic; small noncleaved (Burkitt's and non-Burkitt's);

- **Miscellaneous types** not specifically classified in Working Formulation: cutaneous T-cell lymphoma; adult T-cell leukemia/lymphoma; diffuse intermediately differentiated lymphoma; malignant histiocytosis.

These categories describe how likely the lymphoma is to be life-threatening over a few months or a year. Low grade means not very life-threatening and high grade means very life-threatening. It is important to understand that these grades refer to short-term outlook of people who do not receive treatment. Some people with low-grade NHL live for several years without any treatment, but their cancer may eventually cause fatal complications. On the other hand, some people with high-grade NHL may have a very good response to therapy and live for many years without recurrence.

REAL System

A newer system, called the REAL system (abbreviated from **R**evised **E**uropean **A**merican **L**ymphoma classification), also divides NHL types into categories according to clinical behavior. The REAL system not only uses the appearance of the lymphoma cells for classification, it also uses genetic features of the cells, their chemistry, and finally what happens to people that have these lymphomas—their clinical course. This overview divides the lymphomas into four classes, depending on their prognosis after treatment.

- **Excellent prognosis:** the average five-year survival is over 70 percent—this means that 70 percent of people are alive five years after they first developed signs and symptoms of the lymphoma. This category includes anaplastic large T-/Null cell lymphoma; marginal zone B-cell MALT lymphoma; and follicular lymphoma;

- **Good prognosis:** the average five-year survival is 50 to 70 percent. This category includes marginal zone B-cell nodal lymphoma; lymphoplasmacytoid lymphoma Waldenstrom's Macroglobulinemia; and small lymphocytic lymphoma (Chronic Lymphocytic Leukemia);

- **Fair prognosis:** the average five-year survival is 30 to 49 percent. This category includes primary mediastinal large B-cell lymphoma; diffuse large B-cell lymphoma; Burkitt's lymphoma; and high-grade B-cell Burkitt-like lymphoma;

- **Poor prognosis:** the average five-year survival is below 30 percent. This category includes peripheral T-cell lymphoma; lymphoblastic lymphoma; and mantle cell lymphoma.

The REAL system recognizes thirteen major lymphomas (there are more, but the others are very rare). Only a few of these occur very often. The most common are the diffuse large B-cell lymphoma (31 percent) and follicular lymphoma (22 percent). Small lymphocytic lymphoma, mantle cell lymphoma, and peripheral T-cell lymphoma each represent about 6 percent of NHL cases. All the rest are seen much less often (around 1 to 2 percent of the time).

Signs and Symptoms

- Enlarged lymph nodes close to the surface of the sides of the neck, groin or underarm areas, above the collar bone, and so on;
- Abdominal swelling;
- Abdominal pain due to pressure on the intestine and blockage;
- Cough or shortness of breath caused by swelling of lymph nodes inside the chest;
- Unexplained weight loss;
- Fever;
- Profuse sweating, particularly at night.

Diagnostic Tests

- Fine needle aspiration (FNA)—a thin needle is used to withdraw samples of tissue from the tumor mass so that cells can be examined with a microscope;

- Excisional or incisional biopsy of lymph node—in an excisional biopsy, the entire lesion is removed. An incisional biopsy, which removes only a portion of the affected tissue, is performed on a large or ulcerated lesion or one that appears to grow deeply into the tissue;

- Bone marrow aspiration and biopsy—a bone marrow biopsy uses a large needle to remove a piece of the bone for examination. A bone marrow aspiration uses a thinner needle and syringe to extract cells from the marrow for examination;

- Lumbar puncture (spinal tap)—a needle is placed in the lower back to obtain a small sample of cerebrospinal fluid, which can be examined for cancer cells;

- Immunohistochemistry—cells treated with special laboratory antibodies change color, which distinguishes different types of NHL from one another and from other diseases;

- Flow cytometry—uses lasers and computers to measure the amount of DNA in cancer cells suspended in liquid as they flow past the laser beam;

- Cytogenetics—examination of the chromosomes and genetic material;

- Molecular genetic studies—laboratory tests of the DNA that contains information on each cell's antigen receptors; the most sensitive way to diagnose non-Hodgkin's lymphoma;

- Chest x-ray;

- CT scan—a rotating x-ray beam creates a series of pictures of the body taken from many angles;

- MRI scan—uses magnetic fields and radio waves instead of x-rays to create images of selected areas of the body;

- Gallium scan—a special radioactive substance called gallium is injected into a vein and is taken up by the cancer cells;

- PET scan—images the brain after injection of a very low dose of a radioactive form of a substance.

Treatment

Surgery

Surgery is very rarely used to treat non-Hodgkin's lymphomas, but it may be used sometimes to treat lymphomas that start in certain extranodal organs such as the thyroid or stomach and have not spread beyond these organs.

Radiation Therapy

External beam radiation is rarely used as the primary treatment of early non-Hodgkin's lymphomas. More often, it is used in addition to chemotherapy. Radiation therapy can also be used to ease symptoms caused by lymphoma involving internal organs such as the brain or spinal cord.

Systemic Chemotherapy

Many drugs are useful in the treatment of patients with lymphoma. Usually, several drugs are combined. The most commonly used drugs are cyclophosphamide (Cytoxan), doxorubicin (Adriamycin), vincristine (Oncovin), methotrexate, and corticosteroids.

Biological Therapy

Monoclonal Antibodies. Some monoclonal antibodies can be designed to attack lymphoma cells. The U.S. Food and Drug Administration (FDA) has approved one product called Rituxan or rituximab for treatment of lymphoma. This is sometimes used together with combination chemotherapy for the initial treatment of people with lymphoma and is also used if the lymphoma has relapsed following chemotherapy.

Stem Cell Transplantation

This is an important treatment for patients who have failed their initial chemotherapy. The usual kind of transplant used is autologous, meaning a patient's own stem cells are used and a donor is not needed. (See Chapter 14 for more information on stem cell transplants.)

Multiple Myeloma

Key Statistics

Approximately 14,400 new cases of multiple myeloma (7,500 men and 6,900 women) are diagnosed in the United States each year and about 11,200 people (5,800 men and 5,400 women) die of this disease.

The five-year survival rate is about 45 percent for younger adults (younger than 50) and decreases with age. It is 25 percent for people ages 65 to 74.

> The immune system is composed of several types of cells, including lymphocytes, that work together to fight off infections and other diseases. There are two types of lymphocytes: T cells and B cells. When B cells respond to an infection, they mature and change into plasma cells. Plasma cells produce and release proteins called immunoglobins (antibodies) to attack and help kill disease-causing germs such as bacteria.

Risk Factors

- *Age*. Age is the most significant multiple myeloma risk factor. Only 2 percent of cases are diagnosed in people younger than age 40. The average age at diagnosis is about 70;

- *Race*. Multiple myeloma is about twice as common among African Americans as Caucasians.

Types

Multiple myeloma is a cancer of plasma cells. Normal plasma cells, which are mostly found in the bone marrow, are an important part of the immune system. They produce antibodies that attack specific infectious agents. When plasma cells grow out of control they can produce a tumor. Generally, these tumors grow in multiple sites in the bone marrow, hence the name, multiple myeloma. Instead of producing a variety of antibodies, these cells produce only one kind, called a monoclonal protein that is useless in fighting infection, but often accumulates in large amounts in the blood and is a good marker for the presence of multiple myeloma. This is sometimes called a monoclonal gammopathy. Some parts of these proteins are excreted in the urine. About 20 percent of people with monoclonal gammopathy of undetermined significance (MGUS) or solitary plasma cell tumor will eventually develop multiple myeloma.

Myeloma types range from very well differentiated to very poorly differentiated.

Signs and Symptoms

Some patients with multiple myeloma have no symptoms at all. When symptoms occur, the following are the most common ones:

- Bone pain and often bone fractures;

- Anemia;

- Lowered resistance to infections such as pneumonia;

- Even minor scrapes, cuts, or bruises cause serious bleeding;

- Severe pain, numbness, and/or weakness of limbs due to collapse of spinal bones—the abnormal proteins produced by myeloma cells can be damaging to nerves;

- High blood calcium levels as the minerals from bone are absorbed;

- Weakness and confusion.

Diagnostic Tests

- Blood and urine tests for monoclonal proteins;

- Bone x-rays;

- Bone marrow aspiration and biopsy—a bone marrow biopsy uses a large needle to remove a piece of the bone for examination. A bone marrow aspiration uses a thinner needle and syringe to extract cells from the marrow for examination;

Treatment

Chemotherapy and Other Drugs

The usual treatment for multiple myeloma consists of using melphalan (Alkeran) and Prednisone together. Other chemotherapeutic drugs such as vincristine (Oncovin), cyclophosphamide (Cytoxan), carmustine (BiCNU), and doxorubicin (Adriamycin) are also often used. Dexamethasone is sometimes used instead of prednisone. Some typical combinations are:

- MP: melphalan and prednisone;

- VBMCP: vincristine, carmustine (BiCNU), melphalan, cyclophosphamide, and prednisone;

- VAD: vincristine, doxorubicin (Adriamycin), and dexamethasone.

A nonchemotherapy drug that has been found to be effective is thalidomide (Thalomid). Interferon has also been used.

Another class of drugs used are bisphosphonates such as pamidronate (Aredia) and zoledronate. These help keep the bones intact.

Radiation Therapy

External beam radiation therapy is often given as a treatment for areas of bone damaged by myeloma that have not responded to chemotherapy and are causing serious symptoms. Myeloma responds well to radiation therapy.

Surgery

Although surgery is occasionally used to remove solitary plasmacytomas, it is very rarely used in treating multiple myeloma.

Stem Cell Transplantation

Many patients are treated with autologous stem cell transplant. Although this hasn't proven curative, many believe it prolongs the life of patients with this disease (see Chapter 14 for more information on stem cell transplants).

Plasmapheresis

This treatment removes blood from a vein and separates the blood cells (which are returned into another vein) from the blood plasma (liquid part of the blood). Because plasma contains the abnormal antibody protein produced by the myeloma cells, it is discarded and replaced with a salt solution and blood proteins from donors. Plasmapheresis is helpful when accumulation of certain myeloma proteins causes the blood to become very thick, thereby interfering with circulation to the brain and causing stroke-like symptoms. Although plasmapheresis can relieve some symptoms, it does not kill the myeloma cells.

Bone

Key Statistics

About 2,900 new cases of cancer of the bones and joints (1,600 men and 1,300 women) are diagnosed in the United States each year and about 1,400 people (800 men and 600 women) die from these cancers. Primary cancers of bones account for less than 0.2 percent of all cancers. Because there are so many different types, a five-year survival rate for bone cancers can't be determined.

Risk Factors

- *Genetics.* A very small number of bone cancers (especially osteosarcomas) appear to have a hereditary basis. Children with certain rare inherited cancer syndromes have an increased risk of developing osteosarcoma. Li-Fraumeni syndrome makes people much more likely to develop several types of cancer, including osteosarcoma and other types of sarcoma;

- *Retinoblastoma.* Children who have inherited a tendency to develop retino-blastoma, a rare eye cancer, also have an increased risk for developing osteosarcoma;

- *Radiation.* Exposure to large doses of radiation—for example, radiation therapy to treat another cancer—may increase risk of bone cancer. Being treated at a young age and/or being treated with high doses of radiation increases risk. Exposure to radioactive materials such as radium and strontium may cause bone cancer;

Bone is the supporting framework of the body. Most bones are hollow. The end of the bone is called the epiphyses, and next to it is a zone of cartilage, a softer form of bone-like tissue that acts as a cushion between bones and, together with ligaments and some other tissues, forms the joints between bones. The outside of the bone is covered with a layer of fibrous tissue called periosteum. The portion of a long bone between the ends or extremities is called the diaphysis; it is made up of a tube of compact bone (bone substance that is dense and hard). The bone itself contains two kinds of cells: osteoblasts, which are responsible for forming bone; and osteoclasts, which are responsible for dissolving bone. Bone is very active. New bone is constantly forming and old bone is dissolving.

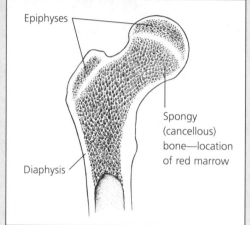

Bone marrow, soft tissue inside the hollow bones, is located in the inside structure of bones, the cancellous (spongy) bone. The marrow of some bones consists only of fatty tissue. The marrow of other bones is a mixture of fat cells and blood-forming cells. These blood-forming cells produce red blood cells, white blood cells, and blood platelets. There are some other cells in the marrow such as plasma cells, fibroblasts, and reticuloendothelial cells.

- *Bone abnormalities.* Conditions such as Paget's disease, a benign condition that affects mostly people over age 50, increase risk of bone cancer. Bone sarcomas (usually osteosarcoma) develop in about 5 to 10 percent of severe cases of Paget's disease, usually when many bones are affected.

The following increase the risk of chondrosarcoma:

- Multiple exostoses (overgrowths of bone tissue);

- Multiple osteochondromas (benign bone tumors);

- Multiple enchondromas (several benign cartilage tumors).

Types of Primary Bone Cancers

There are several different types of primary bone cancer. Their names are based on the area of bone or surrounding tissue that is affected, and the kind of cells forming the malignant tumor. Most bone cancers are called sarcomas, which mostly develop from bone, cartilage, muscle, fibrous tissue, fatty tissue, or nerve tissue.

Osteosarcoma

Osteosarcoma (also called osteogenic sarcoma) is a cancer of the bone itself, and is the most common primary bone cancer (35 percent of cases). It most often occurs in young people between the ages of 10 and 30 and affects men more than women. About 10 percent of cases develop in people in their 60s and 70s. These tumors develop most often in bones of the legs, arms, and pelvis. (See *Osteosarcoma*, pages 589–593, for more information).

Chondrosarcoma

This is a cancer of cartilage, and is the second most common primary bone cancer (26 percent of cases). This cancer is uncommon in people younger than 20 years old. After age 20, the risk of developing chondrosarcoma continues to rise until reaching about 75 years. Men and women are equally likely to get this cancer. Although this cancer usually occurs in bones of the arms, legs, and pelvis, the ribs and some other bones are occasionally affected.

Ewing's Tumor

This cancer (also called Ewing's sarcoma) is named after Dr. James Ewing, the doctor who first described it in 1921. Ewing's tumors usually but not always develop in bones, especially the long bones of the legs and arms, and less than 10 percent develop in other tissues and organs. Ewing's tumor is the third most common primary bone cancer (16 percent of cases). This cancer usually appears in children and adolescents and is uncommon in adults over 30 years old. Ewing's tumors occur most frequently in the white population and are rare among African Americans and Asian Americans.

Fibrosarcoma and Malignant Fibrous Histiocytoma

These cancers rarely start in bones. They usually develop from "soft tissues," such as ligaments, tendons, fat, and muscle. These cancers usually occur in elderly and middle-aged adults. Bones most often affected include those of the legs, arms, and jaw.

Giant Cell Tumor of Bone

This type of primary bone tumor has benign and malignant forms. Approximately 10 percent are cancerous and spread to other parts of the body, but even the benign form can recur locally after surgery. These tumors typically affect the arm or leg bones of young and middle-aged adults.

Chordoma

This tumor usually occurs in the base of the skull and bones of the spine. Surgery and radiation therapy are difficult because of the nearby spinal cord and nerves that may be involved. Long-term follow-up is important because these tumors can come back, even ten or more years after treatment.

Signs and Symptoms

- Pain—may be worse at night or when the affected bone is used. This is the most common complaint;

- A lump or mass—depending on where the tumor is, a lump or mass may be felt.

Diagnostic Tests

- X-rays of the bone;

- CT or MRI scan—a CT scan is a rotating x-ray beam that creates a series of pictures of the body taken from many angles. An MRI scan uses magnetic fields and radio waves instead of x-rays to create images of selected areas of the body;

- Radionuclide scanning or scintigraphy—the patient is given a dose of radioactive substance, which is absorbed by bone containing metastatic EFT. Using special radiation-sensing cameras, doctors can determine whether a mass is cancerous and whether a cancer has spread to other parts of the body;

- Biopsy of the tumor or cancerous area—either a needle biopsy or incisional biopsy may be done.

Treatment

Surgery

Depending on the type and stage of the bone cancer, surgery may be used to remove the cancer and about an inch of tissue surrounding the tumor. It is not always necessary to amputate an entire limb, since segments of the bone can be removed and replaced with bone grafts, and/or metal rods or plates to maintain function in the affected area or limb. This limb-sparing surgery may follow chemotherapy and/or radiation therapy, which shrinks the tumor.

Radiation Therapy

Radiation therapy is sometimes the main treatment, especially in those whose general health is too poor to undergo surgery. Radiation therapy is used as an adjuvant treatment either before or after surgery. It can also be used as a palliative treatment (for symptom relief).

Chemotherapy

Chemotherapy may be a main treatment or given before or after surgery depending on the specific type of bone cancer. It can be used before surgery to shrink a tumor to allow limb-sparing surgery, or after surgery to prevent distant recurrence. It will often be used if the cancer is too advanced to be cured by surgery. The major drugs are doxorubicin (Adriamycin), ifosfamide (IFEX), methotrexate, and cisplatin (Platin). These are given in combinations of two or more drugs.

Kaposi's Sarcoma

Key Statistics

The frequency of KS in AIDS patients has decreased dramatically in the last few years to less than 10 percent. About one in four homosexual or bisexual males with AIDS have KS or will develop it during their illness. About 1 to 3 percent of epidemic KS cases occur among other people with HIV (women and nonhomosexual males), most of whom contract the virus through intravenous drug use.

The incidence has dropped by 90 percent in the last few years so that it is newly diagnosed in only 1 in 100,000 males in the United States each year and far fewer females. The death rate and five-year survival rate are a function of the HIV infection and AIDS rather than the sarcoma, so no survival rates are available for this cancer.

A sarcoma is a cancer that develops in connective tissues such as cartilage, bone, fat, muscle, blood vessels, or fibrous tissues (related to tendons or ligaments). This disease typically causes tumors to develop in the tissues below the skin surface, or in the mucous membranes of the mouth, nose, or anus. These lesions (abnormal tissue areas) appear as raised blotches or nodules that may be purple, brown, or red in color. Although the skin lesions of KS may be disfiguring, they usually are not life-threatening or disabling.

For decades KS was considered a rare disease that mostly affected elderly men of Mediterranean or Jewish heritage, organ transplant patients, or young adult African men. In the last 20 years, however, the vast majority of KS cases have developed in association with human immunodeficiency virus (HIV) infection and the acquired immunodeficiency syndrome (AIDS), especially among homosexual men. It seems to be caused by the transmittal of a second herpes virus called HHV-8.

Risk Factors

- *Gender.* Men are much more likely to get Kaposi's sarcoma than women;

- *HIV infection.* The highest risk of KS occurs among male homosexuals and bisexuals infected with HIV.

Types of Kaposi's Sarcoma

Classic Kaposi's Sarcoma

Classic Kaposi's sarcoma usually develops in elderly Jewish men of Eastern European origin or Mediterranean heritage (primarily Italian). Classic KS is quite rare, even in these ethnic and age groups. The lesions usually start in the feet and legs, progress quite slowly, and are rarely life-threatening.

African (Endemic) Kaposi's Sarcoma

This form of the disease is fairly common among people living in equatorial Africa. In many cases, this disease is identical to classic KS, although it usually strikes at a much younger age. It affects many more men than women. Typically, African (endemic) KS causes skin lesions that do not produce symptoms and do not spread to other parts of the body. There is also a childhood form that is much more virulent.

Transplant-Related (Acquired) Kaposi's Sarcoma

Kaposi's sarcoma is 150 to 200 times more likely to develop in transplant patients than among the general population because these people are taking drugs to suppress their immune system.

AIDS-Related (Epidemic) Kaposi's Sarcoma

This occurs primarily in people who have contracted HIV infection through sexual contact and is thought to be due primarily to infection with the human herpesvirus-8 virus.

Non-Epidemic, Gay-Related Kaposi's Sarcoma

KS can develop in homosexual men who do not show evidence of HIV infection. The lesions usually occur only on the skin of the arms and legs but sometimes develop on the genitals. New lesions may arise every few years.

Signs and Symptoms

- Purplish raised spots on the skin of the face and chest and in the mouth in AIDS patients, and on the skin of the legs in classical KS;

- Local swelling around KS lesions as they get bigger;

- Trouble eating because of KS in the mouth, esophagus, or stomach;

- Bleeding from the intestinal tract;

- Coughing blood because of KS lesions in the lungs.

Diagnostic Tests

- Punch biopsy—removing a small, round piece of tissue;

- Excisional biopsy—removing the entire lesion;

- Endoscopic biopsy in the intestinal tract—involves using a thin, flexible, lighted tube called an endoscope to look for lesions and then using small surgical instruments to biopsy them;

- Sigmoidoscopy—using a slender, flexible, hollow, lighted tube about the thickness of a finger to search for abnormalities in the lower part of the colon;

- Bronchoscopy—involves passing a long, lighted tube called a bronchoscope down the throat to look at the lining of the lung's main airways;

- Chest x-ray;

- CT scan—a rotating x-ray beam creates a series of pictures of the body taken from many angles.

Treatment

In some cases, KS is not a serious condition, and it requires no specific treatment. Sometimes, particularly in AIDS patients, it may be life-threatening.

Treatment of the underlying AIDS is the most important step in treating AIDS-related KS.

Surgery

There are treatments available for people with all types of Kaposi's sarcoma. Types of surgery include:

Surgical excision. This is used to remove KS lesions;

Electrodesiccation and curettage. This uses an electric probe to destroy the tissue with heat; the tissue is then scraped away;

Cryosurgery. This uses a supercold probe to freeze the tissue.

Radiation Therapy

Lesions on the skin can be treated with local external beam radiation therapy.

Chemotherapy

Chemotherapy can be given locally with injection of drugs such as vinblastine (Velban) or interferon directly into KS lesions. Also, a newer treatment, topical application of a drug called alitretinoin (Panretin Gel) has been successful in almost 50 percent of patients.

Usually, a single chemotherapy drug is given for KS in the early stages, and combinations are used in more advanced disease. Among the single chemotherapy drugs given to treat KS are bleomycin (Blenoxane), etoposide (VePesid), paclitaxel (Taxol), vinblastine (Velban), vincristine (Oncovin), and doxorubicin (Adriamycin). Combination regimens include vinblastine + vincristine; bleomycin + vinblastine or vincristine; or bleomycin + doxorubicin + vinblastine or vincristine.

More recently, it was discovered that placing the active molecules of certain drugs into liposomes, protective globules made of lipids (fats), increases their effectiveness. Two liposomal-encapsulated forms of the cancer drugs doxorubicin and daunorubicin are available.

Other promising drugs include the antiretroviral agents (see page 538 of *AIDS-Related Cancers*).

Breast

Key Statistics

Breast cancer is the most common cancer among women, excluding skin cancers. Approximately 193,700 new cases of invasive breast cancer (stages I to IV) are diagnosed among women in the United States each year. Carcinoma in situ, which is not invasive, accounts for another 46,400 new cases. Breast cancer also occurs in men with an estimated 1,400 new cases diagnosed each year.

The incidence of breast cancer is slowly increasing. Breast cancer is the second leading cause of cancer death in women, exceeded only by lung cancer. There are about 40,600 deaths from breast cancer in the United States (40,200 women and 400 men) each year. Death rates from breast cancer have been declining. This is probably the result of earlier detection and improved treatment.

The five-year survival rate for women with localized breast cancer is 97 percent. It is 77 percent if the cancer involved lymph nodes when first diagnosed, and 21 percent if the cancer has spread outside the breast and local lymph nodes.

Risk Factors

- *Age*. Breast cancer incidence increases with age;
- *Inherited gene abnormalities*. Approximately 5 to 10 percent of all breast cancers occur in women who have inherited an abnormal gene. The best known of these are called BRCA1 and BRCA2;

The breasts rest on the major chest muscle, the pectoralis major. Each breast contains fifteen to twenty lobes arranged like wheel spokes around a hub, coming together just under the nipple. Each lobe is comprised of many lobules, at the end of which are glands, or sacs, where milk is produced in response to hormonal signals. Ducts connect the lobes, lobules, and glands. Most cancers start in these ducts. Lymph vessels form a network throughout each breast and drain to lymph nodes under the arm and in the chest.

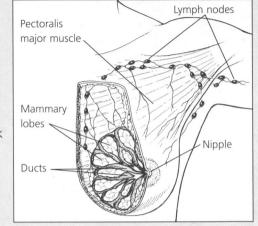

- *Family history.* Having one or more first-degree relatives (mother, sister, or daughter) increases risk considerably;

- *Personal history of breast cancer.* A woman with cancer in one breast has a three- to fourfold increased risk of developing a new cancer in the other breast or in another part of the same breast;

- *Previous breast biopsy.* Women with a history of breast biopsies have a higher risk;

- *Previous breast irradiation.* Women who have had chest area radiation therapy as treatment for another cancer (such as Hodgkin's disease or non-Hodgkin's lymphoma) are at significantly increased risk;

- *Long menstrual history.* Women who started menstruating before age 12 and went through menopause after age 50 have a slightly higher risk of breast cancer;

- *Oral contraceptive use.* Women now using oral contraceptives have a slightly greater risk of breast cancer;

- *Late or no childbearing.* Women who have had no children or who had their first child after age 30 have a slightly higher risk;

- *Postmenopausal hormone replacement therapy.* Taking estrogen and progesterone after menopause increases breast cancer risk;

- *Drinking alcohol* increases risk slightly;

• *Obesity, high fat intake, and physical inactivity* all contribute to increased breast cancer risk.

Types of Breast Cancer

The two main types of breast adenocarcinomas are ductal carcinomas and lobular carcinomas. There are also several subtypes of adenocarcinoma.

Carcinoma In Situ

This is noninvasive breast cancer, meaning that the cancer has not invaded surrounding fatty tissues in the breast or spread to other organs in the body. There are 46,400 cases of carcinoma in situ diagnosed in the United States each year in addition to the invasive cancers. The majority (88 percent) of these are ductal (cancer that begins in the ducts—milk passages), which is called ductal carcinoma in situ (DCIS). Most of the rest are lobular (cancer that begins in the lobules—milk glands), which is called lobular carcinoma in situ (LCIS). Although these don't spread, they may be a precursor of invasive cancer.

Infiltrating (or Invasive) Ductal Carcinoma (IDC)

This is the most common invasive cancer (80 to 85 percent). This cancer starts in a duct, breaks through the wall of the duct, and invades the fatty tissue of the breast.

Infiltrating (or Invasive) Lobular Carcinoma (ILC)

About 10 to 15 percent of invasive breast cancers are invasive lobular carcinomas. This cancer starts in the lobules and can spread to other parts of the body.

Medullary, Tubular, Papillary, and Mucinous Carcinomas

These are all uncommon types of cancer, which generally have a better prognosis than ductal or lobular carcinoma. They have no distinctive clinical features.

Mucinous (or Colloid) Carcinoma

This rare type of invasive breast cancer is formed by mucus-producing cancer cells. The prognosis for mucinous carcinoma is better than for the more common types of invasive breast cancer.

Paget's Disease of the Nipple

This rare type of breast cancer spreads to the skin of the nipple and then to the areola. Paget's disease accounts for only 1 percent of all cases and may be associated with in situ or infiltrating breast carcinoma.

Phyllodes Tumor

This very rare type of breast tumor forms from the connective tissue of the breast. Phyllodes (also spelled phylloides) tumors are usually benign.

Tubular Carcinoma

Tubular carcinomas are a special type of infiltrating breast carcinoma. They account for about 2 percent of all breast cancers.

Signs and Symptoms

- The most common sign of breast cancer is a new lump or mass in breast that is often painless and firm, but can be tender as well as soft;

- Generalized swelling of part of a breast (even if no distinct lump can be felt);

- Skin irritation or dimpling;

- Nipple pain or retraction (turning inward), redness or scaliness of the nipple or breast skin, or a discharge other than breast milk;

- Sometimes a breast cancer can spread to underarm lymph nodes and cause them to be obviously enlarged, even before the original tumor in the breast tissue is large enough to be felt.

Diagnostic Tests

Imaging Tests for Breast Disease Diagnosis

- Diagnostic mammography—an x-ray of the breast;

- Ultrasonography (ultrasound)—uses sound waves and their echoes to produce images of internal organs or outline a part of the body, such as the breast;

- Ductogram—a type of x-ray test in which the shape of the duct on an x-ray image is outlined.

Nipple Discharge Examination

If there is a nipple discharge, some of the fluid may be collected and examined under a microscope to see if any cancer cells are present.

Biopsy

This involves the removal of a sample of tissue so doctors can see whether cancer cells are present.

- *Fine needle aspiration biopsy (FNAB)*—removes fluid from a cyst or cells from a tumor by using a fine needle;

- *Core needle biopsy*—removes a small cylinder of tissue from a breast abnormality;

- *Excisional surgical biopsy*—removal of all or part of the mass.

Laboratory Tests

The tissue removed during the biopsy is examined in the lab to see whether the cancer is in situ (not invasive) or invasive and to determine the cancer's type.

- *Grades of breast cancer*—a pathologist looks at the tissue sample under a microscope and then assigns a grade to it. The histologic tumor grade (sometimes called its Bloom-Richardson grade, Scarff-Bloom-Richardson grade, or Elston-Ellis grade) is based on the arrangement of the cells in relation to each other, as well as features of individual cells. It is used for invasive cancers but not for in situ cancers. Grade 1 cancers have relatively normal-looking cells that do not appear to be growing rapidly and are arranged in small tubules. Grade 3 cancers, the highest grade, lack these features and tend to grow and spread more aggressively;

- *Estrogen and progesterone receptors*—an important step in evaluating a breast cancer is to test for the presence of receptors on cells that recognize the hormones estrogen and progesterone;

- *Tests of ploidy and cell proliferation rate*—the ploidy of cancer cells refers to the amount of DNA they contain. If the amount of DNA is abnormal, the cells are described as aneuploid. Some studies have found that aneuploid breast cancers tend to be more aggressive;

- *Flow cytometry*—uses lasers and computers to measure the amount of DNA in cancer cells suspended in liquid as they flow past the laser beam;

- *HER2/neu testing*—tests whether cancer cells have a growth-promoting protein called HER2/neu.

Treatment

Surgery

Breast conservation therapy. This surgery removes the mass and a ring of surrounding normal tissue. Partial or segmental mastectomy or quadrantectomy removes more breast tissue than a lumpectomy (up to one-quarter or more of the breast). This is almost always followed by about six weeks of radiation therapy;

Mastectomy. In a simple or total mastectomy the surgeon removes the entire breast, but does not remove lymph nodes from under the arm or muscle tissue from beneath the breast. Modified radical mastectomy involves the removal of the entire breast and some of the axillary (underarm) lymph nodes. Radical mastectomy is an extensive operation that is rarely done, removing the entire breast, axillary lymph nodes, and the pectoral (chest wall) muscles under the breast;

Axillary dissection. Some of the lymph nodes from under the arm are removed for microscopic examination. Axillary dissection is part of a surgical treatment of breast cancer;

Sentinel Lymph Node Biopsy (SLNB). (See Chapter 5 for information about SLNB);

Reconstructive surgery and breast implant surgery. Breast reconstruction may be done at the same time as the mastectomy (immediate reconstruction) or later (delayed reconstruction). It may use implants and/or tissue from other parts of the body (autologous tissue reconstruction).

Radiation Therapy

External beam radiation is the usual type of radiation therapy for women with breast cancer. Brachytherapy is sometimes used. Radiation therapy to the breast is given after breast-conserving surgery. It is also used after mastectomy in women who have several axillary lymph nodes involved with cancer.

Chemotherapy

Chemotherapy is recommended for most women after breast cancer surgery to prevent the cancer from coming back. It is also used to treat the cancer if it has come back or spread outside the breast and lymph nodes. Several different combinations of drugs are used. The most common drugs used in these combinations are cyclophosphamide (Cytoxan), fluorouracil (5-FU), doxorubicin (Adriamycin), methotrexate, paclitaxel (Taxol), docetaxel (Taxotere), and vinorelbine (Navelbine).

Hormone Therapy

Most breast cancers are estrogen dependent—that is, they grow in the presence of estrogen. If the estrogen receptor test is positive, the tumor is most likely estrogen dependent. After surgery most women will be given a drug to block the estrogen receptor for five years. The most commonly used drug is tamoxifen (Nolvadex). Tamoxifen can also prevent breast cancer in women at high risk and is used to treat breast cancer when it has spread outside the breast and lymph nodes.

Another type of drug will block the remaining estrogen production from the adrenal gland in postmenopausal women. These drugs, called aromatase inhibitors, are options for postmenopausal women whose advanced breast cancer continues to grow during or after tamoxifen treatment. Anastrozole (Arimidex) and letrozole (Femara) are examples of these.

Other less common hormone therapies for advanced cancer are progestins (other hormones produced in the ovaries) or androgens (male hormones). Oophorectomy, or removal of the ovaries, may eliminate the body's main source of estrogen in premenopausal women.

Stem Cell Transplantation

These are considered experimental therapy. Most studies have shown no benefit and this treatment is not recommended (see Chapter 14 for more information on stem cell transplants).

Immunotherapy with Trastuzumab (Herceptin)

Trastuzumab (Herceptin) is a monoclonal antibody that attaches to a growth-promoting protein known as HER2/neu, present in about one-third of breast cancers. Used together with chemotherapy, Herceptin can shrink some breast cancers that have high levels of HER2/neu protein.

Brain and Spinal Cord

Key Statistics

Approximately 17,200 new cases of brain and spinal cord cancers (9,800 men and 7,400 in women) are diagnosed in the United States each year and about 13,100 people (7,200 men and 5,900 women) die from these malignant tumors. Many types of cancers start in the brain and spinal cord, but they differ in adults and children. The incidence of all these cancers is increasing for unknown reasons.

The five-year survival rates are quite variable depending on age. This is because younger people get different tumors. For people under 45, the five-year survival rate is 60 percent; for those aged 45 to 54 it is 24 percent; and for patients 55 to 64 it is 11 percent. Older patients (aged 65 to 74) have a five-year survival rate of 7 percent. The survival rate drops to 4 percent in those over 75.

Risk Factors

- *Radiation.* People who have radiation to the brain for other reasons have an increased risk of brain cancer;

- *Immune deficiency.* People with impaired immune systems have an increased risk of developing lymphomas of the brain or spinal cord;

- *Genetics.* People with certain family cancer syndromes of nervous tissue have an increased risk of brain cancer.

The brain is the center of thought, memory, emotion, and speech. It also perceives sensation and tells our muscles to move. This is done through nerves directly attached to the brain and through the spinal cord.

The cerebrum is the largest and main portion of the brain. The cerebellum is attached to the back of the brain stem and controls coordination of movement.

The brain and spinal cord are surrounded and cushioned by a special fluid, called cerebrospinal fluid, which is produced in the brain. The spaces around the brain are lined by specialized tissues called the meninges, which help form the spaces through which cerebrospinal fluid travels. The spinal cord carries signals controlling muscles, sensation, and bladder and bowel control.

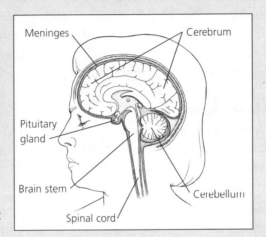

The brain stem contains bundles of very long axons that carry signals controlling muscles and sensation or feeling.

The pituitary is a gland at the base of the brain that produces secretions that affect most basic body functions.

Because the brain is made of different types of cells, different kinds of cancer start in the brain, depending on the cell.

Types of Brain and Spinal Cord Cancers

Tumors of the brain are labeled by the cell from which they develop.

Astrocytomas

Most tumors that arise within the brain start in astrocytes and are called astrocytomas. These range from low grade, which are the slowest growing, to the highest grade, anaplastic astrocytomas or glioblastomas, which are the fastest growing.

Most cannot be cured because they spread widely throughout the surrounding normal brain tissue although they do not spread outside the brain or spinal cord.

There are some special types of astrocytomas that tend to have a particularly good prognosis. These are called noninfiltrating astrocytomas (juvenile pilocytic astrocytomas and subependymal giant cell astrocytomas).

Oligodendrogliomas

These tumors start in brain cells called oligodendrocytes. They spread or infiltrate in a manner similar to astrocytomas and, in most cases, cannot be completely removed by surgery. But they often grow slowly and can be associated with long-term survivals.

Ependymomas

These tumors arise from the ependymal cells, which line the ventricles (fluid-filled spaces in the brain). Ependymomas may block the exit of cerebrospinal fluid from the ventricles, causing the ventricle to become very large—a condition called hydrocephalus. Ependymomas characteristically do not spread or infiltrate into normal brain tissue. As a result, some ependymomas can be completely removed and cured by surgery. Ependymomas may spread along the cerebrospinal fluid pathways but do not spread outside the brain or spinal cord.

Meningioma

Meningiomas arise in cells of the outer covering of the brain, the meninges. They are quite common, accounting for about 50 percent of primary brain and spinal cord tumors, and most (about 85 percent) are benign and curable with surgery.

Medulloblastomas. These rare tumors that develop from neurons of the cerebellum are fast-growing tumors, but they can be treated and are often cured by radiation therapy. Medulloblastomas occur most commonly in children and frequently spread throughout the cerebrospinal fluid pathways. (See the "Brain and Spinal Cord Tumors in Children" section of *Childhood Cancers*, pages 597–601, for more information.)

Ganglioglioma

A tumor containing both neurons and glial cells is called a ganglioglioma. These tumors have a high rate of cure by surgery alone or surgery combined with radiation therapy.

Schwannoma (Neurilemoma)

These usually benign tumors start in Schwann cells, which surround cranial nerves and other nerves. They often form near the cerebellum and in the cranial nerve responsible for hearing and balance.

Chordoma

These tumors usually start in the lower end of the spinal cord. These typically come back many times over ten to twenty years and can spread or metastasize to other organs.

Lymphoma

Lymphomas of the brain are malignancies of lymphoid tissue. They are highly malignant and are often seen in people with immune deficiencies such as AIDS.

Signs and Symptoms

- Headache is often the commonest sign;

- Persistent vomiting;

- Mental changes such as lethargy and persistent drowsiness;

- Sudden onset of bad decision making and confusion;

- Loss of vision;

- Loss of function of a part of the body or loss of sensation (numbness) from a part of the body;

- Epileptic seizures.

Diagnostic Tests

- MRI scan—uses magnetic fields and radio waves instead of x-rays to create images of selected areas of the body. This is the single most important test;

- CT scan—a rotating x-ray beam creates a series of pictures of the body taken from many angles. It may show that a brain tumor is very likely;

- PET scan—images the brain after injection of a very low dose of a radioactive form of a substance in order to evaluate the tumor grade;

- Biopsy—removal of tissue for examination;

- Stereotactic biopsy—removal of a small piece of tissue with a thin needle placed within the tumor with the help of a CT or an MRI scan and a computer;

- Lumbar puncture (spinal tap)—a needle is placed in the lower back to obtain a small sample of cerebrospinal fluid, which can be examined for cancer cells.

Treatment

Although survival may be prolonged by treatment, most malignant brain tumors are not cured by surgery, radiation, or chemotherapy.

Surgery

The first step in most cases is surgical removal of as much of the tumor as possible. Some tumors may be cured by surgical removal alone or by surgery combined with radiation therapy. These tumors include meningiomas, some ependymomas, gangliogliomas, and cerebellar astrocytomas. Others are not cured because cells from the tumor infiltrate into the normal surrounding brain tissue; however, surgery can relieve pressure on the brain.

Radiation Therapy

Up to one half of all medulloblastomas and virtually all germinomas (the most common germ cell tumors of the nervous system) are cured by radiation therapy. Unfortunately, most brain tumors are not cured by radiation. Astrocytomas, oligodendrogliomas, and ependymomas are not cured by radiation therapy, but can be helped by it. Some tumors of children may necessitate radiation therapy for the spinal cord as well.

Techniques such as three-dimensional treatment planning (conformal radiation) and stereotactic radiosurgery (with a "gamma knife" or a linear accelerator, a machine that gives off gamma rays and electron beams) may help spare normal tissue because radiation can damage normal brain tissue. This can lead to memory loss, poor thinking ability, and even confusion and dementia.

Chemotherapy

Often cortisone-like drugs such as dexamethasone (Decadron) are given to reduce the swelling that often occurs around brain tumors. This may help relieve headache and other symptoms. Also, drugs may be prescribed to prevent seizures, usually diphenylhydantoin (Dilantin).

Treatment of Specific Types of Brain and Spinal Cord Tumors

- *Astrocytomas:* are treated with surgery, when possible, often with the addition of radiation and chemotherapy with a drug called BCNU;

- *Lymphomas:* surgery is for biopsy and diagnosis only in this case. Standard treatment is radiation therapy to the whole brain, often combined with chemotherapy with drugs such as methotrexate and procarbazine along with corticosteroids. In addition, chemotherapy must be given into the spinal fluid by spinal taps or a thin tube placed in the skull, because lymphomas spread there;

- *Oligodendrogliomas:* surgery cannot usually cure this tumor but can relieve symptoms and prolong survival. Surgery may be followed by chemotherapy and sometimes radiation therapy when the tumor causes disability;

- *Ependymomas:* these tumors may be cured by surgery alone. If not completely removed by surgery, radiation therapy is given;

- *Meningiomas:* these tumors can usually be cured if completely removed surgically. Radiation therapy may control regrowth of meningiomas that cannot be completely removed or those that recur after surgery;

- *Schwannomas:* these tumors are effectively cured by surgical removal. In some centers small acoustic schwannomas are treated by stereotactic radiosurgery. For malignant schwannomas, radiation therapy is often given after surgery.

Introduction

Approximately 8,600 children under the age of 15 are diagnosed with cancer in the United States each year. Because of significant advances in therapy, 75 percent of these children will survive five years or more, an increase of almost 40 percent since the early 1960s. Nevertheless, cancer is still the leading cause of death (an estimated 1,500 deaths) from disease in children under age 15, second only to accidents in most age groups. Mortality rates have declined 50 percent since 1973.

The types of cancers that occur in children vary greatly from those seen in adults. Leukemias, brain and other nervous system tumors, lymphomas (lymph node cancers), bone cancers, soft tissue sarcomas, kidney cancers, eye cancers, and adrenal gland cancers are the most common cancers of children, while skin, prostate, breast, lung, and colorectal cancers are the most common in adults. The stage of growth and development is another important difference between adults and children; the immaturity of children's organ systems often has important treatment implications.

Many pediatric cancers occur very early in life and many parents want to know why. Some of these cancers are the result of a familial predisposition (cancer runs in family). Radiation exposure contributes to certain types of childhood cancers. Unlike cancers of adults, childhood cancers are not significantly related to lifestyle-related risk factors such as tobacco or alcohol use, poor diet, or not enough physical activity. The cause of most childhood cancers is not known.

Cancers in children often are difficult to recognize. Parents should see that their children have regular medical checkups and should be alert to any unusual signs or symptoms that persist. These include an unusual mass or swelling; unexplained paleness and loss of energy; sudden tendency to bruise;

a persistent, localized pain or limping; prolonged, unexplained fever or illness; frequent headaches, often with vomiting; sudden eye or vision changes; and excessive, rapid weight loss.

Children with cancer and their families have special needs that can be best met by children's cancer centers. Treatment of childhood cancer in specialized centers takes advantage of a team of specialists who know the differences between adult and childhood cancers, as well as the unique needs of children with cancers. This team usually includes pediatric oncologists, surgeons, radiation oncologists, pediatric oncology nurses and nurse practitioners. The treatment of childhood cancer also involves many professionals other than nurses and doctors. Children's cancer centers have psychologists, social workers, child life specialists, nutritionists, rehabilitation and physical therapists, and educators who can support and educate the entire family.

The childhood cancers included in this *Overview* include:

- **Acute lymphocytic (lymphoblastic) leukemia (ALL)** is the most common childhood malignancy and accounts for almost one-third of all childhood cancers;

- **Wilms' tumor** is a cancer that may involve one or both kidneys. It is most often found in children between 2 and 3 years old;

- **Neuroblastoma** is the most common extracranial (outside the brain) solid tumor in children and most often diagnosed during the first year of life;

- **Retinoblastoma** is a cancer of the eye. Although relatively rare, it accounts for 5 percent of childhood blindness;

- **Rhabdomyosarcoma** is the most common soft tissue sarcoma in children. The tumor originates from the same embryonic cells that develop into striated (voluntary) muscles;

- **Central nervous system** (brain and spinal cord) cancers are the second most common cancers in children. Most brain cancers of children involve the cerebellum or brain stem;

- **Bone cancer** is uncommon, comprising approximately 0.2 percent of all new cancer cases in the United States. The incidence of primary bone cancer (cancers starting in bones) is highest in children and adolescents, but cancer that is metastatic (spreading) to the bone is more common than primary bone cancer in all age groups;

- **Osteosarcoma** is the most common type of primary bone cancer in children and young adults;

- **Ewing's sarcoma** is a less common primary bone cancer that occurs mostly in children and adolescents.

Childhood Leukemia

Key Statistics

Approximately 2,700 children are diagnosed with leukemia in the United States each year. Leukemia is the most common cancer in children and adolescents. It accounts for about one-third of all cancers in children under age 15 and one-fourth of cancers occurring before age 20.

Of the 2,700 children diagnosed, approximately 2,000 are diagnosed with ALL. Many of the remaining children will be diagnosed with AML. Leukemia is divided into two types: acute (rapidly growing) and chronic (slowly growing), with the vast majority of childhood leukemia being the acute form. ALL occurs most often between ages 2 and 6.

The five-year survival rate of children with ALL is almost 80 percent. The five-year survival rate of children with AML is about 40 percent.

Risk Factors

Children are unlikely to be exposed to environmental risk factors so that most of the risk factors are genetic.

- *Immune system deficiencies.* Certain genetic diseases cause children to be born with an abnormal or deficient immune system. These children also have an increased risk of developing leukemia. Also prolonged immuno-suppression as in a transplant situation can also increase leukemia risk;

- *Defined genetic disorders.* Disorders such as Li-Fraumeni syndrome, Down's syndrome, Klinefelter's syndrome, neurofibromatosis, ataxia-telangectasia, Wiscott-Aldrich syndrome, and Fanconi's anemia may result in an increased risk of leukemia. There are undefined genetic disorders also, since the sibling of an identical twin who develops ALL or AML before 6 years of age has a 20 to 25 percent chance of developing leukemia. Fraternal (not identical) twins and other brothers and sisters have slightly increased chances (two to four times) of developing leukemia;

- *Chemotherapy.* Children treated for other malignant disease with chemotherapy have a higher risk of AML;

Leukemia begins in the bone marrow. The bone marrow is made up of blood-forming cells and supporting tissues. Bone marrow stem cells continually reproduce and their "offspring" go through a multistep process of maturation, eventually becoming one of three main types of blood cells: red blood cells, white blood cells, or platelets. In infants, bone marrow is found in almost all bones of the body, but by the teenage years, it is found primarily in the flat bones (skull, shoulder blade, ribs, pelvis) and vertebrae (back bones). Red blood cells carry oxygen from the lungs to all other tissues of the body. Platelets are actually fragments that break off from a type of bone marrow cell called the megakaryocyte. Blood platelets are important in plugging small areas of damage to blood vessels caused by cuts or bruises. White blood cells, also known as leukocytes, are important in defending the body against microorganisms (germs).

Lymphoid tissue, also found in the bone marrow as well as elsewhere, is the main component of the immune system. The main cell type that forms lymphoid tissue is the lymphocyte. These are the cells from which acute lymphocytic leukemia (ALL) develops. There are two main types of lymphocytes, B lymphocytes (or B cells) and T lymphocytes (or T cells). Although both can develop into leukemia, B cell leukemias are much more common than T cell leukemias.

- *Race*. Caucasians have a higher rate of ALL;
- *Radiation*. Significant radiation exposure to the fetus within the first months of development may also carry up to a fivefold increased risk of developing ALL.

Types of Leukemia

Almost all leukemia in children is acute. Acute leukemia is divided into acute lymphocytic leukemia (ALL) and acute nonlymphocytic leukemia (ANLL). Acute myelogenous leukemia or acute myeloid leukemia (AML) is another name for ANLL. The only type of chronic leukemia in childhood is chronic myelogenous leukemia (CML). It will not be discussed in this document because it is so rare, accounting for only about 2 percent of leukemias in children.

Most childhood leukemias are classified based on their appearance under the microscope. In acute lymphocytic leukemias, complex testing is needed to decide on the exact type of leukemia a child has. These tests of leukemic cells from a child's blood or bone marrow include: flow cytometry (a test that uses special antibodies to detect specific substances on the cell surface or inside the cell), cytogenetics (studies to detect changes in the chromosomes of cells), and molecular genetic tests (which show changes in the cell's DNA).

Acute Lymphocytic Leukemia (ALL)

ALL is a cancer of the lymphocyte-forming cells called lymphoblasts. It is divided into three types according to the cells' appearance under the microscope: L1, L2, or L3. L1 lymphoblasts, the most common in children, are smaller cells. L2, which account for 10 percent of ALL cases, are larger. L3 lymphoblast is the rarest subtype.

Another way to look at ALL is by its immunologic type (B cell or T cell). About 85 percent of ALL is of B cell origin.

The subtypes of B cell ALL are: 1) early precursor B or early pre-B ALL (the most common), 2) pre-B ALL (less common), and 3) mature B cell leukemia (only 2 percent).

About 13 to 15 percent of ALL is of T cell origin. This type of leukemia is more likely to affect boys than girls and generally affects children at an older age than B cell ALL does.

Acute Myelogenous Leukemia (AML)

AML (also called acute nonlymphocytic leukemia or ANLL) is a cancer of the bone marrow cells that form granulocytes (myeloblasts), monocytes (monoblasts), red blood cells (erythroblasts), and platelets (megakaryoblasts). Like ALL, AML is also divided into several subtypes. Although ancillary tests are often helpful in separating AML from ALL, the subtypes of AML are classified almost exclusively by their appearance under the microscope, using routine and cytochemical stains.

Hybrid or Mixed Lineage Leukemias

There are leukemias in which some features of both ALL and AML are seen.

Signs and Symptoms

- Shortness of breath, excessive tiredness, or pale skin because of anemia;
- High fever, due to infection;
- Bruising and bleeding;
- Bone or joint pain;
- Swelling of abdominal organs or lymph nodes;
- Cough.

Diagnostic Tests

- Blood cell counts and blood cell examination;

- Bone marrow aspiration and biopsy—a needle is used to remove a sample of bone marrow that can be examined for cancer cells; special stains help diagnose the leukemia;

- Lumbar puncture (spinal tap)—a needle is placed in the lower back to obtain a small sample of cerebrospinal fluid, which can be examined for cancer cells;

- Cytochemistry—cells are exposed to stains (dyes) that are attracted to certain chemicals only present in some types of leukemia cells;

- Flow cytometry of blood cells—to determine the type of leukemia using special antibodies to detect specific substances on the cell surface or inside the cell;

- Immunocytochemistry—cells are treated with special laboratory antibodies so that certain types of cells change color. The color change is detectable under a microscope;

- Cytogenetics—in certain types of leukemia, part of one chromosome may be attached to part of a different chromosome. Recognizing these translocations under the microscope helps in identifying certain types of ALL and AML;

- Chest x-ray.

Treatment

Surgery

Because leukemia cells spread so extensively throughout the bone marrow and to many other organs, it is impossible to cure this type of cancer by surgery.

Radiation Therapy

Radiation treatment is used in leukemia treatment only to treat leukemia cells in the brain or in the testes.

Chemotherapy

In general, AML treatment will use higher doses of chemotherapy over a shorter period of time, and ALL will use lower doses of chemotherapy over a longer period of time.

Stem Cell Transplantation

This treatment can be used for children whose chances of being cured are very poor with standard or even intensive chemotherapy. Stem cell transplantation (SCT) is used for patients with ALL who relapse within the first twelve to eighteen months after going into remission. It is more controversial to use SCT for those children with ALL who relapse more than eighteen months after finishing their initial chemotherapy. These children will often do well with another round of standard dose chemotherapy.

On the other hand, because children with AML relapse more readily, some doctors will recommend SCT for some children right after they have gone into remission. If a child with AML relapses after their first round of standard induction chemotherapy, then most doctors will recommend SCT as soon as they go into remission again. (See Chapter 14 for more information on stem cell transplants.)

Treatment of Children with Acute Lymphocytic Leukemia

Treatment of children with ALL is divided into three phases—induction, consolidation or intensification, and maintenance. The total duration of therapy (induction, intensification, and maintenance) for most ALL treatment plans is two to three years.

Induction. Most ALL patients receive three drugs (prednisone, asparaginase [Elspar], and vincristine [Oncovin]) for the first month of treatment. A fourth drug called an anthracycline (daunomycin is the one most often used) will be added if the leukemia looks particularly fast growing.

Consolidation or intensification. The next, most intensive phase of chemotherapy lasts four to eight months. Several new drugs such as cyclophosphamide, thioguanine, and cytarabine may be given. In addition, chemotherapy will be given into the spinal fluid and many children will also have radiation therapy to the brain.

Maintenance. Once the leukemia appears to be in remission, maintenance therapy begins using 6-MP and methotrexate along with vincristine and prednisone. These latter two are just given for brief periods each month. Occasionally, leukemia patients at higher risk may receive more intensive chemotherapy.

If a child with ALL relapses, they will be treated again with chemotherapy. Usually different drugs are added to the standard ones. The most commonly used chemotherapy drugs are anthracyclines, cytosine arabinoside, and drugs called epipodophyllotoxins. They may also receive prednisone and vincristine. Intrathecal chemotherapy will also be given, but not radiation therapy. Also, stem cell transplant will be considered for children whose leukemia comes back within eighteen to thirty months.

Treatment of Children with Acute Myelogenous Leukemia

Treatment of children with AML is divided into the following two phases:

Induction. Treatment for AML uses different combinations of drugs than those used for ALL. They include daunomycin, cytosine arabinoside, and sometimes, etoposide (VePesid). Intrathecal chemotherapy is also given most of the time, but not radiation therapy to the brain.

Intensification. This begins after a remission, when the bone marrow has no more visible leukemia cells. Usually high doses of cytarabine (Cytosar-U) are given in one or two courses. Daunomycin may be added. Sometimes allogeneic or autologous stem cell transplant will be recommended.

Less than 15 to 20 percent of children with AML do not respond to treatment. The outlook for the child who doesn't go into remission or relapses is very poor. Many different drugs in different combinations have been used in these situations, none very successfully. Some doctors will perform an allogeneic stem cell transplant even when there is no remission. This can be sometimes successful.

Osteosarcoma

Key Statistics

Osteosarcoma is the most common bone cancer in children and adults (see *Bone Cancer*, pages 561–565). Approximately 900 new cases of osteosarcoma are diagnosed in the United States each year, and adolescent boys are affected more often than girls. Osteosarcoma occurs most often in teens and young adults, but there is a second peak in those who are in their sixties and seventies.

The five-year survival rate for osteosarcoma is around 60 to 70 percent. The numbers are not exact because of the small number of patients and the wide variation in the age groups affected.

Risk Factors

- *Age.* The risk of osteosarcoma is highest during the teenage "growth spurt." Since children with osteosarcoma are usually tall for their age,

There are several types of living cells in bones. Osteoblasts are responsible for forming bone matrix (connective tissue and mineral that gives bone its strength). Osteoclasts prevent too many bone matrixes from accumulating and help bones maintain their proper shape. By depositing or removing minerals from the bones, osteoclasts help control the amount of these minerals in the blood. Some bones also contain bone marrow, which contains fat cells and, most importantly, hematopoietic cells (the cells that produce blood cells).

There are two main types of bones—flat bones and long bones. The flat bones help to protect the brain and the organs of the chest, abdomen, and pelvis. The skull bones and sternum (chest bone), for example, are flat bones. The long bones support the legs and arms. Muscles that move the arms and legs are attached to these long bones. Osteosarcoma tends to affect bones of the arms or legs.

experts believe there is a relationship between rapid bone growth and risk of tumor formation;

- *Gender.* Osteosarcoma is almost twice as common in males than females;

- *Radiation.* People who have been treated with radiation for cancer have a higher risk of later developing postradiation osteosarcoma (osteosarcoma that occurs after radiation). Being treated at a younger age and/or being treated with higher doses of radiation (usually over 60 Gy) increase the risk;

- *Other bone diseases.* People with certain noncancerous bone diseases—such as Paget's disease of the bone and multiple hereditary osteochondromas—have an increased risk of later developing osteosarcoma, usually as an adult;

- *Genetics.* Children with certain rare inherited cancer syndromes such as Li-Fraumeni syndrome and retinoblastoma have an increased risk of developing osteosarcoma.

Types of Osteosarcoma

There are several subtypes of osteosarcoma that can be recognized by how they look on x-rays and under the microscope. Some of these subtypes have a much better prognosis than others.

Subtypes of Osteosarcoma

Osteosarcoma subtypes are divided into high, intermediate, and low grade. The higher the grade, the more likely it is that the cancer will spread.

High grade: Conventional central; Small cell; High grade surface; Telangiectatic.

Intermediate grade: Periosteal.

Low grade: Parosteal; Intraosseous low grade.

Signs and Symptoms

- Pain in a bone—particularly of the arm or leg—that tends to be worse at night and increases with activity;

- Swelling in a bone;

- A lump or mass;

- Fracture—about 30 percent of telangiectatic osteosarcomas cause a fracture at the tumor site. People with a fracture next to or through an osteosarcoma will describe having had soreness in a limb for a few months and suddenly feeling severe pain in the limb.

Diagnostic Tests

- Bone x-ray—doctors will usually recognize osteosarcoma on regular x-rays of the bone. However, a biopsy is needed to prove that cancer is really present;

- Needle biopsy—removal of tissue by needle for later examination;

- Open excisional or incisional biopsy—the surgeon cuts through the skin, exposes the tumor, and cuts out a piece of tissue for examination;

- MRI scan—uses magnetic fields and radio waves instead of x-rays to create images of selected areas of the body;

- Chest x-ray—this is always obtained, preferably before a biopsy;

- CT scan—a rotating x-ray beam creates a series of pictures of the body taken from many angles;

- Bone scan—in this procedure, a type of radioactive material is injected into a vein. The tumor absorbs this radioactive material and is detected by a special type of camera. The bone scan can also detect spread of the osteosarcoma to the lungs and/or to other bones;

- Thallium-201 scan or PET scan—thallium-201 chloride is a radioactive material that is attracted to living tumor cells. A dead tumor or areas of infection will absorb less of the material. New studies are looking into the usefulness of the thallium-201 scan to assess response of osteosarcoma to chemotherapy;

- Cytogenic and molecular genetic studies—tests of the chromosomes or genes in tissue samples help distinguish osteosarcoma from other cancers.

Treatment

Surgery

It is very important that the biopsy and surgical treatment be planned together and, if possible, that the same orthopedic surgeon does both operations at a cancer center.

The surgical treatment can be amputation (removing the cancer and all or part of an arm or leg) or limb-sparing surgery (removing the cancer without amputation). Patients and/or their parents should ask the surgeon to explain the best approach to removing the cancer and keeping as much use of the involved arm or leg.

Complete removal of osteosarcoma is generally not done until after the biopsy and after chemotherapy has been administered. This is done in an effort to spare as much of the affected area as possible.

Reconstructive Surgery. Sometimes if the leg must be amputated, rotationo-plasty is done. This means that after removing the cancer by a mid-thigh amputation, the lower leg and foot is rotated and attached to the thigh bone and the ankle functions as a knee joint. Of course, the patient will need a prosthetic device to extend the leg. If the osteosarcoma is located in the upper arm, the tumor may be removed and the lower area reattached so that the patient has a functional but much shorter arm. If the osteosarcoma is located in the lower jaw bone, the entire lower half of the jaw may be removed and later engrafted with bones from other parts of the body.

Surgical Treatment of Metastasis. Surgical treatment to remove osteosarcoma metastases to the lungs must be planned very carefully in case more tumors are found during the operation than can be seen in the chest CT scan. Patients who have had a good response to chemotherapy and have tumors in both lungs can have surgery of one side of the chest at a time. Removing tumors from both lungs at the same time represents another alternative. Removal of all the lung metastases will give the patient the only chance for cure. However, some lung metastases are too big or are too close to important structures in the chest (such as large blood vessels) to be removed.

Chemotherapy

Most cases of osteosarcoma are treated with chemotherapy given as an adjuvant (addition) to surgery. The drugs used currently to treat osteosarcoma include high-dose methotrexate, doxorubicin (Adriamycin), cisplatin (Platinol), ifosfamide (IFEX), etoposide (VePesid), carboplatin (Paraplatin), and cyclophosphamide (Cytoxan).

Sometimes chemotherapy is given before surgery to shrink the tumor. For patients whose cancers respond well to chemotherapy (based on biopsies after treatment that show mostly or all dead cancer cells), the survival rate is about 80 to 90 percent.

Radiation Therapy

Osteosarcoma cells are not easily killed by radiation. Radiation is, however, effective in palliation (symptom relief) when tumors can't be surgically removed.

Ewing's Family of Tumors

Key Statistics

Approximately 200 children and adolescents are diagnosed with a Ewing's tumor in the United States each year. About 6 percent of all childhood bone tumors are Ewing's family of tumors (EFT).

The outlook for children with EFT has greatly improved. Almost 60 percent of children with the cancer will survive more than five years. If the tumor is localized to one area (less than ten centimeters or four inches), and can be completely removed by the surgeon, the five-year survival rate is 80 percent or better when radiation therapy and chemotherapy are used after surgery. If the tumor cannot be removed but is still small, the survival rate is still better than 70 percent. If, however, the tumor is large and cannot be removed completely, the five-year survival rate is probably less than 60 percent, even if there is good response to chemotherapy and radiation therapy. When metastases are present at diagnosis, the five-year survival rate is less than 30 percent. Children younger than 10 years of age seem to have a better prognosis than older children and adolescents with EFT.

Another childhood cancer shares many features with Ewing's tumor and extraosseous (not in bone) Ewing's (also called EOE). Primitive neuroecto-dermal tumors (PNETs) are rare cancers found in soft tissue and bone. Ewing's tumor, which is seen in bones, EOE, and PNET have similar abnormalities in their DNA—these cells contain similar proteins that are rarely found in other types of cancers. These three cancers are thought to develop from the same type of normal cells in the body. For these reasons, doctors refer to these cancers as tumors of the Ewing's family (TEF). Of the tumors in this family, Ewing's tumor of bone accounts for most cases (87 percent). EOE and PNET represent 8 percent and 5 percent of cases, respectively.

Most tumors develop in the middle of long bones of the legs or arms. They also occur in the pelvic bones or in the chest near the ribs. (PNET or EOE of the chest wall is also called Askin's tumor.)

Risk Factors

- *Race*. Ewing's occurs most frequently in the white population and is rare among African Americans and Asian Americans;

- *Age*. Most EFT cases occur in children between the ages of 10 and 20. EFT can also affect young adults into their twenties as well as children under age 10.

Signs and Symptoms

- Bone pain—this occurs in about 85 percent of patients. The pain may be caused by the spread of the tumor under the periosteum (tissue covering the bone). Or the pain may be from a fracture (break) of a bone that has been weakened by the tumor;

- Swelling or mass—60 percent of Ewing's tumors of bone and almost all of the Ewing's tumors of soft tissue cause swelling. About 30 percent of the time the bone tumor may be soft and warm to touch;

- Fever—because the above signs and symptoms are also typical of normal bumps and bruises or bone infections, some cases of EFT are not easily recognized. Only after the child's condition does not resolve quickly or is not improved by antibiotics is the diagnosis of a simple bruise or an infection questioned and cancer considered. If the tumor has spread, a patient may feel very tired or even lose weight;

- Fatigue;

- Weight loss;
- If the tumor is near the spine, weakness or paralysis can occur, but this rarely happens.

Diagnostic Tests

- X-rays;
- CT scan—a rotating x-ray beam creates a series of pictures of the body taken from many angles;
- MRI scan—uses magnetic fields and radio waves instead of x-rays to create images of selected areas of the body;
- Radionuclide scanning or scintigraphy—the patient is given a dose of radioactive substance, which is absorbed by bone containing metastatic EFT. Using special radiation-sensing cameras, doctors can determine whether a mass is cancerous and whether a cancer has spread to other parts of the body;
- Biopsy—removal of tissue for examination;
- Immunohistochemistry—a portion of the sample is treated with special laboratory antibodies to identify substances that are found in EFT cells but not in other types of cancer;
- Cytogenetics—close examination of EFT cells usually reveals translocations, meaning that part of one chromosome breaks off and attaches to another chromosome. Observing these translocations often helps distinguish between cases of EFT and other types of cancer;
- Bone marrow aspiration and biopsy—a bone marrow biopsy uses a large needle to remove a piece of the bone for examination. A bone marrow aspiration uses a thinner needle and syringe to extract cells from the marrow. These samples are examined for EFT cells.

Treatment

Most children with EFT are treated according to a national treatment guideline, called a protocol. One of the most successful has been the Pediatric Intergroup Ewing's Sarcoma Study (IESS).

Surgery

Many of the tumors involving soft tissue and some of the bones that are not essential can be removed without causing any disability or deformity. Others, such as those involving most bones of the arms and legs, cannot be completely removed without affecting usefulness of the limb. Today limb-sparing operations are available that can remove portions of a bone and replace this tissue with grafts from other bones or a prosthesis (metal and/or plastic bones and joints). Sometimes an entire bone can be replaced with a prosthesis. Limb-sparing surgery is complex and can be done only by specially trained surgeons. A child may require two or more operations and months of physical therapy before the affected limb functions well.

Some children are not able to undergo limb-sparing surgery because their tumors involve bones that are difficult to replace or because the tumors also involve essential nerves or blood vessels that cannot be removed without severely damaging the limb. These children are usually treated with radiation therapy instead of surgery.

Chemotherapy

Almost all patients with EFT are treated with chemotherapy before treatment of the primary tumor with surgery or radiation therapy. Chemotherapy is continued after the surgery or radiation for a total of about one year of chemotherapy. The standard treatment is vincristine (Oncovin), doxorubicin (Adriamycin), and cyclophosphamide (Cytoxan), alternating with ifosfamide (IFEX) and etoposide (VePesid). The three-to-four-week cycles are repeated four or five times. If the Ewing's sarcoma or PNET has spread, these same drugs are given at higher doses. The same drugs are used for metastatic disease.

Radiation Therapy

External beam radiation therapy is used as primary treatment for Ewing's tumors when surgery isn't feasible. Radiation is thought to be as effective as surgery. It can also be used for palliation (symptom relief) of recurrent tumors.

Brain and Spinal Cord Tumors in Children

Central nervous system tumors of adults and children often form in different areas, develop from different cell types, and may have different prognoses and treatments. This section discusses tumors in children, but because the information in some sections is lengthy and is the same as in the adult brain cancer section under *Central Nervous System,* you will be referred to that section when appropriate.

Key Statistics

Approximately 2,200 children are diagnosed with malignant brain and other nervous system tumors in the United States each year.

Over half of patients with childhood brain tumors (all types combined) survive longer than five years. The outlook varies according to the type of cancer. For example, approximately 90 percent of astrocytomas of the cerebellum are cured by surgery.

Risk Factors

In general, there are no clearly documented risk factors for brain tumors in children. Rare cases of brain and spinal cord cancers run in families. In general, persons with familial cancer syndromes have multiple tumors that occur when they are young. (See the *Brain and Spinal Cord* overview of the *Central Nervous System* section, pages 576–581, for more information.)

Types of Brain and Spinal Cord Tumors in Children

There are some important differences in the types of CNS tumors that affect adults and children. Some common cancers of adults are rare in children and some childhood cancers almost never occur in adults.

Type of Tumor	Percentage of Childhood CNS Tumors
Supratentorial (not involving the cerebellum, brain stem, or spinal cord) astrocytoma	25–40%
Cerebellar astrocytoma	10–20%
Brain stem glioma	10–20%
Medulloblastoma	10–20%
Ependymoma	5–10%
Craniopharyngioma	6–9%
Pineal tumors	0.5–2%
Other	12–14%

(See the *Brain* overview of the *Central Nervous System* section for more details on types of tumors. Only information pertaining specifically to children is included here.)

Astrocytoma

About half of all childhood brain tumors are astrocytomas. Some special types of astrocytomas tend to have a particularly good prognosis. These are noninfiltrating astrocytomas (juvenile pilocytic astrocytomas and subependymal giant cell astrocytomas). Juvenile pilocytic astrocytomas most commonly occur in the cerebellum but also occur in the optic nerve, hypothalamus, brain, or other areas.

Medulloblastoma

This is the second most common tumor in childhood, occurring in younger children around 5 years of age. It usually involves the cerebellum, the part of the brain needed for coordination, and can spread down the spinal canal.

Brain Stem Glioma

This type of tumor involves the brain stem, the part of the brain responsible for controlling our breathing and heartbeat, and the part that connects the brain to the spinal cord.

Ependymoma

This tumor arises in the lining of the ventricles of the brain, fluid-filled spaces in each cerebral hemisphere. They tend to spread throughout the spinal fluid.

Cranipharyngioma

This type of tumor arises near the pituitary gland.

Signs and Symptoms

- Seizures—epileptic seizures are often the first symptom of a brain tumor (although most seizures in children are not caused by brain tumors);

- Headache—this is a common symptom of brain tumor;

- Loss of vision—loss of eyesight, difficulty focusing, or double vision can all signify a brain tumor;

- Mental changes—a decline in school performance, fatigue, personality changes, and complaints of vague, intermittent headaches are common;

- Nausea and vomiting or poor appetite;

- Growth disturbances;

- Swelling of the soft spot of the skull (fontanelle) in infants.

Diagnostic Tests

- CT scan—a rotating x-ray beam creates a series of pictures of the brain taken from many angles;

- MRI scan—uses magnetic fields and radio waves instead of x-rays to create images of the brain;

- PET scan—images the brain after injection of a very low dose of a radioactive form of a substance;

- Magnetic resonance spectroscopy—this test is like an MRI, but measures brain chemistry rather than anatomy. Use of this technique for diagnosing brain and spinal cord tumors is still experimental;

- Angiography—involves injecting a special dye into blood vessels near the tumor, and helps doctors view the blood supply of a tumor;

- Biopsy—opening the skull and removing some of the tumor tissue for examination;

- Stereotactic biopsy—rather than a biopsy, above, a surgeon may use a thin, carefully guided needle placed within the tumor to remove a small piece of tissue;

- Lumbar puncture (spinal tap)—a needle is placed in the lower back to obtain a small sample of cerebrospinal fluid, which can be examined for cancer cells.

Treatment

Children with central nervous system (CNS) tumors may be treated by surgery, radiation therapy, chemotherapy, or a combination of treatments.

Surgery

Surgery alone or combined with radiation therapy may cure some tumors. These tumors include some cerebellar astrocytomas, pleomorphic xanthoastrocytomas, dysembryoplastic neuroepithelial tumors, ependymomas, craniopharyngiomas, gangliogliomas, meningiomas, and many low-grade astrocytomas. Even when surgery doesn't cure, it may help control otherwise uncontrollable epilepsy.

Children with infiltrating tumors, such as anaplastic astrocytomas or glioblastomas, are not cured by surgery. However, surgery reduces the amount of tumor that needs to be treated by radiation or chemotherapy, which improves the results of these treatments. Surgery is not used for brain stem gliomas.

In addition, surgery may improve some of the symptoms caused by brain tumors, particularly those caused by a buildup of pressure within the skull. These symptoms include headache, nausea, vomiting, and blurred vision.

Radiation Therapy

Radiation is used when a tumor cannot be completely removed by surgery. After surgery for medulloblastomas, radiation therapy is usually administered to the tumor bed and spinal cord. Radiation is the mainstay of treatment for brain stem gliomas. It is also used after surgery for ependymomas. Generally, radiation is not needed after surgery for astrocytomas.

Because normal brain cells are rapidly growing within the first several years of life, radiation therapy is not usually given before the age of 2 or 3 in order to avoid damage that might impair the child's future intellectual growth.

Chemotherapy

Chemotherapy drugs are generally used for astrocytomas if they come back after surgery and radiation. Children under 3 years of age who have medulloblastomas are usually treated with chemotherapy instead of radiation therapy, and older children with medulloblastoma sometimes receive chemotherapy with their radiation. This is also true for children with ependymomas. Chemotherapy may be used on other types of tumors, but it is not as successful.

Some of the chemotherapy drugs used to treat children with brain tumors include cyclophosphamide (Cytoxan), melphalan (Alkeran), lomustine (CeeNU), carmustine (BiCNU), etoposide (VePesid), thiotepa, cisplatin (Platinol), carboplatin (Paraplatin), and vincristine (Oncovin). These drugs may be used singly or in various combinations, depending on the specific type of brain tumor.

Often cortisone-like drugs such as dexamethasone (Decadron) are given to reduce the swelling that often occurs around brain tumors. This may help relieve headache and other symptoms. Also, drugs may be prescribed to prevent seizures, which happen often in people with brain tumors. The drug that is most often prescribed is called diphenylhydantoin (Dilantin).

Neuroblastoma

Key Statistics

Approximately 650 new cases of neuroblastoma are diagnosed in the United States each year. It is the third most common type of cancer in children and the most common cancer in infants. Nearly 90 percent of cases are diagnosed in those ages 6 and under.

About one-third of neuroblastomas start in the adrenal glands, another third begin in the sympathetic nervous system ganglia of the abdomen, and most of the rest start in sympathetic ganglia of the chest or neck or the parasympathetic ganglia in the pelvis.

The five-year survival rate for infants is 83 percent; for children ages 1 to 4, it is 55 percent; and for older children it is 40 percent.

> Neuroblastomas are cancers that begin in nerve cells of the sympathetic nervous system. The sympathetic nervous system controls involuntary body functions such as heart rate, blood pressure, and digestion. The sympathetic nervous system, a part of the autonomic nervous system, consists of nerve fibers that run along side the spinal cord, clusters of nerve cells called ganglia (plural of ganglion) present at certain points along their path, and nerve-like cells found in the medulla (center) of the adrenal glands. The adrenals are triangular-shaped glands located above the kidneys.

Risk Factors

- *Family history.* There is evidence suggesting that certain people may very rarely inherit an increased risk of developing neuroblastoma. Children with the familial form of neuroblastoma (those with an inherited tendency to develop this cancer) usually come from families with one or more affected members who often develop neuroblastoma as infants;

- *Gender.* Neuroblastoma is more common in boys than girls.

Types of Neuroblastoma

Ganglioneuroblastoma is a cancerous tumor that contains immature neuroblasts (nerve cells found in the embryo), which can grow and spread abnormally, as well as some mature cells. Sometimes the cancer cells are mixed in with various amounts of spindle-shaped cells called stromal cells.

Signs and Symptoms

- Abdominal swelling or an abdominal tumor;

- A mass in the neck;

- Bone pain;

- Swelling of the eyes and/or black and blue eyes;

- Chronic diarrhea;

- Fever;

- Lumps anywhere in the body;

- Swelling of the legs or face;

- Leg weakness and paralysis.

Diagnostic Tests

- Blood and urine tests for catecholamines—these tests attempt to identify any of these chemicals, which are made by nerve tissues. Other blood studies will check liver and kidney function and the salt balance in the body;

- CT scan—a rotating x-ray beam creates a series of pictures of the body taken from many angles;

- MRI scan—uses magnetic fields and radio waves instead of x-rays to create images of selected areas of the body;

- Ultrasonography (ultrasound)—uses sound waves and their echoes to produce images of internal organs;

- Bone marrow aspiration and biopsy—a bone marrow biopsy uses a large needle to remove a piece of the bone for examination. A bone marrow aspiration uses a thinner needle and syringe to extract cells from the marrow for examination;

- Chest x-ray—a standard chest x-ray is obtained if it is suspected that the tumor has invaded the chest and to rule out metastatic involvement of the lymph nodes in the chest or the lungs;

- Skull x-ray—this is done to be sure cancer has not spread to the skull bones;

- Radionuclide scanning or scintigraphy—the patient is given a dose of radioactive substance, which is absorbed by bone containing metastatic EFT. Using special radiation-sensing cameras, doctors can determine whether a mass is cancerous and whether a cancer has spread to other parts of the body.

Treatment

Surgery

After neuroblastoma is diagnosed, surgery is used to remove the tumor. In some cases, surgery can remove the entire tumor and result in a complete cure. Sometimes surgery is repeated after other treatments (chemotherapy and/or radiation therapy) to check the results of therapy and to remove any remaining cancerous tissue if possible.

During the operation, the surgeon will look carefully for evidence of tumor spread to other organs. If possible, the surgeon will remove the entire tumor. Even if the tumor cannot be completely taken out, additional treatment with radiation or chemotherapy after removing most of the cancer may result in a cure. Chemotherapy is sometimes used before surgery to shrink the tumor and make it easier to remove completely.

Chemotherapy

In most cases, treatment involves a combination of medications. The main drugs used to treat children with neuroblastoma are cyclophosphamide (Cytoxan), cisplatin (Platinol), vincristine (Oncovin), doxorubicin (Adriamycin), etoposide (VePesid), and topotecan (Hycamtin). Overall, these drugs produce a complete or a partial response in up to two-thirds of children.

Among the combinations used today are cyclophosphamide plus doxorubicin, and cisplatin plus teniposide (Vumon). These combinations are sometimes added to other groups of drugs to produce longer responses in children with advanced stages of neuroblastoma.

In some cases, especially when the cancer has spread too far to be completely removed by surgery, chemotherapy is the primary treatment.

Some times high-dose chemotherapy with stem cell transplants is used to treat children with neuroblastoma.

Bone Marrow Transplantation and Peripheral Blood Stem Cell Transplantation

High-intensity chemotherapy can destroy bone marrow completely. Without marrow, new blood cells cannot develop. To solve this problem, a child with neuroblastoma treated with very high intensity chemotherapy will need to undergo bone marrow transplantation or peripheral blood stem cell transplantation. (See Chapter 14 for information about stem cell transplants.)

Radiation Therapy

For many years external beam radiation has been used to destroy neuroblastoma cells that remain behind after surgery in patients with larger tumors. It also works well to shrink tumors before surgery, making them easier to remove at the time of surgery.

Studies show that in some cases, the use of radiation combined with chemotherapy produces better results (in terms of complete cure and long-term survival) than chemotherapy alone. Radiation may have to be used for infants with who have trouble breathing because of a very enlarged liver. Because of the long-term side effects, radiation is avoided when surgery alone is likely to be curative. It can also help relieve pain of children with advanced neuroblastoma.

Retinoblastoma

Key Statistics

Approximately 300 children are diagnosed with retinoblastoma in the United States each year. Retinoblastoma is the only common type of eye cancer in children. About 75 percent of children with retinoblastoma have a tumor in one eye. In about 25 percent of cases, both eyes are affected. Almost all children with retinoblastoma are under 5 years of age and most are younger than 2.

The five-year survival rate for retinoblastoma is over 93 percent.

The eye consists of a sphere called the globe, which is filled with a gelatinous material called vitreous; a lens with an iris like a camera on the front; and the retina in the back. The lens and the iris focus incoming light on the retina. The retina is like the film in a camera and is connected to the brain by the optic nerve.

Risk Factors

- *Genetics*. This is the major risk factor. About 40 percent of cases of retinoblastoma are due to a genetic mutation inherited from one of the child's parents. About 60 percent of hereditary retinoblastomas affect both eyes and about 40 percent affect one eye. Nonhereditary retinoblastomas nearly always affect on eye only. Hereditary retinoblastomas tend to develop in younger children than sporadic ones. Most hereditary retinoblastomas are detected by 1 year of age.

Types of Retinoblastomas

Although other cancers can spread to the eye, the most common in children being leukemia, retinoblastoma is the only cancer that begins in the eyes of children. All retinoblastomas have similar appearances. The only difference is whether they affect one or both eyes.

Retinoblastoma starts in the retina, the very back portion of the eye. When something goes wrong during the development of retinal cells, the cells continue to grow rapidly and out of control, forming this cancer instead of developing into cells specialized for detecting light.

The tumor can fill much of the eyeball, and cells may float through the vitreous to form other tumors. If these tumors block the channels that are important in circulation of fluid within the eye, the pressure inside the eye increases, resulting in glaucoma. Glaucoma is one of the serious complications of retinoblastoma that can lead to loss of vision in the affected eye.

Signs and Symptoms

- Cat's eye reflex—normally when a light is shone in a child's eye, the pupil looks red because the color of the light is changed by blood in vessels that cover the back of the eye. If instead the pupil appears white, this is cause for concern. The medical name for this finding is leucocoria;

- Strabismus—sometimes both eyes do not appear to aim in the same direction;

- A pupil that does not get smaller when exposed to bright light;

- Eye pain;

- Redness of the white part of the eye.

Diagnostic Tests

- Ophthalmology exam—the ophthalmologist will use special lights and magnifying lenses to view the retina. General anesthesia (medication to make the child unconscious) is usually necessary so that the doctor can take a careful and detailed look;

- Ultrasonography (ultrasound)—uses sound waves and their echoes to produce images of internal organs, such as the inner parts of the eye;

- MRI scan—uses magnetic fields and radio waves instead of x-rays to create images of selected areas of the body;

- CT scan—a rotating x-ray beam creates a series of pictures of the body taken from many angles;

- Bone scan—this test involves injecting a small amount of radioactive substance into a vein. The substance accumulates in areas of bone that may be abnormal because of cancer metastasis;

- Lumbar puncture (spinal tap)—spread of cancer to the surface of the brain can often be detected by using a thin needle to remove samples of the fluid that surrounds the brain and spinal cord and examining it under the microscope;

- Bone marrow aspiration and biopsy—a bone marrow biopsy uses a large needle to remove a piece of the bone for examination. A bone marrow aspiration uses a thinner needle and syringe to extract cells from the marrow for examination.

Treatment

Overall, over 90 percent of children can expect to be cured of retinoblastoma. The results are even better when the tumor has not spread beyond the globe and dramatically worse if it has spread.

Surgery

The usual treatment then is to remove the whole eye (enucleation). Within about three to six weeks, the child can be fitted with an artificial eye that has been made to match the size and color of the remaining eye. When tumor occurs in both eyes, enucleation of both eyes would automatically cause complete blindness. If there is any chance of preserving any useful vision in one or both eyes by using more conservative treatments, these should be considered.

Radiation Therapy

Radiation therapy has been known for a long time to be an effective treatment for some patients with retinoblastoma. One advantage over surgery is that it may possibly preserve vision in the eye.

Unfortunately, there are also several potential disadvantages. It may eventually lead to cataracts (areas of damage in the eye's lens that can interfere with vision) and damage to the retina. Radiation therapy can lead to problems with growth of bone and other the tissues near the eye, and it can possibly predispose the patients to develop a different cancer in the normal tissues.

External beam radiation therapy or brachytherapy, in which the radioactive material is temporarily placed inside the eye socket next to the eyeball, may be used.

Laser Therapy

Photocoagulation uses a laser. It is focused on the tumor and destroys the cancer cells by heat caused by the laser beam.

Cryotherapy

Cryotherapy uses a probe that is cooled to very low temperatures to destroy the retinoblastoma cells by freezing. The procedure must be repeated several times to be effective. It is only effective for relatively small tumors and is not used for children with several tumors.

Chemotherapy

Chemotherapy may be used to shrink small tumors, which can then be treated more effectively by photocoagulation, cryotherapy, or brachytherapy. The drugs used include carboplatin (Paraplatin), cisplatin (Platinol), vincristine (Oncovin), etoposide (VePesid), cyclophosphamide (Cytoxan), and doxorubicin (Adriamycin). Combinations of drugs (such as etoposide and carboplatin; or vincristine, teniposide [Vumon], and carboplatin) are often used.

Unfortunately, retinoblastomas tend to be resistant to chemotherapy. Retinoblastoma metastases often shrink for a period of time, but usually begin growing again within a year.

After Treatment

Genetic Counseling

Because about 40 percent of cases of retinoblastoma are due to an inherited genetic mutation, the family of the child with retinoblastoma may be referred for genetic counseling. Once one child is diagnosed, it is important to determine if other children in the family have inherited the same abnormal gene and are at risk of being affected.

Second Cancers

Survivors who have the hereditary form of retinoblastoma also have an increased lifelong risk for developing other types of cancer. Careful exams of the entire body are necessary to avoid missing a second cancer. When people with retinoblastoma develop a second cancer, it is usually a relatively rare type, including osteosarcoma (a type of bone cancer), soft tissue sarcomas (cancers that develop in muscle, tendons and ligaments, and fatty tissue), and malignant melanoma (a type of skin cancer). Children with familial retinoblastoma have about an 8 percent risk of developing a specific type of brain tumor related to retinoblastoma.

Rhabdomyosarcoma

Key Statistics

Approximately 350 children are diagnosed with rhabdomyosarcoma in the United States each year, which makes it the most common type of sarcoma occurring in the soft tissues (which lie between the skin and bone) in children.

The five-year survival rate is 64 percent.

> Rhabdomyosarcoma is a cancer made up of cells which, when viewed under a microscope, resemble developing muscle cells of the fetus. Skeletal muscles first begin to form in embryos about seven weeks after the egg cell is fertilized by a sperm cell. At that time rhabdomyoblasts (cells that will eventually form muscles) begin to produce two special proteins, actin and myosin, which are assembled into overlapping bundles that are responsible for a muscle's ability to contract.
>
> Over 85 percent of rhabdomyosarcomas occur in infants, children, and teenagers. They occur most frequently in areas where skeletal muscles are found: head and neck (35 percent), urinary and reproductive organs (27 percent), arms and legs (18 percent), and trunk (7 percent). However, they can also occur in areas where skeletal muscles are either absent or very inconspicuous, for example, in the top of the head, prostate, and bile duct system.

Risk Factors

Some families have an inherited tendency for developing not only rhabdomyosarcoma, but also other tumors, including breast cancer and brain tumors. This very rare condition is called Li-Fraumeni syndrome. Two other rare inherited conditions are also associated with increased risk of rhabdomyosarcoma. Children with Beckwith-Wiedemann syndrome have a high risk of developing Wilms' tumor, a type of kidney cancer (see pages 612–615), but children with this syndrome may also develop rhabdomyosarcoma. These inherited conditions account for only a small fraction of rhabdomyosarcoma cases.

Types of Rhabdomyosarcoma

There are three main types of rhabdomyosarcomas. The most common type, embryonal rhabdomyosarcoma, tends to occur in the head and neck area, bladder, vagina, and in or around the prostate and testes. It usually affects infants and young children. Cells of embryonal (embryo-like) rhabdomyosarcomas resemble the developing muscle cells of a 6- to 8-week-old fetus. The second type, alveolar rhabdomyosarcoma, occurs more often in large muscles of the trunk, arms, and legs, and typically affects older children or teenagers. This type is called alveolar because the malignant cells form little hollow spaces, or alveoli. Alveolar rhabdomyosarcoma cells resemble the normal muscle cells seen in a 10-week-old fetus. Pleomorphic rhabdomyosarcoma occurs mainly in adults 30 to 50 years of age. It rarely occurs in children.

Many other sarcomas occur in soft tissues of children, but all are rare.

Signs and Symptoms

Many rhabdomyosarcomas are easily detected because they cause visible or palpable symptoms. For example, small tumors developing in the muscles behind the eye cause the eye to bulge out, and tumors in the nasal cavity often cause nosebleeds or a discharge of bloody mucus. When small lumps form near the surface of the body, parents will often see them or feel them. The following symptoms may occur:

- Localized swelling—this is particularly common when the tumor is on the trunk, extremities, or groin. Tumors around the eye cause the eye to bulge or appear to be cross-eyed. In the ear or nasal sinuses, rhabdomyosarcoma can mimic earache or a sinus infection;

- Bleeding—this may occur from masses in the bladder and vagina;

- Difficulty with urination or defecation;

- Vomiting, abdominal pain, or constipation—these symptoms are caused when tumors are in the abdomen or pelvis. Rarely, rhabdomyosarcoma arises in the bile ducts and may cause yellowing of the eyes or skin;

- Enlarged lymph nodes;

- Bone pain;

- Chronic cough;

- Weakness and weight loss.

Diagnostic Tests

- Surgical biopsy—removal of a small piece of tumor, which can then be examined;

- Core biopsy—a rather large needle is inserted directly into a mass to withdraw a cylindrical piece of tissue which can be analyzed;

- Fine needle aspiration (FNA)—a thin needle is used to withdraw fluid or small samples of tissue from the mass so that cells can be viewed with a microscope;

- Immunochemistry—this technique uses special laboratory antibodies that specifically recognize substances present in rhabdomyosarcoma cells but not in other cancers;

- CT scan—a rotating x-ray beam creates a series of pictures of the body taken from many angles;

- MRI scan—uses magnetic fields and radio waves instead of x-rays to create images of selected areas of the body;

- Bone scan—this test involves injecting a small amount of radioactive substance into a vein. The substance accumulates in areas of bone that may be abnormal because of cancer metastasis;

- Bone marrow biopsy— a needle is used to remove a sample of bone marrow that can be examined for cancer cells;

- Angiography—this x-ray procedure examines blood vessels.

Treatment

Surgery

The guiding principle of surgery is to try and remove as much of the tumor as possible without causing any major physical impairment. This means that often, not all the tumor is removed. Additional treatment with chemotherapy and radiation therapy, however, can be curative.

Chemotherapy

All children with rhabdomyosarcoma are treated with chemotherapy. One large study involving multiple institutions showed that even with complete surgical removal followed by radiation therapy to the tumor bed, 80 percent of children had recurrence of their tumor in other parts of the body.

The main drugs used in embryonal rhabdomyosarcoma that is completely resected (removed) are vincristine (Oncovin) and dactinomycin (Cosmegen). Cyclophosphamide (Cytoxan) and sometimes doxorubicin (Adriamycin) and cisplatin (Platinol) may be added for alveolar tumors and for group II and group III tumors. These standard drugs are not as successful in children with metastatic disease. The most promising new drugs being evaluated are ifosfamide (IFEX), etoposide (VePesid), and topotecan (Hycamtin).

Radiation Therapy

Radiation therapy is given to all areas of known disease if possible. Radiation may also be useful even if all the cancer has apparently been surgically removed. Several new techniques, such as hyperfractioned irradiation and brachytherapy, are being evaluated to see if effective doses of radiation can be given more selectively (delivering more radiation to the tumor and less to normal tissues).

Wilms' Tumor

Key Statistics

Approximately 550 new cases of kidney cancer are diagnosed in children and adolescents in the United States each year. About 500 of these are Wilms' tumors and they most often occur in children under age 5. The overall five-year survival rate for children with Wilms' tumor is about 92 percent.

The kidneys are two bean-shaped organs fixed to the back wall of the abdominal cavity. One kidney is just to the left and the other just to the right of the backbone. The lower rib cage protects the kidneys. A kidney of an average 3-year-old child weighs slightly less than two ounces.

The kidney is responsible for maintaining the normal composition of blood plasma by filtering out any excessive salts and waste materials. It is made up of millions of microscopic filtering structures called glomeruli, which are a small bundles of tiny blood vessels arranged in a ball and surrounded by a capsule. These filter fluid and small molecules into tubular structures that reabsorb what the body needs to retain. The rest of the materials, which are essentially waste, are collected into a large structure called the renal pelvis. The waste leaves the kidney as urine through a long slender tube called a ureter that is attached to the pelvis. The ureters connect the kidneys to the bladder. Each kidney has one ureter.

Risk Factors

- *Family history.* Between 1 and 2 percent of children with Wilms' tumors have one or more relatives with the same cancer. Scientists think these children inherit an abnormal gene from one parent that greatly increases their risk of developing Wilms' tumor;

- *Genetics.* Several rare genetic syndromes are associated with Wilms' tumors. About 15 percent of children with Wilms' tumor also have birth defects, most of which occur in syndromes. (Syndromes are groups of symptoms, signs, malformations, or other abnormalities that often occur together.) These are:

  - *WAGR syndrome.* This abbreviation stands for **W**ilms' tumor, **A**niridia (complete or partial lack of the colored area of both eyes), **G**enitourinary tract abnormalities (defects of the kidneys, urinary tract, penis, scrotum, clitoris, testicles, or ovaries), and mental **R**etardation. Children with WAGR syndrome have a 33 percent chance of developing Wilms' tumor;

  - *Beckwith-Wiedemann syndrome.* Children with this syndrome have larger-than-normal internal organs, hemihypertrophy (an oversized arm and/or leg on one side of the body), kidney cysts, and sometimes tumors in the liver, adrenal gland, or pancreas. They have a high risk of developing Wilms' tumor;

  - *Denys-Drash syndrome.* The penis, testicles, and scrotum do not develop. For unknown reasons, the kidneys in these children become diseased and stop working, and Wilms' tumors may grow in the diseased kidneys.

Types of Kidney Cancer

Wilms' Tumor

Most Wilms' tumors affect only one kidney. Between 2 and 5 percent are found in both kidneys.

Wilms' tumors are classified into one of two major types, depending on how they look under the microscope: Wilms' tumor of favorable histology and Wilms' tumor of unfavorable histology.

Tumors lacking anaplasia are called "Wilms' tumors of favorable histology." About 95 percent of Wilms' tumors have favorable histology, which means they have a much better outlook for cure than those of unfavorable histology.

In some Wilms' tumors, the nucleus at the center of some or all cells looks quite distorted or is much too large. A Wilms' tumor that contains large, irregular nuclei or anaplasia is called "a Wilms' tumor of unfavorable histology." The prognosis for cure tends to be worse than that of Wilms' tumors without anaplasia. Also, tumors with many areas of anaplasia have a worse prognosis than tumors with a focal or more limited anaplasia.

Other Types of Kidney Cancer

There are several rare types of kidney tumors that affect children. The most common benign (not cancerous) kidney tumor of children is called mesoblastic nephroma. Clear cell sarcoma of kidney (CCSK) and malignant rhabdoid tumor of kidney are two types of cancerous childhood kidney tumors. They tend to have a poor prognosis if they have spread beyond the kidney. Very rarely, children develop renal cell carcinoma.

Signs and Symptoms

*   Abdominal swelling—this is the most common sign of Wilms' tumor;

*   Abdominal pain—this occurs some of the time in children with this cancer;

*   Blood in the urine—some children with Wilms' tumors experience this symptom;

*   Fever—this can also be a symptom.

Diagnostic Tests

*   CT scan—a rotating x-ray beam creates a series of pictures of the body taken from many angles;

*   MRI scan—uses magnetic fields and radio waves instead of x-rays to create images of selected areas of the body;

*   Ultrasonography (ultrasound)—uses sound waves and their echoes to produce images of internal organs;

*   Chest x-ray—a chest x-ray is used to look for any spread of Wilms' tumor to the lungs;

*   Bone scan—a bone scan involves injecting small amounts of a special radioactive material into a vein. The radioactive substance collects in areas of diseased bone and can help doctors find cancer that has spread to bones.

Treatment

Up until the mid-1960s, almost all children with Wilms' tumors died of this disease. Now, over 90 percent are cured.

Surgery

The first goal of treatment is to remove the primary tumor even if distant metastases (spread) are present. The most common operation for Wilms' tumor is called a radical nephrectomy. Radical nephrectomy removes the cancer along with the whole kidney, the ureter, the adrenal gland that is next to the kidney, and the fatty tissue immediately around the kidney. Regional lymphadenectomy may be done along with the radical nephrectomy. This procedure removes lymph nodes next to the kidney. At the time of surgery, the liver and other kidney are examined and any suspicious areas are biopsied.

Chemotherapy

All cases of Wilms' tumor are treated with chemotherapy given as an adjuvant (addition) to surgery. The drugs used most often in different combinations include dactinomycin (Cosmegen) and vincristine (Oncovin) and, for advanced stages, doxorubicin (Adriamycin), cyclophosphamide (Cytoxan), and/or etoposide (VePesid).

Radiation Therapy

External beam radiation therapy is often used along with surgery in stage III, IV, and V Wilms' tumors and in earlier stages if the tumor is anaplastic, which means it has unfavorable histology.

Esophagus

Key Statistics

Approximately 13,200 new cases of esophageal cancer (9,900 men and 3,300 women) are diagnosed in the United States each year and an estimated 12,500 people (9,500 men and 3,000 women) die of this disease. Because the disease is usually diagnosed at an advanced stage, most people with esophageal cancer eventually die from it. However, survival rates have been improving.

Esophageal cancer is much more common in some other countries such as Iran, northern China, India, and southern Africa.

The five-year survival rate if the cancer is localized is 27 percent. Once it has spread to local lymph nodes the survival rate drops to 13 percent. It drops to 2 percent if the cancer has spread past local lymph nodes.

Risk Factors

- *Age.* The disease is most common in people in their 50s, 60s, and 70s;

- *Gender and race.* Men have a threefold higher rate of esophageal cancer than women and African Americans have a higher rate than Caucasians;

- *Tobacco.* Smoking cigarettes, cigars, and/or pipes, and chewing tobacco increase the risk of esophageal cancer;

- *Alcohol.* Long-term heavy drinking of alcohol is an important risk factor for esophageal cancer. When combined with heavy smoking, the risk increases to forty times normal;

The esophagus is a muscular tube about ten to thirteen inches long and roughly ¾ inch across at its smallest point. It connects the throat to the stomach and carries food into the stomach. The connection to the stomach is called the gastroesophageal or GE junction. This junction has muscle, called the lower esophageal sphincter, which helps to keep food and stomach acid from refluxing back into the esophagus.

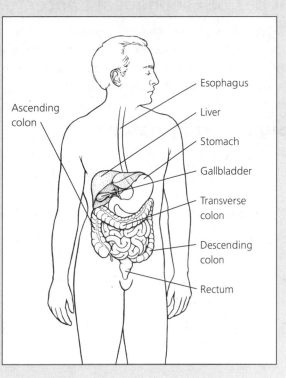

Esophagus

Ascending colon

Liver

Stomach

Gallbladder

Transverse colon

Descending colon

Rectum

- *Barrett's esophagus*. This is a change in the normal cells lining the lower esophagus caused by acid reflux. People with Barrett's esophagus have a much increased risk of esophageal cancer;

- *Heartburn*. Long-standing gastric reflux (heartburn) increases the risk of esophageal cancer;

- *Diet*. Diets that are low in fruits and vegetables as well as certain minerals and vitamins, particularly vitamins A, C, and riboflavin, may increase the risk for esophageal cancer. Overeating, which can lead to obesity, increases the risk of esophageal cancer;

- *Lye ingestion*. Children who accidentally swallow household lye have a high rate of esophageal cancer when they become adults;

- *Achalasia*. This condition causes the lower esophageal sphincter to not relax properly to allow food and liquid to pass into the stomach. About 6 percent of all people with achalasia will develop squamous cell esophageal cancer. This is a rare inherited disease that causes excess growth of the skin on the palms of the hands and soles of the feet. People with this condition also have a very high risk (about 40 percent) for esophageal cancer.

Types of Esophageal Cancer

There are two main types of esophageal cancer: squamous cell carcinoma and adenocarcinoma. Squamous cell cancers make up only about 50 percent of esophageal cancers. Adenocarcinoma, the other type, is increasing in incidence. It mostly occurs in the lower esophagus.

Signs and Symptoms

- Dysphagia—difficulty swallowing with the sensation of food getting stuck in the throat or chest occurs when the opening of the esophagus is about half as narrow as it should be. When swallowing becomes difficult, people often change their diet and eating habits without realizing it;

- Pain—in rare cases, people can have mid-chest pain or discomfort, a slight pressure sensation, or burning;

- Unintended weight loss—the person with this cancer cannot swallow enough food and nutrients to maintain their weight;

- Other symptoms—hoarseness, hiccups, pneumonia, and high blood calcium levels are usually signs of more advanced cancer of the esophagus.

Diagnostic Tests

- Barium swallow—this is a series of x-rays performed while the patient swallows a barium-containing liquid that can be seen on the x-rays;

- Endoscopy—inserting a flexible, lighted tube into the throat and through the esophagus in order to look inside the stomach;

- CT scan—a rotating x-ray beam creates a series of pictures of the body taken from many angles;

- Endoscopic ultrasonography—an internal sonogram done with the transmitter/receiver placed inside a hollow organ such as the esophagus. This is a good way to measure the size of internal tumors;

- Chest x-ray;

- Biopsy—removal of tissue for examination.

Treatment

Surgery

Depending on the stage of esophageal cancer, surgery may be used to remove the cancer and some of the surrounding tissue. Two rather complicated operations are commonly done for cancers of the esophagus.

Surgery can cure some patients whose cancer has not spread beyond the esophagus. Unfortunately, less than 25 percent of all esophageal cancers are discovered early enough for doctors to offer curative surgery as a treatment option. Therefore, it is important to understand that the goal of surgery might be to improve eating.

Esophagectomy. This procedure removes part of the esophagus containing the cancer and connects the upper part of the esophagus to the stomach. Lymph nodes near the esophagus are also removed. This procedure is done for early stage esophageal cancers that have not spread to the stomach.

Esophagogastrectomy. This procedure removes part of the esophagus containing the cancer as well as the upper part of the stomach next to the esophagus. Lymph nodes near the esophagus are also removed. The remaining part of the stomach is then connected to the upper part of the esophagus to allow food to pass into the stomach.

Chemotherapy

While primary chemotherapy alone will not cure esophageal cancer, there are three situations when it is used:

- As palliative therapy, meaning to control symptoms of advanced cancer;

- Preoperatively to reduce the tumor size and possibly allow a more complete surgical removal of the cancer;

- Sometimes used along with radiation before surgery to make surgery easier.

   The chemotherapeutic drugs used to treat esophageal cancer include fluorouracil (5-FU), bleomycin (Blenoxane), cisplatin (Platinol), mitomycin (Mutamycin), doxorubicin (Adriamycin), methotrexate, paclitaxel (Taxol), vinorelbine (Navelbine), topotecan (Hycamtin), and irinotecan (Camptosar).

Radiation Therapy

Although external beam radiation therapy or brachytherapy can cure some small cancers, it is very useful for palliation (symptom relief).

Palliative Therapy

Esophageal Metallic Stents. These metal mesh devices are placed into the esophagus across the width of the tumor. They self-expand to help keep the esophagus open and will relieve dysphagia (difficulty swallowing) in more than 80 percent of people.

Laser Endoscopy. Patients with tumors that are partially blocking the esophagus may benefit from vaporization and coagulation of the cancerous tissues with a laser. About 70 percent to 80 percent of patients will benefit from laser endoscopy. However, the procedure needs to be repeated every six to eight weeks.

Photodynamic Therapy (PDT). This new method begins with the injection of a nontoxic chemical into the blood that concentrates in the cancer. A special type of laser light is then focused on the cancer through an endoscope and causes changes in the chemical that has collected inside the cancer cells and kills them.

Stomach

Key Statistics

Approximately 21,700 new cases of stomach cancer (13,400 men and 8,300 women) are diagnosed in the United States each year and about 12,800 people (7,400 men and 5,400 women) die of this disease. Most people diagnosed with stomach cancer are in their 60s and 70s.

Stomach cancer is most common in certain Asian, Central European, Central American, and South American countries, especially Japan, Chile, Costa Rica, Hungary, and Poland. It is the leading cause of cancer death in many of these countries and is a major cause of cancer death worldwide.

In the United States, stomach cancer is now only one-fourth as common as it was in 1930. The reasons for this dramatic decline but may be related to increased use of refrigeration for food storage and decreased use of salted and smoked foods.

The five-year survival rate for all stages of diagnosis is 22 percent. If the cancer is discovered early and is localized, the five-year survival rate is 59 percent.

Risk Factors

- Helicobacter pylori *infection*. Patients with adenocarcinoma of the stomach have a higher rate of infection with this bacterium than people without this cancer. *Helicobacter* infection is also associated with some types of stomach lymphoma;

The stomach is a sack-like organ that holds food and begins the digestive process by secreting gastric juice. The esophagus joins the stomach just beneath the diaphragm (the breathing muscle under the lungs).

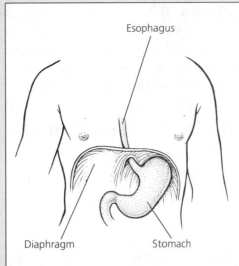

The stomach is divided into five different sections. The upper portion (closest to the esophagus) of the stomach is the proximal stomach. Some cells of this area of the stomach produce acid and pepsin (a digestive enzyme), the ingredients of the gastric juice that help digest food. The lower portion (closest to the intestine) is the distal stomach. This area includes the antrum, where the food is mixed with gastric juice, and the pylorus, which acts as a valve to control emptying of the stomach contents into the small intestine.

- *Diet.* An increased risk is associated with diets containing large amounts of smoked foods, salted fish and meat, certain foods high in starch that are also low in fiber, and pickled vegetables. On the other hand, eating whole grain products and fresh fruits and vegetables that contain vitamins A and C appears to lower the risk of stomach cancer. Nitrates and nitrites are substances commonly found in cured meats, some drinking water, and certain vegetables. They can be converted by certain bacteria, such as *Helicobacter pylori,* into compounds that have been found to cause cancer in animals;

- *Smoking.* This has been shown to increase stomach cancer risk;

- *Previous stomach surgery.* People who have had part of their stomach removed to treat diseases such as ulcers are at increased risk. Risk increases for as long as fifteen to twenty years after surgery;

- *Pernicious anemia.* Certain cells in the stomach lining normally produce a substance essential for absorbing vitamin B_{12} from foods, which leads to B_{12} deficiency and pernicious anemia. This condition is associated with an increased risk of stomach cancer;

- *Gender.* Stomach cancer is about twice as common in men as in women;

- *Age*. There is a sharp increase in stomach cancer after the age of 50;

- *Genetics*. Hereditary nonpolyposis colon cancer (Lynch Syndrome or HNPCC) and Familial Adenomatous Polyposis are inherited genetic disorders that cause a slightly increased risk of stomach cancer in family members. People with several close blood relatives who have had stomach cancer are more likely to develop this disease.

Types of Stomach Cancer

Approximately 90 to 95 percent of the malignant tumors of the stomach are adenocarcinomas. The term gastric cancer almost always refers to adenocarcinoma of the stomach, which develops from the cells that form the inner lining of the stomach.

The following are other, less common tumors that are found in the stomach:

- Lymphomas account for about 4 percent of stomach cancers. Slowly growing lymphoma of mucosa-associated lymphoid tissue is called MALT;

- Gastric stromal tumors develop from the muscle or connective tissue of the stomach wall. Some are benign; others are malignant and are also called gastric sarcomas. They make up about 2 percent of cancers starting in the stomach;

- Carcinoid tumors are tumors of hormone-producing cells of the stomach and account for about 3 percent of stomach cancers.

Signs and Symptoms

Patients who have stomach cancer rarely have symptoms in the early stages of the disease. People who have any of these problems that persist for a long time should check with their doctor, especially if they are over 50 years old or have stomach cancer risk factors.

- Unintended weight loss and lack of appetite;

- Abdominal pain;

- Vague discomfort in the abdomen, usually above the navel;

- A sense of fullness in the upper abdomen, just below the chest bone after eating a small meal;

- Heartburn, indigestion, or ulcer-type symptoms;

- Nausea;

- Vomiting, with or without blood;

- Swelling of the abdomen due to accumulation of fluid and cancer cells.

Diagnostic Tests

- Upper endoscopy—inserting a flexible, lighted tube down the throat to view the lining of the esophagus, stomach, and the first part of the small intestine;

- Barium upper GI radiographs—involves drinking a barium-containing solution that coats the lining of the esophagus, stomach, and first portion of the small intestine so that abnormalities on the linings of these organs will show up on x-ray pictures;

- Endoscopic ultrasonography—an internal sonogram done with the transmitter/receiver placed inside a hollow organ such as the esophagus. This is a good way to measure the size of internal tumors.

Treatment

Surgery

Surgery is the only way to cure stomach cancer. Even when the cancer is too widespread to be completely removed by surgery, most patients are helped by palliative surgery to control bleeding or to allow food to flow through the stomach without being blocked. The particular operation performed usually depends on what part of the stomach is involved (proximal or distal) and how much cancer is in the surrounding tissue.

Distal Subtotal Gastrectomy. This operation removes the lower portion of the stomach closest to the intestines. Sometimes the first part of the small intestine (the duodenum) is also removed.

Proximal Subtotal Gastrectomy. This operation removes the upper portion of the stomach closest to the esophagus. The nearby end of the esophagus may also be removed.

Total Gastrectomy. This operation removes the entire stomach. Usually in curative resections (operations intended to cure the cancer by completely removing it), the nearby lymph nodes and some of the omentum (fatty tissue in the abdomen) are removed.

Chemotherapy

Chemotherapy can be used to palliate advanced disease (relieve symptoms), or it can be used as adjuvant therapy to prevent recurrence after surgery. Chemotherapy for stomach cancer may use one drug such as fluorouracil (5-FU), which is often combined with radiation therapy. Chemotherapy may also use a combination of several anticancer drugs. The most commonly used drugs are cisplatin (Platinol), doxorubicin (Adriamycin), etoposide (VePesid), mitomycin (Mutamycin), and methotrexate. Combinations of two to four drugs are usually used.

Radiation Therapy

External beam radiation therapy, especially when combined with chemotherapy drugs, is used to delay or prevent cancer recurrence after surgery and may help patients to live longer. It also can be used to palliate localized painful areas in patients with advanced disease.

Colon and Rectum

Key Statistics

Approximately 98,200 new cases of colon cancer (46,200 men and 52,000 women) and 37,200 new cases of rectal cancer (21,100 men and 16,100 women) are diagnosed in the United States each year. Colon cancer and rectal cancer are referred to together as colorectal cancer. Colorectal cancer is the third most common cancer in men and women and the second leading cause of death from cancer.

The death rate from colorectal cancer has been going down for the past 20 years. This may be because there are fewer cases, they are found earlier, and treatments have improved. Colon cancer is responsible for approximately 48,100 deaths (23,000 men and 25,100 women) each year. About 8,600 people (4,700 men and 3,900 women) die from rectal cancer each year.

The five-year survival rate for people who are diagnosed with localized colorectal cancer is 90 percent. If the cancer has spread to surrounding lymph nodes, the five-year survival rate drops to 65 percent. It falls to 8 percent if the cancer is widespread when it is first diagnosed.

Risk Factors

- *Polyps or adenomas.* Most colorectal cancers begin as benign growths called polyps or adenomas. Having these increases the risk of colorectal cancer;

The five-foot-long colon (large intestine) has four sections. It begins at the ascending colon, where waste passes from the small intestine into the colon. This ascends upward on the right side of the abdomen and connects to the transverse colon, which goes across the body to the left side and connects to the descending colon, which continues downward on the left side. Finally this becomes the sigmoid colon, which joins the

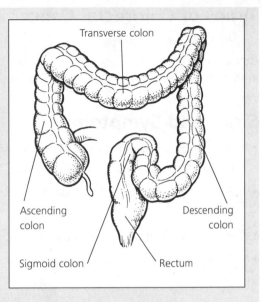

Transverse colon

Ascending colon

Descending colon

Sigmoid colon

Rectum

final six inches or so of the large intestine called the rectum. The anus is the opening where waste matter passes out from the rectum of the body.

- *Ulcerative colitis and Crohn's colitis.* These conditions are associated with a high risk of colorectal cancer;

- *Age.* The risk of colorectal cancer increases with age. Most patients are over 50 years old;

- *Diet.* A high-fat diet, especially fat from animal sources, can increase the risk of colorectal cancer;

- *Physical inactivity.* This increases the risk of developing colorectal cancer as does obesity;

- *Smoking and alcohol.* Both smoking and drinking alcohol increase the risk of colorectal cancer;

- *Genetics.* About 10 percent of colorectal cancers are caused by inherited gene mutations or changes in DNA. One mutation causes the development of multiple polyps in the colon and rectum, which invariably degenerate into cancer. A second mutation causes the development of adenomas that rapidly transform into cancer at a young age. Both of these gene mutations are well defined and can be tested for. Finally, there are patients that have a strong family history of colorectal cancer but in whom a specific gene mutation hasn't been identified;

- *History of colorectal cancer.* Having a history of colorectal cancer increases the risk for a new cancer.

Types of Colorectal Cancer

Over 95 percent of colorectal cancers are adenocarcinomas. These are cancers that develop from the glandular cells that line the colon and rectum. The rest are carcinoid tumors, gastrointestinal stromal tumors, or lymphomas.

Signs and Symptoms

- A change in bowel habits such as diarrhea, constipation, or narrowing of the stool that lasts for more than a few days;

- A feeling that you need to have a bowel movement that is not relieved by doing so;

- Rectal bleeding or blood in the stool;

- Cramping or steady abdominal pain;

- Weakness and fatigue.

Diagnostic Tests

- Colonoscopy or sigmoidoscopy;

- Barium enema x-ray;

- Stool tests for blood;

- CT scan—a rotating x-ray beam creates a series of pictures of the body taken from many angles;

- MRI scan—uses magnetic fields and radio waves instead of x-rays to create images of selected areas of the body;

- Carcinoembryonic antigen (CEA) test—a blood test that searches for CEA, a substance produced by cells of most colon and rectal cancers and released into the bloodstream.

Treatment

Surgery

Surgery is the main treatment for colon cancer.

Colon Surgery. The usual operation is called a segmental resection, in which the cancer and about one-third of the colon as well as the nearby lymph nodes are removed. The remaining sections of the colon are then reattached. Some very large cancers can block the flow of feces. This causes a bowel obstruction that doctors need to treat with a temporary colostomy when they remove the tumor.

Sometimes a very small cancer in the tip of a polyp can be removed through the colonoscope.

Rectal Surgery. Surgery is usually the main treatment for rectal cancer, although radiation therapy may also be used as a primary therapy or in addition to surgery. Very small tumors can be removed through the anus by a local excision.

Larger rectal cancers are removed by one of two surgical procedures. One, called a low anterior resection, uses an abdominal incision and removes the part of the rectum containing the cancer, then reconnects the cut ends of the rectum. A second operation, called abdominal-perineal resection, is used when the cancer is so low in the rectum that the lower rectum and anus must be removed. This operation requires a permanent colostomy.

Surgical Treatment of Colorectal Cancer Metastases. Removing or destroying metastases in the lungs, liver, ovaries, or elsewhere in the abdomen may sometimes be curative if there are a small number of them. Sometimes surgical treatment of metastases can help the patient live longer. Liver metastases may also be destroyed by freezing them (cryosurgery), by heating them with microwaves, by embolization (injection of material into large blood vessels feeding the tumor to block blood flow), or by injection of concentrated alcohol into the tumor.

Radiation Therapy

Radiation Therapy for Colon Cancer. The most beneficial time to use external beam radiation therapy is when the cancer has attached to an internal organ or the lining of the abdomen. Radiation therapy is used to kill the cancer cells remaining after surgery.

Radiation Therapy for Rectal Cancer. External beam radiation therapy or endocavitary radiation therapy, which is aimed through the anus, may be used. Most doctors recommend radiation therapy for large rectal cancers, either before or after surgery. Brachytherapy (internal radiation therapy) is sometimes used in treating people with rectal cancer.

Chemotherapy

The drug most often used to treat colon cancer is fluorouracil (5-FU). It is usually given intravenously, although an oral form, capecitabine (Xeloda), has recently been developed. In adjuvant therapy, chemotherapy is often given together with other drugs, such as leucovorin (Wellcovorin), which increases its effectiveness. Leucovorin and 5-FU are also used for palliative treatment. Irinotecan (Camptosar) is often used as palliative treatment, either combined with fluorouracil (Adrucil) treatment or instead of fluorouracil, if fluorouracil is no longer working. Other drugs, such as oxaliplatin and tomudex, may be used alone or in combination with 5-FU for patients whose cancers do not respond to standard chemotherapy. New clinical trials have begun to study irinotecan as an adjuvant treatment (used right after surgery to prevent recurrence). Although adding irinotecan to the standard chemotherapy combination of 5-FU and leucovorin makes the treatment more effective, it may also increase side effects, particularly severe diarrhea and potentially fatal infections.

Liver

Key Statistics

Approximately 16,200 new cases of primary liver cancer and intrahepatic bile duct cancer (10,700 men and 5,500 women) are diagnosed in the United States each year and about 14,100 people (8,900 men and 5,200 women) die of this disease.

This cancer is relatively rare in most areas of North America and Europe but is about fifty times more common in certain African and east Asian countries. In some areas of Africa and Asia, it is the most common type of cancer.

Since symptoms of liver cancer often do not appear until the disease is advanced, only a small number of liver cancers are found early. Less than 30 percent of the patients having explorative surgery are able to have their cancer completely removed by surgery.

The five-year survival rate is 6 percent overall. It is slightly better in younger patients.

Risk Factors

- *Hepatitis B and hepatitis C*. Chronic infection with hepatitis B virus (HBV) or hepatitis C virus (HCV) are the major risk factors for liver cancer;

- *Aflatoxin*. This carcinogenic substance is produced by a fungus found in tropical and subtropical regions that often contaminates peanuts, wheat, soybeans, ground nuts, corn, and rice;

- *Cirrhosis*. This scarring of the liver is due to damage by viral hepatitis B or C, alcohol abuse, or hemochromatosis (an inherited disorder that causes iron to accumulate and damage the liver). Cirrhosis increases the risk of liver cancer. Alpha-1-antitrypsin deficiency is another inherited

The liver is the largest internal organ of the body, weighing about three pounds and accounting for about 2 percent of a person's body weight. It is sheltered by the lower right ribs and lies underneath the right lung. It is shaped like a pyramid and is divided into right and left lobes, each of which is divided into segments.

The liver processes and stores many of the nutrients absorbed from your intestine that are necessary for your body to function. Some nutrients must be chemically changed (metabolized) in the liver before the rest of the body can use them for energy or use them to build and repair tissue. The liver produces many of the clotting factors that keep you from bleeding too much when you are cut or injured, secretes bile into the intestine to help absorb nutrients, and plays an important role in removing toxic wastes from the body.

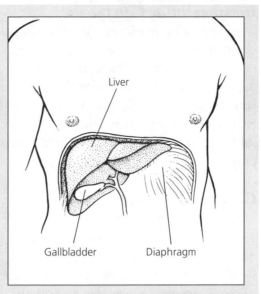

disorder that can cause cirrhosis and slightly raise the risk of hepatocellular carcinoma (HCC). Some other rare inherited liver diseases leading to cirrhosis can also increase risk;

- *Chemicals.* Chemicals such as vinyl chloride or thorium dioxide (Torotrast) are risk factors for angiosarcoma of the liver, cholangiocarcinoma, and HCC;

- *Oral contraception (OC).* These are a cause of benign tumors called hepatic adenomas, which may slightly increase the risk of liver cancer;

- *Anabolic steroids.* These are male hormones, often abused by athletes seeking to increase their strength. They can slightly increase the risk of HCC;

- *Arsenic.* High levels of arsenic in drinking water increase the risk of HCC.

Types of Liver Cancer

The liver is formed by several different types of cells and tumors can start in any of these cell types.

Hepatocellular Carcinoma

Also known as hepatoma or HCC, hepatocellular carcinoma is the most common type of primary liver cancer. HCC develops from hepatocytes (the main type of liver cell) and accounts for about 84 percent of primary liver cancers. For this reason, the remaining sections refer only to HCC. The fibrolamellar subtype of HCC is the most significant. Patients with fibrolamellar HCC are usually women, and they are often younger than those with other subtypes. Most importantly, this subtype is associated with a much better prognosis than other forms of HCC.

Cholangiocarcinoma

This type of adenocarcinoma starts in small bile ducts within the liver. About 13 percent of primary liver cancers are cholangiocarcinomas. People with gallstones or gallbladder inflammation, chronic ulcerative colitis (a long-standing inflammation of the large intestine), or chronic infection with *Clonorchis sinensis* (a parasitic worm found in parts of Asia) have an increased risk of developing this cancer. Jaundice without abdominal pain is most typical of cholangiocarcinomas that start near the hilum of the liver (the area where bile ducts exit the liver on their way to the gallbladder). Cholangiocarcinomas in that area are also known as Klatskin tumors.

Angiosarcomas or Hemangiosarcomas

The risk of developing an angiosarcoma from blood vessels of the liver is greatly increased by exposure to certain chemicals (see page 629). Angiosarcomas of the liver are rare, accounting for about 1 percent of liver cancers.

Hepatoblastoma

This rare liver cancer is usually found in children less than 4 years old. About 70 percent of children with this disease are treated successfully and the survival rate is over 90 percent for early stage hepatoblastomas.

Signs and Symptoms

Although the relatively nonspecific signs and symptoms are usually not present until the late stages of liver cancer, in exceptional cases they may permit an early diagnosis.

- Weight loss;

- Appetite loss;

- Early satiety (feeling full before meal is finished);

- Persistent abdominal pain;

- Increasing swelling of the "stomach" area, with or without breathing difficulty;

- Sudden jaundice with no apparent cause;

- Dramatic deterioration in the overall condition of a person with chronic hepatitis or cirrhosis;

- Liver enlargement or a mass that can be felt in the area of the liver.

Some liver tumors produce hormones that act on organs other than the liver. These hormones may cause high calcium levels, low blood sugar levels, or enlargement of the breasts in men.

Diagnostic Tests

- Ultrasonography (ultrasound)—uses sound waves and their echoes to produce images of internal organs;

- CT scan—a rotating x-ray beam creates a series of pictures of the body taken from many angles;

- MRI scan—uses magnetic fields and radio waves instead of x-rays to create images of selected areas of the body;

- Angiography—an x-ray procedure for examining blood vessels;

- Laparoscopy—this procedure uses a thin, lighted tube through which a doctor can view the liver and other internal organs;

- Biopsy—removal of tissue for examination;

- Alpha-fetoprotein (AFP) blood test—AFP levels are increased in most patients with hepatocellular carcinoma;

- Other blood tests—may include abnormal liver function tests, such as alkaline phosphatase.

Treatment

Surgery

Surgical Resection. Removal of the tumor along with the surrounding part of the liver offers the major chance to cure liver cancer.

Transplantation. In this procedure, the entire liver is removed and replaced with a liver from a deceased donor. The results of this may be as good as surgical resection, but is limited to patients without active hepatitis infection.

For patients whose liver cancer was caused by hepatitis C infection, post-operative treatment with anti-hepatitis C drugs may help prevent the emergence of a new liver cancer.

Tumor Ablation or Embolization. Ablation refers to local (rather than systemic) methods that destroy the tumor without removing it. Methods include cryosurgery (destruction of tumor by freezing it with a very cold metal probe) and ethanol ablation (injecting concentrated alcohol directly into the tumor to kill cancer cells). These treatments are excellent options for patients with multiple areas of cancer, as well as those with cirrhosis, hepatitis, or other serious health problems. With embolization, particles—which are sometimes radioactive—are infused into the blood vessels supplying the tumor.

Chemotherapy

Doxorubicin (Adriamycin) is the most successful single drug against HCC, and cisplatin (Platinol) has been shown to be of slight value. Since systemic chemotherapy has had little or no impact on this cancer, hepatic artery infusion (a type of regional chemotherapy) has been used. This approach involves injecting chemotherapy directly into the artery supplying blood to the liver. It can be helpful in palliating some patients, meaning it can relieve some symptoms, such as pain.

Radiation Therapy

This is rarely of value except to palliate (provide symptom relief) large painful tumors.

Gallbladder

Key Statistics

Approximately 6,900 new cases of gallbladder cancer (3,200 men and 3,700 women) are diagnosed in the United States each year and about 3,300 people (1,200 men and 2,100 women) die of this disease. The risk of developing gallbladder cancer is very different for people living in different parts of the U.S. and in other countries. In this country, the risk is highest in New Mexico, where it accounts for almost 9 percent of all cancers.

The five-year survival rate is only 10 percent for people with this disease.

Risk Factors

- *Gallstones.* Most people with gallbladder cancer have gallstones;

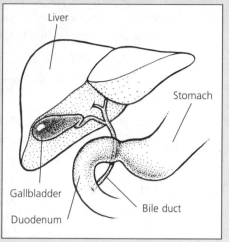

The gallbladder is a small pear-shaped organ that lies underneath the right lobe of the liver. The liver makes bile, which is transported to the gallbladder through the hepatic duct and stored there. During meals the bile is discharged into the small intestine (the duodenum is the upper part of the small intestine) through the common bile duct. The bile helps in digesting fatty foods.

Liver

Stomach

Gallbladder

Bile duct

Duodenum

- *Ethnic origin.* Mexican Americans and Native Americans have higher incidences of gallbladder cancer;

- *Gender.* Women are three times more likely to have gallbladder cancer;

- *Age.* Gallbladder cancer is a disease of older people;

- *Congenital abnormalities* of the bile ducts;

- *Gallbladder polyps;*

- *Obesity.* Obesity is also a risk factor for gallstones.

Types of Gallbladder Cancer

Over 80 percent of gallbladder cancers are adenocarcinomas. A small percentage of these are papillary, which means their cells grow in a fingerlike fashion. These do not tend to spread elsewhere as do nonpapillary kinds. Over 75 percent of gallbladder adenocarcinomas are nonpapillary adenocarcinomas. Almost all the rest are mucinous adenocarcinomas, adenosquamous carcinomas, squamous cell carcinomas, or small cell carcinomas.

Signs and Symptoms

Signs and symptoms are usually not present until the later stages of gallbladder cancer.

- Abdominal pain—more than half of all people with gallbladder cancer have abdominal (stomach area) pain at the time of diagnosis. Most often this is in the right upper abdomen;

- Nausea and/or vomiting—more than half of all people with gallbladder cancer report vomiting as a symptom;

- Jaundice—almost half of all people with gallbladder cancer have jaundice (a yellowish discoloration of the skin and whites of the eyes sometimes accompanied by itching) when they are diagnosed;

- Gallbladder enlargement—this can sometimes be felt by the doctor during a physical exam, and can also be detected by imaging studies such as ultrasound;

- Loss of appetite and weight loss;

- Abdominal swelling.

Diagnostic Tests

- Blood tests—these may test for bilirubin (what gives bile its color). A high bilirubin count may indicate either gallbladder or liver problems. Abnormally high levels of two enzymes—alkaline phosphatase and aspartate aminotransferase—can also indicate gallbladder or liver problems;

- Ultrasonography (ultrasound)—uses sound waves and their echoes to produce images of internal organs;

- CT scan—a rotating x-ray beam creates a series of pictures of the body taken from many angles;

- MRI scan—uses magnetic fields and radio waves instead of x-rays to create images of selected areas of the body;

- Endoscopic retrograde cholangiopancreatography (ERCP)—in this procedure, a doctor passes a long, flexible tube down the patient's throat, through the esophagus and stomach, and into the common bile duct. A small amount of contrast medium (harmless dye) helps outline the bile duct and pancreatic duct in x-ray images;

- Laparoscopy—this procedure uses a thin, lighted tube through which a doctor can view the liver and other internal organs;

- Biopsy—removal of tissue for examination.

Treatment

Surgery

Nearly all doctors agree that surgery offers the only hope for curing people with gallbladder cancer.

When imaging studies indicate a high likelihood that all of the cancer can be removed, the cancer is said to be "resectable."

Simple cholecystectomy. If the entire gallbladder is removed, the operation is called a cholecystectomy or simple cholecystectomy;

Extended cholecystectomy. This operation involves removal of the gallbladder, about an inch or more of liver tissue next to the gallbladder, and all the lymph nodes in the region;

Radical gallbladder resection. This procedure includes at least removal of the gallbladder, a wedge-shaped section of the liver close to the gallbladder, the common bile duct, part or all of the ligament that runs between the liver and the intestines, and/or the lymph nodes around the pancreas, around the vein that brings blood to the liver from the stomach and intestines, and around the artery that brings blood to most of the small intestine and to the pancreas.

If the cancer is suspected to have spread beyond the lymph nodes in the area, the operation may also include, as necessary, removal of the pancreas, the duodenum, more of the liver, and any additional areas of organs to which cancer has spread;

Open cholecystectomy. If the surgeon removes the gallbladder through a large cut in the abdominal wall, it is called an open cholecystectomy;

Laparascopic cholecystectomy. If imaging and/or other diagnostic tests do not lead doctors to think that gallbladder cancer is present, but indicate that the gallbladder should be removed because of gallstones or other problems, the operation may be done with the aid of a laparoscope. If the surgeon sees cancer, he or she will often change the operation to an open cholecystectomy (removal of the gallbladder through a larger cut in the abdomen) to avoid releasing cancer cells into the abdominal cavity while removing the gallbladder.

Radiation Therapy

Because gallbladder cancer is somewhat rare, the value of radiation therapy along with surgery is not known. Some studies suggest that using radiation in that way helps people live longer after potentially curative surgery.

Radiation directed to the tumor can also be used to reduce painful symptoms in people with inoperable or advanced gallbladder cancer.

Chemotherapy

Drugs such as mitomycin (Mutamycin) or a combination of fluorouracil (5-FU), doxorubicin (Adriamycin), and mitomycin can shrink gallbladder cancers in a small number of people, but they cannot cure the disease. There is no chemotherapy regimen known to prolong life, but chemotherapy can help palliate (relieve) symptoms.

Because chemotherapy is not very effective, most doctors will not recommend it as an adjuvant to surgery.

Thyroid

Key Statistics

Approximately 19,500 new cases of thyroid cancer (4,600 men and 14,900 women) are diagnosed in the United States each year and an estimated 1,300 people (500 men and 800 women) die of this disease. Although the incidence of this cancer has been slowly increasing, the death rate has been decreasing.

The five-year survival rate for all patients is 95 percent.

Risk Factors

- *Radiation*. This is the single most important risk factor. Radiation to the face and neck in children, done in the past for acne and to shrink tonsils or adenoids, is one source. The other is radioactive contamination such as from Chernobyl;

- *Iodine*. A very low iodine intake may increase the risk slightly. This is not seen in this country because iodine is added to table salt and other foods;

- *Genetics*. Families exist in which the incidence of thyroid cancer is high; and genetic conditions may create increased risk;

- *Gender*. Women have a much higher rate of thyroid cancer than men.

Types of Thyroid Cancer

Although many people have nodules on their thyroid, less than 5 percent of these are cancerous. Papillary carcinoma and follicular carcinoma are the

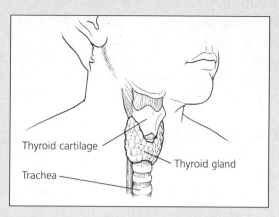

The thyroid gland is found under the Adam's apple in the front part of the neck. (Thyroid cartilage is firm tissue that separates the thyroid gland from the front of the larynx.) The thyroid gland has two lobes—the right lobe and the left lobe—united by a narrow isthmus. This gland takes up iodine from the diet and the blood and makes thyroid hormone that is important for many body functions. The thyroid gland contains mainly two types of cells. Thyroid follicle cells actually make and store thyroid hormone. The other type of cells, called C-cells, make another hormone, calcitonin.

most common types. They are grouped together by some doctors and called differentiated thyroid cancer or well-differentiated thyroid cancer. Medullary carcinoma, Hurthle cell carcinoma (a subtype of follicular carcinoma), anaplastic carcinoma, and thyroid lymphoma are less common.

Papillary Carcinoma

The most common type of thyroid cancer is papillary carcinoma (also called papillary cancer or papillary adenocarcinoma). Papillary cancers develop from the thyroid follicle cells and typically grow very slowly. Usually they occur in only one lobe of the thyroid gland, but about 10 to 20 percent of the time both lobes are involved.

Follicular Carcinoma

Follicular cancer—follicular carcinoma or follicular adenocarcinoma—is much less common than papillary thyroid cancer. Hurthle cell carcinoma, also known as oxyphil cell carcinoma, is thought to be a subtype of follicular cancer.

Anaplastic Carcinoma

This rare and very aggressive form of thyroid cancer is believed to develop from an existing papillary or follicular cancer. Anaplastic carcinoma is sometimes called undifferentiated thyroid cancer.

Medullary Carcinoma (MTC)

This is a moderately aggressive form of thyroid cancer that develops from the C-cells of the thyroid gland. These cancers usually make calcitonin, which is a hormone that normally helps control the amount of calcium in blood, and a protein called carcinoembryonic antigen (CEA). About one-fourth of these cases occur on a genetic or familial basis called Multiple Endocrine Neoplasias (MEN).

Thyroid Lymphoma

Lymphoma can develop in the thyroid gland, but is very uncommon in that location. Most thyroid lymphomas occur in people who have a disease called chronic lymphocytic thyroiditis (also known as Hashimoto's thyroiditis).

Signs and Symptoms

- A "lump" in the neck, sometimes growing rapidly;

- Pain in the neck, sometimes going up to the ears;

- Hoarseness;

- Trouble swallowing;

- Breathing problems like feeling as if one were "breathing through a straw";

- A cough that persists and is not due to a cold.

Diagnostic Tests

- Fine needle aspiration (FNA)—a thin needle is used to withdraw fluid or small samples of tissue from the tumor mass so that cells can be examined with a microscope;

- Blood tests—a thyroid stimulating hormone (TSH) blood test may be useful in checking the overall condition of the thyroid gland. If medullary thyroid cancer is suspected, a blood calcitonin test will be done. This test can help predict whether a MTC is present;

- Thyroid scan—uses a small amount of radioactive iodine and a special camera placed in front of the neck to identify abnormal areas;

- Ultrasonography (ultrasound)—uses sound waves and their echoes to produce images of internal organs;

- CT scan—a rotating x-ray beam creates a series of pictures of the body taken from many angles;

- MRI scan—uses magnetic fields and radio waves instead of x-rays to create images of selected areas of the body;

- Octreotide scan—sometimes an octreotide scan, which uses a radioactively tagged hormone, may be done to evaluate the spread of medullary thyroid cancer.

Treatment

Surgery

Surgery is the main treatment for all types of thyroid cancer and is used in nearly every case. Surgeons will remove almost all of the thyroid gland. This operation is called sub-total or near-total thyroidectomy. Only in the case of papillary cancers smaller than 1 cm (about ½ inch) that show no signs of invasion beyond the thyroid gland, is it likely that the surgeon will perform a lobectomy (remove only the affected side of the thyroid gland). When cancer has spread outside the thyroid gland, surgery is always used to debulk the tumor (remove as much cancer as possible) that has invaded the neck. This is especially true for treatment of medullary thyroid cancer and anaplastic cancer.

One major concern is that if too much of the gland is removed, all the parathyroid glands, which are imbedded in the gland, will also be removed. These glands control calcium metabolism and it is difficult to control calcium balance in their absence.

Because thyroid cancer may spread to nearby lymph nodes, these lymph nodes may need to be removed.

Radioactive Iodine Therapy

Just like nonradioactive iodine, radioactive iodine concentrates almost exclusively in the thyroid gland and can destroy all the cells. This treatment is used to destroy any thyroid tissue not removed by surgery, and to treat thyroid cancer that has spread to lymph nodes and other parts of the body.

Before treatment, thyrotropin is given by injection to help stimulate the uptake of the radioactive iodine by the thyroid cells.

Thyroid Hormone Therapy

All people with thyroid cancer are treated with thyroid hormone to replace what was previously produced by the gland. It also inhibits the body's normal stimulus to thyroid gland growth and may suppress any cancer regrowth.

Radiation Therapy

If cancers do not respond to radioiodine therapy, external beam radiation therapy may be used to treat local neck recurrences or distant metastases that are causing pain or other symptoms.

Chemotherapy

Papillary and follicular thyroid cancer have been treated with the drug doxorubicin (Adriamycin), either alone or combined with other agents, with some responses. In cases of metastatic medullary thyroid carcinoma, doxorubicin or dacarbazine (DTIC-Dome) have been used with some response. Doxorubicin has also been used with radiation therapy to treat anaplastic thyroid cancer, but the results have been poor. Thyroid lymphomas require treatment with the same combinations of chemotherapy drugs commonly used to treat lymphomas.

Pancreas

Key Statistics

Approximately 29,200 people (14,200 men and 15,000 women) are diagnosed with cancer of the pancreas in the United States each year and an estimated 28,900 people (14,100 men and 14,800 women) die of this disease. Pancreatic cancer is the fourth leading cause of cancer death in men and in women.

The five-year survival rate is 4 percent for all patients with this disease. For those people in whom it is caught early, the five-year survival rate is 16 percent.

Risk Factors

- *Age*. People over 60 years old are most likely to get this cancer;

- *Gender.* Men are about 30 percent more likely to develop cancer of the pancreas than are women;

- *Race*. African Americans are at higher risk than white or Asian Americans;

- *Smoking*. Smokers have a higher risk;

- *Diet*. People who eat a diet high in meats and fat have an increased risk. Fruits, vegetables, and dietary fiber appear to have a protective effect;

- *Diabetes*. People with diabetes are at higher risk;

- *Genetics*. Some people with a family history may have an inherited tendency to develop this cancer. This may be a factor in about 5 to 10 percent of cases.

The pancreas is located behind the stomach. Shaped a little bit like a fish with a wide head, a tapering body, and a narrow pointed tail, it is about six inches long but less than two inches wide, and extends horizontally across the abdomen. The head of the pancreas is located on the right side of the abdomen, behind the junction of the stomach and the duodenum (the first part of the small intestine). The body of the pancreas is located behind the stomach, and the tail of the pancreas is on the left side of the abdomen next to the spleen.

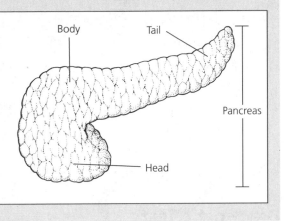

Types of Pancreatic Cancer

The pancreas functions as two separate glands. Exocrine cells in the gland produce pancreatic enzymes that are secreted into the intestine and help digest fats, proteins, and carbohydrates. Endocrine cells in the pancreas are known as islets of Langerhans. They release two hormones into the blood that help control blood sugar and others that affect different body functions. The exocrine cells and endocrine cells of the pancreas form completely different types of tumors.

Exocrine cells of the pancreas can form benign tumors; these occur much less frequently than cancers. About 95 percent of cancers of the exocrine pancreas are adenocarcinomas that usually begin in the ducts of the pancreas, but sometimes may develop from the cells that actually produce the pancreatic enzymes (the acinar cells). Less common cancers of the exocrine pancreas include adenosquamous carcinomas, squamous cell carcinomas, and giant cell carcinomas.

Tumors of the endocrine pancreas—neuroendocrine tumors, or, more specifically, islet cell tumors—are much less common. Islet cell tumors that produce insulin are known as insulinomas, and tumors that produce glucagon are called glucagonomas. Less often, islet cell tumors may produce other hormones. Most islet cell tumors are benign. Those that are malignant are called islet cell cancers or islet cell carcinomas.

A special type of cancer that occurs where the bile duct and pancreatic duct empty into the duodenum is called ampullary cancer or carcinoma of the ampulla of Vater.

Signs and Symptoms

- Jaundice;

- Abdominal (stomach) pain and/or pain in the middle to upper back;

- Unintended weight loss;

- Loss of appetite;

- Severe tiredness;

- Difficulty digesting fat (stools may be pale, bulky, greasy, and float in the toilet);

- Blood clots. Rarely, substances released by cancer cells may cause formation of blood clots or other problems with fatty tissue under the skin;

- Enlargement of the gallbladder or liver.

Diagnostic Tests

- Fine needle aspiration (FNA)—a thin needle is used to withdraw fluid or small samples of tissue from the tumor mass so that cells can be examined with a microscope;

- CT scan—a rotating x-ray beam creates a series of pictures of the body taken from many angles;

- MRI scan—uses magnetic fields and radio waves instead of x-rays to create images of selected areas of the body;

- Endoscopic retrograde cholangiopancreatography (ERCP)—a long flexible tube is passed through the throat, esophagus, and stomach, into the first part of the small intestine. A small amount of dye is then injected through the tube and outlines the pancreatic duct in x-ray images. The doctor doing this test can also remove cells for examination under a microscope;

- Blood tests—tumor markers CA 19-9 and/or by carcinoembryonic antigen (CEA) may be elevated.

Treatment

Surgery

Two general types of surgical treatments are used to treat cancer of the pancreas: curative surgery, performed when it is possible to remove all of the cancer, and palliative surgery to relieve symptoms or prevent complications such as blockage of the bile ducts.

Curative Procedures

- *Distal pancreatectomy*. This operation removes only the tail of the pancreas or the tail and a portion of the body of the pancreas. The spleen is usually removed as well. This operation is used more often with islet cell tumors found in the tail and body of the pancreas, but it is rarely used for cancers of the exocrine pancreas;

- *Total pancreatectomy*. This operation removes the entire pancreas and the spleen;

- *Pancreaticoduodenectomy (Whipple procedure)*. This is the most commonly used operation for attempting to completely remove a cancer of the exocrine pancreas. It removes the head of pancreas and sometimes removes the body of the pancreas as well. It also removes part of the stomach, the entire duodenum (first part of the small intestine), a small part of the jejunum (second part of the small intestine), and lymph nodes near the pancreas. The gallbladder and part of the common bile duct are removed and the remaining bile duct is attached to the small intestine so that bile from the liver can continue to enter the small intestine. It cannot be emphasized too strongly that for patients to have the most successful outcomes, they must be treated by a surgeon who has performed many of these operations and at a hospital that has had a large experience with pancreatic surgery.

Palliative Procedures

- *Surgery to reroute* the flow of bile from the common bile duct directly into the small intestine without the need to pass through the head of the pancreas. Bypassing the duodenum when the other palliative procedure is done can often avoid a second operation;

- *Placement of a stent* (tube) through an endoscope. This stent helps keep the bile duct open and resists compression from the surrounding cancer.

Chemotherapy

Until recently, fluorouracil (5-FU) was the chemotherapy drug most often used in treating cancer of the pancreas. Recent studies have found gemcitabine (Gemzar) to be more effective than 5-FU in treating metastatic cancer of the pancreas. Other drugs that are used include cisplatin (Platinol) and streptozotocin. These drugs may relieve symptoms and therefore are useful when the cancer is incurable.

Radiation Therapy

Patients may receive external beam radiation therapy treatment before or after surgery. Radiation therapy, often combined with chemotherapy (chemo-radiation), may be used for patients whose tumors are too widespread to be removed by surgery.

Intraoperative electron beam radiation therapy is a new approach to treating patients with cancers of the pancreas that is being studied at some cancer centers. With this treatment, external beam radiation therapy using electrons is delivered from a machine in the operating room.

Eye

Key Statistics

Although intraocular melanoma is the most common cancer of the eye, it is an extremely rare cancer. Approximately 2,100 new cases of eye cancer (1,100 men and 1,000 women) are diagnosed in the United States each year and an estimated 200 people (100 men and 100 women) die from this disease. This type of cancer can occur at any age, but most cases occur in people over age 50. Caucasians have eight times greater the risk of intraocular melanoma than African Americans, and three times greater risk than those of Asian descent.

Today, it is possible in many cases to treat the cancer without having to remove it. However, it may be necessary to use a treatment that results in partial vision loss.

The five-year survival rate is hard to estimate accurately because of the small number of cases, but it is around 65 percent. This figure is much higher if the tumor is found early.

Risk Factors

- *Race*. This cancer rarely occurs in African Americans;
- *Hormones*. In women, pregnancy and estrogen replacement therapy may slightly increase the risk;
- *Sunlight*. Exposure to excessive amounts of sunlight may increase risk.

Ocular melanoma begins in the uvea, a part of the eye. The uvea has three parts: 1) the iris (the colored or pigmented part), 2) the choroid (a thin, pigmented layer that underlies and nourishes the retina and the forward portion of the eye with blood), and 3) the ciliary body (a thickened portion of tissue that connects the choroid and the iris).

The anterior chamber is the area in front of the iris and behind the cornea (the thin transparent membrane that covers the front of the eye). The retina contains specialized nerve cells that are sensitive to light. These cells are connected to the brain by the optic nerve. The lens is a flattened sphere of transparent fibers connected to the ciliary muscle. A thin protective membrane called the conjunctiva doubles over to cover the visible sclera.

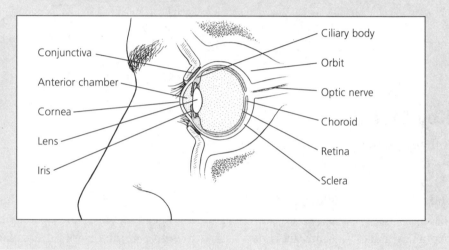

Types of Eye Cancer

Intraocular Melanoma

This rare cancer is found within the globe of the eye, in the uvea. Approximately 90 percent of intraocular melanomas occur in the choroid. Two types of cells exist in intraocular melanoma tumors: spindle cells and nonspindle cells, which include mixed-cell and epithelioid cell tumors. Non-spindle cell tumors are more difficult to treat. Melanomas of the iris are the easiest for a physician to see, are relatively slow-growing, and, because they rarely spread, are less threatening. These are more likely to be noted by the patient, because they often arise in a pigmented spot on the iris that has been present for many years and then begins to grow. Intraocular melanoma is *not* usually related to melanomas of the skin.

Lymphomas may involve parts of the eye, but usually as part of a systemic lymphoma. Other cancers may metastasize to the eye.

Signs and Symptoms

Because the eye is surrounded by bone on all sides but one, a growing tumor is soon crowding against the other structures in the eye, and therefore will cause symptoms, including:

- Change in position of the globe of the eye within its socket;
- Bulging of the eye;
- A change in the way the eye moves within the socket;
- Pain, in or around the eye;
- Changes in vision, such as loss of ability to see to the left and right or up and down while looking straight ahead or floaters that look like spots or squiggles drifting in the field of vision;
- Decreased vision;
- Pain in the eye.

Diagnostic Tests

- Visual inspection;
- Eye photographs;
- CT scan—a rotating x-ray beam creates a series of pictures of the body taken from many angles;
- MRI—uses magnetic fields and radio waves instead of x-rays to create images of selected areas of the body;
- Ultrasonography (ultrasound)—uses sound waves and their echoes to produce images of internal organs;
- Fluorescein angiography—involves injecting a special dye into a blood vessel in order to highlight details of blood vessels on an x-ray image;
- Chest x-ray;
- Blood tests of liver function.

Treatment

Your doctor or ophthalmologist may decide to wait until the tumor shows signs of growth before beginning treatment. In many cases, it is possible to treat the tumor effectively, without loss of the eye. Because these are so rare, it is important to be treated by someone with experience in treating uveal melanomas.

Small Melanomas

Surgery. Small melanomas can be removed and still preserve a functioning eye. Surgery may involve removal of the tumor, portions of the eye, or the entire eye, depending on the size of the tumor;

Radiation therapy. Either external beam or a kind of brachytherapy, where a radioactive source is placed near the tumor, can be used;

Photocoagulation. Use of a tiny laser beam to remove cancerous cells can be used on very small tumors;

Observation. Small tumors can be observed without treatment. If the tumor grows, it may be removed along with a portion of the eye.

Medium Melanomas

It is less clear how to treat medium melanomas, and many options are available. The specific options include the following:

Watch carefully. If the tumor is not growing, treatment may not be necessary;

Radiation therapy. Internal or external radiation, as for small melanomas;

Surgery. Removing the tumor and part of the eye, but preserving vision;

Enucleation. This method is used if the other approaches aren't feasible.

Large Melanomas

Enucleation. This is the most widely accepted treatment for large melanomas;

Enucleation with radiation therapy. Preoperative or postoperative radiation therapy is recommended by some physicians in the hope of reducing spread and local recurrence.

Recurrent Intraocular Melanoma

The choice of treatment will depend on the treatment that was used in the past, the person's age and general health, the site of the recurrence, and how far the cancer has spread.

Chemotherapy is not used to treat this disease unless the melanoma has become widespread. Then the drugs used are the same as those used to treat skin melanomas.

Vagina

Key Statistics

Vaginal cancer is rare. Approximately 2,100 new cases of vaginal cancer are diagnosed in the United States each year and an estimated 600 women die of this disease. Because there are so few cases, the five-year survival rate isn't precisely known. In large studies, the five-year survival rate was 40 to 80 percent if the cancer hadn't spread outside the pelvis. The smaller cancers had the best results.

Risk Factors

The risk factors for vaginal cancer are similar to those for cervical cancer.

- *Age*. Approximately half of women diagnosed are 60 years old or older. Most cases of the disease are diagnosed in women between the ages of 50 and 70;

- *Human papillomavirus (HPV) infection*. This virus, transmitted by sexual contact, is present in many patients with vaginal cancer;

- *Cervical cancer*. Having cervical cancer increases the risk of developing vaginal cancer;

- *Smoking*. Smoking may increase the risk of this cancer;

- *Diethylstilbesterol (DES)*. About 1 out of every 1,000 women whose mothers took diethylstilbestrol (DES) when pregnant with them between 1940 and 1971 develop clear-cell adenocarcinoma of the vagina or cervix. Some studies suggest that DES daughters are also at somewhat increased

The vagina is a three- to four-inch tube that joins the cervix, the lower part of the uterus, at one end, and at the other end opens onto the vulva, the external genitalia. The walls of the vagina are lined by a thin layer called the epithelium. The epithelium is formed by squamous epithelial cells. The part of the vaginal wall underneath the epithelium contains connective tissue, involuntary muscle tissue, and lymph vessels and nerves. Glands in the cervix secrete mucus to keep the vaginal lining moist.

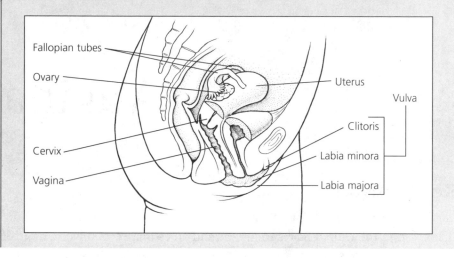

risk of developing squamous cell cancer of the cervix and precancerous changes of cervical squamous cells.

Types of Vaginal Cancer

Squamous Cell Carcinoma

From 85 to 90 percent of vaginal cancers begin in the epithelial lining of the vagina. They tend to occur in the upper area of the vagina near the cervix. Vaginal squamous cell carcinomas do not appear suddenly—they develop over a period of many years from precancerous changes called vaginal intraepithelial neoplasia (often abbreviated as VAIN).

Verrucous carcinoma is a rare type of squamous cell carcinoma that tends to grow slowly. It grows mostly toward the inside of the vagina, and often appears as warty or cauliflower-like lumps.

Adenocarcinoma

About 5 to 10 percent of vaginal cancers are adenocarcinomas. The usual type typically develops in women older than age 50. Clear cell adenocarcinoma occurs more often in young women who were exposed to diethylstilbestrol (DES) when they were in their mothers' wombs.

Malignant Melanoma

These cancers account for about 2 to 3 percent of all vaginal cancers. Melanoma tends to affect the lower or outer portion of the vagina. The tumors show considerable variation in size, color, and growth pattern.

Sarcomas

Two to three percent of vaginal cancers form deep in the wall of the vagina, not on its surface (the epithelium). The most common type of vaginal cancer, leiomyosarcoma, typically affects women older than age 50. Leiomyosarcomas resemble the involuntary muscle cells of the vaginal wall. Rhabdomyosarcoma is a childhood cancer. It is usually detected in children younger than 3 years old. Its cells resemble voluntary muscle cells, which are not normally found in the vaginal wall.

Signs and Symptoms

* Vaginal bleeding, often after intercourse;

* Vaginal discharge;

* Pain with intercourse;

* Pelvic pain—this is not as common as other signs and symptoms.

Diagnostic Tests

* Colposcopy—in this procedure the cervix is viewed through a colposcope, an instrument with magnifying lenses, in order to identify any abnormal areas;

* Biopsy—removal of tissue for examination;

* Cystoscopy—a thin tube with a lens and light is inserted into the bladder through the opening called the urethra to check for spread of vaginal cancer to the bladder;

* Proctosigmoidoscopy—a slender, flexible, hollow, lighted tube is placed into the rectum to check for spread of vaginal cancer to the rectum or colon. This is done when patients have large vaginal cancers and/or cancers that are located in the part of the vagina next to the rectum and colon.

* Barium enema—this test is rarely performed except in patients with gastrointestinal symptoms;

* Chest x-ray—done to check for any signs that the vaginal cancer has spread through the bloodstream to the lungs;

- CT scan—a rotating x-ray beam creates a series of pictures of the body taken from many angles.

Treatment

Surgery

Surgical procedures are usually reserved for small stage I lesions, radiation therapy failures, stage I clear cell adenocarcinomas, nonepithelial tumors (sarcomas), and melanomas. The extent of the surgery depends on the size and stage of the cancer. It can range from laser surgery or local excision needed to remove a precancer (VAIN) to radical vaginectomy (removal of the vagina and adjacent tissues), sometimes together with radical hysterectomy (removal of the uterus with adjacent connective tissue) and lymphadenectomy (removal of lymph nodes from the groin area or from inside the pelvis near the vagina).

If a woman has already had radiation for cervical cancer, it may be necessary to perform pelvic exenteration (an operation that combines a radical hysterectomy with removal of the vagina and possibly the bladder, rectum, and part of the colon).

Radiation Therapy

Radiation therapy using external beam radiation therapy and/or brachytherapy is the preferred method of treating most cancers of the vagina.

Chemotherapy

Systemic chemotherapy has not been very successful in treating vaginal cancer. Its use is generally limited to clinical trials for patients with distant metastases.

Treatment of Vaginal Precancers (VAIN)

The lesions can be treated by laser surgery, loop electroexcision procedure (abbreviated LEEP or LLETZ), or topical chemotherapy. Because low-grade VAIN will often disappear without any treatment, some doctors treat only intermediate or high-grade VAIN.

Vulva

Key Statistics

Approximately 3,600 new cases of vulvar cancer are diagnosed in the United States each year and about 800 people die of this disease.

The five-year survival rate for patients whose cancers are small (less than one inch) is around 95 percent. If the tumor is between one and three inches, the five-year survival rate is 73 percent. It is lower for larger tumors and also if the cancer has spread to many lymph nodes.

> The vulva is the external portion of the female reproductive system. The vulva includes two prominent skin folds known as the labia majora, two more barely visible, hairless skin folds called the labia minora, the clitoris, and the "vestibule" of the vagina.
>
> Cancer of the vulva is a malignancy that can occur on any part of the female external reproductive system, but most often affects the inner edges of the labia majora or the labia minora. Less often, cancer occurs on the clitoris or in Bartholin's glands (small mucus-producing glands on either side of the vaginal opening).

Risk Factors

- *Age*. Most patients are in their 70s or older; however, a small but increasing number of people diagnosed with vulvar cancer are younger;

- *Human papillomavirus infection (HPV)*. This sexually transmitted virus is associated with about 30 to 50 percent of vulvar cancers;

- *Smoking*. This may increase the risk;

- *Inflammation or scarring*. Chronic inflammation or a scarring condition called lichen sclerosus can increase the risk of vulvar cancer.

Types of Vulvar Cancer

Squamous Cell Carcinoma

Over 90 percent of cancers of the vulva begin in squamous cells, the main cell type of the skin. This type of cancer usually forms slowly over many years and is usually preceded by precancerous changes that may last for several years. The medical term most often used for this precancerous condition is vulvar intraepithelial neoplasia (VIN) or dysplasia. It is not possible to predict which women with VIN or dysplasia will develop vulvar cancer, so treatment of all cases is very important.

Melanoma

The second most common type of vulvar cancer (about 4 percent) is melanoma (see *Melanoma*, pages 697–700). From 5 to 8 percent of melanomas in women occur on the vulva, usually on the labia minora and clitoris.

Adenocarcinoma

Some vulvar cancers develop from Bartholin's glands, which are found at the opening of the vagina and produce a mucus-like lubricating fluid. Since a tumor in the Bartholin's gland is easily mistaken for a cyst (accumulation of fluid in the gland), delay in accurate diagnosis is common. Rarely, adenocarcinomas form in the sweat glands of the vulvar skin.

Paget's Disease

This is a condition in which adenocarcinoma cells are found in the vulvar skin. Between 20 and 25 percent of patients with vulvar Paget's disease also have an invasive adenocarcinoma of a Bartholin's gland or sweat gland. In the remaining 75 to 80 percent, the malignant cells are found only in the skin's top layer and do not involve the tissues under that layer.

Signs and Symptoms

- Roughening of the vulvar area or bumps in the area or a lump;
- Itching;
- Bleeding;
- Tenderness of the vulva;
- Scaliness of the vulva.

Diagnostic Tests

- Biopsy—this can be either excisional (removing the entire abnormal area) or incisional (removing a small piece of tissue from the suspicious area to examine under the microscope);

- Colposcopy—treating the skin with a dilute solution of acetic acid that causes areas of VIN (preinvasive vulvar cancer) and cancer to turn white, making them easier to see through the colposcope;

- Cystoscopy—using a lighted tube to check the inside surface of the bladder for cancer that may have metastasized there;

- Proctoscopy—a visual inspection of the rectum using a lighted tube;

- Examination of the pelvis under anesthesia—this permits a thorough examination that can better evaluate the extent of cancer spread to internal organs of the pelvis;

- Chest x-ray—this is done to see if vulvar cancer has spread to the lungs;

- CT scan—a rotating x-ray beam creates a series of pictures of the body taken from many angles. It is useful in predicting whether the vulvar cancer is likely to spread to lymph nodes in the pelvis or along the major blood vessels;

- MRI scan—uses magnetic fields and radio waves instead of x-rays to create images of selected areas of the body. This is rarely used in place of a CT scan to evaluate vulvar cancer.

Treatment

Surgery

When cancer is detected early, it's not necessary to remove a large amount of surrounding normal tissue and regional lymph nodes in order to achieve a cure. When cancer is more advanced, a more extensive procedure may be necessary.

The following types of surgery are performed depending upon how much tissue needs to be removed:

Laser surgery. This is used as a treatment for VIN (preinvasive vulvar cancer). It is not a treatment for invasive cancer;

Excision. The cancer and a margin of normal-appearing skin around it (usually about ½ inch) are excised by a wide local excision. If extensive, it may be called a simple partial vulvectomy;

Vulvectomy. There are several operations in which part of the vulva or the entire vulva is removed. A skinning vulvectomy means only the top layer of skin affected by the cancer is removed. That procedure is rarely done. A simple vulvectomy removes the entire vulva. A radical vulvectomy can be complete or partial. When part of the vulva, including the deep tissue, is removed, the operation is called a partial vulvectomy. A complete radical vulvectomy removes the entire vulva and deep tissues, including the clitoris. An operation to remove the lymph nodes near the vulva, called a groin dissection, is sometimes done for larger tumors.

Pelvic Exenteration. This operation includes vulvectomy and removal of the pelvic lymph nodes, as well as removal of one or more of the following structures: the lower colon, rectum, bladder, uterus, cervix, and vagina.

Treatment for Adenocarcinoma. If Paget's disease is present and there is no associated invasive carcinoma, treatment is wide local excision or simple vulvectomy. If an invasive adenocarcinoma of a Bartholin's gland or of vulvar skin sweat glands is present, radical vulvectomy is recommended with removal of inguinal (groin) lymph nodes on one or both sides of the body.

Treatment for Melanoma. Treatment options depend on how deeply the melanoma has invaded. If the depth is less than $3/4$ millimeter, partial vulvectomy with two-centimeter (about $3/4$-inch) margins is the usual treatment. Radical vulvectomy may rarely be used when the lesion extensively involves the vulva.

Radiation Therapy

Radiation may be combined with surgery to kill more cancer cells in advanced cases. In patients too frail for surgery, radiation is sometimes the primary treatment. It can also be used to help preserve sexual function when the tumor is involving a sensitive area such as the clitoris, or used to palliate when the cancer can't be surgically removed.

Chemotherapy

Drugs most often used in treating vulvar cancer include cisplatin (Platinol), mitomycin (Mutamycin), and fluorouracil (5-FU). Vulvar cancers that have spread to other organs tend to be resistant to chemotherapy, so it has little role in those situations.

Cervix

Key Statistics

Approximately 12,900 new cases of invasive cervical cancer are diagnosed in the United States each year and about 4,400 women die of this disease.

Some researchers estimate that noninvasive cervical cancer (carcinoma in situ) is about four times more common than invasive cervical cancer.

The five-year survival rate for all patients is 70 percent, but when the cancer is found early it is 92 percent.

> The cervix is the lower part of the uterus (womb), which connects the body of the uterus to the vagina (birth canal). The part of the cervix closest to the body of the uterus is called the endocervix. The part next to the vagina is the ectocervix.
>
> Cancer of the cervix develops when the lining of the cervix gradually changes from a normal state to a precancerous state, then to a cancerous state. This process usually takes several years but can sometimes happen in less than a year. For some women, precancerous changes may disappear without any treatment. If these precancers are treated, true cancers can often be prevented.

Risk Factors

- *Sexual activity.* Sexual activity is the major risk factor for cervical cancer. The earlier the activity begins in a woman's life, the higher is the risk. Likewise, the risk increases with increasing number of sexual partners. The accepted cause of cervical cancer is infection with viruses called human papillomaviruses (HPV), which are transmitted by sexual contact. There are many types of HPV. Some only cause genital warts. These are called "low-risk" viruses. However, other sexually transmitted HPVs have been linked with genital or anal cancers in both men and women. These are called "high-risk" HPV types and include HPV 16, HPV 18, HPV 33, HPV 35, and HPV 45, as well as others;

- *Smoking.* Smoking increases the cancer-causing effect of HPV;

- *Immune deficiency.* HIV infection as well as any defect in the body's immunity will increase the chance that HPV infection will lead to cancer;

- *Oral contraceptives.* These may increase the risk of cervical cancer after five or more years of use;

- *Race.* The death rate for African Americans is over twice the national average. Hispanics and American Indians also have above average cervical cancer death rates.

Types of Cervical Cancer

Approximately 85 to 90 percent of cervical cancers are squamous cells carcinomas. They begin in the ectocervix (outer part of the cervix), most often at its border with the endocervix. The remaining 10 to 15 percent of cervical cancers are adenocarcinomas, which develop from the mucus-producing gland cells of the endocervix. Less commonly, cervical cancers have features of both squamous cell carcinomas and adenocarcinomas. These are called adenosquamous carcinomas or mixed carcinomas.

Signs and Symptoms

Cervical precancers and early cancers rarely show symptoms or signs of cervical cancer. A woman usually develops symptoms when the cancer has become invasive. When symptoms occur, the following are the most common ones:

- An unusual discharge such as blood spots or light bleeding from the vagina (separate from the normal monthly menstrual period);

- Bleeding following intercourse;

- Pain during intercourse.

Diagnostic Tests

- Pap smear—this is the single most important diagnostic test for detecting early cancer. It can also find precancerous lesions that can be treated and prevent the development of cancer;

- Colposcopy—in this procedure the cervix is viewed through a colposcope, an instrument with magnifying lenses, in order to identify any abnormal areas;

- Colposcopic biopsy—if when a doctor examines the cervix with a colposcope he or she finds an abnormal area, a small section of the abnormal area is removed for examination;

- Endocervical curettage (endocervical scraping)—a narrow instrument (the curette) is inserted into the endocervical canal (the passage between the outer part of the cervix and the inner part of the uterus) and removes some tissue for examination;

- Cone biopsy—two methods are commonly used for cone biopsies, the loop electrosurgical excision procedure (LEEP or LLETZ) and the cold knife cone biopsy:

     The LEEP (LLETZ) removes tissue with a wire that is heated by electrical current. This short procedure uses a local anesthetic, and can be done in your doctor's office.

     The cold knife cone biopsy uses a surgical scalpel or a laser to remove tissue.

- Cystoscopy, proctoscopy, and examination under anesthesia—during cystoscopy, a slender tube with a lens and a light is placed into the bladder through the urethra in order to check the bladder and urethra for possible cancers and possibly remove small tissue samples for testing. Proctoscopy is a visual inspection of the rectum through a lighted tube to check for spread of cervical cancer. Examination of the pelvis under anesthesia can help to find out whether the cancer has spread beyond the cervix;

- CT scan—a rotating x-ray beam creates a series of pictures of the body taken from many angles;

- MRI scan—uses magnetic fields and radio waves instead of x-rays to create images of selected areas of the body;

- Intravenous urography (also known as intravenous pyelogram or IVP)—an x-ray of the urinary system, taken after injecting a special dye into a vein. This procedure can identify abnormalities of the urinary tract, such as changes caused by spread of cervical cancer to the pelvic lymph nodes.

Treatment

Surgery

Laser surgery. Used as treatment for preinvasive cervical cancer;

Cone biopy. Using a surgical or laser knife (cold knife cone) or using the LEEP (LEETZ) procedure can be used as the sole treatment in those women with early (stage IA) cancer who might want to have children;

Simple hysterectomy;

Radical hysterectomy and pelvic lymph node dissection;

Pelvic exenteration.

Radiation Therapy

External beam radiation therapy combined with internal brachytherapy directly on the cervix can be used instead of surgery for some patients. External beam is also used for some high-risk patients after surgery.

Chemotherapy

Drugs most often used in treating cervical cancer include cisplatin (Platinol), ifosfamide (IFEX), and fluorouracil (Adrucil). Usually they are given in some combination of these. Chemotherapy is used for treating widespread cancer. It is also used combined with radiation therapy for women with more advanced disease.

Treatment in Pregnancy

Most doctors feel that if the cancer is at a very early stage, such as stage IA, it is safe to continue the pregnancy to term. Several weeks after delivery, a hysterectomy is recommended. If the cancer is stage IB, then the patient and her doctor must decide whether to continue the pregnancy. If not, treatment would be hysterectomy and/or radiation. If they decide to continue the pregnancy, the baby should be delivered by cesarean section as soon as it is able to survive outside the womb. For more advanced cancers, immediate treatment is the safest option.

Uterus

Key Statistics

Approximately 38,300 new cases of cancer of the uterine body are diagnosed in the United States each year, and more than 95 percent of these are endometrial cancers. It is estimated that 6,600 women die of this disease. Cancer of the endometrium is the most common cancer of the female reproductive organs in this country.

The five-year survival rate for all patients is 84 percent. It is 96 percent when the cancer is detected early.

The uterus is divided into two parts. The upper part, or the corpus, is the body of the uterus, where a fetus grows (this discussion is about cancers that begin in this part of the uterus). The cervix is the lower part of the uterus (womb), which connects the body of the uterus to the vagina (birth canal). (See *Cervix*, pages 657–660, for more information about cancer of the cervix.)

Risk Factors

- Estrogen exposure. Estrogens are the major risk factor for uterine cancer. Excess estrogen exposure can come about because of a combination of early menarche and/or late menopause, or taking estrogens as hormone replacement therapy in menopause. Never becoming pregnant also increases estrogen exposure;

- *Obesity*. Having more fat tissue can increase a woman's estrogen levels, which may explain why being obese increases a woman's risk of endometrial cancer two to five times, depending on how overweight she is;

- *Tamoxifen*. This is a drug that acts like estrogen and is given to women with breast cancer. It increases the risk of uterine cancer;

- *Diabetes*. Women with diabetes have a higher risk of endometrial cancer;

- *Hypertension*. This increases the risk of endometrial cancer. It is not known why;

- *Radiation*. Prior pelvic radiation increases the risk of endometrial cancer;

- *Age*. Ninety-five percent of endometrial cancers occur in women age 40 or older. The average age at diagnosis is 60;

- *Family history*. Endometrial cancer tends to run in some families who also have an inherited tendency to develop colon cancer called hereditary nonpolyposis colon cancer (HNPCC).

Risk Factors for Sarcomas

Several factors have been found that increase a woman's risk of developing a uterine sarcoma.

- *Prior pelvic radiation therapy*. This increases the risk of sarcomas;

- *Race*. Sarcomas are more common in African-American women;

- *Age*. Uterine sarcomas tend to occur in middle-aged and elderly women, although they may affect younger women as well.

Signs and Symptoms

- Vaginal bleeding—this is the major symptom of uterine cancer. Any irregular bleeding in a premenopausal woman or any bleeding whatsoever in a postmenopausal woman should be evaluated by a doctor.

Types of Uterine Cancers

Over 90 percent of cancers of the uterus start in the lining and are adenocarcinomas. The rest are sarcomas or mixed Mullerian tumors.

These fall into one of three categories, based on the type of cell from which they developed:

- Endometrial stromal sarcomas—develop in the stroma (supporting connective tissue) of the endometrium;

- Uterine leiomyosarcomas—start in the muscular wall of the uterus;

- Uterine carcinosarcomas—also known as malignant mixed mesodermal tumors or malignant mixed Mullerian tumors (abbreviated as MMMT), include features of both sarcomas and carcinomas.

Diagnostic Tests

- Endometrial biopsy—a sample of endometrial tissue is obtained through a very thin, flexible tube inserted into the uterus through the cervix;

- Dilation and curettage (D&C)—involves using a special surgical instrument to scrape tissue from inside the uterus for testing;

- Testing of endometrial tissue;

- Transvaginal ultrasound—uses sound waves to create images of the uterus. A probe inserted into the vagina releases sound waves that echo off the tissues of the pelvic organs. A computer analyzes the pattern of echoes to create images on a computer screen, used to help determine whether a tumor is present;

- Ultrahysterosonogram or saline infusion sonogram—saline (salt water) is introduced into the uterus through a catheter before the transvaginal ultrasound so the doctor can see abnormalities of the uterine lining more clearly;

- CT scan—a rotating x-ray beam creates a series of pictures of the body taken from many angles;

- MRI scan—uses magnetic fields and radio waves instead of x-rays to create images of selected areas of the body;

- Chest x-ray.

Treatment

Surgery

Simple hysterectomy;

Radical hysterectomy. This operation also removes the entire uterus. The tissues next to the uterus (parametrium and uterosacral ligaments), and the upper part (about one inch) of the vagina next to the cervix are also removed;

Bilateral salpingo-oophorectomy (BSO). This operation removes both fallopian tubes and both ovaries;

Pelvic lymph node dissection;

Laparoscopic lymph node sampling.

Radiation Therapy

The amount of the pelvis that needs to be exposed to radiation therapy depends on the extent of the disease. If the disease was at an early stage, none is needed. If the stage is advanced, then external beam radiation will be given to the pelvis. In cases where only the upper third of the vagina, the vaginal cuff, needs to be treated, a radioactive application is inserted through the vagina. This internal application of radiation therapy is called brachytherapy. In some situations, both brachytherapy (internal radiation therapy) and external beam radiation therapy are given.

Chemotherapy

Chemotherapy is effective in shrinking endometrial cancers. Combination chemotherapy is sometimes more effective in treating cancer than one drug alone. Drugs used in treating endometrial cancer may include doxorubicin (Adriamycin), cisplatin (Platinol), and paclitaxel (Taxol). Chemotherapy is used primarily for treating recurrent or advanced disease that cannot be successfully treated with surgery or radiation therapy. It is not curative.

Drugs used in treating uterine sarcomas may include doxorubicin, cyclophosphamide (Cytoxan), ifosfamide (IFEX), and cisplatin.

Hormone Therapy

Hormone therapy uses medications such as progesterone to slow the growth of cancer cells. Progesterone-like drugs are very effective in shrinking advanced cancers in some women. These are not curative. This approach is sometimes used for endometrial cancer and endometrial stromal sarcomas but is rarely used for other types of uterine sarcomas. Tamoxifen (Nolvadex), an antiestrogen drug often used to treat breast cancer, may also be helpful in treating advanced or recurrent endometrial cancer.

Ovary

Key Statistics

Ovarian cancer is the sixth most common cancer among women, excluding skin cancers, accounting for 4 percent of all cancers in women. Approximately 23,400 new cases of ovarian cancer are diagnosed in the United States each year and about 13,900 women die from this disease.

The five-year survival rate for all women is 50 percent. For the 25 percent of women whose disease is diagnosed when it is still confined to the ovary, the rate is 95 percent. But for distant disease, the five-year survival rate is 28 percent.

> One ovary is located on each side of the uterus in the pelvis. The ovaries produce eggs (ova). The ovaries are also the main source of the female hormones estrogen and progesterone.

Risk Factors

These risk factors do not apply to other, less common types of ovarian cancer, such as germ cell tumors and stromal tumors.

- *Age.* The incidence of ovarian cancer increases with age and peaks in women in their 70s;

- *Reproductive history.* Women who haven't had children or had their first child after age 30, haven't taken oral contraceptives, started menstruating at an early age (before age 12), and/or experienced menopause after age 50, may have an increased risk;

- *Family history.* A family history of ovarian cancer or breast cancer increases the risk, particularly if the cancers involve mutations in the BRCA1 or BRCA2 genes. Women with a family history of inherited colon cancer because of a mutation of the HNPCC gene are also at increased risk.

Types of Ovarian Cancer

In general, ovarian tumors are named according to the kind of cells (epithelial, stromal, or germ cell) from which the tumor began.

Epithelial Ovarian Cancers

Approximately 85 percent of ovarian cancers are epithelial ovarian carcinomas. They are classified as serous, mucinous, endometriod, and clear cell types. Undifferentiated epithelial ovarian carcinomas don't look like any of these four subtypes, and they tend to grow and spread more quickly.

Primary Peritoneal Carcinoma

Primary peritoneal carcinoma—also called extraovarian primary peritoneal carcinoma (EOPPC) and serous surface papillary carcinoma—is a cancer closely related to epithelial ovarian cancer. It develops from cells that line the pelvis or abdomen, which are very similar to epithelial cells on the surface of the ovaries. Because EOPPC tends to spread along the surfaces of the pelvis and abdomen, it is often difficult to tell exactly where the cancer first started. Under a microscope, EOPPC looks just like epithelial ovarian cancer. Women who have had their ovaries removed can still develop this type of cancer.

Germ Cell Tumors

Germ cells are the cells that usually form the ova or eggs. There are several subtypes of germ cell tumors. Most are benign, although some are cancerous and may be life threatening. Malignant germ cell tumors account for about 15 percent of ovarian cancers. The different types are teratomas (they can be benign or malignant), dysgerminomas, and endodermal sinus tumors. These mostly occur in young women.

Stromal Tumors

These tumors account for about 5 percent of ovarian cancers. They start from connective tissue cells that hold the ovary together and produce the female hormones estrogen and progesterone. More than half are found in women over age 50, but some occur in young girls. Some of these tumors produce female hormones or, less often, male hormones. They can cause menstrual periods and breast development in young girls. If male hormones are produced, the tumors can disrupt normal periods and cause facial and body hair to grow. Types of malignant (cancerous) stromal tumors include granulosa cell tumors, granulosa-theca tumors, and Sertoli-Leydig cell tumors, which are usually considered low-grade cancers.

Signs and Symptoms

- Prolonged swelling of the abdomen—due to a mass or accumulation of fluid;
- Digestive problems, including gas, loss of appetite, bloating, long-term abdominal pain, or indigestion;

- Unusual vaginal bleeding;
- Pelvic pressure (feeling as though you have to urinate or defecate all the time);
- Pelvic pain;
- Leg pain or swelling due to blood clots in the leg;
- Back pain.

Diagnostic Tests

- Ultrasonography (ultrasound)—uses sound waves and their echoes to produce images of internal organs;
- CT scan—a rotating x-ray beam creates a series of pictures of the body taken from many angles;
- Chest x-ray—this test may be done to determine whether ovarian cancer has spread to the lungs;
- MRI scan—uses magnetic fields and radio waves instead of x-rays to create images of selected areas of the body;
- Biopsy—removal of tissue for examination.

Treatment

Surgery

For women of childbearing age who have small tumors confined to a single ovary, an effort will be made to treat the disease without removing both ovaries and the uterus. Otherwise, for most epithelial tumors, a more extensive procedure will be done. This usually includes removing both ovaries and tubes, the uterus, and the omentum (a fatty layer covering the organs), lymphadenectomy (also called lymph node biopsy or dissection), and removing the lymph nodes. In addition, the surgeon will do biopsy sampling throughout the abdominal cavity to look for cancer. The surgeon will also take washings from the abdominal cavity to look for stray cancer cells that may be floating about.

The other important surgical procedure is cytoreduction or debulking. This is done for more advanced cancer. In this procedure, the surgeon removes as much tumor as possible, even though all of it can't be removed.

Chemotherapy

Combination therapy using a platinum compound, such as cisplatin (Platinol) or carboplatin (Paraplatin), and a taxane such as paclitaxel (Taxol), is the standard approach. This is used in most women whose cancer isn't confined to the ovary.

Tumor recurrence is sometimes treated with additional cycles of a platinum compound and/or a taxane. In other cases, recurrence is treated with second-line agents such as topotecan (Hycamtin), anthracyclines such as doxorubicin (Adrimycin) and liposomal doxorubicin (Doxil), gemcitabine (Gemzar), cyclophosphamide (Cytoxan), vinorelbine (Navelbine), altretamine (Hexalen), ifosfamide (IFEX), etoposide (VePesid), and fluorouracil (Adrucil).

Most patients with germ cell cancers receive combination chemotherapy with a frequently used treatment called BEP, combining the three drugs **b**leomycin (Blenoxane), **e**toposide, and cisplatin (**P**latinol).

Intraperitoneal chemotherapy is injected directly into the abdomen. This approach concentrates the dose of chemotherapy reaching the cancer cells on the abdominal lining and limits the amount that reaches the rest of the body, thereby reducing some side effects.

Radiation Therapy

Although in the past it was often used, radiation therapy is now only rarely used as the primary treatment for ovarian cancer. It can be used to treat the whole pelvis, which has cured some women in the past.

Larynx

Key Statistics

Approximately 10,000 new cases of laryngeal cancer (8,000 men and 2,000 women) are diagnosed in the United States each year and about 4,000 people (3,100 men and 900 women) die of this disease. An estimated 2,500 cases of hypopharyngeal cancer are diagnosed per year.

When patients newly diagnosed with larynx and hypopharynx cancers are carefully examined, about 15 percent will have another cancer in nearby areas such as the mouth, esophagus, or lung. Another 10 to 20 percent will develop a cancer in one of these organs at a later time. It is very important that these people have follow-up examinations for the rest of their lives and avoid risk factors like smoking and drinking.

The five-year survival rate is 70 percent.

The larynx, also called the voice box or Adam's apple, is divided into three levels: the glottis (or the vocal cords), the supraglottis (the area above the vocal cords including the epiglottis), and the subglottis (the area below the vocal cords).

Sound for speaking is produced in the larynx and it protects the airway during swallowing. The vocal cords come together to change the sound and pitch of the voice and close tightly during swallowing to keep food and saliva from entering the lungs.

The hypopharynx is the part of the esophagus or food pipe that immediately surrounds the larynx.

Risk Factors

- *Smoking.* The risk of developing cancer in the larynx area is five to thirty-five times greater in smokers than in nonsmokers;

- *Alcohol use.* Heavy drinkers have a risk of laryngeal cancer two to five times that of nondrinkers. The combined risks of tobacco and alcohol may be up to 100 times more than people with neither habit;

- *Poor nutrition.* Nutritional deficiencies with specific vitamin deficiencies may play a role in increased risk;

- *Occupational exposures.* Exposures to wood dust and paint fumes, for example, and to certain chemicals as well as asbestos may increase laryngeal cancer risk;

- *Gender.* Men are more likely to develop laryngeal cancer;

- *Age.* Most patients with these cancers are in their 60s when the cancers are first found;

- *Race.* African Americans are about 50 percent more likely to get this cancer than Caucasians.

Types of Laryngeal and Hypopharyngeal Cancers

Several types of cancers can develop in the larynx and hypopharynx. About 95 percent of these are squamous cancers, developing from the squamous cells that form the lining of the larynx and hypopharynx. They begin as precancers that are called dysplasia, squamous intraepithelial neoplasia, or laryngeal intraepithelial neoplasia (LIN). Most of these precancers never develop into actual cancers, but go away without any treatment, especially if the factors (such as smoking) that cause precancers and cancers are stopped.

Some precancers eventually develop into carcinoma in situ (CIS). The cells of this form of cancer replace the lining layer but do not spread to deeper areas of the tissue or to other parts of the body. If CIS is not treated, about 30 percent will become an invasive squamous cell cancer. Rarely, cancer develops from the mucus- and saliva-secreting glands beneath the lining layer of the larynx and hypopharynx. These cancers are called adenocarcinomas, adenoid cystic carcinomas, and mucoepidermoid carcinomas.

Cancers such as chondrosarcomas or synovial sarcomas can develop from connective tissues of the larynx or hypopharynx, but this is very, very rare.

Signs and Symptoms

- Hoarseness that lasts more than two weeks;

- Persistent cough;

- Persistent sore throat;

- Difficulty swallowing or pain with swallowing;

- Difficulty breathing;

- Persistent ear pain;

- A lump or mass in the neck;

- Unintended weight loss.

Diagnostic Tests

- Complete head and neck exam (including nasopharyngoscopy and laryngoscopy)—fiberoptic scopes (flexible, lighted, narrow tubes inserted through the mouth or nose) and mirrors are used to examine the larynx and hypopharynx. The nasopharynx (area behind the nose) and mouth, tongue, floor of the mouth, the rest of the oral cavity, and the neck are carefully viewed and felt for any evidence of cancer;

- Panendoscopy—a surgeon views the larynx, hypopharynx, esophagus, trachea and bronchi, and breathing tubes through a scope to determine the size of the tumor and how much it has spread to surrounding areas. This examination is performed in the operating room, with the patient under general anesthesia;

- CT scan—a rotating x-ray beam creates a series of pictures of the body taken from many angles;

- MRI scan—uses magnetic fields and radio waves instead of x-rays to create images of selected areas of the body;

- Barium swallow—this is a series of x-rays performed while the patient swallows a barium-containing liquid that can be seen on the x-rays.

- Chest x-ray—a chest x-ray is routine because smoking causes lung cancer and emphysema as well as laryngeal and hypopharyngeal cancers;

- Endoscopic biopsy—the surgeon operates special instruments through an endoscope to remove small tissue samples;

- Fine needle aspiration (FNA)—a thin needle is used to withdraw fluid or small samples of tissue from the tumor mass so that cells can be examined with a microscope.

Treatment

The treatment options for most laryngeal and hypopharyngeal cancers are surgery and radiation therapy either alone or in combination, depending on the stage of the tumor. Advances in reconstructive surgery have improved the quality of life after surgical treatment of these cancers. Chemotherapy is usually reserved for tumors that have spread too far for surgery or radiation therapy to treat the entire cancer.

Surgery

There are several operations commonly used in treating patients with laryngeal and hypopharyngeal cancers.

Total laryngectomy. More advanced laryngeal and hypopharyngeal cancers usually require removal of the entire voice box. The windpipe is then brought up to the skin of the neck as a stoma (or hole) that the patient can breathe through. Artificial devices can be implanted to help with speech;

Artial laryngectomy. There are various procedures for removing different areas of the larynx while keeping as much of the natural larynx as possible and removing the cancer;

Neck dissection. There are several forms of neck dissections to remove lymph nodes that may contain cancer cells, ranging from the radical neck dissection which also removes some muscle, to a selective neck dissection that only removes the lymph nodes;

Total or partial pharyngectomy. Surgery for cancers of the hypopharynx will remove a portion or all of the hypopharynx. Several reconstruction procedures can be used to rebuild the pharynx and improve the ability to swallow;

Tracheotomy. A hole may be placed in the neck to bypass a large tumor and allow more comfortable breathing;

Gastrostomy tube. A feeding tube inserted through the skin and muscle of the abdomen directly into the stomach can provide extra nutrition when cancer prevents the person from swallowing.

Radiation Therapy

External beam radiation therapy for laryngeal and hypopharyngeal cancer is usually given in daily fractions (doses), but other options are being studied. For example, hyperfractionation refers to dividing the radiation over a larger number of doses (two treatments per day instead of one, for example). Accelerated fractionation indicates that the radiation treatment is completed more quickly (6 weeks instead of 7 weeks, for instance).

Chemotherapy

The two drugs used most often for cancers of the larynx and hypopharynx are cisplatin (Platinol) and fluorouracil (5-FU). Additional drugs that may be used include methotrexate, bleomycin (Blenoxane), and carboplatin (Paraplatin). Several other drugs are being studied but are only used on rare cases. Chemoradiotherapy (chemotherapy given at the same time as radiation) has been shown in a few studies to cure some patients with head and neck cancers and allow them to keep their larynx even in advanced disease.

Oral Cavity

Key Statistics

Approximately 30,100 new cases of oral cavity and pharyngeal cancer (20,200 men and 9,900 women) are diagnosed in the United States each year and an estimated 7,800 people (5,100 men and 2,700 women) die of this disease. Both the incidence and death rate for this cancer have been decreasing.

The five-year survival rate for all patients is 56 percent, but it is 82 percent if the cancer is found early.

Risk Factors

- *Smoking.* Smokers are six times more likely than nonsmokers to develop these cancers. Smoking cigarettes, cigars, and pipes all increase risk for these cancers. Smokeless tobacco ("snuff" or chewing tobacco) increases the risk of cancers of the cheek, gingiva (gums), and inner surface of the lips by about fifty times;

- *Alcohol use.* These cancers are about six times more common in drinkers than in nondrinkers. People who smoke and also drink alcohol have a much higher risk of cancer than those using alcohol or tobacco alone;

- *Sun exposure.* More than 30 percent of patients with cancers of the lip have outdoor occupations associated with prolonged exposure to sunlight;

- *Diet.* A poor diet that leads to vitamin A deficiency is associated with an increased risk;

- *Human papillomavirus (HPV).* HPV infection may be a factor that contributes to the development of oral cavity and oropharyngeal cancers in approximately 20 percent of people;

The oral cavity starts at the skin edge of the lips and includes the lips, the inside lining of the lips and cheeks, the teeth, the gums, the front two-thirds of the tongue, the floor of the mouth below the tongue, the bony roof of the mouth, and the area behind the wisdom teeth.

The oropharynx is the part of the throat just behind the mouth. It begins where the oral cavity stops and includes the base or back third of the tongue, the soft palate, the tonsils and tonsillar pillars, and the back wall of the throat.

Minor salivary glands located throughout the oral cavity and oropharynx make saliva that keeps the mouth moist and helps digest food.

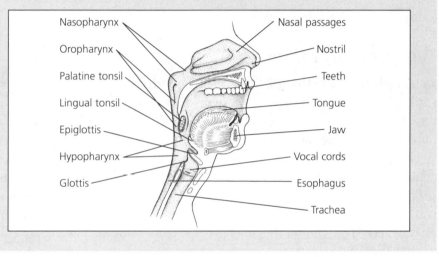

- *Age.* The number of people with oral and oropharynx cancer increases with age. The incidence of this cancer is especially high in those over age 40;

- *Gender.* Oral and oropharyngeal cancer is twice as common in men as in women.

Signs and Symptoms

It is important to keep in mind that about 15 percent of patients with oral cancers will have another cancer in a nearby area such as the larynx, esophagus, or lung, in addition to the oral cancer symptoms below:

- A sore in the mouth that does not heal (most common symptom);

- Pain in the mouth that doesn't go away (also very common);

- A persistent lump or thickening in the cheek;

- A persistent white or red patch on the gums, tongue, tonsil, or lining of the mouth;

- A sore throat or a feeling that something is caught in the throat that doesn't go away;

- Difficulty chewing or swallowing;

- Difficulty moving the jaw or tongue;

- Numbness of the tongue or other area of the mouth;

- Swelling of the jaw that causes dentures to fit poorly or become uncomfortable;

- Loosening of the teeth or pain around the teeth or jaw;

- Voice changes;

- A lump or mass in the neck.

Types of Oral Cancer

Leukoplakia, Erythroplakia, and Dysplasia

Leukoplakia and erythroplakia are terms that describe an abnormal area in the mouth or throat. Leukoplakia is a white area. Erythroplakia is a slightly raised, red area that bleeds easily if scraped.

These white or red areas may be a cancer, dysplasia—a precancerous condition—or some relatively harmless condition. About 5 percent of leukoplakias are cancerous or are precancerous changes that progress to cancer within ten years if not properly treated. Erythroplakia is usually more serious. As much as 51 percent of these nonspecific red lesions are malignant.

Malignant Oral Cavity and Oropharyngeal Tumors

More than 90 percent of cancers of the oral cavity and oropharynx are squamous cell cancer. Verrucous carcinoma is a low-grade type of squamous cell carcinoma that makes up less than 5 percent of all oral cavity tumors. It metastasizes rarely but can spread deeply into surrounding tissue.

There are several types of minor salivary gland cancers, including adenoid cystic carcinoma, mucoepidermoid carcinoma, and polymorphous low-grade adenocarcinoma. The tonsils and base of the tongue contain lymphoid (immune system) tissue that can develop into a cancer.

The treatments for minor salivary gland cancers and lymphomas are different from those for squamous cell carcinoma and are not discussed in this section.

Diagnostic Tests

- Complete head and neck exam (including nasopharyngoscopy, pharyngoscopy, and laryngoscopy)—special fiberoptic scopes (flexible, lighted, narrow tubes inserted through the mouth or nose) and mirrors are used to examine the oropharynx;

- Panendoscopy (including laryngoscopy, esophagoscopy, and possible bronchoscopy)—this very thorough exam of the oral cavity, oropharynx, larynx, esophagus, and the trachea and bronchi is performed in the operating room, with the patient under general anesthesia;

- Exfoliative cytology—the doctor scrapes a suspicious lesion and smears it onto a slide for examination under the microscope;

- Incisional biopsy—involves removing small tissue samples for examination;

- Fine needle aspiration (FNA)—a thin needle is placed into the mass so that cells can be withdrawn and viewed with a microscope if a patient has a neck mass that can be felt;

- CT scan—a rotating x-ray beam creates a series of pictures of the body taken from many angles;

- MRI scan—uses magnetic fields and radio waves instead of x-rays to create images of selected areas of the body;

- Panorex—a panorex is a rotating x-ray of the maxilla (upper jawbone) and mandible (lower jaw bone);

- Chest x-ray—because smoking causes lung cancer and emphysema as well as oral and oropharyngeal cancers, a chest x-ray is routinely done;

- Barium swallow—this is a series of x-rays performed while the patient swallows a barium-containing liquid that can be seen on x-rays.

Treatment

Surgery

Primary tumor resection. The primary tumor and a zone of normal-appearing tissue surrounding it can be removed by several different ways. If it is small and easily accessible, surgery can be done through the mouth. Larger tumors, especially those involving the oropharynx, may be removed through an incision in the neck or through a mandibulotomy (splitting the jaw bone with a saw to provide access to the tumor). Sometimes either the upper or lower jaw bone is partly removed. Reconstructive surgery may be required if the surgery causes a large defect. If the lip is involved, only a small amount of tissue may be removed;

Neck dissection. There are several forms of neck dissections to remove lymph nodes that may contain cancer cells, ranging from the radical neck dissection to a selective neck dissection;

Dental extraction and implants. Depending on the expected radiation plan and condition of the patient's teeth, it may be necessary to remove some or even all the teeth. When a portion of the mandible is removed and recon-structed with bone from another part of the body, dental implantation (implantation of hardware that will support prosthetic teeth) can be performed at the same time or later.

Radiation Therapy

External beam radiation therapy is often used postoperatively to prevent local recurrence. It can also be used for palliation when surgery is not feasible. Brachy-therapy also has a role in treating inoperable tumors as well as recurrent ones.

Chemotherapy

Chemotherapy is generally used for cancers that have spread, but may be used for shrinking local tumors, often in combination with radiation. The two chemotherapy drugs used most often for cancers of the oral cavity and oropharynx are cisplatin (Platinol) and fluorouracil (5-FU). Other drugs that may be used include methotrexate, bleomycin (Blenoxane), and carbo-platin (Paraplatin). These drugs are usually used in combination to have a stronger effect.

Salivary Gland

Key Statistics

Salivary gland cancers are uncommon cancers that account for less than 1 percent of all cancers, and about 7 percent of cancers of the head and neck area. The five-year survival rate isn't precisely known because there are many different types of this cancer, but it is approximately 50 to 75 percent.

Risk Factors

There are no clear-cut, proven risk factors for salivary gland cancers, but some studies have suggested that the following may be risk factors:

* *Radiation treatment* to the head and neck area;

* *Industrial exposure to certain radioactive substances.* These include nickel alloy dust or silica dust;

Major salivary glands and minor salivary glands produce saliva. There are 600–1,000 minor salivary glands, which are too small to see without a microscope, located beneath the lining of the lips, tongue, hard and soft palate, and inside the cheeks, nose, sinuses, and larynx (voicebox).

The three types of major salivary glands are the parotid glands, submandibular glands, and sublingual glands. There are two glands of each type—one on the left side and one on the right. The parotid glands are the largest salivary glands and are found on each side of the face, just in front of the ears. They overlie the jaw joint. The submandibular glands are the next largest salivary glands and are found on either side of the

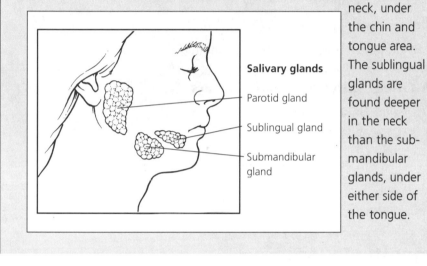

Salivary glands

Parotid gland

Sublingual gland

Submandibular gland

neck, under the chin and tongue area. The sublingual glands are found deeper in the neck than the sub- mandibular glands, under either side of the tongue.

- *Poor diet.* A diet that is deficient in vegetables and high in animal fat may increase risk.

Signs and Symptoms

- A mass or lump in the area of the salivary glands;

- Ongoing pain in the area of the salivary glands;

- Asymmetry of the salivary glands (difference between the size and/or shape of glands on the left and right sides);

- Numbness of part of the face;

- New weakness of the muscles on one side of the face.

Types of Salivary Gland Cancer

About 80 percent of all salivary gland tumors begin in the parotid glands, 10 to 15 percent start in the submandibular glands, and the remainder are located in the sublingual and minor salivary glands. Tumors of the parotids are usually benign (noncancerous). Masses in the minor salivary glands (the smallest of salivary glands) are usually malignant (cancerous). Even so, because there are so many more parotid gland tumors, there are a greater number of cancers found in the parotid glands than any other salivary glands. The malignant tumors listed below are classified by whether they are low grade (meaning they grow slowly and don't tend to spread) or high grade (faster growing and more likely to spread to other parts of the body).

Low-Grade Salivary Gland Cancers

- Acinic cell carcinoma;

- Mucoepidermoid carcinoma (grade 1 or 2);

- Polymorphous low-grade adenocarcinoma.

High-Grade Salivary Gland Cancers

- Mucoepidermoid carcinoma (grade 3);

- Adenoid cystic carcinoma;

- Adenocarcinoma (usual type), poorly differentiated carcinoma;

- Malignant mixed tumor;

- Squamous cell carcinoma.

Diagnostic Tests

- CT scan—a rotating x-ray beam creates a series of pictures of the body taken from many angles.

- MRI scan—uses magnetic fields and radio waves instead of x-rays to create images of selected areas of the body;

- Fine needle aspiration (FNA)—a thin needle is used to withdraw fluid or small samples of tissue from the tumor mass so that cells can be examined with a microscope;

- Chest x-ray—this x-ray can help detect cancer that has spread to the chest.

Treatment

Surgery

Salivary Gland Surgery. Most parotid cancers can be treated by removing only the superficial lobe of the gland. This operation is called a superficial parotidectomy. If the cancer involves deeper tissues, a total parotidectomy will remove the entire gland and might also remove the facial nerve, which passes through the gland. This nerve is responsible for facial movement and without it, that side of the face will droop. Cancers of the submandibular or sublingual glands are treated by removing the entire gland and, when needed, some of the surrounding tissue or bone. Several important nerves pass through or near these glands. These nerves control movements of the tongue as well as sensation and taste of certain parts of the tongue.

Minor salivary gland cancers can occur in the lips, tongue, hard and soft palate, entire oral cavity, throat, voicebox, nose, and sinuses. Usually the cancer and some surrounding tissue will need to be removed by an operation called a wide local excision.

Neck Dissection. A neck dissection removes the lymph nodes, lymph vessels, connective tissue, and sometimes muscle, nerve, and some blood vessels from one side of the neck. A partial or selective neck dissection removes only a few lymph nodes.

Pedicle or Free Flap Reconstruction. Reconstructive surgery may be needed to repair defects in the mouth, throat, or neck caused by removal of very large salivary gland cancers that have spread extensively to nearby tissues.

Dental Extraction

Depending on the expected radiation plan and condition of the patient's teeth, it may be necessary to remove some or even all of the teeth.

Radiation Therapy

External beam radiation is often used postoperatively, particularly when the tumor cannot be completely removed or is likely to come back. Alternatively, it can be used as palliative treatment for recurrent disease. Brachytherapy (internal radiation) is also be used in certain situations.

Chemotherapy

Chemotherapy is only used to palliate recurrent disease. Salivary gland cancers are not very responsive to chemotherapy. Some of the chemotherapy drugs used alone or in combination to treat salivary cancers include cisplatin (Platinol), doxorubicin (Adriamycin), fluorouracil (5-FU), cyclophosphamide (Cytoxan), and methotrexate.

Lung

Key Statistics

Approximately 169,500 new cases of lung cancer (90,700 men and 78,800 women) are diagnosed in the United States each year and an estimated 157,400 people (90,100 men and 67,300 women) die from this disease, accounting for 28 percent of all cancer deaths. Lung cancer is the leading cause of cancer death among both men and women. More people die of lung cancer than of colon, breast, and prostate cancers combined.

Lung cancer accounts for approximately 13 percent of all new cancers. The average age of people diagnosed with lung cancer is 60.

The five-year survival rate averages 15 percent for all patients with this disease. If the cancer is found very early without any spread to lymph nodes, the five-year survival rate is 48 percent. If cancer has invaded the lymph nodes, this drops to 21 percent.

Risk Factors

- *Smoking.* Most lung cancer occurs as a result of exposure to tobacco (as well as marijuana), therefore most lung cancers occur in smokers. The more cigarettes a person smokes, the greater the risk is of developing lung cancer. If a person stops smoking, the risk of cancer gradually recedes, but it does not return to that of someone who has never smoked. Nonsmokers exposed to secondhand smoke are also at increased risk for lung cancer. A nonsmoker who is married to a smoker has a 30 percent greater risk of developing lung cancer than the spouse of a nonsmoker;

The lungs are two sponge-like organs found in the chest cavity. The right lung has three sections, called lobes. The left lung has two lobes. The lining that surrounds the lungs and helps to protect them and to facilitate the sliding motion during breathing is called the pleura. The chest cavity is called the pleural cavity. The trachea (windpipe) brings air down into the lungs. It divides into tubes called the

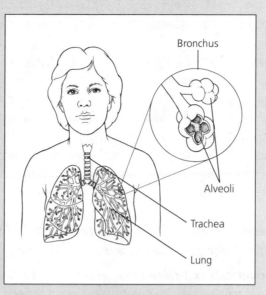

bronchi, which divide into smaller branches called the bronchioles. At the end of the bronchioles are tiny air sacs known as alveoli. Lung cancer usually begins in the lining of the bronchi.

- *Asbestos*. Workers who handle asbestos have a much higher rate of lung cancer. If they smoke, their risk is considerably higher—up to fifty to ninety times that of the general population;

- *Environmental and occupational exposures*. Workers exposed to other cancer-causing agents such as radioactive ores like uranium and chemicals such as arsenic, vinyl chloride, nickel chromates, coal products, mustard gas, and chloromethyl ethers have a higher risk of lung cancer. Even working with fuels such as gasoline may increase a person's risk of developing lung cancer;

- *Radon*. People who have large amounts of radon in their homes from underground seepage are at higher risk;

- *Previous lung damage*. People with scarring in their lungs from old infections such as tuberculosis or exposure to certain mineral dusts such as silica have a higher risk of developing lung cancer;

- *Family history*. People with a strong family history of lung cancer have a higher risk of developing lung cancer.

Types of Lung Cancer

Most lung cancers start in the lining of the bronchi. Less often, cancers begin in the trachea, bronchioles, or alveoli. Lung cancer is usually divided into two major types: small cell lung cancer (SCLC) and non–small cell lung cancer (NSCLC). A mixed small cell/large cell carcinoma may have characteristics of both types.

Small Cell Lung Cancer (SCLC)

About 20 to 30 percent of all lung cancers are SCLC, so named for the size of the cancer cells. Other names for SCLC are oat cell carcinoma and small cell undifferentiated carcinoma. Although each of the cells is small, they can multiply quickly and form large tumors, and they can spread to lymph nodes and other organs such as the bones, brain, adrenal glands, and liver. This type of cancer often starts in the bronchi and metastasizes toward the center of the lungs. Small cell lung cancer is almost always caused by smoking.

Non–Small Cell Lung Cancer (NSCLC)

These subtypes of cancer account for between 70 to 80 percent of lung cancers.

Squamous cell carcinoma. Accounting for approximately 30 percent of all lung cancers, this type of cancer is associated with a history of smoking and tends to be found centrally, near a bronchus;

Adenocarcinoma. This type accounts for about 40 percent of lung cancers and is usually found in the outer region of lung;

Large-cell undifferentiated carcinoma. This type of cancer accounts for about 10 percent of lung cancers. It may appear in any part of the lung.

Other Types of Lung Cancer

Carcinoid tumors of the lung account for less than 5 percent of lung tumors. Most are slow-growing tumors. Other, even more rare lung tumors include adenoid cystic carcinomas, hamartomas, lymphomas, and sarcomas.

Signs and Symptoms

Since symptoms of lung cancer often do not appear until the disease is advanced, only about 15 percent of lung cancer cases are found in the early stages before the cancer has spread to nearby lymph nodes or elsewhere. Lung cancer may cause these signs and symptoms:

- A cough that does not go away;
- Chest pain, often aggravated by deep breathing;
- Hoarseness;
- Weight loss and loss of appetite;
- Bloody or rust-colored sputum;
- Shortness of breath;

- Fever without a clear reason;

- Recurring infections such as bronchitis and pneumonia;

- Wheezing.

  When lung cancer spreads to distant organs, it may cause:

- Bone pain;

- Neurologic changes such as weakness or numbness of a limb or dizziness;

- Jaundice;

- Masses near the surface of the body, due to cancer spreading to the skin or to lymph nodes in the neck or above the collarbone;

- Severe shoulder pain and drooping or weakness of one eyelid, reduced or absent perspiration on the same side of the face, and a smaller pupil in the eye of that side can be caused by a cancer at the top of the lung;

- Weakness can be due to high serum calcium or low serum sodium levels caused by certain hormone-like substances that the tumor produces;

- Excess growth of certain bones is often found in the fingertips (hypertrophic osteoarthropathy);

- Excess breast growth in men.

Diagnostic Tests

- CT scan—a rotating x-ray beam creates a series of pictures of the body taken from many angles;

- MRI scan—uses magnetic fields and radio waves instead of x-rays to create images of selected areas of the body;

- PET scan—images the brain after injection of a very low dose of a radioactive form of a substance;

- Bone scan—this test involves injecting a small amount of radioactive substance into a vein. The substance accumulates in areas of bone that may be abnormal because of cancer metastasis;

- Sputum cytology—a sample of phlegm is examined under a microscope to see if cancer cells are present;

- Needle biopsy—a needle removes a sample of the mass, which can then be examined;

- Bronchoscopy—a flexible, fiberoptic, lighted tube is passed through the mouth into the bronchi to help find some tumors or blockages in the lungs or to take biopsies to be examined under a microscope;

- Mediastinoscopy—a small cut is made in the neck and a hollow lighted tube is inserted behind the sternum (breast bone). Special instruments, operated through this tube, can be used to take a tissue sample from the mediastinal lymph nodes (along the windpipe and the major bronchial tube areas);

- Bone marrow biopsy—a needle is used to remove a sample of bone marrow that can be examined for cancer cells under the microscope;

- Blood tests—certain blood tests can help determine if the lung cancer has spread to the liver or bones and to help diagnose certain paraneoplastic syndromes.

Treatment

Surgery

Surgery may be used to remove the cancer and some of the surrounding lung tissue. If a lobe (section) of the lung is removed, it is called a lobectomy. If the entire lung is removed, the surgery is called a pneumonectomy. Removing part of a lobe is known as a segmentectomy or wedge resection.

Radiation Therapy

Radiation therapy is sometimes used as the primary treatment for lung cancer, especially in some patients whose general health is too poor for them to undergo surgery. External beam radiation therapy is most often used to treat a primary lung cancer or its metastases to other organs. Brachytherapy can be used to help relieve blockage of large airways by cancer.

After surgery, radiation therapy can be used to kill very small deposits of cancer that cannot be seen and removed during surgery. Radiation therapy can also be used to relieve symptoms of lung cancer such as pain, bleeding, difficulty swallowing, and problems caused by brain metastases.

Chemotherapy

Cisplatin (Platinol) or a related drug, carboplatin (Paraplatin), are the chemotherapy drugs most often used in treating both kinds of lung cancer. Usually these drugs are combined with others such as gemcitabine (Gemzar), paclitaxel (Taxol), docetaxel (Taxotere), etoposide (VePesid), or vinorelbine (Navelbine), doxorubicin (Adriamycin), or cyclophosphamide (Cytoxan).

Testes

Key Statistics

Approximately 7,200 new cases of testicular cancer are diagnosed in the United States each year and an estimated 400 men die of this disease. The testicular cancer rate has more than doubled among Caucasians in the past 40 years but has remained the same for African Americans.

Testicular cancer is one of the most curable forms of cancer, with a cure rate of more than 90 percent in all stages combined. The five-year survival rate is over 95 percent.

Each of the two testicles is somewhat smaller than a golf ball. Both are contained within a sac of skin called the scrotum, which hangs below either side of the penis. The testicles manufacture the male hormones, the most abundant of which is testosterone. They also produce sperm, the male reproductive cells. Sperm cells are carried from the testicle by the vas deferens to the seminal vesicles, where they are mixed with fluid produced by the prostate gland.

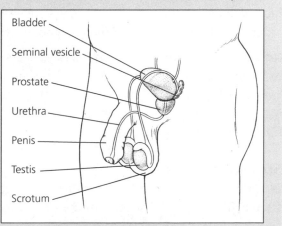

Bladder

Seminal vesicle

Prostate

Urethra

Penis

Testis

Scrotum

Risk Factors

- *Age.* Most testicular cancers occur between the ages of 15 and 40;

- *Cryptorchidism.* About 14 percent of cases of testicle cancer occur in men with a history of cryptorchidism, making this condition the main risk factor. Cryptorchidism occurs when testicles, which develop in the pelvic cavity and then descend into the scrotum, fail to descend. Often they eventually do descend during childhood, which reduces the risk. Men with a cryptorchid testis on one side also have a higher rate of testicular cancer in the normally descended testicle;

- *Family history.* This increases the risk;

- *Cancer of one testicle.* This increases the risk for cancer in the other testicle;

- *Race.* Caucasians have a much higher incidence than any other group.

Types of Testicular Cancer

The testicles contain several types of cells, each of which may develop into one or more types of cancer.

Germ Cell Tumors

Over 90 percent of testicular cancers develop in germ cells. The two main types are seminomas and nonseminomas, but many tumors contain features of both types. Because of the way these "mixed" tumors grow, spread, and respond to treatment, they are classified as being nonseminomas.

Seminoma. About half of all testicle germ cell cancers are seminomas, which develop from the sperm-producing germ cells of the testicle. The main subtypes of these tumors are typical (or classic) seminomas and spermatocytic seminomas. Over 90 percent of seminomas are typical. Most spermatocytic tumors grow very slowly and usually do not metastasize. The average age of men who are diagnosed with spermatocytic seminoma is 65, about 15 years older than the average age of men diagnosed with typical seminoma.

Nonseminoma Germ Cell Cancer. These cancers usually occur in men who are in their 20s. The main types of nonseminoma germ cell cancers are embryonal carcinoma, yolk sac carcinoma, choriocarcinoma, and teratoma. Most tumors are mixed and contain at least two different types of nonseminoma germ cell cancers.

Stromal Tumors

Tumors can also arise in the supportive and hormone-producing tissues, or stroma. These gonadal stromal tumors account for 4 percent of adult testicle tumors and 20 percent of childhood testicular tumors. The two main types are Leydig cell tumors and Sertoli cell tumors.

Leydig Cell Tumors. These develop from normal Leydig cells (also called interstitial cells), which normally produce androgens (male sex hormones). Seventy-five percent of cases develop in adults; 25 percent of cases occur in children. They often produce androgens, but in some cases produce estrogens (female sex hormones).

Sertoli Cell Tumors. These tumors develop from the normal testicular cells of the same name, which support and nourish the sperm-producing germ cells.

Secondary Testicular Tumors

Secondary testicular tumors are those that begin in another organ and then spread to the testicle. Lymphoma is the most common secondary testicular cancer. Among men over 50 years of age, testicular lymphoma is more common than primary testicular tumors.

Signs and Symptoms

- A lump or swelling in a testicle—this occurs in over 90 percent of men and can be painless or cause some discomfort. Men may notice testicular enlargement or swelling. Men with testicular cancer often report a sensation of heaviness or aching in the lower abdomen or scrotum;

- Breast tenderness or breast growth—this is due to hormone production by the tumor;

- Back pain—low back pain is a frequent symptom of later-stage testicle cancer.

Diagnostic Tests

- Ultrasonography (ultrasound)—uses sound waves and their echoes to produce images of internal organs;

- Blood tests—many testicular cancers secrete high levels of certain proteins such as alpha-fetoprotein (AFP) or human chorionic gonadotropin (HCG); blood tests can identify these proteins;

- CT scan of the pelvis and abdomen—this test uses a rotating x-ray beam to create a series of pictures of the body from many angles;

- MRI scan—uses magnetic fields and radio waves instead of x-rays to create images of selected areas of the body;

- Chest x-ray—chest x-rays may be performed if metastasis is suspected.

Treatment

Surgery

Surgery to remove testicular cancer is known as a radical inguinal orchiectomy. An incision is made in the groin and the testicle is withdrawn from the scrotum through the opening. A cut is made through the spermatic cord that attaches the testicle to the abdomen.

Depending on the type and stage of the cancer, lymph nodes may also be removed during a second, more extensive operation. This operation, called retroperitoneal lymph node dissection, can be a major operation.

Radiation Therapy

External beam radiation therapy may follow surgery for seminoma tumors because these tend to spread to local lymph nodes in the abdomen, and radiation can prevent recurrence. Radiation therapy is generally not used for nonseminoma tumors. Radiation will be used to treat the cancer, seminoma, or nonseminoma if it recurs in the brain.

Chemotherapy

Chemotherapy treatment has a very high cure rate even if the cancer is widespread. It is used for anyone with a high risk of spread outside the testis or someone who has demonstrated cancer in lymph nodes or other tissues away from the tumor. It is also used if the cancer recurs after initial surgery.

The main drugs used in various combinations to treat testicle cancer are cisplatin (Platinol), vinblastine (Velban), bleomycin (Blenoxane), cyclophosphamide (Cytoxan), etoposide (VePesid), and ifosfamide (IFEX).

Stem Cell Transplantation

High-dose combination chemotherapy combined with stem cell transplantation is used to treat some patients with advanced germ cell cancer who have not been cured with standard chemotherapy. (See Chapter 14 for more information on stem cell transplants.)

Prostate

Key Statistics

Approximately 198,100 new cases of prostate cancer are diagnosed in the United States each year and about 31,500 men die of this disease. One man in six will be diagnosed with prostate cancer during his lifetime, but only one man in thirty will die of this disease.

Prostate cancer is the second leading cause of cancer death in men in the United States, exceeded only by lung cancer. Prostate cancer accounts for about 11 percent of male cancer-related deaths. It is the cancer that most commonly affects American men, excluding skin cancers.

The five-year survival rate for all stages combined is 96 percent.

> The prostate, found only in men, is a walnut-sized gland located in front of the rectum, at the outlet of the bladder. It contains gland cells that produce some of the seminal fluid, which protects and nourishes sperm cells in semen. Just behind the prostate gland are the seminal vesicles that produce most of the fluid for semen. The prostate surrounds the first part of the urethra, the tube that carries urine and semen through the penis.

Risk Factors

- *Age.* The chance of having prostate cancer increases rapidly after age 50. More than 80 percent of all prostate cancers are diagnosed in men over the age of 65;

- *Race.* Prostate cancer occurs almost 70 percent more often in African-American men than it does in Caucasian men;

- *Diet.* A high-fat diet may increase risk;

- *Family history.* A strong family history of prostate cancer increases the risk;

- *Genetic changes.* Changes in the HPC gene and CAPB gene appear to be responsible for about 5 to 10 percent of prostate cancers.

Types of Prostate Cancer

Ninety-nine percent of prostate cancers are adenocarcinomas that develop from the glandular cells. Other cancers in the prostate are rare. Most prostate cancers grow very slowly.

Prostatic intraepithelial neoplasia (PIN) is a condition in which there are changes in the microscopic appearance (the size, shape, or the rate at which they multiply) of prostate gland cells. PIN is classified as either low grade or high grade and may lead to the development of prostate cancer.

Signs and Symptoms

Early prostate cancer usually causes no symptoms. When symptoms occur, the following are the most common ones:

- Slowing or weakening of the urinary stream or the need to urinate more often may occur, but these symptoms are not specific and are most often caused by benign diseases of the prostate;

- Blood in the urine, difficulty having an erection, and pain in the pelvis, spine, hips, or ribs are symptoms of advanced prostate cancer.

Diagnostic Tests

- Core needle biopsies—samples of tissue are taken from different areas of the prostate and then examined under a microscope. This is the main method used to diagnose prostate cancer;

- CT scan—this x-ray procedure produces detailed cross-sectional images of the body;

- MRI scan—uses magnetic fields and radio waves instead of x-rays to create images of selected areas of the body;

- Radionuclide bone scan—an intravenous injection of radioactive material settles in damaged bone tissue throughout the entire skeleton. This procedure helps show whether the cancer has spread from the prostate gland to bones;

- ProstaScint scan—like the bone scan, the ProstaScint scan uses low-level radioactive material that attaches only to prosatate cells to find cancer that has spread beyond the prostate. The test may also be used if the blood PSA level begins to rise after a period of remission following therapy and other tests are not able to find the exact location of the recurrent cancer;

- Lymph node biopsy—a surgeon or radiologist removes cells from lymph nodes or removes lymph nodes for examination.

Treatment

Surgery

Radical Prostatectomy. In this procedure, the entire prostate gland plus some tissue around it is removed. There are two main types of radical prostatectomy, radical retropubic prostatectomy and radical perineal prostatectomy.

Radical perineal prostatectomy removes the prostate through an incision in the perineum, the skin between the anus and scrotum. This procedure is used less often than retropubic surgery because the nerves cannot be spared and lymph nodes can't be removed during radical perineal prostatectomy. Retropubic surgery involves making an incision in the pelvis and can allow the surgeon to avoid damaging the nerves responsible for erections as well as making it possible to biopsy lymph nodes.

Cryosurgery. Cryosurgery (also called cryotherapy or cryoablation) is used to treat localized prostate cancer by freezing the cells with a metal probe. Warm salt water is circulated through a catheter in the urethra to keep it from freezing. The probe is placed through a skin incision located between the anus and scrotum and is guided into the cancer using transrectal ultrasound.

Radiation Therapy

Radiation is also used to treat cancer that is still confined within the prostate gland or that only has spread to nearby tissue. If the disease is more advanced, radiation may be used to reduce the size of the tumor and to provide relief from present and future symptoms. Radiation usually eliminates the need for surgery. Men who do not respond well to radiation therapy can sometimes still have surgery ("salvage prostatectomy") at a later date.

External Beam Radiation Therapy. Radiation is directed at the prostate gland from an external source. A new approach, three-dimensional conformal radiation therapy, uses sophisticated computers to precisely map the location of the cancer within the prostate, and radiation beams are then aimed at the tumor from several directions. Conformal proton beam radiation therapy uses a similar approach in focusing proton beams on the cancer. Both may reduce the side effects of radiation.

Brachytherapy. Radioactive materials are placed inside thin needles, which are inserted through the skin of the perineum (area between the scrotum and anus) into the prostate. These can be left in for a very short time and then removed and often combined with external beam radiation, or they can be left in permanently.

Strontium 89. This palliative treatment injects a radioactive substance into a vein, where it settles in areas of bone containing cancer. The radiation given off by the strontium 89 kills the cancer cells and relieves the pain caused by bone metastases. About 80 percent of prostate cancer patients with painful bone metastases are helped by this treatment.

Hormone Ablation Therapy

Because prostate cancer is often stimulated to grow by a man's naturally occurring testosterone, removing testosterone will often cause the cancer to shrink. Although this is mostly used to palliate widespread cancer, it is often used temporarily during initial treatment.

Orchiectomy. Removing the testicles—the main source of male hormones— can shrink most prostate cancers.

Luteinizing Hormone–Releasing Hormone (LHRH) Analogs. Leuprolide (Lupron), and goserelin (Zoladex) lower testosterone levels as effectively as orchiectomy by decreasing the androgens produced by a man's testicles. LHRH analogs (also called LHRH agonists) are injected either monthly or every three to four months.

Anti-Androgens. Even after orchiectomy or during treatment with LHRH analogs, a small amount of androgen is still produced by the adrenal glands. Drugs such as flutamide (Eulexin), bicalutamide (Casodex), and nilutamide (Nilandron) block the body's ability to use androgens.

Chemotherapy

Chemotherapy is sometimes used when prostate cancer has spread outside the prostate gland and hormone therapy isn't working. This treatment may slow the cancer's growth and reduce pain. Chemotherapy is not recommended as a treatment for early prostate cancer.

Some of the chemotherapy drugs used to treat prostate cancer that has returned or continued to grow and spread after treatment with hormonal therapy are doxorubicin (Adriamycin), estramustine (Emcyt), etoposide (VePesid), mitoxantrone (Novantrone), vinblastine (Velban), and paclitaxel (Taxol).

Expectant Therapy (Watching and Waiting)

Because prostate cancer often spreads very slowly, older men or those with serious health problems may never need treatment. Some men choose watchful waiting because they think the side effects of aggressive treatment outweigh their benefits. Follow-up care is still necessary and if bothersome symptoms develop or the cancer begins to grow more quickly, active treatment may be considered.

Penis

Key Statistics

Penile cancer is rare in this country; however, it is much more common in other parts of the world. Approximately 1,200 new cases of penile cancer are diagnosed in the United States each year and an estimated 300 men die of this disease.

The five-year survival rate for men with localized disease is 80 percent for local disease, 52 percent if lymph nodes are involved, and 18 percent if the cancer has spread elsewhere.

The penis is the external male genital organ and contains several types of tissue, including skin, nerves, smooth muscle, and blood vessels. Inside the penis is the urethra, the tube through which urine and semen exit the body. The head of the penis is called the glans. At birth, the glans is covered by a loose piece of skin called the foreskin or prepuce.

Risk Factors

- *Foreskin.* Men who were circumcised at birth rarely develop this disease;

- *Human papillomavirus infection.* This sexually transmitted infection is associated with penile cancer. The likelihood of developing this infection is increased if a man has unprotected sexual relations with multiple partners or has a partner with this infection;

- *Smoking.* The cancer-causing chemicals in tobacco are believed to damage the DNA of cells in the penis and contribute to the development of penile cancer, especially in men who also have HPV infections;

- *Ultraviolet light exposure.* There is a higher rate of penile cancer among men who have a skin disease called psoriasis and who have been treated with a combination involving a drug called psoralen and exposure to ultraviolet light.

Types of Penile Cancer

Different types of penile cancer can develop in each kind of cell the structure contains. The differences are important, because they determine the seriousness of the cancer and the type of treatment needed.

Squamous Cell Cancer

About 95 percent of penile cancers develop from flat, scale-like skin cells called squamous cells. Squamous cell penile cancers can develop anywhere on the organ, but most develop on the foreskin (in men who have not been circumcised) or on the glans.

Signs and Symptoms

Most penile cancers do not cause pain. When symptoms occur, the following are the most common ones:

- A painless ulcer or growth on the penis—especially on the glans or foreskin, but also sometimes developing on the shaft. In most cases, this is the first sign of penile cancer;

- Rash-like symptoms—a reddish, velvety rash, small crusty bumps, or flat growths that are bluish-brown in color. They may not be visible unless the foreskin is pulled back;

- A persistent discharge—usually with a foul odor, may be present beneath the foreskin;

- Changes in color, skin thickening, or accumulation of tissue;

- Ulceration and bleeding;

- Swollen lymph nodes in the groin—if cancer has progressed to a more advanced stage.

Diagnostic Tests

- Excisional or incisional biopsy—in an excisional biopsy, the entire lesion is removed. An incisional biopsy, which removes only a portion of the affected tissue, is performed on a large or ulcerated lesion or one that appears to grow deeply into the tissue;

- CT scan—a rotating x-ray beam creates a series of pictures of the body taken from many angles;

- MRI scan—uses magnetic fields and radio waves instead of x-rays to create images of selected areas of the body;

- Fine needle aspiration (FNA)—a thin needle is used to withdraw fluid or small samples of tissue from the tumor mass so that cells can be examined with a microscope;

- Sentinel lymph node biopsy—a radioactive tracer and/or a blue dye is injected into the region of the tumor and is carried by the lymphatic vessels to a lymph node. If this node contains cancer, more lymph nodes are removed. If the node is free of cancer, additional lymph node surgery may be avoided.

Treatment

Surgery

Surgery is the most common treatment for all stages of penile cancer.

Excision (Excisional Biopsy). Simple excision of the tumor along with some surrounding normal skin. The remaining skin is carefully stitched back together.

Electrodesiccation and Curettage. Curettage involves removing the cancer by scraping with a curette (a long, thin instrument with a scraping edge, similar in appearance to a vegetable peeler). Electrodesiccation is then done on the area. An electric current delivered through a needle destroys any remaining cancer cells. Electrodesiccation and curettage is a good treatment for small basal cell and squamous cell (skin) cancers on the penis.

Cryosurgery. Liquid nitrogen is used to freeze and kill abnormal cells in precancerous conditions and small basal cell and squamous cell carcinomas. After the dead tissue thaws, blistering and crusting may occur.

Mohs' Surgery (Microscopically Controlled Surgery). During this highly specialized procedure, the surgeon removes a layer of the skin that the tumor may have invaded and then carefully marks its location with colored dyes. The surgeon checks the sample under a microscope immediately. If it is malignant, more pieces of the tumor will be removed in a similar fashion and examined until the skin samples are found to be free of cancerous cells.

Laser Surgery. This process, in which a beam of laser light vaporizes cancer cells, is useful for squamous cell carcinoma in situ (involving only the outer layer of the skin or epidermis) and for very superficial basal cell carcinomas (types of skin cancer).

Other Procedures

- Amputation or penectomy removes part or all of the penis;

- Partial penectomy removes only the end of the penis. The surgeon leaves enough of the shaft to allow the man to direct his stream of urine away from his body;

- A total penectomy removes the entire penis, including the roots that extend into the pelvis. The surgeon creates a new opening for the urethra (tube from the bladder) between the man's scrotum (sac for the testicles) and his anus. The man can still control his urination, because the "on-off" valve in the urethra is above the level of the penis;

- Lymphadenectomy. In this procedure, lymph nodes may be surgically removed from both groins since they may contain cancer. Lymphadenectomy is performed on larger cancers.

Radiation Therapy

External beam radiation therapy or brachytherapy may be used as an alternative to surgery and may help some men avoid partial or complete amputation of the penis. Radiation therapy of groin and pelvic lymph nodes may be used as an alternative to their surgical removal or to reduce the risk of penile cancer coming back.

Chemotherapy

Topical chemotherapy using fluorouracil (5-FU) generally is used only for premalignant conditions or CIS. Systemic chemotherapy using cisplatin (Platinol), vincristine (Oncovin), methotrexate, and bleomycin (Blenoxane) can temporarily delay the spread of advanced penile cancers and relieve some symptoms. These drugs are also being studied as an adjuvant therapy to prevent or delay cancer recurrence after surgery.

Melanoma

Key Statistics

Approximately 51,400 new cases of melanoma (29,000 men and 22,400 women) are diagnosed in the United States each year and about 7,800 people (5,000 men and 2,800 women) die of this disease. Although melanoma accounts for only 4 percent of skin cancer cases, it causes about 79 percent of skin cancer deaths.

The number of new melanomas diagnosed in the United States is increasing. Since 1973, the incidence rate for melanoma has more than doubled from approximately 6 to 14 percent and the mortality rate has increased by about 44 percent.

The five-year survival rate of all patients is 89 percent. It is 96 percent when the melanoma is discovered early.

Melanoma is a cancer that begins in the melanocytes, the cells that produce the skin coloring or pigment known as melanin. Other names for this cancer include malignant melanoma, melanoma skin cancer, and cutaneous melanoma.

Melanoma most often appears on the trunk of fair-skinned men and on the lower legs of fair-skinned women, but people with other skin types are commonly affected, as are other areas of the skin. Rarely, melanomas can form in parts of the body not covered by skin, such as the eyes, mouth, vagina, large intestine, and other internal organs.

Risk Factors

- *Ultraviolet light exposure.* This is the major risk factor. Sunlight as well as light from tanning lamps and booths are sources. People with excessive exposure are at greater risk for skin cancer, including melanoma. People who suffer severe, blistering sunburns, particularly in their childhood or teenage years, are also at increased risk of developing melanoma. Intermittent, intense exposures are more associated with melanoma risk than lower level, chronic exposures, even if the total dose of UV is the same;

- *Moles.* Someone with many moles, particularly with dysplastic nevi (an atypical mole; nevus is the medical name for a mole, and dysplastic means atypical), has a higher risk—6 to 10 percent. If two or more of a person's close relatives have melanoma, a person's risk goes to 50 percent;

- *Genetics.* As many as 10 percent of melanomas occur in people with a strong family history of melanoma. Several changes in chromosome have been described in these families. Many of these people have congenital melanocytic nevi, where the average lifetime risk of developing melanoma may be about 6 percent;

- *Race.* The risk of melanoma is about twenty times higher for Caucasians than for African Americans. This is due to the protective effect of skin pigment. Whites with red or blond hair and fair skin that freckles or burns easily are at especially high risk.

Types of Melanoma

Of the four types of melanoma, superficial spreading melanoma is the most common (70 percent) and tends to be flat. Nodular melanomas are smooth nodules and are the next most common. Lentigo maligna melanoma, a kind that tends to occur in highly sun-exposed areas such as the hands and the back of neck, is the next most common. Acral lentiginous melanomas occur on palms, soles, and nail beds.

Signs and Symptoms

Most people have moles, and almost all moles are harmless. But it is important to recognize changes in a mole that can suggest a melanoma may be developing. The ABCD rule can help distinguish a normal mole from a melanoma.

- Asymmetry—one half of the mole does not match the other half;

- Border irregularity—the edges of the mole are ragged or notched;

- Color—the color over the mole is not the same. It may include differing shades of tan, brown, or black, and sometimes patches of red, blue, or white;

- Diameter:—the mole is wider than six millimeters, or about ¼ inch (although doctors are finding more melanomas between three and six millimeters in recent years).

Some melanomas do not fit the ABCD rule described above, so it is particularly important to be aware of *changes* in the shape, size, and color of skin lesions.

Diagnostic Tests

Skin Biopsy

- Punch biopsy—removes a sample of skin. It cuts through all the layers of the skin, including the dermis, epidermis, and the upper parts of the subcutis;

- Incisional and excisional biopsies—an incisional biopsy removes only a portion of the tumor. Removal of the entire tumor is called an excisional biopsy;

- Lymph node biopsy—this procedure involves removing an abnormally large lymph node surgically, through a small skin incision;

- Chest x-rays—chest x-rays can detect lung metastases.

Treatment

Surgery

Simple Excision. Thin melanomas can be completely cured by a relatively minor surgery called simple excision. The tumor is cut out, along with a small amount of normal, noncancerous skin at the edges.

Re-Excision (Wide Excision). When the diagnosis of melanoma is established by biopsy, the site will need to be excised again. More skin will be cut away from the melanoma site and the tissue from the final excision will be examined to make sure that no cancer cells remain in the skin.

Amputation. If the melanoma is on a finger or toe, the treatment is to amputate as much of that digit as necessary.

Therapeutic Lymph Node Dissection. This procedure removes most of the lymph nodes in the area of the melanoma for microscopic examination. It is often done if fine needle aspiration biopsy (FNA) or excisional lymph node biopsy shows evidence of melanoma.

Some doctors recommend a lymph node dissection for all patients who might have melanoma in their lymph nodes. If the lymph nodes are not enlarged, then a sentinel node biopsy procedure may be done. If the sentinel lymph node does not show cancer, then it is unlikely the melanoma has spread to the lymph nodes; there is no need for a lymph node dissection.

Surgery for Metastatic Melanoma

Sometimes removing a melanoma deposit that has come back in another organ can be life-saving. However, if there are many lesions, surgery will not be effective.

Chemotherapy

Chemotherapy drugs used to treat melanoma that has become widespread include dacarbazine (DTIC-Dome), carmustine (BiCNU), and cisplatin (Platinol). These are often used in combination. About 20 to 30 percent of people treated will have a temporary remission of their melanoma.

Radiation Therapy

The main role of external beam radiation therapy for melanoma is palliation (to relieve symptoms) of metastases to the brain or perhaps bone.

Immunotherapy

Two cytokines, interferon-alpha and interleukin-2, are used to treat patients with melanoma. Both drugs can help shrink metastatic melanomas in about 10 to 20 percent of patients. Interferon-alpha is also used after surgery in patients with particularly high-risk melanomas to prevent recurrence.

Nonmelanoma

Key Statistics

Cancer of the skin is the most common cancer, accounting for more than 40 percent of all cancers. Approximately 1.3 million cases of nonmelanoma skin cancer are diagnosed in the United States each year. Men have a slightly higher incidence of basal cell carcinomas than women. Approximately 2,000 people die from nonmelanoma skin cancer each year. (These figures are estimates because doctors are not required to report cases of nonmelanoma skin cancer to cancer registries.)

The five-year survival rate is over 99 percent.

The skin has three layers called the epidermis, dermis, and subcutis. The top layer is the epidermis. This is where skin cancer forms. The two major cell types are the squamous cells, called keratinocytes, which are the outer layer, and the basal cells that lie below the keratinocytes. Basal cells continually divide to form new keratinocytes, which replace older keratinocytes that wear off of the skin surface. Melanocytes are also present in the epidermis. These skin cells produce the protective pigment called melanin.

The middle layer of the skin is called the dermis. It contains hair follicles, sweat glands, blood vessels, and nerves that are held in place by a protein called collagen, which gives the skin its resilience and strength.

The last and deepest layer of the skin is called the subcutis. The subcutis and the lowest part of the dermis form a network of collagen and fat cells.

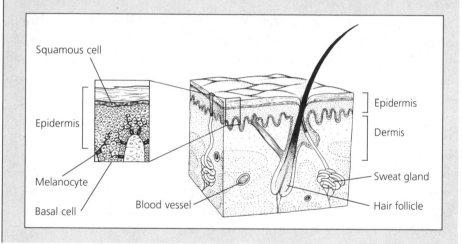

Risk Factors

* *Exposure to ultraviolet (UV) light.* UV light is the major risk factor for this cancer. People who are often exposed to strong sunlight (the main source of UV radiation) without protection have a greater risk of developing nonmelanoma skin cancer. Tanning lamps and tanning booths also increase the risk of nonmelanoma skin cancer;

* *Fair skin.* The fairer the skin, the higher the risk of developing this cancer;

* *Radiation.* People who have had radiation treatment have a higher risk of developing nonmelanoma skin cancer in the area that received the treatment;

* *Arsenic.* Excess arsenic exposure, either by ingestion or directly to the skin, increases the risk of skin cancer;

- *Psoriasis treatment.* Psoralen and ultraviolet light treatments (PUVA) given to some patients with psoriasis can increase the risk of developing squamous cell skin cancer, and probably other skin cancers;

- *Immune deficiency.* This increases the rate of skin cancer;

- *Genetic disorders.* Xeroderma pigmentosa, a rare inherited condition, reduces the skin's ability to repair damage to DNA caused by sun exposure and basal cell nevus syndrome, a disorder that is usually inherited and leads to multiple basal cell carcinomas.

Types of Nonmelanoma Skin Cancer

The two most common types of nonmelanoma skin cancer are basal cell carcinoma and squamous cell carcinoma.

Basal Cell Carcinoma

About 75 percent of all skin cancers begin in the deepest layer of the epidermis, the basal cell layer. These basal cell carcinomas usually develop on sun-exposed areas, especially the head and neck. Basal cell carcinoma is slow-growing and rarely spreads unless left untreated. It tends to recur in the original site as well as elsewhere on the skin.

Squamous Cell Carcinoma

Squamous cell carcinomas develop in higher levels of the epidermis and account for about 20 to 25 percent of all skin cancers. They commonly appear on sun-exposed areas of the body such as the face, ear, neck, lip, and back of the hands. They can also develop within scars or skin ulcers elsewhere. Squamous cell carcinomas tend to be more aggressive than basal cell cancers and more likely to spread.

Less Common Types of Nonmelanoma Skin Cancer

Because the skin contains cells other than basal cells and squamous cells, other cancers can develop as well. These are lymphomas, sarcomas, Merkel cell carcinomas, adnexal carcinomas, sebaceous carcinomas, and atypical fibroxanthomas. Together, they account for less than 1 percent of non-melanoma skin cancers.

Precancerous and Preinvasive Skin Conditions

Actinic Keratosis. Overexposure to the sun causes these small (usually less than ¼ inch) rough spots that may be pink-red or flesh-colored to develop on the face, ears, back of the hands, and arms of middle-aged or older people with fair skin. However, they can arise on other sun-exposed areas as well.

People with one actinic keratosis will usually develop many more. These occasionally develop into squamous cell carcinomas.

Squamous Cell Carcinoma In Situ. The cells of these early cancers, also called Bowen's disease, are entirely within the epidermis and have not invaded the dermis. Compared with actinic keratoses, Bowen's disease patches tend to be larger (often over ½ inch), redder, more scaly, and crusted. (Bowen's disease of the anal and genital skin is often related to sexually transmitted HPV infection.)

Signs and Symptoms

- A new growth, spot, or bump that's getting larger (over a few months or one to two years)—this is the major sign of nonmelanoma skin cancer. Generally, the surface of these growths is rough, the shape is irregular, and the spot is often reddish in color;

- A sore that doesn't heal within three months.

Diagnostic Tests

- Shave biopsy—the doctor "shaves" off the top layers of the skin (the epidermis and the most superficial part of the dermis) with a surgical blade;

- Punch biopsy—a punch biopsy removes a sample of skin. It cuts through all the layers of the skin, including the dermis, epidermis, and the upper parts of the subcutis;

- Excisional or incisional biopsy—in an excisional biopsy, the entire lesion is removed. An incisional biopsy, which removes only a portion of the affected tissue, is performed on a large or ulcerated lesion or one that appears to grow deeply into the tissue.

Treatment

The treatments described in this section apply to actinic keratosis, squamous cell carcinoma, basal cell carcinoma, and Merkel cell carcinoma. Cutaneous lymphoma, Kaposi's sarcoma (see pages 565–568), and other sarcomas are treated differently.

Surgery

Fortunately, most basal cell and squamous cell carcinomas can be completely cured by fairly minor surgery.

Simple Excision. Thin lesions can be completely cured by a relatively minor surgery called simple excision. The area is cut out, along with a small amount of skin at the edges.

Curettage and Electrodesiccation. Curettage involves scraping the cancer off the skin, and electrodesiccation involves using a slight electric current to kill any remaining cells.

Cryosurgery. Liquid nitrogen freezes and kills abnormal cells. Cryosurgery is often used for precancerous conditions such as actinic keratosis and for small basal cell and squamous cell carcinomas.

Mohs' Surgery (Microscopically Controlled Surgery). This is used for cancers of cosmetically important areas such as the face because it minimizes the amount of normal tissue removed. Thin slices of the tumor are removed and each slice is examined immediately under the microscope. The surgeon continues to remove more slices until the cancer is completely removed.

Laser Surgery. This relatively new approach uses a beam of laser light to vaporize cancer cells. It is useful for squamous cell carcinoma in situ (which involves only the epidermis) and for very superficial basal cell carcinomas.

Lymph Node Surgery. If lymph nodes near a nonmelanoma skin cancer (especially a squamous cell or Merkel cell carcinoma) are growing larger, doctors will remove them.

Chemotherapy

Topical Chemotherapy. An anticancer medication such as fluorouracil (5-FU) is placed directly onto the skin. It is generally used only for premalignant conditions such as actinic keratosis.

Systemic Chemotherapy. One or more chemotherapy drugs may be used to treat squamous cell carcinoma or Merkel cell carcinoma that has metastasized (spread) to other organs. Some chemotherapy drugs such as cisplatin (Platinol), doxorubicin (Adriamycin), fluorouracil (5-FU), or mitomycin (Mutamycin) can temporarily delay the spread of these cancers and relieve some symptoms. However, systemic chemotherapy (alone or together with radiation therapy) is not able to cure metastatic nonmelanoma skin cancer.

Radiation Therapy

If a tumor is very large or is located on an area of the skin that makes surgery difficult, external beam radiation therapy may be used as the primary treatment instead of surgery. Primary radiation therapy is often useful for some elderly patients who, because of poor general health, cannot tolerate surgery. It can cure small cancers and delay the growth of more advanced ones. It may also be used to treat nonmelanoma skin cancer that has spread to lymph nodes or other organs. In some cases, radiation can be used after surgery as adjuvant therapy.

Kidney

Key Statistics

Approximately 30,800 new cases of kidney cancer (18,700 men and 12,100 women) are diagnosed in the United States each year and about 12,100 people (7,500 men and 4,600 women) die from this disease. These statistics include both adults and children.

The five-year survival rate for all patients with kidney cancer is 62 percent. It is 89 percent if the cancer has not spread outside the kidney.

Risk Factors

- *Smoking*. About 30 percent of renal cell carcinoma (RCC; the most common type of kidney cancer) in men and 25 percent in women may be due directly to smoking. Smoking doubles the risk of developing RCC;

- *Analgesic abuse*. The overuse of phenacetin-containing pain killers (no longer available in the United States) increases the risk for kidney cancer;

- *Occupational exposures*. Exposure to materials such as asbestos, petroleum products, cadmium, and some organic solvents increases risk;

- *Genetic disorders of the kidney*. Disorders such as tuberous sclerosis, von Hippel-Lindau disease, or a strong family history of kidney cancer increase risk;

- *Obesity*. A very overweight person has a much higher risk of developing renal cell cancer;

The kidneys are two large bean-shaped organs fixed to the upper back wall of the abdominal cavity on either side of the backbone. Both are protected by the lower ribcage.

The kidneys' main job is to filter the blood and rid the body of excess water, salt, and waste products. The filtered waste products are concentrated into urine. Urine leaves the kidneys through long slender tubes called ureters that connect to the bladder. Urine flows down the ureters into the bladder, where it is stored until urination. The bladder empties the urine through a tube called the urethra.

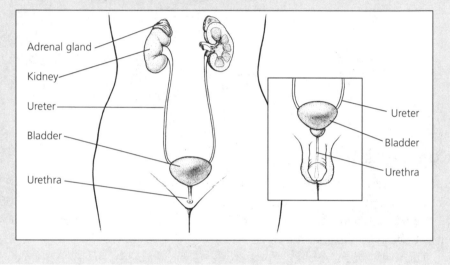

- *Long-term kidney failure*. This can lead to cyst formation in the kidney and can increase the cancer risk;

- *Age*. Most renal cell carcinomas occur in adults between the ages of 50 and 70;

- *Gender*. RCC is about twice as common in men as in women.

Types of Kidney Cancer

Kidney Cancer or Renal Cell Carcinoma (RCC)

This is the most common kidney cancer and accounts for more than 85 percent of malignant kidney tumors. RCC begins small and usually grows as a single mass. Sometimes a kidney may contain more than one tumor, or tumors may be found in both kidneys at the same time.

Clear Cell Type. These cancer cells, which contain fat or sugar, look almost invisible or clear.

Granular Cell Type. These tumor cells are full of tiny pink granules called mitochondria. Mitochondria are like tiny power plants that provide energy for a cell. The mixed type of RCC contains both clear and granular cells. The spindle cell type of RCC means that the tumor contains long cells with pointed ends.

Other Types of Kidney Tumors

About 7 percent of all kidney tumors are transitional cell carcinomas. Transitional cell carcinomas begin in the renal pelvis, the junction of the ureter and the kidney. They are made up of cells different from RCC and therefore look very different under the microscope. Studies have shown that these cancers are highly linked to cigarette smoking. About 90 percent of transitional cell carcinomas of the kidney are curable if they are found early enough.

Renal sarcomas are a rare type of kidney cancer (less than 1 percent of all kidney tumors) that begins within the kidney's connective tissue.

Signs and Symptoms

- Blood in the urine (hematuria);
- Low back pain not associated with injury;
- A mass or lump in the abdomen (belly);
- Fatigue;
- Weight loss that is rapid or not intentional;
- Fever not associated with a cold, flu, or other infection;
- Swelling of ankles and legs (edema);
- High blood pressure.

Diagnostic Tests

- CT scan—a rotating x-ray beam creates a series of pictures of the body taken from many angles;
- MRI scan—uses magnetic fields and radio waves instead of x-rays to create images of selected areas of the body;
- Ultrasonography (ultrasound)—uses sound waves and their echoes to produce images of internal organs;
- Intravenous pyelogram (IVP)—in this older x-ray procedure a special contrast dye is injected into a vein. The dye is concentrated in and secreted by the kidneys into the urine. IVP can help identify a cancer or show kidney damage caused by the tumor;

- Angiography—contrast dye is injected into an artery leading to the kidney to outline blood vessels. It helps diagnose renal cancers since they have a special appearance with this test;

- Chest x-ray—a chest x-ray is used to see if the cancer has spread to the lungs;

- Bone scan—uses small amounts of a special radioactive material that is injected into the blood stream and helps doctors identify diseases;

- Urinalysis—special microscopic examination of urine samples can show actual cancer cells in the urine;

- Blood tests—a complete blood count and chemical test of the blood can detect some findings associated with renal cell cancer;

- Fine needle aspiration (FNA)—a thin needle is used to withdraw fluid or small samples of tissue from the tumor mass so that cells can be examined with a microscope.

Treatment

Surgery

The chances of surviving a RCC without having surgery are poor. Depending on the type and stage, surgery may be used to remove the cancer together with some of the surrounding kidney tissue or the entire kidney. Sometimes it is necessary to remove the adrenal gland above the each kidney, depending on the location of the tumor.

Radical Nephrectomy. This commonly performed surgery removes the whole kidney (along with its cancer), the attached adrenal gland, and the fatty tissue immediately around the kidney. Regional lymphadenectomy to remove nearby lymph nodes is usually done along with the radical nephrectomy.

Partial Nephrectomy. This procedure removes only the part of the kidney containing cancer the cancer, leaving the rest of the organ behind. Partial nephrectomies are often done in patients with cancer in both kidneys, or in patients with only one kidney who develop RCC. More and more partial nephrectomies are being done in patients with small RCCs (smaller than three centimeters or about 1¼ inches) in one of their kidneys.

Removal of Metastases. About one-third of patients with RCC already have metastatic spread of their cancer. Sometimes surgical removal of the metastases will temporarily relieve the pain and some other symptoms of metastatic disease. Occasionally, removal of metastases, if there are only a few, can be curative.

Arterial Embolization. A very small catheter (tube) is placed in an artery in the groin and pushed through the vessel until it reaches the kidney's artery. Material is then injected into the artery to block it. This procedure, while rarely performed, is sometimes done before nephrectomy to reduce bleeding during the operation.

Chemotherapy

RCC is very resistant to chemotherapy. There is no standard way to treat it with drugs. Some drugs, such as vinblastine (Velban), floxuridine (FUDR), and fluorouracil (5-FU), are mildly effective.

Radiation Therapy

RCC is not very sensitive to radiation. Use of radiation therapy before or after removing the cancer is not routinely recommended. However, radiation may be useful to palliate or ease symptoms such as pain, bleeding, or problems caused by metastases.

Immunotherapy

Several types of immunotherapy are used to treat patients with metastatic RCC.

Cytokines. These proteins activate the immune system. Interleukin-2 (IL-2) and interferon-alpha have become two of the standard treatments for metastatic RCC. Both cytokines cause these cancers to shrink to less than half their original size in about 20 percent of patients. Patients who respond to IL-2 tend to have lasting responses. Cytokines are also used to stimulate immune system cells that have been removed from the patient.

Bladder

Key Statistics

Approximately 54,300 new cases of bladder cancer (39,200 men and 15,100 women) are diagnosed in the United States each year and about 12,400 people (about 8,300 men and 4,100 women) die of this disease. Bladder cancer is the sixth most common cancer in the United States, excluding skin cancers.

The five-year survival rate for all patients is 81 percent. It is 94 percent for patients with localized cancer.

> The bladder is a hollow pelvic organ with flexible, muscular walls. It stores urine, which is made by the kidneys and is carried to the bladder by two tubes called ureters. The bladder empties the urine through another tube called the urethra. In women, the urethra is a very short tube that ends just in front of the vagina. In men, the urethra is longer. It passes through the prostate gland and the penis and ends at the tip of the penis.
>
> The wall of the bladder has several layers. A layer of cells lines the inside of the kidney, ureter, bladder, and urethra. This layer is called the urothelium or transitional epithelium. Beneath the urothelium is a thin zone of connective tissue called the lamina propria. The next deeper layer is a wider zone of muscle tissue called the muscularis propria. Beyond this muscle, another zone of fatty connective tissue separates the bladder from other nearby organs.

Risk Factors

- *Smoking.* Smokers are more than twice as likely to get bladder cancer as nonsmokers. Smoking causes about half of the deaths from bladder cancer among men and over one-third of bladder cancer deaths in women. Cancer-causing substances in tobacco smoke are absorbed from the lungs and get into the blood where they are filtered by the kidneys and concentrated in the urine;

- *Occupational exposure to certain chemicals.* Industrial chemicals called aromatic amines, such as benzidine and beta-naphthylamine, which are sometimes used in the dye industry, can cause bladder cancer. Other industries in which certain organic chemicals are used may also put workers at risk for bladder cancer, including the makers of rubber, leather, textiles, and paint products as well as printing companies. Smoking further increases the risk;

- *Race.* Caucasians are two times more likely to develop bladder cancer than are African Americans;

- *Age.* Risk increases with age. The average age at diagnosis is 68 to 69 years. Less than 1 percent of bladder cancers occur among people under age 40;

- *Chronic bladder inflammation.* Urinary infections, kidney and bladder stones, and other causes of chronic bladder irritation have been linked with bladder cancer (especially squamous cell carcinoma of the bladder). A parasitic worm found mostly in northern Africa, called *Schistosoma hematobium,* which can get into the bladder, is also a risk factor for bladder cancer.

Types of Bladder Cancer

Three main types of cancers affect the bladder. Urothelial carcinoma (also known as transitional cell carcinoma or TCC) is by far the most common form of bladder cancer, accounting for more than 90 percent of these cancers. Squamous cell carcinomas account for only about 3 to 8 percent of bladder cancers, but nearly all of them are invasive. Adenocarcinomas account for only about 1 to 2 percent of bladder cancers, and nearly all of them are invasive.

Urothelial Tumors

Not all urothelial tumors are the same. They are divided into subtypes according to whether they are noninvasive or invasive and whether their shape is papillary or flat.

Papillary. Papillary tumors have slender finger-like projections that grow into the hollow center of the bladder. Some grow only toward the center of the bladder. They can be noninvasive, which means that the cancer involves only the innermost layer of the bladder, the urothelium, or they can be invasive, which means they have spread to deeper layers of the bladder.

Nonpapillary or Transitional Cell Carcinoma. These are flat tumors that can be noninvasive or invasive.

Signs and Symptoms

- Blood in the urine—this is the single most important sign of bladder cancer;

- Change in bladder habits—feeling a need to urinate more often than usual can be a sign of bladder cancer.

Diagnostic Tests

- Cystoscopy—a slender tube with a lens and a light is placed into the bladder through the urethra to check for possible cancers;

- Urine cytology—urine is examined under a microscope to find any cancerous or precancerous cells;

- Biopsy—a sample of tissue is removed for examination;

- Bladder tumor marker studies—these chemical or immunologic (using antibodies) tests to detect specific substances are released by bladder cancer cells into the urine;

- Intravenous pyelogram (IVP)—a dye that concentrates in the kidneys is injected through a vein into the bloodstream. An x-ray of the kidneys is taken, and any tumor or other abnormality that is causing the blood in the urine can then be seen;

- Retrograde pyelography—uses special dye to outline the lining of the bladder, ureters, and kidneys on x-rays;

- Chest x-ray—is done to look for any mass or spot on the lungs, if it is suspected that the bladder cancer has spread distantly;

- CT scan—a rotating x-ray beam creates a series of pictures of the body taken from many angles;

- MRI scan—uses magnetic fields and radio waves instead of x-rays to create images of selected areas of the body;

- Ultrasonography (ultrasound)—uses sound waves and their echoes to produce images of internal organs;

- Bone scan—involves injecting a small amount of radioactive substance into a vein. The substance accumulates in areas of bone that may be abnormal because of cancer metastasis (spread).

Treatment

Surgery

Transurethral Surgery. For early stage or superficial bladder cancers, a transurethral resection (TUR) is the most common operation. It is done using a cystoscope. Any remaining cancer may be treated using the cystoscope by fulguration burning the base of the tumor. Cancer can also be destroyed using the cystoscope and a high-energy laser.

Cystectomy. When invasive bladder cancer is present, it is usually necessary to remove the diseased area by cutting completely through the bladder wall. In rare cases if the cancer is not very large, it may be possible to remove it by a partial cystectomy. In this operation, only a part of the bladder is removed. If the cancer is larger or if more than one area of cancer is present, a radical cystectomy is done to remove the entire bladder and nearby lymph nodes. In men, the prostate is also removed. In women, the uterus (womb), ovaries, a small portion of the vagina, and fallopian tubes are routinely removed with the bladder.

Reconstructive Surgery. If the whole bladder is removed, a urostomy may be needed. A short piece of intestine is separated and attached to the ureters. Urine from the ureters flows into this small sac, which is connected to the skin of the abdomen.

Another option is a continent diversion. Urine is stored in the intestinal sac and emptied only when the patient places a drainage tube (catheter) into the hole. There is no bag on the outside. Sometimes a diversion is made without removing the bladder to relieve blockage of urine flow when a tumor has spread or cannot be removed.

Intravesical Therapy

Intravesical Chemotherapy. A medication placed directly into the bladder can reach cancer cells near the bladder lining but does not reach cancer cells in the kidneys, ureters, and urethra. This treatment uses drugs such as mitomycin (Mutamycin), doxorubicin (Adriamycin), epirubicin (Ellence), and thiotepa (Thiotepa can be absorbed from the bladder and cause toxicity in the rest of the body).

Intravesical Immunotherapy

Intravesical immunotherapy uses Bacillus Calmette-Guerin (BCG), a tuberculosis vaccine, which is thought to stimulate an immune response in the bladder and eliminate small tumors.

Systemic Chemotherapy. The chemotherapy combinations used most often for bladder cancer are M-VAC (methotrexate, vinblastine, doxorubicin [Adriamycin], and cisplatin) and MCV (methotrexate, cisplatin, and vinblastine). Other drugs sometimes used in systemic chemotherapy of bladder cancer include cyclophosphamide (Cytoxan), gemcitabine (Gemzar), and paclitaxel (Taxol).

Radiation Therapy

External beam radiation therapy or interstitial radiation therapy after surgery can kill small deposits of cancer cells that may not be visible during surgery. The combination of radiation therapy and chemotherapy given after transurethral bladder surgery is sometimes able to completely destroy cancers that would otherwise require cystectomy for complete removal.

Resources

AMERICAN CANCER SOCIETY RESOURCES

The American Cancer Society (ACS) provides educational materials and information on cancer, offers a variety of patient programs, and directs people to services in their community. To find your local office, contact us at 800-ACS-2345 or visit our web site (*http://www.cancer.org*).

National Home Office
1599 Clifton Road NE
Atlanta, GA 30329-4251
Toll-Free: 800-ACS-2345 (800-227-2345)
Web site: *http://www.cancer.org*

American Cancer Society Programs and Services
The ACS programs and services listed below may be of special interest to those with cancer and their loved ones. Contact the American Cancer Society for more information about services in your area.

CANCER SURVIVORS' NETWORK. This network provides both a telephone-based and an online community that welcome cancer survivors, friends, and families to share and communicate with others with similar interests and experiences. The program offers a vibrant community of real people supporting one another and sharing personal experiences with cancer. The web site enables registered members to have live, private chats, to create personal web pages to share experiences, thoughts, and wisdom, to help people create personal support communities of people who share common concerns and interests, and offers information about resources. The telephone component uses an interactive voice response system and consists of pre-recorded discussions among survivors and family. Users can navigate from discussion to discussion or leave a comment or question twenty-four hours a day, seven days a week, at 877-333-HOPE (877-333-4673).

HOPE LODGES. Hope Lodges are temporary residential facilities providing sleeping rooms and related facilities for people with cancer who are undergoing outpatient treatment and their family members. Approval from a doctor or referring agency is necessary. (See *Transportation and Accommodation Services*, pages 747–749, for more information.)

I CAN COPE. This program addresses the educational and psychological needs of people with cancer and their families. A series of eight classes discusses the disease, coping with daily health problems, controlling cancer-related pain, nutrition for the person with cancer, expressing feelings, living with limitations, and local resources. Through lectures, group discussions, and study assignments, the course helps people with cancer regain a sense of control over their lives.

LOOK GOOD...FEEL BETTER. Toll-Free: 800-395-LOOK (800-395-6005) Founded in partnership with the National Cosmetology Association and the Cosmetic, Toiletry, and Fragrance Association (CTFA) Foundation as a free national public service program dedicated to teaching women with cancer how to restore a healthy appearance and self-image during and after chemotherapy and radiation therapy.

MAN TO MAN. This program provides accurate, factual information to men and their partners about prostate cancer in a supportive environment following essential guidelines that ensure program integrity and credibility. Man to Man is an ideal vehicle by which new relationships are formed between patients/survivors and care providers with a two-way exchange of information, trust, and respect.

REACH TO RECOVERY. This program is designed to help patients with breast cancer cope with their diagnosis, treatment, and recovery. The volunteers for this program are women who have had breast cancer and are specially trained to share their knowledge and experiences in a supportive and nonintrusive manner. Ongoing support groups are available to help deal with the challenges of breast cancer. Reach to Recovery also provides early support to women who may have breast cancer or have just been diagnosed with cancer.

Chartered Divisions of the American Cancer Society

California Division (California)
California Division, Inc.
1710 Webster Street, Suite 210
Oakland, CA 94612
Phone: 510-893-7900

Eastern Division (New Jersey, New York)
Eastern Division, Inc. *(Northern Office)*
6725 Lyons Street
P.O. Box 7
East Syracuse, NY 13057
Phone: 315-437-7025

Eastern Division, Inc. *(Southern Office)*
2600 U.S. Highway 1
North Brunswick, NJ 08902-6001
Phone: 732-297-8000

Florida Division (Florida, Puerto Rico)
Florida Division, Inc.
3709 West Jetton Avenue
Tampa, FL 33629-5146
Phone: 813-253-0541

Puerto Rico Division, Inc.
Calle Alverio #577
Esquina Sargento Medina
Hato Rey, PR 00918
Phone: 787-764-2295

Great Lakes Division (Indiana, Michigan)
Great Lakes Division, Inc.
1205 East Saginaw Street
Lansing, MI 48906
Toll-Free: 800-723-0360

Heartland Division (Kansas, Missouri,
Nebraska, Oklahoma)
Heartland Division, Inc.
1100 Pennsylvania Avenue
Kansas City, MO 64105
Phone: 816-842-7111

Illinois Division (Illinois)
Illinois Division, Inc.
77 East Monroe Street, 13th floor
Chicago, IL 60603-5795
Phone: 312-641-6150

Mid-Atlantic Division (Delaware,
Maryland, Washington, DC, Virginia,
West Virginia)
Mid-Atlantic Division, Inc.
1875 Connecticut Avenue NW, Suite 730
Washington, DC 20009
Phone: 202-483-2600

Mid-South Division (Alabama, Arkansas,
Kentucky, Louisiana, Mississippi,
Tennessee)
Mid-South Division, Inc.
1100 Ireland Way, Suite 300
Birmingham, AL 35205
Phone: 205-879-2242

Midwest Division (Iowa, Minnesota,
South Dakota, Wisconsin)
Midwest Division, Inc.
3316 Sixty-Sixth Street
Minneapolis, MN 55435
Phone: 612-925-2772

New England Division (Connecticut,
Maine, Massachusetts, New Hampshire,
Rhode Island, Vermont)
New England Division, Inc. *(Framingham)*
30 Speen Street
Framingham, MA 01701-1800
Phone: 508-270-4600

New England Division, Inc. *(Meriden)*
Meriden Executive Park
538 Preston Avenue
Meriden, CT 06450-1004
Phone: 203-379-4700

Northwest Division (Alaska, Oregon,
Washington, Montana)
Northwest Division
2120 First Avenue North
Seattle, WA 98109-1140
Phone: 206-283-1152

Ohio Division (Ohio)
Ohio Division, Inc.
5555 Frantz Road
Dublin, OH 43017
Toll-Free: 800-686-4357

Pennsylvania Division (Pennsylvania)
Pennsylvania Division, Inc.
Route 422 and Sipe Avenue
Hershey, PA 17033-0897
Phone: 717-533-6144

Rocky Mountain Division (Colorado,
  Idaho, North Dakota, Utah, Wyoming)
Rocky Mountain Division, Inc.
2255 South Oneida
Denver, CO 80224
Phone: 303-758-2030

Southeast Division (Georgia, North
  Carolina, South Carolina)
Southeast Division, Inc.
2200 Lake Boulevard
Atlanta, GA 30319
Phone (Call Center): 404-816-4994

Southwest Division (Nevada, Arizona,
  New Mexico)
Southwest Division, Inc.
2929 East Thomas Road
Phoenix, AZ 85016
Phone: 602-224-0524

Texas Division (Hawaii, Texas)
Hawaii Pacific Division, Inc.
2370 Nuuanu Avenue
Honolulu, HI 96817
Phone: 808-595-7500

Texas Division, Inc.
2433 Ridgepoint Drive A
Austin, TX 78754
Phone: 512-919-1800

OTHER ORGANIZATIONS

Listings in this section represent organizations that operate on a national level and provide some type of service or resource to consumers related to cancer. This list is designed to give you a starting point for seeking information, support, and needed resources. If you have a question that cannot be answered by one of the sources listed here, do not give up. Many of these organizations provide referrals, and your questions may be directed to other organizations or individuals.

Most of the organizations listed here can be contacted via phone, fax, or e-mail, and some through their web site. Many of the web sites provide much of the same information that is available by postal mail. Some organizations are solely web-based and will require Internet access. Keep in mind that new web sites appear daily while old ones expand, move, or disappear entirely. Some of the web sites or content may change. Often, a simple Internet search will point you to the new web site for a given organization. The American Cancer Society web site provides links to outside sources of cancer information as well (*http://www.cancer.org*).

Health Information on the Internet

There is a vast amount of information about cancer on the Internet. This information can be very valuable to those facing cancer in making decisions about their illness and treatment. However, since any group or individual can publish on the Internet, it is important to consider the credentials and reputation of the organization providing information. Always discuss information you find on the Internet with your health care team. Internet information should not be a substitute for medical advice.

The agencies, organizations, corporations, and publications represented in this resource guide are not necessarily endorsed by the American Cancer Society. This guide is provided for assistance in obtaining information only.

Cancer and Health Information

The listings in this section include resources for general and specific information about cancer and cancer-related health concerns and conditions. Contact the ACS for additional resources, including resources for specific cancer types. See also Patient Education, Support, and Advocacy, *pages 742–746.*

AARP

601 E Street NW • Washington, DC 20049
Toll-Free: 800-424-3410
E-mail: member@aarp.org
Web site: *http://www.aarp.org*
Web site (for Pharmacy Service): *http://www.aarppharmacy.com*
This organization offers membership to anyone over age 50 for a small yearly fee. It focuses on addressing the needs of older people on a national level. The web site includes information on a member pharmacy service that offers discounts on drugs.

AIDS Clinical Trials Information Service (ACTIS)

P.O. Box 6421 • Rockville, MD 20849-6421
Toll-Free: 800-TRIALS-A (800-874-2572)
Toll-Free (TTY): 888-480-3739
Phone: 301-519-0459
Fax: 301-519-6616
E-mail: ACTIS@actis.org
Web site: *http://www.actis.org*
The AIDS Clinical Trials Information Service (ACTIS) is federally supported and sponsored. It provides up-to-date information about clinical trials that evaluate experimental drugs and other therapies for HIV infection and AIDS-related conditions.

AMC Cancer Research Center & Foundation

1600 Pierce Street • Denver, CO 80214
Toll-Free: 800-321-1557
Toll-Free (Counseling): 800-525-3777
Phone: 303-233-6501
Web site: *http://www.amc.org*
Through the counseling line of this nonprofit research center, you can request free publications and receive answers to questions about cancer. The web site contains an area about ongoing research and general information about specific types of cancer.

American Brain Tumor Association

2720 River Road • Des Plaines, IL 60018
Phone: 847-827-9910
Fax: 847-827-9918
E-mail: info@abta.org
Web site: *http://www.abta.org*
Offers publications and services to people with brain tumors and their families, including information about treatments, coping mechanisms, support resources, research updates, a pen pal program, and a section for kids.

American Institute for Cancer Research (AICR)

1759 R Street NW • Washington, DC 20009

Toll-Free: 800-843-8114

Phone: 202-328-7744

E-mail: aicrweb@aicr.org

Web site: *http://www.aicr.org*

Focuses on the relationship between diet and nutrition and cancer prevention and treatment. Creates public health education programs, funds research, and provides information to the public and health care professionals.

American Medical Association (AMA)

515 North State Street • Chicago, IL 60610

Phone: 312-464-5000

Web site: *http://www.ama-assn.org*

The AMA develops and promotes standards in medical practice, research, and education. Under the consumer health information section, the web site contains databases on doctors and hospitals, which can be searched by medical specialty. A pull-down menu of specific conditions (such as breast cancer) is also provided.

American Society of Clinical Oncology (ASCO)

1900 Duke Street, Suite 200 • Alexandria, VA 22314

Phone: 703-299-0150

Fax: 703-299-1044

E-mail: asco@asco.org

Web site: *http://www.asco.org*

An international medical society representing about 10,000 cancer specialists involved in clinical research and patient care. The web site is a resource for cancer patients, doctors, and researchers and includes patient guides, a glossary of cancer terms, an ASCO member oncologist locator, news and information about different cancers and drug treatments, information about cancer legislation, summaries of government reports, and links to related sites.

The American Society for Therapeutic Radiology and Oncology (ASTRO)

12500 Fair Lakes Circle, Suite 375 • Fairfax, VA 22033-3882

Toll-Free: 800-962-7876

Phone: 703-227-0187

Fax: 703-502-7852

Web site: *http://www.astro.org*

Focusing on the use of radiation therapy for the treatment of cancer, this society's web site includes an overview of radiation therapy and a list of frequently asked questions. Some breast cancer–specific information is also available.

Association of Community Cancer Centers (ACCC)

11600 Nebel Street, Suite 201 • Rockville, MD 20852

Phone: 301-984-9496

Fax: 301-770-1949

Web site: *http://www.accc-cancer.org*

This national organization includes over 650 hospitals, cancer centers, group practices, and free-standing clinics. This web site contains a searchable database of cancer centers listed by state as well as information about oncology drugs (registration is required) and specific cancers.

Breast Cancer Awareness

U.S. Department of Defense

Web site: *http://www.tricaresw.af.mil/breastcd/index.html*

This interactive web site provides information about breast cancer diagnosis and treatment. The site contains detailed downloadable text on breast cancer as well as movies illustrating some of the steps involved in detection and treatment.

Department of Defense Breast Cancer Decision Guide

Breast Cancer Prevention, Education and Diagnosis Program Initiative

Web site: *http://www.bcdg.org*

The U.S. Department of Defense Breast Cancer Prevention, Education and Diagnosis Program Initiative developed this web site for individuals diagnosed with breast cancer and their family members. The site provides information for patients, doctors, and family members on breast cancer diagnosis, treatment, and decision-making. A glossary of terms and a section dealing with military-specific issues is also provided.

Canadian Cancer Society (CCS)

10 Alcorn Avenue, Suite 200 • Toronto, Ontario • M4V 3B1

Phone: 416-961-7223

Fax: 416-961-4189

E-mail: info@cis.cancer.ca

Web site: *http://www.cancer.ca*

This organization provides facts about cancer, treatment, prevention, and Canadian units of the CCS, in English and French.

CancerGuide

E-mail: steve.dunn@cancerguide.org

Web site: *http://cancerguide.org*

Information about cancer assembled by a computer-literate layperson: cancer fundamentals, recommended books, clinical trials, how to research medical literature, and alternative therapies.

Cancer Research Institute (CRI)

681 Fifth Avenue • New York, NY 10022

Toll-Free: 800-99-CANCER (800-992-6237)

Phone: 212-688-7515

E-mail: info@cancerresearch.org

Web site: *http://www.cancerresearch.org*

An institute funding cancer research and providing public information on cancer immunology and cancer treatment, the CRI helps locate immunotherapy clinical trials, and offers a cancer reference guide and other informational booklets.

Center for Devices and Radiological Health

Food and Drug Administration • CDRH/FDA Consumer Staff

1350 Piccard Drive • HFZ-210 • Rockville, MD 20850

Toll-Free: 888-463-6332

Phone: 301-827-3990

Fax: 301-443-9535

Web site (breast implant information): *http://www.fda.gov/cdrh/breastimplants/indexbip.html*

Women considering or who have had breast reconstruction using implants can obtain an information package from this organization. The text of the package can also be viewed on the web site.

Centers for Disease Control and Prevention (CDC)
Cancer Prevention and Control Program
CDC/DCPC • 4770 Buford Highway NE • MS K64 • Atlanta, GA 30341
Toll-Free: 888-842-6355
Fax: 770-488-4760
E-mail: cancerinfo@cdc.gov
Web site: *http://www.cdc.gov/cancer*
The CDC is an agency of the United States Department of Health and Human Services. Their mission is to promote health and quality of life by preventing and controlling disease, injury, and disability. The CDC provides information about chronic diseases such as cancer. The web site contains a searchable map of centers, information about cancer, downloadable publications, and links to related sources. *Spanish-speaking staff and Spanish materials are available.*

Consumer Products Safety Commission
Washington, DC 20207-0001
Toll-Free: 800-638-2772
Toll-Free (TTY): 800-638-8270
Fax: 301-504-0124
Web site: *http://www.cpsc.gov*
Releases information about unsafe products and product recall lists.

DES Action USA
610 Sixteenth Street, Suite 301• Oakland, CA 94612
Toll-Free: 800-337-9288
Phone: 510-465-4011
Fax: 510-465-4815
E-mail: desaction@earthlink.net
Web site: *http://www.desaction.org*
Publishes information and a newsletter about the effects of diethylestilbestrol (DES) exposure.

DES Cancer Network
514 Tenth Street NW, Suite 400 • Washington, DC 20004
Toll-Free: 800-DES-NET4 (800-337-6384)
Fax: 202-628-6217
E-mail: desnetwrk@aol.com
Web site: *http://www.descancer.org*
A network for women and men exposed to DES, with a special focus on cancer. Supports referrals, education, research advocacy, and an annual conference for cancer survivors and publishes a newsletter.

Environmental Protection Agency (EPA)
Ariel Rios Building • 1200 Pennsylvania Avenue NW • Washington, DC 20460
Phone: 202-260-2090
Web site: *http://www.epa.gov*
The EPA implements the federal laws designed to promote public health by protecting our nation's air, water, and soil from harmful pollution. The web site offers environmental news, community concerns, information about laws and other regulations, and links to other sources of information.

HealthScout

Web site: *http://www.healthscout.com*

Healthscout is a general health web site that provides health care news and medical information. It also provides connections to other health resources.

International Agency for Research on Cancer (IARC)

World Health Organization • 150 cours Albert Thomas • F-69372 Lyon cedex 08, France

Phone: 33-4-72-73-84-85

Fax: 33-4-72-73-85-75

Web site: *http://www.iarc.fr*

IARC coordinates and conducts research on the causes of human cancer and the mechanisms of carcinogenesis. The IARC Monographs, available on the IARC web site, are critical reviews and evaluations of evidence on the carcinogenicity of a wide range of human exposures. The IARC web site contains: three databases with information on the occurrence of cancer worldwide, a database including carcinogenic risks to humans, a list of publications, and links to related cancer sites.

International Association of Laryngectomees

8900 Thornton Road • Box 99311 • Stockton, CA 95209

Toll-Free: 866-IAL-FORU (866-425-3678)

Fax: 209-472-0516

Web site: *http://www.larynxlink.com*

This voluntary organization is dedicated to the total rehabilitation of laryngectomees. Promotes exchange and dissemination of ideas and information to laryngectomee clubs and to the public.

International Myeloma Foundation

12650 Riverside Drive, Suite 206 • North Hollywood, CA 91607

Toll-Free: 800-452-CURE (800-452-2873)

Phone: 818-487-7455

Fax: 918-487-7454

E-mail: TheIMF@myeloma.org

Web site: *http://www.myeloma.org*

Dedicated to improving quality of life for myeloma patients, while working toward prevention and a cure.

Let's Face It USA

P.O. Box 29972 • Bellingham, WA 98228-1972

Phone: 360-676-7325

E-mail: letsfaceit@faceit.org

Web site: *http://www.faceit.org*

Information and support network for people with head and neck cancer and others with facial disfigurement.

Leukemia & Lymphoma Society

1311 Mamaroneck Avenue, Third floor • White Plains, NY 10605

Toll-Free: 800-955-4572

Phone: 914-949-5213

Web site: *http://www.leukemia-lymphoma.org/hm_lls*

This national voluntary health agency, which was formerly known as the Leukemia Society of America, offers a variety of service programs and resources related to leukemia, lymphoma, Hodgkin's disease, and myeloma, including improving quality of life. Contact the national office for a listing of local chapters.

Lymphoma Research Foundation of America
8800 Venice Boulevard, Suite 207 • Los Angeles, CA 90034
Phone: 310-204-7040
Fax: 310-204-7043
Web site: *http://www.lymphoma.org*
Funds medical research devoted to improving lymphoma treatments, and offers a newsletter and support system to patients and their families.

MayoClinic.com
Web site: *http://www.mayohealth.org*
This web site contains a database searchable by keyword and topic. It also offers a question and answer link to a doctor at the Mayo Clinic, as well as links to reference articles and cancer organizations.

Medscape
Web site: *http://www.medscape.com*
Although registration is required to view some of the content, this web site offers a great deal of information on prescription drugs as well as medical articles. There are also links to several organizations, cancer centers, database and education web sites, journals, and government sites. The web site is also searchable by key word. Registration is free.

MedWatch
Toll-Free: 800-332-1088
Web site: *http://www.fda.gov/medwatch*
Through MedWatch, the FDA maintains an adverse event and product reporting program. The organization accepts reports of problems with food, drugs, or devices from the general public. The web site includes medical product safety alerts as well as searchable FDA safety databases and FDA medical bulletins.

National Alliance of Breast Cancer Organizations (NABCO)
9 East Thirty-Seventh Street, Tenth floor • New York, NY 10016
Toll-Free: 888-80-NABCO (888-806-2226)
Phone (emergencies only): 212-889-0606
Fax: 212-689-1213
E-mail: nabcoinfo@aol.com
Web site: *http://www.nabco.org*
This nonprofit organization includes a network of more than 400 organizations. The NABCO web site includes information about breast cancer and breast health, a directory of nation-wide events, a resource list, a list of local support groups, and a directory of clinical trials. The site also allows women to register for a mammography e-mail reminder.

National Brain Tumor Foundation
414 Thirteenth Street, Suite 700 • Oakland, CA 94612-2603
Toll-Free: 800-934-CURE (800-934-2873)
Phone: 510-839-9777
Fax: 510-839-9779
E-mail: nbtf@braintumor.org
Web site: *http://www.braintumor.org*
Raises funds for research and provides information and support services to people with brain tumors and their families.

The National Breast Cancer Coalition
1707 L Street NW, Suite 1060 • Washington, DC 20036
Toll-Free: 800-622-2838
Phone: 202-296-7477
Fax: 202-265-6854
Web site: *http://www.natlbcc.org*
Strives to involve women with breast cancer and those that care about them in changing public policy. Goals include increasing breast cancer research funding and improving access to screening, increasing the influence that breast cancer survivors have over research, clinical trials, and national policy.

National Cancer Institute (NCI)
NCI Public Inquiries Office • Building 31, Room 10A31
31 Center Drive, MSC 2580 • Bethesda, MD 20892-2580
Toll-Free: 800-4-CANCER (800-422-6237)
Web site: *http://www.cancer.gov*
This government agency provides information on cancer research, diagnosis, and treatment through several services (see list below). People with cancer, caregivers, and health care professionals may call the NCI's toll-free telephone service for cancer-related information. *Spanish-speaking staff and Spanish materials are available.*

For more information about or area listings of Community Clinical Oncology Programs, Comprehensive Cancer Centers, or Clinical Cancer Centers, call NCI at 800-4-CANCER. Or go to: http://www.nci.nih.gov/cancercenters/centerslist.html *for information about the listings in your area.*

See also listings for NCI's CancerTrials *and* Clinical Trials Cooperative Group Program *in the* Clinical Trials *section (pages 732–733).*

CancerFax
Toll-Free Fax: 800-624-2511
Fax: 301-402-5874
CancerFax includes information about cancer treatment, screening, prevention, and supportive care. To obtain a contents list, dial the fax number from a fax machine hand set and follow the recorded instructions.

Cancer Information Service (CIS)
Toll-Free: 800-4-CANCER (800-422-6237)
Toll-Free (TTY): 800-332-8615
Web site: *http://cis.nci.nih.gov*
The CIS provides information to consumers and health care professionals. Call CIS for a referral to a pain control clinic or support group in your area. The web site contains a wealth of information including pamphlets and brochures on cancer diagnosis, treatment, research, and prevention. *Spanish-speaking staff is available.*

CANCERLIT (Bibliographic Database)
Web site: *http://cnetdb.nci.nih.gov/cancerlit.html*
This searchable site is maintained by the NCI and contains cancer and pain articles published in medical and scientific journals, books, government reports, and articles that were presented at national meetings. A link to the PDQ (CancerNet/NCI database) search engine is provided, which allows you to search for clinical trials by state, city, and type of cancer.

CancerNet

Web site: *http://cancernet.gov*

Web site (Spanish version): *http://cancernet.gov/sp_menu.htm*

Web site (On-line ordering): *http://publications.nci.nih.gov*

A comprehensive web site that contains information on diagnosis, treatment, support, resources, literature, clinical trials, prevention and risk factors, and testing. Up to twenty publications can be ordered on-line. The publications list is searchable. *Some publications are available in Spanish.*

National Center for Complementary and Alternative Medicine

National Institutes of Health • NCCAM Clearinghouse

P.O. Box 8218 • Silver Spring, MD 20907-8218

Toll-Free: 888-644-6226

Phone outside the U.S.: 301-231-7537, ext. 5

Fax: 301-495-4957

Web site: *http://nccam.nih.gov*

This site provides information on complementary and alternative methods being promoted to treat different diseases.

National Comprehensive Cancer Network (NCCN)

50 Huntingdon Pike, Suite 200 • Rockledge, PA 19046

Toll-Free: 888-909-NCCN (800-909-6226)

Phone: 215-728-4788

Fax: 215-728-3877

E-mail: information@nccn.org

Web site: *http://www.nccn.org*

The NCCN is a nonprofit organization that is an alliance of cancer centers. The American Cancer Society has partnered with NCCN to translate the NCCN Clinical Practice Guidelines into patient-friendly resources. The Clinical Practice Guidelines are available to doctors by contacting NCCN. The *Treatment Guidelines for Patients,* which are available on-line, offer the latest information for a variety of cancers and cancer-related conditions (e.g., breast cancer, prostate cancer, colon and rectal cancer, pain control, nausea and vomiting). The guidelines offer easy-to-understand information for patients and family members about treatment options, and printed copies of the guidelines are available through the ACS.

National Consumers League

1701 K Street NW, Suite 1201• Washington, DC 20006

Phone: 202-835-3323

Fax: 202-835-0747

Web site: *http://www.nclnet.org*

Experts in law, business, and labor provide consumer protection and advocacy. Publishes education brochures about general health issues, including cancer screening tests.

National Council Against Health Fraud

P.O. Box 141 • Fort Lee, NJ 07024

Phone: 201-723-2955

E-mail: ncahf@worldnet.att.net

Web site: *http://www.ncahf.org*

Focuses on health misinformation, fraud, and quackery, and provides information on unusual methods of cancer management. Can refer people to lawyers and help those who have had negative experiences to share their story.

National Institutes of Health (NIH)
Bethesda, MD 20892
Phone: 301-496-4000
E-mail (please submit questions and requests via e-mail): nihinfo@od.nih.gov
Web site: *http://www.nih.gov*
The NIH is an agency of the Public Health Services, which in turn is part of the U.S. Department of Health and Human Services. The NIH mission is to uncover new knowledge that will lead to better health for everyone. NIH conducts research in its own laboratories, supports the research of non-Federal scientists, helps in the training of research investigators, and fosters communication of medical information.

National Institutes of Health Consensus Program
P.O. Box 2577• Kensington, MD 20891
Toll-Free: 800-644-2667
E-mail: consensus@od.nih.gov
Web site: *http://consensus.nih.gov*
Updates practicing doctors and the public with current responsible information on the pros and cons of various medical technologies.

U.S. National Library of Medicine
National Institutes of Health • Department of Health and Human Services
8600 Rockville Pike • Bethesda, MD 20894
Web site: *http://www.nlm.nih.gov*
Provides a search engine for health, medical, scientific literature, and research as well as links to other government resources.

Internet Grateful Med
Web site: *http://igm.nlm.nih.gov*
Provides access to millions of literature references and abstracts in Medline and other databases, with links to on-line journals. The site is searchable by key words.

NLM Gateway
Web site: *http://gateway.nlm.nih.gov/gw/Cmd*
Offers links to searchable databases and allows users to search simultaneously in multiple retrieval systems.

PubMed
Web site: *http://www.ncbi.nlm.nih.gov/PubMed*
Provides access to millions of literature references and abstracts in Medline and other databases, with links to on-line journals. The site is searchable by key word.

National Kidney Cancer Association
1234 Sherman Avenue, Suite 20 • Evanston, IL 60202-1375
Toll-Free: 800-850-9132
Phone: 847-332-1051
Fax: 847-332-2978
E-mail: office@kidneycancerassociation.org
Web site: *http://www.nkca.org*
Provides information to patients and doctors, sponsors research on kidney cancer, gives referrals to doctors, publishes a newsletter, and acts as a patient advocate.

National Toxicology Program (NTP)

National Institutes of Health

National Institute of Environmental Health Sciences • Durham, NC 27704

Web site: *http://ntp-server.niehs.nih.gov*

The NTP's Report on Carcinogens identifies substances and mixtures or exposure circumstances that are *"known"* or are *"reasonably anticipated"* to cause cancer, and to which a significant number of Americans are exposed. The *Report on Carcinogens* is published every two years and is available on the NTP web site.

National Women's Health Information Center

The Office on Women's Health • U.S. Department of Health and Human Services

8550 Arlington Boulevard, Suite 300 • Fairfax, VA 22031

Toll-Free: 800-994-WOMAN (800-994-9662)

Toll-Free (TDD): 888-220-5546

Web site: *http://www.4woman.gov*

Web site (Spanish version): *http://www.4woman.gov/Spanish/index.htm*

This web site has a searchable database of information on various women's health issues, including breast cancer. Documents accessible through this site include information from the NCI, the CDC, and several other government agencies. The site contains a section for special groups, which separates breast cancer and other health information by specific minority group. It also contains links to on-line medical dictionaries and journals.

OncoLink

University of Pennsylvania Cancer Center

E-mail: editors@oncolink.upenn.edu

Web site: *http://www.oncolink.com*

Sponsored by the University of Pennsylvania Cancer Center Resource, this web site provides information on cancer, including clinical trials, support groups, educational materials, cancer screening and prevention, financial questions, and other resources for people with cancer.

Physicians Data Query (PDQ)

National Cancer Institute

Toll-Free: 800-4-CANCER (800-422-6237)

Web site: *http://cancernet.nci.nih.gov/pdqfull.html*

Computerized listing of up-to-date and accurate information for people with cancer and health care professionals on the latest treatments, research studies, and clinical trials.

Quackwatch

Web site: *http://www.quackwatch.com*

Quackwatch, Inc. is a nonprofit corporation whose purpose is to combat health-related frauds, myths, fads, and fallacies. The Quackwatch web site is a comprehensive source of information regarding fraudulent claims. *Information is offered in German, Spanish, French, and Portuguese as well as in English.*

Skin Cancer Foundation

245 Fifth Avenue, Suite 1403 • New York, NY 10016

Toll-Free: 800-SKIN-490 (800-754-6490)

Fax: 212-725-5751

E-mail: info@skincancer.org

Web site: *http://www.skincancer.org*

Conducts educational programs for the public and medical communities; supports medical training, cancer screening, and prevention programs; provides information about safe sun exposure for children and adults; and publishes a journal.

The Susan G. Komen Breast Cancer Foundation
5005 LBJ Freeway, Suite 250 • Dallas, TX 75244
Toll-Free (Breast Care Helpline): 800-IM-AWARE (800-462-9273)
Phone: 972-855-1600
Fax: 972-855-1605
E-mail: helpline@komen.org
Web site: *http://www.komen.org*
This organization promotes research, education, screening, and treatment. The web site contains the latest news and information regarding breast health, drug therapies, treatment options, educational events and meetings, survivor stories, and other breast cancer-related information.

US TOO! International, Inc.
5003 Fairview Avenue • Downers Grove, IL 60515
Toll-Free: 800-80-US-TOO (800-808-7866)
Phone: 630-795-1002
Fax: 7630-795-1602
E-mail: ustoo@ustoo.com
Web site: *http://www.ustoo.com*
This independent group provides prostate cancer survivors and their families with emotional and educational support.

Y-ME National Breast Cancer Organization
212 West Van Buren, Suite 500 • Chicago, IL 60607
Toll-Free Hotline: 800-221-2141
Toll-Free Hotline (Spanish): 800-986-9505
Phone: 312-986-8338
Fax: 312-294-8597
Web site: *http://www.y-me.org*
Web site (Spanish version): *http://www.y-me.org/spanish.htm*
This organization focuses on providing information and support to people with breast cancer and their families. Y-ME provides a national hotline, public meetings and seminars, workshops for professionals, referral services, support groups, a newsletter, a resource library, a teen program, and advocacy information.

Cancer Registries

A cancer registry identifies and tracks cancer cases. Hospital registries may be part of a facility's cancer program, while population-based registries are usually associated with state health departments. Hospital registries may evaluate care within a hospital, compare patterns of care, and provide state registries with data. Population-based registries record information about all cases diagnosed within a specific geographic area.

Gilda Radner Familial Ovarian Cancer Registry
Roswell Park Cancer Institute
Elm and Carlton Streets • Buffalo, NY 14263
Toll-Free: 800-OVARIAN (800-682-7426)
Fax: 716-845-8266
Web site: *http://www.ovariancancer.com/grwp.html*
A registry for women with two or more first-degree relatives with ovarian cancer, for research purposes. The registry is also a source of public education and information regarding diagnostic tests, risk factors, and warning signs.

Hereditary Cancer Institute
Creighton University School of Medicine • 2500 California Plaza • Omaha, NE 68178
Toll-Free: 800-648-8133
Web site: *http://www.fascrs.org/registry/creighton.html*
Evaluates families in order to identify possible hereditary cancer syndromes. Will send educational material upon request. Provides recommendations for surveillance.

The Hereditary Colorectal Cancer Registry
The Johns Hopkins Hospital • 550 North Broadway, Suite 108 • Baltimore, MD 21205-2011
Toll-Free: 888-77-COLON (888-772-6566)
Phone: 410-955-3875
Fax: 410-614-9544
E-mail: hccregistry@jhmi.edu
Web site: *http://www.hopkins-coloncancer.org/subspecialties/heredicolor_cancer/overview.htm*
Provides information about hereditary colorectal cancer as well as an opportunity to participate in research on hereditary colon cancer. A separate site exists for kids at risk for Familial Adenomatous Polyposis (FAP).

Intestinal Multiple Polyposis and Colorectal Cancer
P.O. Box 11 • Conynghan, PA 18219
Phone: 570-788-1818
Fax: 570-788-4046
E-mail: impacc@epix.net
Clearinghouse of registries, support groups, and information for those affected by polyposis. Genetic counseling is available. When calling, indicate that you wish to reach IMPACC.

Registry for Research on Hormonal Transplacental Carcinogenesis
University of Chicago • 5841 South Maryland Avenue • MC2050 • Chicago, IL 60637
Phone: 773-702-6671
Fax: 773-702-0840
E-mail: registry@babies.bsd.uchicago.edu
Web site: *http://obgyn.bsd.uchicago.edu/registry.html*
This registry is for women with clear-cell adenocarcinoma of the genital tract, with or without diethylstilbestrol (DES) exposure.

Children's Cancers

The listings in this section include resources for children with cancer. (Note: The majority of children with cancer are treated at large pediatric cancer centers in clinical trials of the Children's Oncology Group. For information about this group, see Clinical Trials, *pages 732–733.) For more information about children's cancers, see* Children's Cancers *in* Overview of Specific Cancers *(pages 582–615). Contact ACS for a list of children's cancer camps in the United States.*

Candlelighters Childhood Cancer Foundation
3910 Warner Street • Kensington, MD 20895
Toll-Free: 800-366-2233
Phone: 301-962-3520
Fax: 301-962-3521
E-mail: info@candlelighters.org
Web site: *http://www.candlelighters.org*
Provides information, support, and advocacy to families of children with cancer, survivors of childhood cancer, and professionals who work with them.

Chai Lifeline/Camp Simcha

151 West Thirtieth Street • New York, NY 10001

Toll-Free: 877-CHAI-LIFE (877-242-4543)

Phone: 212-465-1301

Fax: 212-465-0949

Web site: *http://www.chailifeline.org*

Provides a kosher camp for children with cancer or hematological conditions, free of charge, including transportation from anywhere in the world. Open to children of any religion who meet the medical approval of the director.

Children's Hospice International

901 North Pitt Street, Suite 230 • Alexandria, VA 22314

Toll-Free: 800-24-CHILD (800-242-4453)

Phone: 703-684-0330

Fax: 703-684-0226

Web site: *http://www.chionline.org*

Creates hospice support for children and provides medical and technical assistance, research, and education to their families and health care professionals.

Children's Oncology Camping Association International

P.O. Box 35 • Mountain Center, CA 92561

Toll-Free: 800-737-2667

Web site: *http://www.coca-intl.org*

Provides international directory of oncology camps.

The Children's Organ Transplant Association (COTA)

2501 COTA Drive • Bloomington, IN 47403

Toll-Free: 800-366 2682

E-mail: jennifer@cota.org

Web site: *http://www.cota.org*

Helps families and communities raise funds for children needing transplants and transplant-related expenses.

Federation for Children with Special Needs

1135 Tremont Street, Suite 420 • Boston, MA 02120

Toll-Free in MA: 800-331-0688

Phone: 617-236-7210

Fax: 617-572-2094

E-mail: fcsninfo@fcsn.org

Web site: *http://www.fcsn.org*

This information and referral agency provides training for parents on understanding their rights under special education laws, and helping parents become health care advocates.

Make-A-Wish Foundation of America

3550 North Central Avenue, Suite 300 • Phoenix, AZ 85012

Toll-Free: 800-722-WISH (800-722-9474)

Phone: 602-279-WISH (602-279-9474)

Fax: 602-279-0855

E-mail: mawfa@wish.org

Web site: *http://www.wish.org*

This organization grants wishes to children between the ages of 2 and 18 who have life-threatening illnesses.

Ronald McDonald House Charities
1 Kroc Drive • Oak Brook, IL 60523
Web site: *http://www.rmhc.com*
Supports temporary lodging facilities for the families of seriously ill children being treated at
nearby hospitals.

Starlight Children's Foundation
5900 Wilshire Boulevard, Suite 2530 • Los Angeles, CA 90036
Phone: 323-634-0080
E-mail: info@starlight.org
Web site: *http://www.starlight.org*
Provides entertainment and recreational activities for seriously ill children ages 4–18 through
mobile "fun centers," PC Pal computers, hospital events, and wish-granting activities in
chapter areas.

The Sunshine Foundation
1041 Mill Creek Drive • Feasterville, PA 19053
Phone: 215-396-4770
Fax: 215-396-4774
Web site: *http://www.sunshinefoundation.org*
Grants wishes to chronically or terminally ill and handicapped children whose families are
under a financial strain due to their child's illness.

The Sunshine Kids
2814 Virginia • Houston, TX 77098
Toll-Free: 800-594-5756
Web site: *http://www.sunshinekids.org*
Offers sports, cultural events, and group activities, free of charge, to children receiving cancer
treatment.

Wigs for Kids
Executive Club Building • 21330 Center Ridge Road, Suite C • Rocky River, OH 44116
Phone: 440-333-4433
Fax: 440-333-0200
E-mail: info@wigsforkids.org
Web site: *http://www.wigsforkids.org*
Wigs for Kids is a nonprofit organization providing hair replacement solutions for children
affected by hair loss due to chemotherapy, radiation therapy, alopecia, burns, or other
medical conditions.

Clinical Trials

*The organizations listed in this section may help you understand clinical trials, identify
ongoing clinical trials, or explore the findings of closed clinical trials.*

CancerTrials
National Cancer Institute
Web site: *http://cancertrials.nci.nih.gov*
This site offers information about ongoing cancer clinical trials and explanations of what a
trial is and what is involved. A link to the PDQ (CancerNet/NCI database) search engine
allows you to search for clinical trials by state, city, and type of cancer.

Clinical Trials and Insurance Coverage: A Resource Guide
Web site: *http://cancertrials.nci.nih.gov/understanding/indepth/insurance/index.html*
Part of the NCI's CancerTrials web site, this site offers information regarding the cost of clinical trials and how to determine if you will be covered under your health plan. Information about financial assistance programs for the needy is also available.

Children's Oncology Group (COG)
440 East Huntington Drive • P.O. Box 60012 • Arcadia, CA 91066-6012
Toll-Free: 800-458-NCCF (800-458-6223)
Fax: 626-447-6359
Web site: *http://www.nccf.org*
This international collaborative group develops protocols, conducts clinical trials, and reviews treatment results. Member institutions are located in almost every state and province, at over 235 medical centers. The group is affiliated with the National Childhood Cancer Foundation, which runs all fundraising for COG.

ClinicalTrials.gov
U.S. National Institutes of Health • National Library of Medicine
Web site: *http://clinicaltrials.gov/ct/gui/c/r*
ClinicalTrials.gov provides current information about clinical research studies.

Clinical Trials Cooperative Group Program
National Cancer Institute
Web site: *http://cis.nci.nih.gov/fact/1_4.htm*
This program promotes and supports clinical trials of new cancer treatments. The cooperative groups are composed of academic institutions and cancer treatment centers throughout the United States, Canada, and Europe.

Family Support

The listings in this section include resources that offer support for family members or those who have loved ones with cancer.

Cancer Family Care
2421 Auburn Avenue • Cincinnati, OH 45219
Phone: 513-731-3346
Fax: 513-458-3582
Web site: *http://www.cancerfamilycare.org*
A nonprofit psychosocial counseling agency for people with cancer and their families in Ohio and Kentucky.

Centering Corporation
P.O. Box 4600 • Omaha, NE 68104
Phone: 402-553-1200
Fax: 402-553-0507
E-mail: center@centering.org
Web site: *http://www.centering.org*
This group offers resources for bereavement and coping with loss and sells over 100 books for children and adults.

The Compassionate Friends
P.O. Box 3696 • Oakbrook, IL 60522-3696
Toll-Free: 877-969-0010
Phone: 630-990-0010
Fax: 630-990-0246
E-mail: marion@compassionatefriends.org
Web site: *http://www.compassionatefriends.org*
This nonprofit organization's nationwide and international chapters offer support for
bereaved parents and siblings.

GriefNet
Web site: *http://griefnet.org*
This nonprofit site offers support for people dealing with grief, death, and major loss. Links
to a companion site where children and parents can pose questions and concerns.

National Association of Hospital Hospitality Houses, Inc.
P.O. Box 18087 • Asheville, NC 28814-0087
Toll-Free: 800-542-9730
Phone: 828-253-1188
Fax: 828-253-8082
E-mail: helpinghomes@nahhh.org
Web site: *http://www.nahhh.org*
This membership organization of facilities coordinates lodging and accommodations for
people receiving medical care.

National Family Caregivers Association
10400 Connecticut Avenue, #500 • Kensington, MD 20895-3944
Toll-Free: 800-896-3650
Fax: 301-942-2302
E-mail: info@nfcacares.org
Web site: *http://www.nfcacares.org*
Provides research, education, support, advocacy, and respite care to caregivers.

Ronald McDonald House Charities
1 Kroc Drive • Oak Brook, IL 60523
Web site: *http://www.rmhc.com*
Supports temporary lodging facilities for the families of seriously ill children being treated at
nearby hospitals.

VHL Family Alliance
171 Clinton Road • Brookline, MA 02445-5815
Toll-Free: 800-767-4VHL (800-767-4845)
Phone: 617-277-5667
Fax: 617-734-8233
E-mail: info@vhl.org
Web site: *http://www.vhl.org*
Provides literature and information, referrals, and research resources to von Hippel-Lindau
(VHL) syndrome patients and their families.

Well Spouse Foundation
30 East Fortieth Street PH • New York, NY 10016
Toll-Free: 800-838-0879
Phone: 212-685-8815
Fax: 212-685-8676
Web site: *http://www.wellspouse.org*
Offers support to husbands, wives, and partners of people who are chronically ill and/or disabled.

Home Health Care

Amherst H. Wilder Foundation
919 Lafond Avenue • St. Paul, MN 55104-2198
Phone: 651-642-4000
Web site: *http://www.wilder.org*
Offers services such as psychiatric clinics for children and the elderly, community services, and senior housing.

Gentiva Health Services
3 Huntington Quadrangle, 2S • Melville, NY 11747-8943
Toll-Free: 888-GENTIVA (888-436-8482)
Web site: *http://www.gentiva.com*
Provides community home health care services, including the coordination of health care services, home medical equipment, and infusion therapy. Professionals specialize in areas such as physical therapy, speech pathology, pediatric and geriatric care, and general nursing services.

Home Care Guide for Advanced Cancer
American College of Physicians-American Society of Internal Medicine (ACP-ASIM)
190 North Independence Mall West • Philadelphia, PA 19106-1572
Toll-Free: 800-523-1546, x2600
Phone: 215-351-2600
E-mail: custserv@mail.acponline.com
Web site: *http://www.acponline.org/public/h_care/index.html*
The ACP-ASIM offers this free online book to help caregivers deal with the complex issues involved in caring for a person with cancer. The entire contents of the book can be downloaded.

National Association for Home Care
228 Seventh Street SE • Washington, DC 20003
Phone: 202-547-7424
Fax: 202-547-3540
Web site: *http://www.nahc.org*
The NAHC provides a state-by-state database of phone numbers for home care and hospice agencies.

Oley Foundation
214 Hun Memorial, A-28 • Albany Medical Center • Albany, NY 12208-3478
Toll-Free: 800-776-OLEY (800-776-6539)
Phone: 518-262-5079
Fax: 518-262-5528
E-mail: bishopj@mail.amc.edu
Web site: *http://www.wizvax.net/oleyfdn*
Support for home parenteral and/or enteral nutrition therapy through a newsletter, conferences, meetings, and outreach activities.

Visiting Nurse Associations of America
11 Beacon Street, Suite 910 • Boston, MA 02108
Phone: 617-523-4042
Fax: 617-227-4843
Web site: *http://www.vnaa.org*
This organization's web site contains a visiting nurse locator, caregiver information, and related links to other organizations.

Hospice and Supportive Services
Foundation for Hospice and Home Care
National Association for Home Care • 228 Seventh Street SE • Washington, DC 20003
Phone: 202-547-7424
Fax: 202-547-3540
Web site: *http://www.nahc.org*
This diverse organization offers a broad array of programs to serve the dying, disabled, and disadvantaged.

Hospice Association of America (HAA)
228 Seventh Street SE • Washington, DC 20003
Phone: 202-546-4759
Fax: 202-547-9559
Web site: *http://www.nahc.org/HAA/home.html*
This national trade association represents more than 2,800 hospices and thousands of caregivers and volunteers who serve terminally ill patients and their families. The HAA web site provides general information about hospice care, including a consumer's guide and a Bill of Rights for hospice patients.

Hospice Education Institute/Hospicelink
190 Westbrook Road • Essex, CT 06426
Toll-Free: 800-331-1620
Phone: 860-767-1620
Fax: 860-767-2746
E-mail: hospiceall@aol.com
Web site: *http://www.hospiceworld.org*
This not-for-profit organization provides general information and materials about hospice care and referrals to the hospice nearest you.

Hospice Foundation of America (HFA)
2001 S Street NW, Suite 300 • Washington, DC 20009
Toll-Free: 800-854-3402
Fax: 202-638-5312
E-mail: hfa@hospicefoundation.org
Web site: *http://www.hospicefoundation.org*
HFA offers information and materials on hospice care, a hospice locator service, and educational programs. The web site contains this information as well as links to related sites.

Hospice Net
Suite 51, 401 Bowling Avenue • Nashville, TN 37205
E-mail: comments@hospicenet.org
Web site: *http://www.hospicenet.org*

This nonprofit organization that works exclusively through the Internet provides articles regarding end-of-life issues. Hospice nurses, social workers, bereavement counselors, and chaplains are available to answer questions via e-mail. The web site includes information for patients and caregivers, information about grief and loss, and a hospice locator service.

Joint Commission on Accreditation of Healthcare Organizations (JCAHO)
One Renaissance Boulevard • Oakbrook Terrace, IL 60181
Toll-Free (questions regarding complaints only): 800-994-6610
Phone: 630-792-5000
Fax: 630-792-5005
Web site: *http://www.jcaho.org*
This nonprofit organization evaluates and accredits more than 19,500 health care organizations in the United States, including hospitals, health care networks and health care organizations that provide home care, long-term care, behavioral health care, laboratory, and ambulatory care services. JCAHO makes performance reports of accredited organizations and guidelines for choosing a health care facility available to the public.

Medicare Helpline
Department of Health and Human Services
Toll-Free: 800-MEDICAR (800-633-4227)
Web site: *http://www.medicare.gov*
Call the toll-free number to receive information about local Medicare services.

National Association for Home Care (NAHC)
228 Seventh Street, SE • Washington, DC 20003
Phone: 202-547-7424
Fax: 202-547-3540
Web site: *http://www.nahc.org*
The NAHC provides a state-by-state database of phone numbers for home care and hospice agencies.

National Hospice and Palliative Care Organization
1700 Diagonal Road, Suite 300 • Alexandria, VA 22314
Phone: 703-837-1500
E-mail: info@nhpco.org
Web site: *http://www.nhpco.org*
This organization is dedicated to providing information about hospice care. The web site contains related links, a hospice locator database by state, a newsletter, and other general information.

Partnership for Caring, Inc.
Program Office • 475 Riverside Drive, Suite 1825 • New York, NY 10115
Toll-Free: 800-989-WILL (800-989-9455)
Phone: 212-870-2003
Fax: 212-870-2040
E-mail: pfc@partnershipforcaring.org
Web site: *http://www.choices.org*
Partnership for Caring, Inc., formerly called Choice in Dying, is concerned with protecting the rights and serving the needs of people who are dying of any illness as well as the needs of their families. The organization distributes free information on living will and power of attorney and offers a free counseling service on end-of-life issues.

Visiting Nurse Associations of America (VNAA)
11 Beacon Street • Boston, MA 02108
Phone: 617-523-4042
Fax: 617-227-4843
Web site: *http://www.vnaa.org*
This organization's web site contains a visiting nurse locator, caregiver information, and related links to other organizations.

Money and Insurance

Blue Cross Blue Shield Association
300 E. Randolph Street • Chicago, IL 60601-5099
Phone: 312-653-7500
Web site: *http://www.bcbs.com*
This health insurance provider's web site provides both general and specific health insurance information.

Certified Financial Planner (CFP) Board of Standards
1700 Broadway, Suite 2100 • Denver, CO 80290-2101
Toll-Free: 888-CFP-MARK (888-237-6275)
Fax: 303-860-7388
E-mail: mail@CFP-Board.org
Web site: *http://www.cfp-board.org*
This board regulates Certified Financial Planner licensees.

Communicating for Agriculture (CA) and the Self-Employed, Inc.
P.O. Box 677 • Fergus Falls, MN 56538
Toll-Free: 800-432-3276
Phone: 218-739-3241
Fax: 218-739-3832
Web site: *http://www.cainc.org*
Organization of ranchers, farmers, and self-employed people that offers many services that do not relate to cancer. However, each year it publishes the *Guide to Comprehensive Health Insurance for High-Risk Individuals: A State by State Analysis,* which may be useful to people with cancer.

CPA/PFS
American Institute of CPAs • 1211 Avenue of the Americas • New York, NY 10036-8775
Phone: 212-596-6200
Fax: 212-596-6213
Web site: *http://www.cpapfs.org*
Personal Financial Specialist (PFS) is the financial planning specialty accreditation held by certified public accountants (CPAs) who are members of the American Institute of CPAs (AICPA). At this site, you can locate local CPAs who have earned PFS accreditation, as well as learn about other financial topics.

Disabled American Veterans
807 Maine Avenue SW • Washington, DC 20024
Phone: 202-554-3501
Web site: *http://www.dav.org*
This nonprofit organization aids veterans who have been disabled in war or armed conflict, including those who were exposed to nuclear weapon testing and have since developed a cancer caused by radiation.

Health Insurance Association of America
1201 F Street, Suite 500 • Washington, DC 20004
Phone: 202-824-1600
Fax: 202-824-1722
Web site: *http://www.hiaa.org*
This association represents most U.S. health insurance companies. The web site contains
insurance guides and general insurance information, and an annual directory and survey of
hospitals, along with other information.

Hill-Burton Program
Parklawn Building • 5600 Fishers Lane, Room 10C-16 • Rockville, MD 20854
Toll-Free: 800-638-0742
Toll-Free in MD: 800-492-0359
Phone: 301-443-5656
Fax: 301-443-0619
Web site: *http://www.hrsa.gov/osp/dfcr*
Hill-Burton is a government program whereby hospitals, nursing homes, and other medical
facilities receiving funds from the government (usually for construction costs) are required by
law to provide a reasonable amount of services to persons unable to pay. Their hotline
defines the guidelines and fulfills requests for local Hill-Burton facilities.

Medicare Hotline
Department of Health and Human Services
Toll-Free: 800-MEDICAR (800-633-4227)
Web site: *http://www.medicare.gov*
This toll-free number offers information about local services. The web site offers information on
health plans, nursing homes, dialysis facilities, Medigap policies, contacts, Medicare activities,
participating doctors, and prescription drug assistance programs.

MIB, Inc.
P.O. Box 105 • Essex Station • Boston, MA 02112
Phone (voice mail): 617-426-3660
E-mail: infoline@mib.com
Web site: *http://www.mib.com*
This association of U.S. and Canadian life insurance companies aims to prevent insurance
fraud. Call or follow the instructions on their web site to request a copy of your MIB file and,
if necessary, request corrections.

National Association of Insurance Commissioners (NAIC)
2301 McGee, Suite 800 • Kansas City, MO 64108-2604
Phone: 816-842-3600
Web site: *http://www.naic.org/consumer.htm*
If you think you might buy insurance through a financial planner, check with the State
Insurance Commission. This group, which usually can be found in your state's capital, can
make sure the planner is licensed to sell insurance. Check the phone book or contact the NAIC.

National Association of Personal Financial Advisors
355 West Dundee Road, Suite 200 • Buffalo Grove, IL 60089
Toll-Free: 800-366-2732
Fax: 847-537-7740
E-mail: info@napfa.org
Web site: *http://www.napfa.org*
This group promotes and provides financial advice on a "fee-only" basis, without compensation contingent on the purchase or sale of a financial product.

National Association of Securities Dealers
1735 K Street NW • Washington, DC 20006-1500
Phone: 202-728-8000
Inquiries: 301-590-6500
Fax: 202-293-6260
Web site: *http://www.nasd.com*
This group regulates people who sell mutual funds, annuities, and stocks.

The National Underwriter Company
P.O. Box 14367 • Cincinnati, OH 45250-0367
Toll-Free: 800-543-0874
Fax: 859-692-2246
Web site: *http://www.nuco.com*
This company publishes products for the insurance and financial services industries, including *National Underwriter, Life & Health/Financial Services*.

National Viatical Association
1030 Fifteenth Street, Suite 870 • Washington, DC 20005
Toll-Free: 800-741-9465
Phone: 202-347-7361
Fax: 202-393-0336
Web site: *http://nationalviatical.org*
This organization provides information on the pre-death purchase of life insurance policies. The web site offers information on member organizations, the latest news in the industry, and information on the ethics behind this kind of transaction.

North American Securities Administrators Association (NASAA)
10 G Street NE, Suite 710 • Washington, DC 20002
Phone: 202-737-0900
Fax: 202-783-3571
Toll-Free Fax-On-Demand: 888-84-NASAA (888-846-2722)
E-mail: info@nasaa.org
Web site: *http://www.nasaa.org*
The State Securities Agency enforces the rules on how stocks and bonds are sold. It usually can be found in your state's capital. To find your agency, check the phone book or contact the NASAA.

Pension and Welfare Benefits Administration
U.S. Department of Labor • Division of Technical Assistance and Inquiries, Room N-5619
200 Constitution Avenue NW • Washington, DC 20210
Toll-Free (to order publications only): 800-998-7542
Phone: 202-219-8776
Fax: 202-219-8141
Web site: *http://www.dol.gov/dol/pwba*

The Pension and Welfare Benefits Administration (PWBA) aims to protect the integrity of pensions, health plans, and other employee benefits. The PWBA web site includes: fact sheets on COBRA, ERISA, and HIPA; questions and answers about recent changes in health care law; information about employee benefit laws and regulations; and information on other PWBA programs.

Securities and Exchange Commission (SEC)

450 Fifth Street NW • Washington, DC 20549
Phone: 202-942-7040
E-mail: help@sec.gov
Web site: *http://www.sec.gov*
This federal agency oversees "registered investment advisors"—anyone who is paid for giving investment advice.

Society of Financial Service Professionals

270 S. Bryn Mawr Avenue • Bryn Mawr, PA 19010-2195
Toll-Free (for orders or products only): 800-392-6900
Phone: 610-526-2500
Fax: 610-527-1499
Web site: *http://www.financialpro.org*
This organization offers information about estate, retirement and financial planning; employee benefits; business and compensation planning; and life, health, disability, and long-term care insurance.

State Board of Accountancy

Some financial planners are certified public accountants, or CPAs. CPAs are supervised by their state board of accountancy. Look in the phone book for contact information.

TAKING CHARGE OF MONEY MATTERS

American Cancer Society (ACS)
Toll-Free: 800-ACS-2345
This is an ACS workshop offered through the I CAN COPE program. This workshop offers financial guidance for cancer survivors and their families. Topics include the fundamentals of insurance, estate planning, returning to work, disability insurance, how to improve your financial planning, financial resources, and how to create a budget. Call ACS for more information.

TRICARE

Department of Defense
Web site: *http://www.tricare.osd.mil*
TRICARE, formerly called CHAMPUS, is part of the military health care system. The web site offers a link to TRICARE regional offices and a list of phone numbers.

Viatical and Life Settlement Association of America

800 Mayfair Circle • Orlando, FL 32803
Phone: 407-894-3797
Fax: 407-897-1325
E-mail: viatical@mpinet.net
Web site: *http://www.viatical.org*
This nonprofit trade association is composed of viatical settlement brokers and funding companies. The web site offers contact information on the companies that belong to the association as well as information on viatical settlements.

Pain

Agency for Healthcare Research and Quality (AHRQ)

Office of Health Care Information, Executive Office Center

2101 E. Jefferson Street, Suite 501 • Rockville, MD 20852

Phone: 301-594-1360

Web site: *http://www.ahrq.gov*

The AHRQ, an office within the U.S. Department of Health and Human Services, provides consumers with science-based, easily understandable information that will help them make informed decisions about their own personal health care. They offer a number of clinical practice guidelines on common health problems in consumer versions for the public.

American Pain Society

4700 W. Lake Avenue • Glenview, IL 60025

Phone: 847-375-4715

Toll-Free Fax: 877-734-8758

E-mail: info@ampainsoc.org

Web site: *http://www.ampainsoc.org*

This organization of clinicians and researchers serves people in pain by advancing research, education, treatment, and professional practice.

American Society of Clinical Hypnosis (ASCH)

130 East Elm Court, Suite 201 • Roselle, IL 60172-2000

Phone: 630-980-4740

Fax: 630-351-8490

E-mail: info@asch.net

Web site: *http://www.asch.net*

The American Society of Clinical Hypnosis is an association of 2,400 health care and mental health care professionals who use hypnosis to treat a wide variety of medical, dental, and psychological conditions. ASCH provides referral lists of ASCH members upon request.

City of Hope Pain/Palliative Care Resource Center

1500 E. Duarte Road • Duarte, CA 91010

Phone: 626-359-8111, ext. 63829

Fax: 626-301-8941

E-mail: prc@coh.org

Web site: *http://prc.coh.org*

The City of Hope Pain/Palliative Care Resource Center serves as a clearinghouse to disseminate information and resources to assist health professionals with improving the quality of pain management. They offer information on a variety of topics including pain assessment tools, patient education materials, quality assurance materials, research instruments, and end-of-life resources. The web site provides a list of publications and other materials available for order. Some publications are available online. *Some Spanish materials are available.*

Patient Education, Support, and Advocacy

See also the American Cancer Society Resources, pages 715–718.

American Board of Medical Specialties

1007 Church Street, Suite 404 • Evanston, IL 60201-5913

Phone Verification: 866-ASK-ABMS (866-275-2267)

Phone: 847-491-9091

Fax: 847-328-3596

Web site: *http://www.abms.org*

The American Board of Medical Specialties (ABMS) is the umbrella organization for the twenty-four approved medical specialty boards in the United States. This organization provides information about specialization and certification in medicine. Their web site includes the Doctor Verification Service.

American Self-Help Group Clearinghouse

Northwest Covenant Medical Center

100 Hanover Avenue, Suite 202 • Cedar Knolls, NJ 07927-2020

Phone: 973-326-6789

Fax: 973-306-9467

E-mail: njshc@bc.cybernex.net

Web site: *http://www.selfhelpgroups.org*

This group maintains a searchable database of over 1,000 self-help groups, including those concerning specific illnesses, caregivers, disabilities, and bereavement. It provides a referral service and helps people form their own groups.

Burger King Cancer Caring Center

4117 Liberty Avenue • Pittsburgh, PA 15224

Phone: 412-622-1212

Fax: 412-622-1216

E-mail: cancercr@sgi.net

Web site: *http://trfn.clpgh.org/cancercaring*

This center is dedicated to providing psychological support to people diagnosed with cancer and their families and friends. The Cancer Caring Center is now handling calls for the Cancer Guidance Hotline.

Cancer Care, Inc.

275 Seventh Avenue • New York, NY 10001

Toll-Free: 800-813-HOPE (800-813-4673)

Phone: 212-221-3300

Fax: 212-719-0263

E-mail: info@cancercare.org

Web site: *http://www.cancercare.org*

Cancer Care provides emotional and financial support for people with cancer and their families and educational programs for the general public. Free counseling, outreach programs, and information about and referrals for home care and child care, hospice, and other services are also available. *Spanish information is available on the web site.*

Cancer Research Institute (CRI)

681 Fifth Avenue • New York, NY 10022

Toll-Free: 800-99-CANCER (800-992-2623)

E-mail: info@cancerresearch.org

Web site: *http://www.cancerresearch.org*

An institute funding cancer research and providing public information on cancer immunology and cancer treatment, the CRI helps locate immunotherapy clinical trials, and offers a cancer reference guide and other informational booklets.

Cancervive
11636 Chayote Street • Los Angeles, CA 90049
Toll-Free: 800-4-TO-CURE (800-486-2873)
Phone: 310-203-9232
Fax: 310-471-4618
E-mail: cancervivr@aol.com
Web site: *http://www.cancervive.org*
Cancervive offers several services to people with cancer, including telephone counseling, referrals, and education.

Coping with Cancer Magazine
P.O. Box 682268 • Franklin, TN 37068-2268
Phone: 615-790-2400
Fax: 615-794-0179
E-mail: copingmag@aol.com
Web site: *http://www.copingmag.com*
This bimonthly publication is the only nationally distributed consumer magazine for people whose lives have been touched by cancer.

Make Today Count
Care of Neil O'Connor • K4-B100, CSC • UW Hospital and Clinics
600 Highland Avenue • Madison, WI 53792
Phone: 608-263-8521
E-mail: njoconnor@hosp.wisc.edu
Web site: *http://userpages.itis.com/lemoll/index.html*
This support organization is for people affected by cancer or other life-threatening illness.

The Mautner Project for Lesbians with Cancer
1707 L Street NW, Suite 500 • Washington, DC 20036
Phone (TTY): 202-332-5536
Fax: 202-332-0662
E-mail: mautner@mautnerproject.org
Web site: *http://www.mautnerproject.org*
This group provides vital services and support, including education, information, and advocacy for health issues relating to lesbians with cancer and their families.

The National Coalition for Cancer Research (NCCR)
426 C Street NE • Washington, DC 20002
Phone: 202-544-1880 (ask for NCCR)
Web site: *http://www.cancercoalition.org*
Through NCCR, cancer survivors and researchers track cancer research and monitor legislation and funding.

National Coalition for Cancer Survivorship (NCCS)
1010 Wayne Avenue, Suite 770 • Silver Spring, MD 20910-5600
Toll-Free: 877-NCCS-YES (877-622-7937)
Phone: 301-650-9127
Fax: 301-565-9670
Web site: *http://www.cansearch.org*
Web site (Spanish version): *http://www.cansearch.org/spanish/index.html*
The NCCS is a network of independent organizations working in the area of cancer survivorship and support. The web site offers links to on-line cancer resources, support groups, survivorship programs, advocacy education, and a newsletter.

National Self-Help Clearinghouse
Graduate School and University Center of the City University of New York
365 Fifth Avenue, Suite 3300 • New York, NY 10016
Phone: 212-817-1822
Fax: 212-817-2990
Web site: *http://www.selfhelpweb.org*
This nonprofit organization provides access to regional self-help services.

National Women's Health Network
514 Tenth Street NW, Suite 400 • Washington, DC 20004
Phone: 202-628-7814
Fax: 202-347-1168
Web site: *http://www.womenshealthnetwork.org*
This organization provides advocacy and maintains a clearinghouse on women's health issues.

Oncolink's Coping with Cancer
Web site: *http://www.oncolink.upenn.edu/psychosocial*
Maintained by the University of Pennsylvania Cancer Center, this web site includes information about several different kinds of support groups and other issues that many people with cancer may encounter.

People Living Through Cancer
323 Eighth Street SW • Albuquerque, NM 87102
Toll-Free: 888-441-4439
Phone: 505-242-3263
Fax: 505-242-6756
Web site: *http://www.pltc.org*
Programs and activities to help members make informed choices and interact with other people who have been treated for cancer. Services include a publication, one-to-one matching, support groups and individual counseling, and training for Native Americans who would like to start their own groups.

Pharmaceutical Research and Manufacturers Association of America (PhRMA)
1100 Fifteenth Street NW, Suite 900 • Washington, DC 20005
Phone: 202-835-3400
Fax: 202-835-3414
Web site: *http://www.phrma.org*
The PhRMA provides information about member pharmaceutical companies and drugs that are currently available, in clinical trials, or under development. The web site includes a directory of patient assistance programs for prescription drugs and a database of new medications for cancer and other diseases.

Social Security Administration
Office of Public Inquiries
6401 Security Boulevard, Room 4-C-5 Annex • Baltimore, MD 21235-6401
Toll-Free: 800-772-1213
Toll-Free (TTY): 800-325-0778
Web site: *http://www.ssa.gov*
Call the toll-free number to receive information about local services. *Spanish-speaking staff is available.*

The Wellness Community
35 E. Seventh Street, Suite 412 • Cincinnati, OH 45202-2420
Toll-Free: 888-793-WELL (888-793-9355)
Phone: 513-421-7111
Fax: 513-421-7119
Web site: *http://www.wellness-community.org*
This free program offers support for people with cancer and their loved ones. The nonprofit organization provides professional support services as an adjunct to conventional medical treatment in twenty-six facilities nationwide. Services include support groups, networking groups for specific types of cancer, educational workshops, stress management sessions, lectures, and social gatherings. Support groups are led by licensed psychotherapists.

Rehabilitation

National Lymphedema Network (NLN)
Latham Square • 1611 Telegraph Avenue, Suite 1111 • Oakland, CA 94612
Toll-Free (Hotline): 800-541-3259
Phone: 510-208-3200
Fax: 510-208-3110
Web site: *http://www.lymphnet.org*
The web site for this nonprofit agency offers information about lymphedema, a referral service to medical and therapeutic treatment centers, and information on locating or establishing local support groups. It publishes a newsletter, which contains articles about lymphedema and a resource guide of treatment centers, doctors, therapists, and suppliers.

Plastic Surgery Information Service
American Society of Plastic Surgeons
444 East Algonquin Road • Arlington Heights, IL 60005
Toll-Free: 888-4-PLASTIC (888-475-2784)
Web site: *http://www.plasticsurgery.org*
This service provides a list of board-certified plastic surgeons to women interested in breast reconstruction.

United Ostomy Association
19772 MacArthur Boulevard, Suite 200 • Irvine, CA 92612
Toll-Free: 800-826-0826
Web site: *http://www.uoa.org*
This volunteer-based health organization provides education, information, support, and advocacy for people who have had or will have intestinal or urinary diversions.

Wound, Ostomy and Continence Nurses Society (WOCN)
1550 South Coast Highway, Suite 201 • Laguna Beach, CA 92651
Toll-Free: 888-224-WOCN (888-224-9626)
Fax: 949-376-3456
Web site: *http://www.wocn.org*
This group refers patients to enterostomal nurses in their area.

Smoking

The American Lung Association (ALA)
1740 Broadway • New York, NY 10019
Toll-Free: 800-LUNG-USA (800-586-4872)
Phone: 212-315-8700

Fax: 212-265-5642

Web site: *http://www.lungusa.org*

The mission of the American Lung Association is to prevent lung disease and promote lung health. ALA fights lung disease in all its forms, with special emphasis on asthma, tobacco control, and environmental health.

Office on Smoking and Health

Centers for Disease Control and Prevention (CDC)

4770 Buford Highway NE • Mail Stop K50 • Atlanta, GA 30341-3724

Toll-Free: 800-CDC-1311 (800-232-1311)

Phone: 770-488-5705

This CDC office offers public education and information on smoking and how to stop.

Transportation and Accommodation Services

Air Care Alliance

6202 South Lewis Avenue, Suite F2 • Tulsa, OK 74136-1064

Toll-Free: 888-260-9707

Phone: 918-745-0384

Fax: 918-745-0879

E-mail: mail@aircareall.org

Web site: *http://www.aircareall.org*

Provides a flight to the ambulatory and medically stable person who is unable to travel on public transportation. Call for your local organization.

AirLifeLine

50 Fullerton Court, Suite 200 • Sacramento, CA 95825

Toll-Free: 877-AIR-LIFE (877-247-5433)

Phone: 916-641-7800

Fax: 916-641-0600

Web site: *http://www.airlifeline.org*

This national nonprofit charitable organization of private pilots flies ambulatory patients who cannot afford transportation to medical facilities for diagnosis and treatment. There is no charge for patients who qualify. AirLifeLine and the American Cancer Society have formed a partnership with the goal of making people across the United States aware of this transportation service.

Corporate Angel Network, Inc.

Westchester County Airport • 1 Loop Road • White Plains, NY 10604

Phone: 914-328-1313

Web site: *http://www.corpangelnetwork.org*

Provides free transportation to or from a hospital or treatment center for people with cancer and family members, using corporate airlines. Travelers must be ambulatory and self-sufficient. People who are donating bone marrow or blood to the cancer patient may also travel free.

Hope Lodges

American Cancer Society

Toll-Free: 800-ACS-2345

Hope Lodges are temporary residential facilities providing sleeping rooms and related facilities for people with cancer who are undergoing outpatient treatment and their family members. Approval from a doctor or referring agency is necessary.

Alabama

Joe Lee Griffin Hope Lodge
 (*Birmingham*)
1104 Ireland Way
Birmingham, AL 35205
Toll-Free: 888-513-9933
Phone: 205-558-7860
Fax: 205-558-7862

Arkansas

Hope Lodge (*Little Rock*)
2122 S. Broadway
Little Rock, AR 72206
Phone: 501-374 5869
Fax: 501-372 6995

Florida

ACS Winn-Dixie Hope Lodge
 (*Gainesville*)
2121 SW Sixteenth Street
Gainesville, FL 32608-1417
Phone: 352-338-0601
Fax: 352-378-7792

ACS Winn-Dixie Hope Lodge (*Miami*)
1121 Northwest Fourteenth Street
Miami, FL 33136
Phone: 305-547-2210
Fax: 305-547-4187

Georgia

Winn-Dixie Hope Lodge
 (*Decatur/Atlanta*)
1552 Shoup Court
Decatur, GA 30033
For Reservations: 404-816-4994
Phone: 404-327-9200
Fax: 404-841-9808

Indiana

Hope Lodge (*Indianapolis*)
1795 West Eighty-Sixth Street
Indianapolis, IN 46260
Phone: 317-415-5000
Fax: 317-415-5050

Maryland

Hope Lodge (*Baltimore*)
636 West Lexington Street
Baltimore, MD 21201
Phone: 410-547-2522
Fax: 410-539-8890

Massachusetts

Hope Lodge (*Worcester*)
7 Oak Street
Worcester, MA 01609
Phone: 508-792-2985
Fax: 508-753-3986

Minnesota

Hope Lodge (*Rochester*)
411 Second Street NW
Rochester, MN 55901
Phone: 507-529-4673
Fax: 507-529-4666

Missouri

ACS Hope Lodge (*St. Louis*)
4215 Lindell Boulevard
St. Louis, MO 63108
Toll-Free: 800-489-9730
Phone: 314-286-8150
Fax: 314-286-8155

New York

Buffalo Hope Lodge (*Buffalo*)
197 Summer Street
Buffalo, NY 14222
Toll-Free: 800-489-9730
Phone: 716-882-9244
Fax: 716-882-4436

Rochester Hope Lodge (*Rochester*)
1400 North Winton Road
Rochester, NY 14609
Phone: 716-288-1950
Fax: 716-288-6467

Ohio

Cleveland Hope Lodge (*Cleveland*)
11432 Mayfield Road
Cleveland, OH 44106-2364
Phone: 216-844-4673
Fax: 216-844-2959

Pennsylvania

Hope Lodge (*Hershey*)
125 Lucy Avenue
Hummelstown, PA 17036-9134
Phone: 717-533-5111
Fax: 717-533-2587

Puerto Rico
Hope Lodge *(San Juan; Children only)*
1552 Victoria Street
San Juan, PR 00912
Phone: 787-725-0233
Fax: 787-723-3277

South Carolina
Hope Lodge *(Charleston)*
P.O. Box 573
Charleston, SC 29402-0573
Phone: 843-723-3618
Fax: 843-577-4644

Vermont
Hope Lodge *(Burlington)*
183 East Avenue
Burlington, VT 05401
Phone: 802-658-0649
Fax: same as phone number

National Patient Travel Helpline (NPATH)
Mercy Medical Airlift • 4620 Haygood Road, Suite 1 • Virginia Beach, VA 23455
Toll-Free: 800-296-1217
Phone: 757-318-9174
Fax: 757-318-9107
Web site: *http://www.patienttravel.org*
NPATH is a service provided by Mercy Medical Airlift, a national charity. NPATH maintains data on over 40 organizations providing long and short distance air medical transportation and can provide referrals to charitable and patient discount commercial services. NPATH also provides referrals to sources of help available through the Angel Flight America Network.

Westin Hotel Guestroom for Cancer Patients
Toll-Free: 800-ACS-2345 (800-227-2345)
Web site: *http://www.cancer.org*
In cooperation with the ACS, participating Westin hotels provide overnight accommodations when cancer patients must travel considerable distances from their homes to receive treatment. All accommodations are subject to availability. Some rooms are free; others are offered at reduced rates. Work through the local office of your American Cancer Society to obtain reservations and information.

Treatments

Chemotherapy

Cancer Hope Network
2 North Road, Suite A • Chester, NJ 07930
Toll-Free: 877-HOPE-NET (877-467-3638)
Phone: 908-879-4039
Fax: 908-879-6518
E-mail: info@cancerhopenetwork.org
Web site: *http://www.cancerhopenetwork.org*
This organization, formerly known as CHEMOCare, matches cancer patients with trained volunteers who have undergone and recovered from similar cancer experiences. Volunteers provide free and confidential one-on-one telephone support. Support for family members is also available.

The Chemotherapy Foundation

183 Madison Avenue, Suite 403 • New York, NY 10016
Phone: 212-213-9292
Fax: 212-213-3831
Web site: *http://www.chemotherapyfoundation.org*
Supports laboratory and clinical research to develop more effective methods of cancer diagnosis and therapy. Conducts professional and public education programs and publishes free patient/public information booklets.

Radiation

American Society for Therapeutic Radiology and Oncology (ASTRO)

12500 Fair Lakes Circle, Suite 375 • Fairfax, VA 22033-3882
Toll-Free: 800-962-7876
Phone: 703-502-1550
Fax: 703-502-7852
Web site: *http://www.astro.org*
ASTRO is a professional organization of doctors and scientists. The ASTRO web site includes: an overview of radiation therapy, specific information about radiation therapy for prostate and breast cancer, and links to other health web sites.

Surviving!

Department of Radiation Oncology, Stanford University Medical Center
Division of Radiation Therapy, Room A035 • Stanford, CA 94305-5304
Phone: 650-723-7881
E-mail: socserv@reyes.stanford.edu
Web site: *http://www-radonc.stanford.edu/surviving.html*
Surviving! is a newsletter written and created by cancer survivors for the benefit of cancer patients, their friends, and families. Its goal is to share common experiences and to help recovering patients manage their challenges.

Stem Cell Transplants

Bone Marrow & Transplant Information Network (BMT InfoNet)

2900 Skokie Valley Road, Suite B • Highland Park, IL 60035
Toll-Free: 888-597-7674
Phone: 847-433-3313
Fax: 847-433-4599
E-mail: help@bmtinfonet.org
Web site: *http://www.bmtnews.org*
This not-for-profit organization provides publications and support services to bone marrow, stem cell, and cord blood transplant patients and survivors. It publishes handbooks that explain what is involved in transplants, a book for children, and a quarterly newsletter, which is also available on their web site. Support services include Patient-to-Survivor Link, help with insurance difficulties, and organization referrals.

The Caitlin Raymond International Registry

University of Massachusetts Medical Center
55 Lake Avenue North • Worcester, MA 01655
Toll-Free: 800-726-2824
Phone: 508-334-8969

Fax: 508-334-8972

E-mail: Info@CRIR.org

Web site: *http://www.crir.org*

The Caitlin Raymond International Registry is a resource for patients and doctors conducting a search for unrelated bone marrow or cord blood donors.

Living Bank

P.O. Box 6725 • Houston, TX 77265-6725

Toll-Free: 800-528-2971

Phone: 713-528-2971

Fax: 713-961-0979

E-mail: info@livingbank.org

Web site: *http://www.livingbank.org*

Attempts to motivate and facilitate organ and tissue donor commitment. *Spanish-speaking staff is available.*

National Bone Marrow Transplant Link (NBMT Link)

20411 West 12 Mile Road, Suite 108 • Southfield, MI 48076

Toll-Free: 800-546-5268

Phone: 248-358-1886

Fax: 248-932-8483

E-mail: nmbtlink@mciworld.com

Web site: *http://www.comnet.org/nbmtlink*

Primarily serving as an information center for prospective bone marrow transplant patients, this site contains a BMT resource guide and a survivor's guide, both of which can be printed directly from your computer. Resources for health care professionals are also available.

National Foundation for Transplants

1102 Brookfield, Suite 200 • Memphis, TN 38119-3810

Toll-Free: 800-489-3863

Phone: 901-684-1697

Fax: 901-684-1128

E-mail: NatFoundTX@aol.com

Web site: *http://www.transplants.org*

Provides health care support services, financial services, and advocacy programs for transplantation candidates, recipients, and their families.

National Marrow Donor Program

3001 Broadway Street NE, Suite 500 • Minneapolis, MN 55413

Toll-Free: 800-MARROW2 (800-627-7692)

Fax: 612-627-8195

Web site: *http://www.marrow.org*

This nonprofit group's registry matches unrelated donors and patients. The patient advocacy department offers information regarding insurance, choosing a hospital, and other concerns. The MARROW line answers general calls and explains how to become a marrow donor.

755

ABOUT THE AUTHORS

Harmon J. Eyre, M.D.
Chief Medical Officer
Executive Vice President for Research and Cancer Control

Dr. Eyre is a former president of the American Cancer Society and has been an ACS volunteer for more than twenty-two years. He also served as a medical oncologist at the University of Utah, and has been recognized for his service to numerous professional societies, government groups, and voluntary health agencies in the United States and abroad.

Dianne Partie Lange
Editorial Director

Trained as a nurse, Dianne Partie Lange is a medical journalist and author currently residing in Carnelian Bay, California. She has been the editor-in-chief of *Health* magazine, executive editor for *Self*, and health editor for *Mirabella* and *Allure* magazines. She has written about cancer for the *New York Times*, WebMD.com, and several magazines. She is a contributing editor and "Body News" columnist for *Allure*.

Lois B. Morris
Executive Editor

Lois B. Morris is a New York–based author and journalist whose work appears frequently in magazines and newspapers. She has written or coauthored seven books on health and behavior, and she served as editorial director of *The Columbia University College of Physicians and Surgeons Complete Home Guide to Mental Health*. She is a *More* magazine contributing editor and writes the "Mood News" column for *Allure* magazine.